Preventive Oncology for the Gynecologist

Sumita Mehta • Anshuja Singla
Editors

Preventive Oncology for the Gynecologist

Springer

Editors
Sumita Mehta
Department of Obstetrics and Gynecology
Babu Jagjivan Ram Memorial Hospital
New Delhi, India

Anshuja Singla
Department of Obstetrics and Gynecology
University College of Medical Sciences
and Guru Teg Bahadur Hospital
New Delhi, India

ISBN 978-981-13-3437-5 ISBN 978-981-13-3438-2 (eBook)
https://doi.org/10.1007/978-981-13-3438-2

This Springer imprint is published by the registered company Springer Nature Singapore Pte Ltd.
The registered company address is: 152 Beach Road, #21-01/04 Gateway East, Singapore 189721, Singapore

To our beloved parents, Capt. Sham Sunder and Rashmi Sharma and Sh Surinder and the late Mrs. Swaran Singla, for your unconditional love and support. You are our biggest inspiration.

Preface

"An ounce of prevention is worth a pound of cure."
Benjamin Franklin

Cancer is the most dreadful of all diseases and is likely to be a global pandemic by 2050. Fifty percent of cancers are preventable because of the causal association with modifiable risk factors and early detection of precursor lesions. We need to realize that curing cancer starts with preventing cancer in the first place. Preventive oncology is not given its due and is restricted to a chapter in books on oncology. This book is our earnest endeavour to highlight the preventive aspect of cancers in women and discuss the various measures that can be followed to decrease invasive genital cancers.

The book has been divided into six parts for the reader's convenience. Part I discusses the epidemiology and screening for endometrial cancer. There is a chapter dedicated to prevention and management of endometrial hyperplasias before they turn malignant. The role of chemoprevention in endometrial cancer is discussed and supported with the latest evidence and research.

Cervical cancer is the fourth most common cancer in women, affecting them in their prime. Part II is dedicated to chapters that discuss the diagnosis and treatment of cervical intraepithelial lesions, including a chapter dedicated to HPV infection and its role in cervical carcinogenesis.

Ovarian cancer is the eighth leading cause of cancer deaths in the world, and its prevention is critical in reducing the mortality and morbidity for patients with ovarian cancer. Part III focusses on the prevention of ovarian cancer through risk-reducing salpingo-oophorectomy. Serum tumour markers, which have a pivotal role in screening and risk stratification of ovarian cancers, also have been discussed in detail.

Part IV is dedicated to preventive oncology of the vulva and vagina, where the incidence of high-grade preinvasive disease is increasing in the younger women. The precancerous lesions are often overlooked and are treated as nonspecific dermatologic conditions, with the patients seeking multiple opinions from different specialists for symptom relief. Keeping this in mind, the chapters in this part deal with detection and management of intraepithelial lesions of the vulva and vagina.

Part V deals with the preventive aspect of breast cancer, which is the most frequently diagnosed cancer and the leading cause of cancer death among females worldwide. Chapters in this part elaborate on different imaging modalities used for screening and diagnosis of breast cancer, role of clinical examination and biomarkers and the various risk factors that act individually or in combination to contribute to pathogenesis of breast cancer.

Part VI focusses on infection as a cause of gynaecological cancers. The role of gut and vaginal microbiota in gynaecological malignancies is discussed and supported by the latest evidence and research. Identifying a causal infectious agent helps not only in understanding the biology of the cancers but also in the development of vaccines for its prevention, which is aptly detailed with respect to cervical cancer in another chapter in the part.

All the authors who have contributed to the book are experts in their respective fields and have written chapters that are comprehensive, educative and supported by the latest evidence. The book will be useful to those pursuing the field of gynaecology oncology, general gynaecology practitioners, undergraduates and postgraduates in obstetrics and gynaecology, as well as our colleagues in general surgery.

We hope the book is well read and appreciated and finds a place on the shelves of all those who care and work for the preventive aspect of women's health. It is time we realize that treatment without prevention is simply unsustainable.

New Delhi, India Sumita Mehta
New Delhi, India Anshuja Singla

Contents

About the Editors

Sumita Mehta is a specialist and heads the department of obstetrics & gynecology at Babu Jagjivan Ram Memorial Hospital, Delhi. She is a graduate of Lady Hardinge Medical College, Delhi, and received her diplomate national board of examinations (obstetrics & gynecology) from Sir Ganga Ram hospital, Delhi. She has edited eight books, published numerous articles, and delivered many guest lectures. She also a reviewer for many international journals. She has previously served as secretary of the Indian Society of Colposcopy and Cervical Pathology (ISCCP) and as an executive member and editor for the Association of Obstetricians & Gynecologists of Delhi. She is the state resource person for training of doctors in preventive oncology and a National Expert for project ECHO (Extension for Community Healthcare Outcomes) at the National Institute of Cancer Prevention & Research, Delhi. She is also an IFCPC-IARC (International Federation of Cervical Pathology and Colposcopy–International Agency for Research on Cancer) certified National Trainer for colposcopy. Her primary area of interest is gynecologic oncology.

Anshuja Singla is Associate professor in the department of obstetrics & gynaecology at University College of Medical Sciences and Guru Teg Bahadur Hospital, Delhi. She is actively involved in departmental academic and administrative work. Her areas of interest are gynae oncology and endoscopy. She has many chapters and publications, national and international to her credit.

Contributors

Geeta Acharya Department of Gynaecological Oncology, St. John's Medical College and Hospital, Bangalore, Karnataka, India

Pakhee Aggarwal Department of Obstetrics and Gynaecology, Fortis Memorial Research Institute, Gurugram, Haryana, India

Saman Ahmad Content Department, Applect Learning Systems Pvt. Ltd., New Delhi, India

Sarfraz Ahmad Department of Gynecologic Oncology, Florida Hospital Cancer Institute, Florida State University, Orlando, FL, USA

Department of Gynecologic Oncology, Colleges of Medicine, University of Central Florida, Florida State University, Orlando, FL, USA

Begum Rokey Anwar Department of Gynaecological Oncology, National Institute of Cancer Research and Hospital, Dhaka, Bangladesh

Nidhi Arora Department of Fetal Medicine, Rainbow Hospital, New Delhi, India

Dipanwita Banerjee Department of Gynaecological Oncology, Chittaranjan National Cancer Institute, Kolkata, West Bengal, India

Partha Basu Screening Group, International Agency for Research on Cancer, Lyon, France

Shirin Akter Begum Department of Obstetrics and Gynaecology, Bangabandhu Sheikh Mujib Medical University (BSMMU), Dhaka, Bangladesh

Bharti Bharani Dysplasia Clinic, Indore, Madhya Pradesh, India

Vani Bharani Dysplasia Clinic, Indore, Madhya Pradesh, India

Shruti Bhatia Department of Gynaecological Oncology, Action Cancer Hospital, New Delhi, India

Rani Bhat Department of Gynaecological Oncology, Healthcare Global Enterprises Ltd., Bangalore, Karnataka, India

Vishakha Chandrakant Bidkar Department of Gynaecological Oncology, St. John's Medical College and Hospital, St. John's National Academy of Health Sciences, Bangalore, Karnataka, India

Lorna A. Brudie Department of Gynecologic Oncology, Orlando Health UF Health Cancer Center, Orlando, FL, USA

Alpana Chhetri Department of Obstetrics and Gynaecology, Chittaranjan Seva Sadan College of Obstetrics, Gynaecology and Child Health, Kolkata, West Bengal, India

Neha Gami Department of Obstetrics and Gynecology, Healthplus Clinic and Danat al Emarat Hospital, Abu Dhabi, UAE

Sumit Goyal Department of Medical Oncology, Rajiv Gandhi Cancer Institute and Research Centre, New Delhi, India

Anshul Grover Department of Obstetrics and Gynaecology, Baba Jagjivan Ram Memorial Hospital, New Delhi, India

Bindiya Gupta Department of Obstetrics and Gynaecology, UCMS & GTB Hospital, New Delhi, India

Kanika Gupta Department of Obstetrics and Gynecology, Medcare Multispeciality Hospital, Sharjah, UAE

Monisha Gupta Department of Gynaecologic Oncology, Max Super Speciality Hospital, Shalimar Bagh, New Delhi, India

Department of Surgical Oncology, Max Super Speciality Hospital, Pitampura, New Delhi, India

Sarika Gupta Department of Gynecology, Indraprastha Apollo Hospital, New Delhi, India

Tony Hollingworth Department of Women's Health, Whipps Cross University Hospital, London, UK

Department of Gynaecology, Barts Health NHS Trust, London, UK

Centre for Cancer Prevention, Wolfson Institute for Preventive Medicine, QMUL, London, UK

Robert W. Holloway Florida Hospital Gynecologic Oncology, Orlando, FL, USA

Shilpa Jamwal Department of Gynae-Oncology, Dharamshila Narayana Superspeciality Hospital, New Delhi, India

R. S. Jayshree Center for Molecular Oncology, Kidwai Cancer Institute, Bangalore, Karnataka, India

Smita Joshi Department of Preventive Oncology, Prayas and HCJMRI, Pune, India

Satinder Kaur Department of Gynae-Oncology, Dharamshila Narayana Superspeciality Hospital, New Delhi, India

Ritu Khatuja Department of Obstetrics and Gynaecology, ANIIMS, Port Blair, Andaman and Nicobar Islands, India

Grace N. Kim Department of Pathology, LAC+USC Medical Center, Los Angeles, CA, USA

Department of Pathology, Keck Hospital of USC, Los Angeles, CA, USA

Kiran Abhijit Kulkarni Department of Gynaecological Oncology, St. John's Medical College and Hospital, Bangalore, Karnataka, India

Anshuman Kumar Department of Surgical Oncology, Dharamshila Narayana Superspeciality Hospital, New Delhi, India

Rajesh Kumar Dysplasia Clinic, Indore, Madhya Pradesh, India

Rekha V. Kumar Department of Oncopathology, Kidwai Cancer Institute, Bangalore, Karnataka, India

Shashikant Lele Department of Gynecologic Oncology, Roswell Park Cancer Institute, Buffalo, NY, USA

Sarah Lynam Department of Gynecologic Oncology, Roswell Park Cancer Institute, Buffalo, NY, USA

Angelito Magno Department of Obstetrics and Gynecology, Section of Gynecologic Oncology, De La Salle Health Sciences Institute, De La Salle University Medical Center, Dasmariñas City, Philippines

Ranajit Mandal Department of Gynaecological Oncology, Chittaranjan National Cancer Institute, Kolkata, West Bengal, India

Kerry-Ann McDonald Breast Surgery Division, Department of Surgical Oncology, Roswell Park Comprehensive Cancer Center, Buffalo, NY, USA

Sumita Mehta Department of Obstetrics and Gynecology, Babu Jagjivan Ram Memorial Hospital, New Delhi, India

Ashrafun Nessa Department of Obstetrics and Gynaecology, Bangabandhu Sheikh Mujib Medical University (BSMMU), Dhaka, Bangladesh

Md Kausar Neyaz Department of Research and Development, DSS Imagetech Pvt. Ltd., New Delhi, India

Samuel George Oxley Department of Women's Health, Whipps Cross University Hospital, London, UK

Divya Pandey Department of Obstetrics and Gynecology, Vardhman Mahavir Medical College and Safdarjung Hospital, New Delhi, India

T. Parvathi Department of Gynaecological Oncology, St. John's Medical College and Hospital, Bangalore, Karnataka, India

Bijal M. Patel Department of Gynaecological Oncology, Gujarat Cancer and Research Institute, Ahmedabad, Gujarat, India

Usha Poli MNJ Institute of Oncology & Regional Cancer Center, Hyderabad, India

T. S. Premalatha Department of Gynaecological Oncology, St. John's Medical College and Hospital, Bangalore, Karnataka, India

Swati Rai Department of Obstetrics and Gynaecology, Maulana Azad Medical College and Lok Nayak Hospital, New Delhi, India

Niti Raizada Department of Medical Oncology and Hemato-Oncology, Health Care Global Enterprises, Bangalore, Karnataka, India

Charanjeet Singh Department of Pathology, Florida Hospital, Orlando, FL, USA

Department of Pathology, University of Central Florida, Orlando, FL, USA

Harnoor Singh Department of Radiology, Texas Oncology, Amarillo, TX, USA

Anshuja Singla Department of Obstetrics and Gynaecology, University College of Medical Sciences and Guru Teg Bahadur Hospital, New Delhi, India

G. Sumangala Department of Gynaecological Oncology, St. John's Medical College and Hospital, Bangalore, Karnataka, India

Tien Anh Nguyen Tran Department of Pathology, Florida Hospital Orlando, Orlando, FL, USA

Elizabeth Vallikad Department of Gynaecological Oncology, St. John's Medical College and Hospital, Bangalore, Karnataka, India

Fredric Willmott Department of Women's Health, Whipps Cross University Hospital, London, UK

Garima Yadav Department of Obstetrics and Gynaecology, All India Institute of Medical Sciences, Jodhpur, Rajasthan, India

Jessica Young Breast Surgery Division, Department of Surgical Oncology, Roswell Park Comprehensive Cancer Center, Buffalo, NY, USA

Xingnan Zhou Department of Obstetrics and Gynecology, Peking Union Medical College Hospital, Peking Union Medical College, Chinese Academy of Medical Sciences, Beijing, China

Part I

Endometrium

1 Endometrial Carcinoma: Epidemiology and Risk Factors

Ritu Khatuja and Swati Rai

1.1 Epidemiology

Endometrial carcinoma is a malignant tumor, arising from the inner lining of the uterine corpus, i.e., the endometrium which can invade the layers of the uterus and also spread to distant sites.

Uterine cancer is one of the most common gynecologic malignancies in developed countries, with the incidence of 14.7 per 100,000 women and the mortality rate of 2.3 per 100,000. After cancer of the breast, lung, and colon, it is the fourth most common cancer diagnosed among American women. Recently, due to varied factors, its incidence has also increased in developing countries. After cervical cancer, it is the second most common gynecologic malignancy, with an incidence of 5.5 per 100,000 and a mortality rate of 1.15 per 100,000 [1].

The estimated incidence of endometrial cancer worldwide is 320,000, and it is responsible for 7600 deaths annually. Because of the early detection and reasonable prognosis associated with the disease, newer cases are more (320,000 or 4.8% of cancers in women and 2.3% of the total) as compared to mortality (76,000 deaths or 2.1% of cancer deaths in women). The incidence rate is highest in Northern America and Northwestern Europe, whereas it is low in South and Central Asia and most of Africa. Mortality rates ranged 0.9 to 3.8 per 100,000 in various countries [2]. In spite of low prevalence in developing countries, the mortality rate is still high as compared to developed countries due to low quality of medical services [3]. Data from different agencies has predicted that it will continue to rise in the next 15 years worldwide [4, 5].

The commonest types of endometrial cancers are estrogen-dependent neoplasm that accounts for 80–85% of cases and the non-estrogen-dependent tumors comprising of the remaining 10–15%. The estrogen-dependent tumors are frequently associated with obesity, diabetes, hypertension, nulliparity, early menarche, or late menopause. It is rightly stated that endometrial cancer is a disease of affluent class with high incidence among developed countries. The prevalence of endometrial cancer in developing countries is low, probably due to less incidence of obesity in these countries. Environmental factors play an important role in the pathogenesis of endometrial cancer. The prevalence and the progression of the disease are not effectively related

R. Khatuja (✉)
Department of Obstetrics and Gynaecology, ANIIMS, Port Blair, Andaman and Nicobar Islands, India

S. Rai
Department of Obstetrics and Gynaecology, Maulana Azad Medical College and Lok Nayak Hospital, New Delhi, India

S. Mehta, A. Singla (eds.), *Preventive Oncology for the Gynecologist*,
https://doi.org/10.1007/978-981-13-3438-2_1

with the early detection and treatment. Thus, due to change in lifestyle and dietary habits in both developed and developing nations, the rates are likely to increase [6, 7].

On the other hand, women with large order of births, old age at first child birth, and a short delivery-free period have decreased risk of endometrial cancer, emphasizing the protective role of progesterone in this disease.

The median age of diagnosis of uterine cancer is 62 years. After menopause, it is the commonest malignancy, but it is not common in women with age less than 45 years. Its prevalence is very high between the age group of 55 and 64 years, i.e., 34.5%, and least between the age group of 20 and 34 years (1.7%) [8]. Its incidence is stable in white women but is increased in black, Asian, Pacific, and Hispanics [9]. It is not due to racial differences per se but due to the risk factors associated with the disease.

Endometrial cancer is classified in two different categories on the basis of histology, and they have completely different incidence, response to estrogen therapy, and prognosis [10, 11].

Type I—Type I tumor accounts for 80% of the total endometrial cancer. Most of the tumors are of endometrioid histology (grade 1 or 2). As these tumors are estrogen-responsive and associated with an intraepithelial neoplasm (atypical and/or complex endometrial hyperplasia), thus they have a better outcome. The disease is more prevalent in women of premenopausal to early menopausal state, who are accompanied with obesity and high estrogen levels. There is superficial muscle layer invasion in 69.4% of cases, with high progesterone sensitivity found in almost 80.2% of cases. The 5-year survival rate is 85.6% with good prognosis (Table 1.1) [10, 11].

Type II—Around 10–20% of endometrial carcinomas come under type II category. They are prevalent in late postmenopausal women. There is no correlation with endocrine disorder or atypical endometrial hyperplasia. It comprises of endometrioid tumors of grade 3 type and tumors of non-endometrioid histology such as serous, squamous, mucinous clear cell, mesonephric, transitional cell, and undifferentiated. Its association with estrogen is still debatable. It has low sensitivity to progesterone found in 42.5% of this type. They are usually high-grade carcinomas with a poor outcome. Deep muscle layer invasion is seen almost in 65.7% of type II cases. It has a poor prognosis with 5-year survival rate of 58.8% (Table 1.1) [10].

Table 1.1 Types and characteristics of endometrial cancer

Characteristics	Type I	Type II
Role of estrogen	Present	Absent
Age group	Premenopausal to early menopausal period	Late postmenopausal period
Body mass index (BMI)	High	Low
Parity	Mostly nulliparous	Mostly multiparous
Atypical endometrial hyperplasia	May be present	Absent
Histology	Well differentiated	Poorly differentiated
Racial distribution	Mostly white women	Mostly black women
Muscular invasion	Superficial	Deep
Progesterone treatment	Mostly responsive	No response
Prognosis	Good	Poor

1.2 Risk Factors

Type I of endometrial carcinoma is mainly responsive to estrogen. The long-term exposure to excess endogenous or exogenous estrogen without adequate progesterone support is the most important risk factor for this malignancy. Some factors like nulliparity, diabetes mellitus, and hypertension, which invariably lead to excessive estrogen exposure, are almost always associated with the disease. There are some protective factors which prevent the disease by decreasing the estrogenic effect. Various factors associated with endometrial cancer are described in Table 1.2.

Table 1.2 Various factors associated with endometrial cancer

Endogenous risk factors	Exogenous risk factors	Associated factors
Increasing age	Diet	Infertility
Obesity	Unopposed estrogen therapy	Nulliparity
Chronic anovulation	HRT	Diabetes
Polycystic ovarian syndrome	Tamoxifen	Hypertension
Early menarche, late menopause		Breast cancer
Estrogen-secreting tumor		Tubal ligation
Family history		Socioeconomic status
Genetic factors: Lynch syndromes (HNPCC), BRCA		

Protective Factors

- Hormonal contraceptives for at least 1 year
- Grand multiparity
- Breast feeding
- Smoking
- Exercise
- Coffee/tea

1.3 Endogenous Risk Factors

The most important risk factor repeatedly said is excessive estrogen exposure which may be endogenous or exogenous. Chronic anovulation and excessive endogenous conversion of adrenal precursors to estrone and estradiol by adipose cells in obese women are among the common causes of endogenous estrogen production [12]. Zeleniuch studied the risk of developing endometrial carcinoma in a postmenopausal female and its correlation with higher circulating estrogen and androgen levels without progesterone protection [13].

1.3.1 Age

Endometrial carcinoma occurs most commonly in postmenopausal women. Its prevalence gradually increases from premenopausal stage, and maximum risk is seen in postmenopausal women; the risk decreases after 70 years of age [14]. This type of pattern is mostly in endometrial cancer type I. Obesity and chronic anovulation are associated risk factors in the women who develop endometrial cancer at less than 50 years of age.

1.3.2 Obesity

Obesity is a long-recognized risk factor for endometrial carcinoma which has been validated in many studies. A recent meta-analysis documented a strong association of onset of endometrial cancer with an increase of BMI by 5 kg/m^2 [15]. Even in younger age (less than 45 years), high BMI is correlated with the development of endometrial carcinoma [16]. The effect of obesity on different races is similar. In obese women, androstenedione produced in the ovary and adrenal gland gets converted into estrone, and the testosterone produced by the ovaries gets converted into estradiol in adipose tissues leading to hyperestrogenic state. Also in obesity the level of circulating serum sex hormone-binding globulin is low, and so there is increase in activated estrogen that leads to the endometrial hyperplasia and cancer. Study by Calle et al. showed positive correlation between obesity and mortality with endometrial carcinoma [17].

1.3.3 Chronic Anovulation

In anovulatory women, sex steroid hormones are produced, but not cyclically, so it leads to irregular uterine bleeding. Also, chronic estrogen production not opposed by progesterone causes proliferation of the endometrium. This can cause endometrial hyperplasia and eventually carcinoma. Anovulation mostly occurs during menarche and menopausal transition. Polycystic ovary syndrome is the most common endocrine disorder associated with chronic anovulation followed by thyroid dysfunction and elevated serum prolactin levels.

1.3.4 PCOS (Stein-Leventhal Syndrome)

PCOS is a disorder comprising of chronic anovulation and menstrual irregularities in the form of oligomenorrhea and hyperandrogenism. The main physiology that plays a pivotal role in producing endometrial hyperplasia is the continuous estrogen stimulation unopposed by progesterone. There is a strong relationship between endometrial cancer and anovulation associated with PCOS. However, women with PCOS had other risk factors which are related to endometrial cancer. Also the diagnostic criteria for PCOS were also not consistent; thus, it is difficult to make a risk assessment in PCOS group. Hence, these results provide little support for PCOS being a risk factor for endometrial cancer [18, 19].

1.3.5 Early Menarche and Late Menopause

Early age at menarche is a risk factor associated with endometrial carcinoma in some studies, but evidence is less supportive that late menopause is associated with an increased risk of the disease [20–22]. Both these factors result in long duration of estrogen exposure during which anovulatory cycles are common. A study by Pettersson et al. had shown the relation between the effect of "menstruation span" (years between menarche and menopause, excluding pregnancy-related time) and endometrial cancer. He found that cases which had a span longer than 39 years had 4.2 times the risk compared to the women with span shorter than 25 years. Long or irregular menstrual cycles had also positive relation with endometrial cancer [23].

1.3.6 Estrogen-Secreting Tumors

Some ovarian tumors produce estrogen and may lead to endometrial carcinoma. Granulosa cell tumors are the most likely to be associated with endometrial neoplasia. Granulosa cell tumor of the ovary is associated with 25–50% of endometrial hyperplasia and 5–10% of endometrial carcinoma. The carcinomas associated with granulosa-stromal cell tumors are usually early stage and well differentiated [24].

1.3.7 Family History of Endometrial Cancer

A familial history has been suggested for first-degree relatives, but no candidate genes have been identified till yet [25, 26]. Family history of endometrial cancer and colorectal cancer has high risk for the disease. They develop endometrial cancer at an early age (<50 years) [25]. The collective risk of endometrial cancer up to 70 years of age in women with a first-degree relative with endometrial cancer was considered to be 3.1% compared to less than 2% in the general population.

1.3.8 Genetic Factors

1.3.8.1 Lynch Syndrome

Lynch syndrome is a familial tumor syndrome and also known as hereditary nonpolyposis colorectal cancer (HNPCC). It is an autosomal dominant disorder. The women with Lynch syndrome are more at risk of developing endometrial cancer at a young age as well as higher risk of colon, endometrial, ovarian, biliary tract, gastric, small intestinal, and ureteropelvic cancer and brain tumors with respect to general population [27].

There is significant lifetime risk of endometrial cancer in women with Lynch syndrome ranging from 25 to 60%. The mean age of diagnosis of endometrial carcinoma in women in general population is 61 years, whereas it is 46–54 years in women with Lynch syndrome. The histology of the majority of Lynch syndrome-associated endometrial carcinomas is endometrioid, and it presents at an early stage, similar to sporadic endometrial carcinoma.

Lynch syndrome is caused by germline mutation in one of the DNA mismatch repair genes. The mutation of MLH1, MSH2, MSH6, and PMS2 genes is related with Lynch syndrome [28], but the mutation of gene MSH6 is significantly associated with the risk for endometrial cancer [29].

1.3.8.2 BRCA Mutation

Association of carriers of mutations in the BRCA genes with breast and ovarian cancers is known, but it was also suggested that endometrial cancer has some correlation with mutation in BRCA 1 genes as well as endometrial carcinoma [30]. However, in cases of BRCA mutation carriers on tamoxifen, it was also found that the risk of endometrial carcinoma was much higher [31].

1.3.8.3 Other Genetic Factors

Cowden syndrome (CS) and Peutz-Jeghers syndrome (PJS) are other genetic diseases which are related with endometrial cancer. Hereditary uterine cancers are discussed in detail in Chap. 4.

Cowden syndrome is an autosomal dominant disorder, and mutation in the PTEN tumor suppressor gene leads to this disease. The person suffering from Cowden syndrome may have characteristic formation of multiple hamartomas, distinctive dermal findings, and increased leiomyomas and is susceptible for malignant tumors [32].

Cowden syndrome is associated with breast, thyroid, and endometrial cancers. The cumulative risk of cancer is 85% at the age of 70 years, while the prevalence of endometrial cancer is 48.7% in this disease [33]. The data for this disease is very less, but still lifetime risk of endometrial cancer was noted 13–19% by different studies [34, 35].

PJS is an autosomal dominant disorder. It is identified by pigmentary lesions in the labium and buccal mucosa and multiple gastrointestinal polyposis. In 60% of cases of PJS patients, the mutation of STK11 gene is found in 60%. Patients with this syndrome are associated with more risk for developing of malignant tumors. The accumulated risk of all cancers is 93% until 64 years of age. The patients with PJS are at high risk of breast cancer and gynecological malignant tumors especially the sex cord-stromal ovarian cancer and cervical adenocarcinoma [36, 37].

1.4 Exogenous Risk Factors

1.4.1 Dietary Factors

There is no specific food or beverages that are related with endometrial carcinoma [38]. There are studies which found an association between a high-glycemic diet and endometrial carcinoma, but this is mostly related with obesity [39].

Alcohol use is associated with elevated estrogen levels, but it is uncertain whether alcohol consumption increases the risk of endometrial carcinoma [40]. A meta-analysis of 20 studies found no overall association between alcohol intake and endometrial carcinoma, but it is suggested that the type of beverage may be important, with an increase found for liquor intake, but not wine or beer [41].

1.4.2 Unopposed Estrogen Therapy

Systemic (oral, patch, or vaginal ring) estrogen therapy without an opposing progestin in a woman with a uterus may lead to markedly increased chances of hyperplasia of the endometrium or development of cancer. When a woman uses systemic estrogen therapy without a progestin for 1 year, it was found that endometrial hyperplasia developed in 20–50% of women [42]. This risk can be significantly reduced by the concomitant administration of a progestin [43]. An increased incidence of endometrial carcinoma between 1 and 1.5% has been seen with estrogen exposure which is associated with the dose and duration of the use of estrogen [44, 45].

It appears that most regimens of combined estrogen-progestin postmenopausal hormone therapy are not going to increase the chances of endometrial carcinoma. Women's Health Initiative randomized trial had illustrated this when they compared continuous estrogen-progestin therapy with placebo [46].

1.4.3 Tamoxifen

Tamoxifen, an antiestrogen used in the treatment of breast cancer, is a risk factor for endometrial cancer, but this is still not clear. Tamoxifen use increases the risk of endometrial cancer in postmenopausal women, whereas the risk in premenopausal women is unproven till date [47].

Tamoxifen is a selective estrogen receptor modulator and has both agonist and antagonist properties. The affectivity depends on the individual target organ and serum estrogen level. In breast tissue, it blocks estrogen stimulation and is used for prevention and treatment of breast cancer. Women on the standard tamoxifen dose (20 mg/day) who develop endometrial carcinoma do not differ from other women with endometrial carcinoma in terms of stage and histology [48].

The American College of Obstetricians and Gynecologists does not recommend routine screening for endometrial carcinoma in women on tamoxifen but advises that women be counseled about the risks associated with tamoxifen and should be monitored closely for symptoms of endometrial hyperplasia or carcinoma and undergo evaluation if symptoms of endometrial carcinoma are present [49].

1.4.4 Phytoestrogens

The effect of phytoestrogens on endometrial carcinoma risk is not established [50]. Phytoestrogens are nonsteroidal compound found in many plants, fruits, and vegetables. They have both estrogenic and antiestrogenic properties. Studies are not consistent with the ability of their association with endometrial hyperplasia or carcinoma. Some authors found they are not associated with increased risk of endometrial hyperplasia or carcinoma, and others found they decrease the risk [51, 52].

1.5 Associated Factors

1.5.1 Nulliparity and Infertility

The relation of parity with risk of endometrial cancer is inverse [53]. Nulliparity and infertility are not independently associated with endometrial carcinoma. The more frequent anovulatory cycles in infertile women are likely to be associated with endometrial cancer. Infertility is associated with 3.5-fold increase in risk [54]. Data are inconsistent regarding whether ovulation induction for treatment of infertility is associated with an increased risk of endometrial carcinoma.

1.5.2 Hypertension and Diabetes

The risk of endometrial cancer is increased in women with hypertension and diabetes [55]. Obesity is one of the important comorbid factors for this risk, but some studies have found both hypertension and diabetes with independent effects as well [52, 56]. Women with type 2 diabetes are more at risk of developing endometrial cancer than type 1 diabetes. Diets with high carbohydrates and hyperinsulinemia and elevated levels of insulin-like growth factors can cause proliferation of endometrium and may lead to endometrial cancer; however, the mechanism is not clear.

Corpus cancer syndrome includes diabetes and hypertension in association with endometrial carcinoma. All the three are markers of obesity and hence are associated.

1.5.3 Breast Cancer

Women with breast cancer on tamoxifen are at risk of developing endometrial cancer. This is probably due to common risk factors (e.g., obesity, nulliparity) in both malignancies. Some data suggest that serous endometrial type of endometrial cancer is in women with breast cancer who develop endometrial cancer [57].

1.5.4 Tubal Ligation

There are few conflicting studies regarding tubal ligation and its association with endometrial carcinoma. Opportunistic salpingectomy (performed concomitant with a surgery for another indication) has been proposed to decrease risk of ovarian cancer, but its association to decrease risk of endometrial carcinoma is not clear. The Women's Health Initiative Observational Study found no significant decrease in risk of endometrial carcinoma among women who had undergone tubal ligation [58]. But another study with 211 women with serous endometrial carcinoma found that tubal ligation may play a protective role in reducing the chances of positive cytology and stage IV disease [59].

1.5.5 Socioeconomic Status

Earlier studies reported increased risk of endometrial cancer in women of higher socioeconomic status probably due to more awareness and use of estrogen replacement therapy among educated women [60].

1.6 Protective Factors

1.6.1 Hormonal Contraception

The use of combined estrogen-progestin oral contraceptives decreases the risk of endometrial carcinoma by 30% [61]. Long-term use reduces the risk, and its protective effect lasts for 20 or more years even after discontinuation [62]. The presence of progestin is the cause of beneficial effect of hormonal contraceptives as it plays a preventive role. Studies have found that progestin-only contraceptives (e.g., depot medroxyprogesterone acetate, progestin implants, progestin-releasing intrauterine devices) provide protective effect against the development of endometrial neoplasia [63, 64].

1.6.2 Increasing Age at Last Birth

Childbearing at an older age, independent of parity and other factors, was associated with a decreased risk of endometrial carcinoma in a meta-analysis of 17 studies that included over 8000 cases of endometrial cancer [65].

1.6.3 Breastfeeding

Breastfeeding appears to be associated with a decrease in the risk of endometrial carcinoma. At least mean duration of 3 months of breastfeeding per child is required, to decrease endometrial cancer risk. But the degree of risk did not continue to decrease after 6 to 9 months [66].

1.6.4 Smoking

Cigarette smoking plays a protective role in decreasing the risk of developing uterine carcinoma in postmenopausal women due to its antiestrogenic effect. But the major health risks associated with tobacco far outweigh this single benefit. The effect in premenopausal women is uncertain. The mechanism suggested for this effect is that smoking stimulates hepatic metabolism of estrogens, leading to lowering of estrogen which eventually lead to reduction of incidence of endometrial abnormalities. Thus, smoking has been found to have a protective effect on endometrial carcinoma [67].

1.6.5 Physical Activity

When physical activity is increased, there will be decreased risk of endometrial carcinoma. The mechanism involved is possible association between high levels of physical activity and reduced cancer risk as it leads to decreased obesity as well as central adiposity and favorable changes in immune function and in endogenous sexual and metabolic hormone levels [68].

1.6.6 Coffee/Tea

A meta-analysis found a decreased risk of uterine cancer is directly proportional to the amount of coffee consumption [69]. Another meta-analysis reported a decreased risk of uterine cancer proportional to the quantity of tea consumed; however, the correlation was statistically significant with consumption of green tea only [70].

1.6.7 Other Factors

There is no association between vitamin D and endometrial carcinoma risk; some data suggest that the use of calcium supplements may be protective. Studies have also found association of aspirin with a decreased risk of endometrial cancer [71, 72].

1.6.8 Risk Factors for Type II Endometrial Carcinoma

Type 2 endometrial carcinoma accounts for 10–20% of all cases. There are fewer epidemiologic data about them than type I carcinomas. Type II endometrial carcinomas tend to present at an advanced stage. Approximately 70% of patients with uterine serous cancer (USC) and 50% with clear cell cancers present with stage III or IV disease [73]. It develops in elderly patients, and the probable mechanism involved is mutation of the p53 gene in endometrial cells [74].

1.7 Conclusion

Endometrial cancer is the commonest gynecological malignancy in women with varied incidence worldwide. The number of endometrial cancer is increasing day by day, due to changing lifestyle, increasing obesity, and extended life expectancy. Here, in this chapter we have tried to discuss various factors related with endometrial cancer. However, still there are many potential factors without definite evidence which required further studies.

Key Points

- Endometrial cancer is the fourth most common cancer in women and ranks eighth in terms of cancer mortality.
- The incidence has wide variation across countries with higher incidence among western population although it is increasing worldwide due to change in lifestyle.
- Type I endometrial cancer is most common accounting for 80–90% of cancers with well-known risk factors, whereas the risk factors associated with Type II endometrial cancer are not clear.
- Estrogen whether endogenous or exogenous is a well-established risk factor for endometrial cancer especially type I cancer.
- Clinical conditions like PCOS, unopposed estrogen therapy, diabetes, hypertension, obesity, and tamoxifen use increase the risk of endometrial carcinoma, while oral contraceptive pills, breast feeding, exercise, and coffee/tea are protective.

References

1. Siegel RL, Miller KD, Jemal A. Cancer statistics, 2017. CA Cancer J Clin. 2017;67(1):7–30. https://doi.org/10.3322/caac.21387.
2. Ferlay J, Soerjomataram I, Dikshit R, Eser S, Mathers C, Rebelo M, Parkin DM, Forman D, Bray F. Cancer incidence and mortality worldwide: sources, methods and major patterns in GLOBOCAN 2012. Int J Cancer. 2015;136(5):E359–86. https://doi.org/10.1002/ijc.29210.
3. Terri M, David S, Sherman AJ, Ann GS, Stephen BG. Endometrial cancer: socioeconomic status and racial/ethnic differences in stage at diagnosis, treatment, and survival. Am. J Public Health. 2014;94:2104–11.
4. Rahib L, Smith BD, Aizenberg R, et al. Projecting cancer incidence and deaths to 2030: the unexpected burden of thyroid, liver, and pancreas cancers in the United States. Cancer Res. 2014;74(11):2913–21. https://doi.org/10.1158/0008-5472.CAN-14-0155.
5. Sheikh MA, Althouse AD, Freese KE, et al. USA endometrial cancer projections to 2030: should we be concerned? Future Oncol. 2014;10(16):2561–8. https://doi.org/10.2217/fon.14.192.
6. Smith RA, Cokkinides V, Eyre HJ. American Cancer Society guidelines for the early detection of cancer, 2003. CA Cancer J Clin. 2003;53:27–43.
7. Zeleniuch-Jacquotte A, Lundin E, et al. Circulating enterolactone and risk of endometrial cancer. Int J Cancer. 2006;119:2376–81.
8. http://seer.cancer.gov/statfacts/html/corp.html. Accessed 28 Jan 2018
9. Eheman C, Henley SJ, Ballard-Barbash R, et al. Annual report to the nation on the status of cancer, 1975-2008, featuring cancers associated with excess weight and lack of sufficient physical activity. Cancer. 2012;118(9):2338–66. https://doi.org/10.1002/cncr.27514.
10. Bokhman JV. Two pathogenetic types of endometrial carcinoma. Gynecol Oncol. 1983;15:10.
11. Felix AS, Weissfeld JL, Stone RA, et al. Factors associated with type I and type II endometrial cancer. Cancer Causes Control. 2010;21:1851.
12. Siiteri PK. Adipose tissue as a source of hormones. Am J Clin Nutr. 1987;45:277.
13. Zeleniuch-Jacquotte A, Akhmedkhanov A, Kato I, et al. Postmenopausal endogenous oestrogens and risk of endometrial cancer: results of a prospective study. Br J Cancer. 2001;84:975.

14. Siegel R, Ward E, Brawley O, et al. Cancer statistics, 2011: the impact of eliminating socioeconomic and racial disparities on premature cancer deaths. CA Cancer J Clin. 2011;61:212–36.
15. Renehan AG, Tyson M, Egger M, et al. Body-mass index and incidence of cancer: a systematic review and meta-analysis of prospective observational studies. Lancet. 2008;371:569.
16. Pellerin GP, Finan MA. Endometrial cancer in women 45 years of age or younger: a clinicopathological analysis. Am J Obstet Gynecol. 2005;193:1640.
17. Calle EE, Rodriguez C, Walker-Thurmond K, Thun MJ. Overweight, obesity, and mortality from cancer in a prospectively studied cohort of U.S. Adults. N Engl J Med. 2003;348:1625–38.
18. Pillay OC, Te Fong LF, Crow JC, et al. The association between polycystic ovaries and endometrial cancer. Hum Reprod. 2006;21:924–9.
19. Hardiman P, Pillay OC, Atiomo W. Polycystic ovary syndrome and endometrial carcinoma. Lancet. 2003;361:1810–2.
20. Brinton LA, Berman ML, Mortel R, et al. Reproductive, menstrual, and medical risk factors for endometrial cancer: results from a case-control study. Am J Obstet Gynecol. 1992;167:1317.
21. Xu WH, Xiang YB, Ruan ZX, et al. Menstrual and reproductive factors and endometrial cancer risk: results from a population-based case-control study in urban Shanghai. Int J Cancer. 2004;108:613.
22. Karageorgi S, Hankinson SE, Kraft P, de Vivo I. Reproductive factors and postmenopausal hormone use in relation to endometrial cancer risk in the Nurses' Health Study cohort 1976–2004. Int J Cancer. 2010;126:208.
23. Pettersson B, Adami HO, Bergstrom R, Johansson ED. Menstruation span ± a time-limited risk factor for endometrial carcinoma. Acta Obstet Gynaecol Scand. 1986;65:247–55.
24. Schumer ST, Cannistra SA. Granulosa cell tumor of the ovary. J Clin Oncol. 2003;21:1180.
25. Lucenteforte E, Talamini R, Montella M, et al. Family history of cancer and the risk of endometrial cancer. Eur J Cancer Prev. 2009;18:95.
26. Mucci LA, Hjelmborg JB, Harris JR, et al. Familial risk and heritability of cancer among twins in Nordic countries. JAMA. 2016;315:68.
27. Lynch HT, de la Chapelle A. Hereditary colorectal cancer. N Engl J Med. 2003;348:919–32.
28. Dunlop MG, Farrington SM, Carothers AD, Wyllie AH, Sharp L, Burn J, Liu B, Kinzler KW, Vogelstein B. Cancer risk associated with germline DNA mismatch repair gene mutations. Hum Mol Genet. 1997;6:105–10. J Med Genet 2013; 50, 255–263
29. Hendriks YM, Wagner A, Morreau H, et al. Cancer risk in hereditary nonpolyposis colorectal cancer due to MSH6 mutations: impact on counseling and surveillance. Gastroenterology. 2004;127:17–25.
30. Thompson D, Easton DF. Breast cancer linkage consortium. Cancer incidence in BRCA1 mutation carriers. J Natl Cancer Inst. 2002;94:1358.
31. Beiner ME, Finch A, Rosen B, et al. The risk of endometrial cancer in women with BRCA1 and BRCA2 mutations. A prospective study. Gynecol Oncol. 2007;104:7.
32. Hanssen AM, Fryns JP. Cowden syndrome. J Med Genet. 1995;32:117–9.
33. Bubien V, Bonnet F, Brouste V, et al. High cumulative risks of cancer in patients with PTEN hamartoma tumour syndrome. J Med Genet. 2013;50:255–63.
34. Heald B, Mester J, Rybicki L, et al. Frequent gastrointestinal polyps and colorectal adenocarcinomas in a prospective series of PTEN mutation carriers. Gastroenterology. 2010;139:1927.
35. Riegert-Johnson DL, Gleeson FC, Roberts M, et al. Cancer and Lhermitte-Duclos disease are common in Cowden syndrome patients. Hered Cancer Clin Pract. 2010;8:6.39: 1927
36. Lim W, Hearle N, Shah B, et al. Further observations on LKB1/STK11 status and cancer risk in Peutz–Jeghers syndrome. Br J Cancer. 2003;89:308–13.
37. Giardiello FM, Brensinger JD, Tersmette AC, et al. Very high risk of cancer in familial Peutz-Jeghers syndrome. Gastroenterology. 2000;119:1447–53.
38. Bandera EV, Kushi LH, Moore DF, et al. Consumption of animal foods and endometrial cancer risk: a systematic literature review and meta-analysis. Cancer Causes Control. 2007;18:967.
39. Mulholland HG, Murray LJ, Cardwell CR, Cantwell MM. Dietary glycaemic index, glycaemic load and endometrial and ovarian cancer risk: a systematic review and meta-analysis. Br J Cancer. 2008;99:434.
40. Loerbroks A, Schouten LJ, Goldbohm RA, van den Brandt PA. Alcohol consumption, cigarette smoking, and endometrial cancer risk: results from the Netherlands Cohort Study. Cancer Causes Control. 2007;18:551.
41. Sun Q, Xu L, Zhou B, et al. Alcohol consumption and the risk of endometrial cancer: a meta-analysis. Asia Pac J Clin Nutr. 2011;20:125.
42. Furness S, Roberts H, Marjoribanks J, et al. Hormone therapy in postmenopausal women and risk of endometrial hyperplasia. Cochrane Database Syst Rev. 2009;2:CD000402.
43. Voigt LF, Weiss NS, Chu J, et al. Progestagen supplementation of exogenous oestrogens and risk of endometrial cancer. Lancet. 1991;338:274.
44. Persson I, Adami HO, Bergkvist L, et al. Risk of endometrial cancer after treatment with oestrogens alone or in conjunction with progestogens: results of a prospective study. BMJ. 1989;298:147.
45. Beral V, Bull D, Reeves G, Million Women Study Collaborators. Endometrial cancer and hormone-replacement therapy in the Million Women Study. Lancet. 2005;365:1543.

46. Anderson GL, Judd HL, Kaunitz AM, et al. Effects of estrogen plus progestin on gynecologic cancers and associated diagnostic procedures: the Women's Health Initiative randomized trial. JAMA. 2003;290:1739.
47. Iqbal J, Ginsburg OM, Wijeratne TD, et al. Endometrial cancer and venous thromboembolism in women under age 50 who take tamoxifen for prevention of breast cancer: a systematic review. Cancer Treat Rev. 2012;38:318.
48. Barakat RR, Wong G, Curtin JP, et al. Tamoxifen use in breast cancer patients who subsequently develop corpus cancer is not associated with a higher incidence of adverse histologic features. Gynecol Oncol. 1994;55:164.
49. Committee Opinion No. 601: Tamoxifen and uterine cancer. Obstet Gynecol. 2014; 123:1394.
50. Horn-Ross PL, John EM, Canchola AJ, et al. Phytoestrogen intake and endometrial cancer risk. J Natl Cancer Inst. 2003;95:1158.
51. Myung SK, Ju W, Choi HJ, et al. Soy intake and risk of endocrine-related gynaecological cancer: a meta-analysis. BJOG. 2009;116:1697.
52. North American Menopause Society. The role of soy isoflavones in menopausal health: report of The North American Menopause Society/Wulf H. Utian Translational Science Symposium in Chicago, IL (October 2010). Menopause. 2011;18:732.
53. Parazzini F, Negri E, La Vecchia C, et al. Role of reproductive factors on the risk of endometrial cancer. Int J Cancer. 1998;76:784.
54. Henderson BE, Casagrande JT, Pike MC, et al. The epidemiology of endometrial cancer in young women. Br J Cancer. 1983;47:749–56.
55. Friberg E, Orsini N, Mantzoros CS, Wolk A. Diabetes mellitus and risk of endometrial cancer: a meta-analysis. Diabetologia. 2007;50:1365.
56. Lindemann K, Vatten LJ, Ellstrøm-Engh M, Eskild A. Body mass, diabetes and smoking, and endometrial cancer risk: a follow-up study. Br J Cancer. 2008;98:1582.
57. Liang SX, Pearl M, Liang S, et al. Personal history of breast cancer as a significant risk factor for endometrial serous carcinoma in women aged 55 years old or younger. Int J Cancer. 2011;128:763.
58. Winer I, Lehman A, Wactawski-Wende J, et al. Tubal ligation and risk of endometrial cancer: findings from the Women's Health Initiative. Int J Gynecol Cancer. 2016;26:464.
59. Ayeni TA, Bakkum-Gamez JN, Mariani A, et al. Impact of tubal ligation on routes of dissemination and overall survival in uterine serous carcinoma. Gynecol Oncol. 2013;128:71.
60. Elwood JM, Cole P, Rothman KJ, Kaplan SD. Epidemiology of endometrial cancer. Br J Hosp Med. 1997;59:1055–60.
61. Collaborative Group on Epidemiological Studies on Endometrial Cancer. Endometrial cancer and oral contraceptives: an individual participant meta-analysis of 27 276 women with endometrial cancer from 36 epidemiological studies. Lancet Oncol. 2015;16:1061.
62. Iversen L, Sivasubramaniam S, Lee AJ, et al. Lifetime cancer risk and combined oral contraceptives: the Royal College of General Practitioners' Oral Contraception Study. Am J Obstet Gynecol. 2017;216:580.e1.
63. Soini T, Hurskainen R, Grénman S, et al. Cancer risk in women using the levonorgestrel-releasing intrauterine system in Finland. Obstet Gynecol. 2014;124:292.
64. Montz FJ, Bristow RE, Bovicelli A, et al. Intrauterine progesterone treatment of early endometrial cancer. Am J Obstet Gynecol. 2002;186:651.
65. Setiawan VW, Pike MC, Karageorgi S, et al. Age at last birth in relation to risk of endometrial cancer: pooled analysis in the epidemiology of endometrial cancer consortium. Am J Epidemiol. 2012;176:269.
66. Jordan SJ, Na R, Johnatty SE, et al. Breastfeeding and endometrial cancer risk: an analysis from the epidemiology of endometrial cancer consortium. Obstet Gynecol. 2017;129:1059.
67. Zhou B, Yang L, Sun Q, et al. Cigarette smoking and the risk of endometrial cancer: a meta-analysis. Am J Med. 2008;121:501.
68. Friedenreich CM, Orenstein MR. Physical activity and cancer prevention: etiologic evidence and biological mechanisms. J Nutr. 2002;132:3456S.
69. Bravi F, Scotti L, Bosetti C, et al. Coffee drinking and endometrial cancer risk: a meta-analysis of observational studies. Am J Obstet Gynecol. 2009;200:130.
70. Butler LM, Wu AH. Green and black tea in relation to gynecologic cancers. Mol Nutr Food Res. 2011;55:931.
71. McCullough ML, Bandera EV, Moore DF, Kushi LH. Vitamin D and calcium intake in relation to risk of endometrial cancer: a systematic review of the literature. Prev Med. 2008;46:298.
72. Matsuo K, Cahoon SS, Yoshihara K, et al. Association of low-dose aspirin and survival of women with endometrial cancer. Obstet Gynecol. 2016;128:127.
73. Podratz KC, Mariani A. Uterine papillary serous carcinomas: the exigency for clinical trials. Gynecol Oncol. 2003;91:461.
74. Kaaks R, Lukanova A, Kurzer MS. Obesity, endogenous hormones, and endometrial cancer risk: a synthetic review. Cancer Epidemiol Biomark Prev. 2002;11:1531–43.

Role of Screening Modalities in Endometrial Cancer Detection

2

Angelito Magno and Nidhi Arora

2.1 Introduction

Carcinoma endometrium is the most common gynecologic cancer in developed countries; for women through age 74 years, the incidence is 14.7 per 100,000 and the mortality rate is 2.3 per 100,000. In developing nations, this is the second most common gynecologic cancer (cancer of the cervix being more common); for women through age 74 years, the incidence is 5.5 per 100,000 and mortality rate is 1.5 per 100,000. Among the developed countries, endometrial cancer is the fourth most common cancer ($n = 167{,}900$) compared to 151,700 cases in the developing countries (seventh leading cancer cases) [1]. In the United States, 61,380 new cases have been reported in 2017 [2]. An increasing trend is seen in many countries and is more pronounced in some Asian countries (China, Japan, the Philippines, Singapore, and India), Belarus, Lithuania, Costa Rica, and New Zealand [3]. In China, the annual percent change of cases from 2000 to 2011 was observed as 3.7%. This increasing trend is attributed to increased use of exogenous hormones, reproductive factors, and older menopausal age [4]. Most of the patients with endometrial cancer are diagnosed at an early stage: limited to the primary site (67%), regional organ and lymph node involvement (21%), and distant metastases (8%) [5].

This disease is more common in perimenopausal and postmenopausal women (50–65 years). Only 10–15% of women are aged below 50 years, and 5% developed the cancer younger than 40 years [6]. Risk factors include unopposed estrogen, tamoxifen use, increasing age, obesity, nulliparity, irregular menstrual cycles, smoking (type II endometrial cancer), and Lynch syndrome [7].

The most common clinical presentation is abnormal uterine bleeding, and majority of women presenting with endometrial cancer have pathology confined to the uterus with a 5-year survival rate more than 90% [8]. The majority of the cancer cases are diagnosed at the early stage, thereby favoring a better prognosis. The 5-year relative survival rates of endometrial cancer from 1975 to 2009 are stable at 80% (1975–1977 = 87%, 1987–1989 = 82%, and 2003–2009 = 84%) [9, 10].

2.2 Types of Endometrial Cancer

Endometrial cancer has been divided mainly into two types based on their difference in incidence in the population, the genetics involved, their

A. Magno (✉)
Department of Obstetrics and Gynecology, Section of Gynecologic Oncology, De La Salle Health Sciences Institute, De La Salle University Medical Center, Dasmariñas City, Philippines

N. Arora
Department of Fetal Medicine, Rainbow Hospital, New Delhi, India

S. Mehta, A. Singla (eds.), *Preventive Oncology for the Gynecologist*,
https://doi.org/10.1007/978-981-13-3438-2_2

presentation, prognosis, and the treatment strategies. The two types are the endometrioid (type I) and the non-endometrioid carcinoma (type II) [11]. The more common type is the endometrioid adenocarcinoma (type I) and contributes to almost three-fourths of the endometrial cancers. They usually present as FIGO (International Federation of Gynecology and Obstetrics) grade 1 or 2, have a good prognosis, are estrogen responsive, and may be preceded by an intraepithelial neoplasm. The precursor lesion is the atypical endometrial hyperplasia (also known as endometrial intraepithelial neoplasia) [7]. Endometrial hyperplasia is the proliferation of endometrial glands and stroma primarily due to hyperestrogenism. It has been classified by different systems.

The latest WHO endometrial hyperplasia classification, 2015 (replacing the 1994 classification), has now only two categories. These are (1) hyperplasia without atypia (nonneoplastic) and (2) atypical hyperplasia (endometrial intraepithelial neoplasm) [12].

The earlier 1994 WHO system classification [13] classified endometrial hyperplasia as simple hyperplasia without atypia, complex hyperplasia without atypia, simple atypical hyperplasia, and complex atypical hyperplasia. It was intended to correlate the risk of progression of endometrial hyperplasia to endometrial carcinoma. However, there was a lot of inter-observer variability between different pathologists for the nuclear atypia that was the main feature described for the progression. The new system has helped in avoiding the confusion between the various terms and stresses on the fact that *hyperplasia without atypia is nonneoplastic*. On the contrary, hyperplasia with atypia is seen to be associated with the cellular and genetic changes that are observed with the invasive carcinoma and is thus a precursor lesion for the invasive carcinoma.

Type II tumors comprise FIGO grade 3 endometrioid carcinomas along with tumors of non-endometrioid histology: serous, clear cell, mucinous, squamous, transitional cell, mesonephric, and undifferentiated. Carcinosarcomas also fall in this category [11]. These typically present as high-grade tumors and have poor survival rates. They usually occur in the atrophic endometrium and are so common in the postmenopausal age group. Estrogen stimulation is not a risk factor for type II tumors, and precursor lesions are not identified with this subtype.

2.3 Risk Factors

Risk stratification of endometrial cancer divides individuals into low risk, moderate risk, and high risk.

Low-risk individuals are those with no risk factors [14].

Moderate-risk (other terms: average or increased risk) individuals are those with risk factors like unopposed estrogen use, late menopause, tamoxifen therapy, nulliparity, infertility, chronic anovulation, obesity, and diabetes [15].

High-risk individuals are those who carry hereditary non-polyposis colon cancer (HNPCC)-associated mutations, substantial likelihood of being a mutation carrier (family history of gene mutation), or absence of genetic testing result in families with suspected autosomal dominant predisposition to colon cancer [16]. HNPCC or Lynch syndrome is an autosomal dominant inherited disorder with germline mutations in DNA mismatch repair genes MLH1, PMS2, MSH2, and MSH6. These genetic mutations increase the risk of an individual to develop gastrointestinal, gynecologic, upper urinary tract, pancreatobiliary tract, brain, and sebaceous gland malignancies. Carriers of the genetic mutations have a lifetime risk of developing endometrial cancer of 60% [17]. Lynch syndrome contributes to 2–5% of all endometrial carcinomas [18].

2.4 Clinical Presentation and Diagnosis

The most common symptom of endometrial cancer is vaginal bleeding [19]; however, up to 20% of patients with endometrial cancer are asymptomatic. The amount of bleeding has no correlation with the risk of having the endometrial cancer. The asymptomatic women may present with abnormal findings on cervical cytology. Another presentation is of thickened endometrium as an incidental finding on imaging performed for other indications.

The diagnostic tools available for symptomatic patients are transvaginal sonography and endometrial sampling.

2.4.1 Transvaginal Ultrasound (TVUS)

TVUS is the most common diagnostic modality to evaluate symptomatic patients both in the premenopausal and the postmenopausal age groups. This helps to evaluate for other pathologies associated with abnormal uterine bleeding specially in the premenopausal age group.

Endometrial thickness (ET) is measured in the sagittal view of the uterus. The double layer of the endometrium measured in an anteroposterior dimension from one basalis layer to the other, excluding any fluid within the cavity, is reported as the endometrial thickness. Any focal endometrial lesion requires a biopsy.

2.4.1.1 Symptomatic Postmenopausal Women

Postmenopausal women who are not on any hormonal therapy, an endometrial thickness of less than or equal to 4 or 5 mm is associated with a minimal risk of endometrial disease [20, 21]. The cutoff for endometrial thickness has been studied by various authors. A cutoff value of endometrial thickness of 3, 4, and 5 mm has sensitivity of 98%, 95%, and 90%, respectively, in symptomatic postmenopausal women [22].

The American College of Obstetrics and Gynecology defines this cutoff as ≤4 mm, and the Society of Radiologists in Ultrasound (SRU) defines it as ≤5 mm. Both these bodies state that either TVUS with abovementioned endometrial thickness, respectively, or endometrial sampling is effective as the first procedure in postmenopausal symptomatic women [23, 24]. Also, ACOG states that TVUS can be useful as a second-line diagnostic test when insufficient tissue is obtained after endometrial sampling yielded. If the endometrial thickness is ≤4 mm, then malignancy is rare. Focal pathologies can be visualized on TVUS as mentioned above. To conclude, biopsy can be avoided if the thickness is <4 mm.

However, if a patient continues to be symptomatic on follow-up, biopsy must be performed.

2.4.1.2 Asymptomatic Postmenopausal Women

Yasa et al. assessed the diagnostic accuracy of endometrial thickness measurement of transvaginal ultrasound (TVU) in 276 asymptomatic postmenopausal women in the detection of endometrial carcinoma. Women with endometrial thickness of >4 mm underwent hysteroscopy and dilatation and curettage (D&C). Out of the 276 women, only nine patients (3.3%) had endometrial hyperplasia with atypia, and only eight patients had endometrial adenocarcinoma. The area under the ROC curve was 0.52 (95% CI 0.44–0.57), which indicated a poor accuracy of endometrial thickness of TVU for carcinoma in asymptomatic women [25]. Another study evaluated the endometrial thickness threshold for endometrial sampling in asymptomatic postmenopausal women. A total of 462 women were included, and only nine cases of carcinoma and seven cases of atypical hyperplasia were identified. Atypical hyperplasia is significantly associated with an endometrial thickness of or more than 14 mm (odds ratio 4.29; 95% CI 1.30–14.20; $P = 0.02$), with negative predictive value of 98.3%. Endometrial thickness of 15 mm or more is significantly associated with endometrial carcinoma (odds ratio 4.53; 95% CI 1.20–17.20; $P = 0.03$), with a negative predictive value of 98.5% [26].

At times, TVUS done for postmenopausal women for another indication (other than vaginal bleeding) shows presence of the endometrial fluid with minimal endometrial thickening. The most common cause for this is cervical stenosis. It has been seen in numerous studies that if the endometrial thickness is less than 3 mm with presence of fluid, the chances of endometrial cancer are less. However, the risk increases when it is greater than 3 mm. In such cases, biopsy should be done in postmenopausal asymptomatic women [27–29].

2.4.1.3 Premenopausal Women

The role of TVUS as a diagnostic method for endometrial cancer in premenopausal women has not been clearly defined. In a study of 200 premenopausal women presenting with abnormal uterine bleeding, 20% of women with an endometrial thickness measuring as <5 mm was eventually given the diagnosis of an endometrial polyp or a submucosal leiomyoma as the cause of AUB [30].

The timing of the TVUS is also important in premenopausal women. It must be on day 4, 5, or 6 of the bleeding cycle, the reason being that the endometrium is the thinnest at this time of the menstrual cycle, 4–8 mm in the proliferative phase while 8–14 mm in the secretory phase [31].

Since there is no defined threshold cutoff in premenopausal women with AUB for endometrial thickness on TVUS, it cannot be used as an alternative to endometrial sampling other than as a first-line imaging method to evaluate for other causes of this presentation. Also, it should be clear that in asymptomatic premenopausal women, only the endometrial thickness cannot be used as an indication for the diagnostic biopsy. The clinical history and risk stratification are more important in such cases.

In women on hormonal therapy whether on unopposed estrogen therapy or when estrogen is given with cyclic progestogen, TVUS cannot be used as a screening or diagnostic modality for endometrial cancer [32, 33], the reason again being a lack of threshold cutoff for endometrial thickness. So, endometrial sampling becomes the procedure of choice for this group of women when presenting with abnormal bleeding patterns. They should be assessed clinically and explained that bleeding does occur when they are put on the hormonal therapy and should report if it is persistent or occurs after a long phase of amenorrhea.

2.4.2 Endometrial Sampling

This is the gold standard diagnostic modality for evaluation of any symptomatic woman with suspected endometrial carcinoma. Office endometrial biopsy, dilatation and curettage (D&C), and hysteroscopy with directed biopsy are the various methods to get tissue samples for confirmatory evaluation of the endometrium. The sensitivity for endometrial sampling is more than or equal to 90%. False-negative endometrial sampling is encountered if there is a personal history of colorectal cancer, presence of endometrial polyps, and also in morbidly obese women [34].

The choice of the procedure depends upon the clinical situation.

2.4.2.1 Office Endometrial Biopsy

Endometrial sampling is routinely done with an office endometrial biopsy that can be performed as an outpatient procedure with either no anesthesia or local anesthesia and is the least invasive approach. This can be done by various suction devices or with the use of endometrial brush. The suction devices can be low-pressure (e.g., pipelle, Endocell) or high-pressure devices (e.g., Vabra aspirator, Karman cannula). The low-pressure devices are more commonly used for office endometrial biopsy as they are more flexible, and do not require cervical dilatation making them more comfortable for an outpatient procedure. The endometrial brush (Tao brush) works similar to the Pap brush used for endocervical sampling.

Among all the devices being used for endometrial sampling, the pipelle (Fig. 2.1) has been studied the most. It is less painful and is able to obtain more tissue when compared to Vabra aspirator [35, 36]. It can be used without cervical dilatation in the outpatient department and is also more cost-effective. In a study by [37] Abdelazim

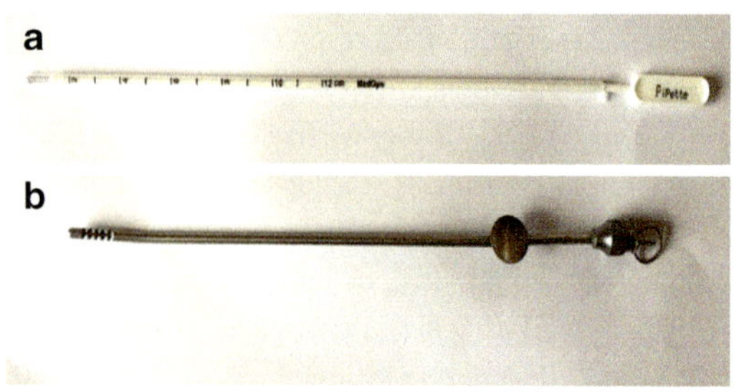

Fig. 2.1 (**a**) Pipelle endometrial sampling device (Pipette MedGyn, RB Medical Herefordshire, UK). (**b**) Novak Endometrial Curette

et al. 2013, its sensitivity for endometrial hyperplasia as well as carcinoma was 100%. Several observational studies are there to support office endometrial biopsy with pipelle as a screening tool in comparison to D&C with and without hysteroscopy. The specimen satisfaction rate varies from 73.9% to 100% and the pathological accuracy between 62.0% and 96.9% for endometrial lesions with greater acceptability for patients than D&C [38–47].

However, a few limitations of pipelle have also been reported. It is not effective in sampling focal pathology like polyps [45], and since theoretically only a small portion of endometrium is sampled, it may not be a good screening tool.

In the systematic review by Du et al. [48] comparing the various endometrial sampling devices, Tao brush was found to be the most effective method for screening endometrial pathology but with the limitations of higher cost and unsuccessful insertion rate [48].

2.4.2.2 Dilatation and Curettage

At times, one may choose to do a D&C as the initial procedure especially in women for whom the office biopsy is intolerable, for patients with heavy bleeding since D&C acts as both a diagnostic and a therapeutic procedure, and in women in the high-risk group, i.e., with Lynch syndrome. The other indications are cervical stenosis, inadequate specimen with office biopsy, or when done along with some other diagnostic/operative procedure.

2.4.2.3 Hysteroscopic-Directed D&C

Hysteroscopy with D&C becomes the procedure of choice when there is suspicion of focal lesions like polyps. It is helpful in visualizing the endometrial cavity completely, and simultaneous therapy can be initiated.

A systematic review and meta-analysis consisting of 45 studies with 12,459 patients was done to assess the agreement between the three preoperative endometrial sampling techniques (office endometrial biopsy, dilatation and curettage, and hysteroscopy with directed biopsy) with the final histopathologic diagnosis of endometrial carcinoma [49]. Of the 45 studies, nine analyzed office endometrial biopsy technique, three analyzed hysteroscopic biopsies, and 16 studies included analyzed D&C. Hysteroscopic technique has a significantly higher agreement with the final diagnosis (0.89, 95% CI 0.80–0.98) than D&C (0.70, 95% CI 0.60–0.79; $P < 0.02$). There was no significant difference in agreement between hysteroscopic biopsies and office endometrial biopsy (agreement of 0.73 (95% CI 0.60–0.86) ($p = 0.08$). In clinical practice, hysteroscopic biopsy and office endometrial biopsy have higher accuracy of getting the final diagnosis than D&C. Another finding of this study was the 8% clinically relevant upgrading rate from low grade in preoperative endometrial sampling to high-grade tumor in final diagnosis.

Figure 2.2 represents a suggested algorithm to decide whether the sample obtained from the endometrium by any technique (office biopsy or curettage) is adequate and if there is any need to resample the endometrium [50].

2.5 Screening for Endometrial Cancer

As mentioned previously, most of the women with endometrial cancer have their first symptom as abnormal bleeding. Earlier symptomatic presentation is able to detect most but not all endometrial cancers at an earlier stage. Also, since the survival is good if diagnosed early, it is questionable to adopt a definite screening protocol. So, for such a disease, the early presentation with abnormal bleeding provides an evidence of secondary prevention, i.e., diagnosis of a disease when its treatment can halt its progression. An important hindrance to make a screening guideline for this cancer is that there is no screening test which is sensitive, specific, and acceptable to the population to be screened or to the physicians.

Thereby, the primary prevention (screening for a disease before the symptomatic presentation) becomes less cost-effective.

Endometrial sampling is no doubt a sensitive and specific test, but at the cost of being invasive and also uncomfortable to the individual. On the

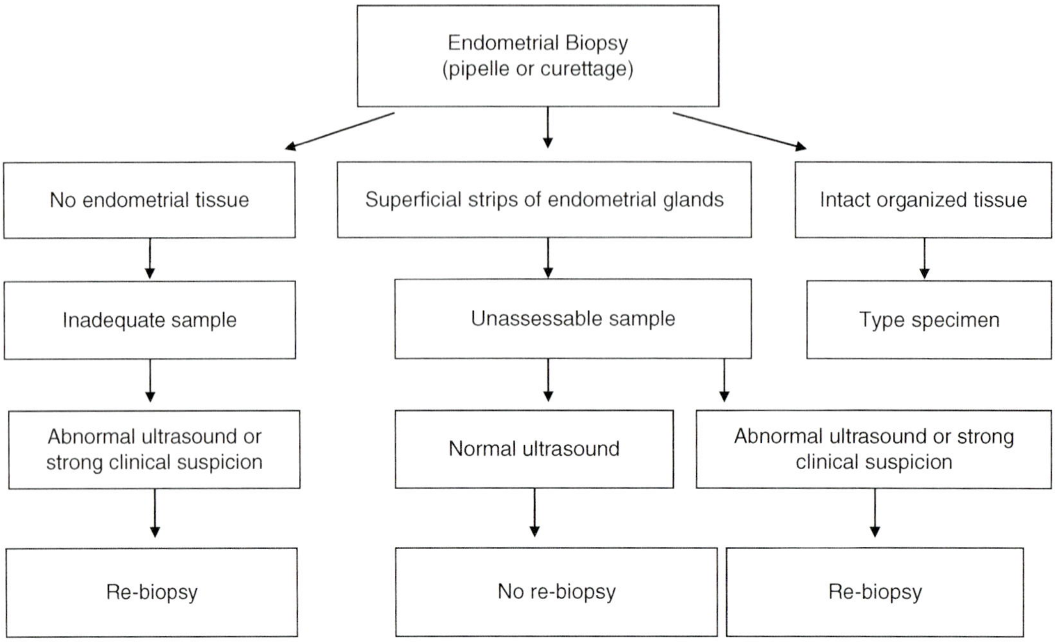

Fig. 2.2 Algorithm for assessment of the adequacy of an endometrial biopsy specimen. Reproduced from Journal of Clinical Pathology, McCluggage WG, 59(8), 801–12, Copyright 2006, with permission from BMJ Publishing Group Ltd

contrary, measurement of endometrial thickness on transvaginal ultrasound, though a sensitive test in picking up endometrial cancer postmenopause, its sensitivity is roughly 20% lower in asymptomatic postmenopausal women as compared to the symptomatic women, with the drawback of low specificity and high false-positive rate. This eventually leads to the option of the invasive endometrial biopsy. Though there is a subgroup of patients who are diagnosed incidentally on conventional Pap smear routinely done for cervical cancer, its sensitivity for endometrial cancer is only 40–55%. On the contrary, the sensitivity of liquid-based preparations is 60–65% [51, 52].

2.5.1 Asymptomatic Women at Average or Increased Risk

Routine screening of asymptomatic women at average or increased risk of endometrial cancer is not advisable due to the lack of satisfactory quality evidence in favor of screening to reduce the mortality from endometrial cancer. The exception to this includes women with the Lynch syndrome (hereditary non-polyposis colon cancer) and other genetic association (Cowden syndrome) who have a substantially increased risk of development of endometrial cancer and should therefore go for routine screening and finally a hysterectomy to reduce the risks.

2.5.2 American Cancer Society

The ACS recommends that low-risk and moderate-risk women at the time of menopause should be informed about the risks and symptoms of endometrial cancer and strongly encouraged to report any unexpected bleeding or spotting.

2.5.3 ACOG Practice Bulletin for Endometrial Cancer [7]

According to ACOG, evidences on the use of imaging tools to evaluate premenopausal women with abnormal uterine bleeding are not clear. Ultrasound measurement of endometrial thickness in this age group should not be performed due to poor diagnostic value. Symptomatic postmenopausal women should be initially evaluated either by endometrial biopsy or transvaginal ultrasound. Symptomatic women with endometrial thickness of greater than 4 mm warrant further evaluation by doing endometrial sampling. Office endometrial biopsy is the method of choice for endometrial evaluation due to its reliability and accuracy in endometrial cancer detection.

2.5.4 Women with Lynch Syndrome

Women with Lynch syndrome who are asymptomatic are advised yearly endometrial sampling, beginning at 30–35 years of age or 5–10 years earlier than the age at which the first diagnosis of the syndrome-related cancer in the family [53].

Some experts have suggested the use of TVUS for screening for endometrial cancer; however, there is no added increase in the sensitivity when combined with endometrial sampling in comparison to sampling alone. Its main use has been seen in screening for the ovarian cancer in these women. There is no sufficient data to differentiate between the endometrial sampling and TVUS as screening modalities for this subgroup of patients. Studies are required to determine their sensitivity in both premenopausal and postmenopausal asymptomatic patients with Lynch syndrome. For now, only endometrial sampling is considered the procedure of choice; though being invasive, it must be performed annually.

2.5.5 Cowden Syndrome

For Cowden syndrome (autosomal dominant syndrome with mutation in PTEN tumor suppressor gene, lifetime risk of endometrial cancer—13–28%), no guidelines are given at present for screening of endometrial cancer. However, this should be managed like Lynch syndrome, i.e., endometrial sampling and risk-reducing hysterectomy [54, 55].

2.5.6 Tamoxifen Users

Women who are on tamoxifen should be explained thoroughly at the time of initiation of therapy for the symptom of vaginal bleeding and endometrial evaluation by transvaginal ultrasound, and endometrial sampling should only be reserved to symptomatic patients. These women have thickened endometrium on TVUS or may have cystic appearance due to activation of adenomyotic foci. There is no threshold cutoff for endometrial thickness for women on tamoxifen. Evaluation of asymptomatic tamoxifen users will result in low incidence of endometrial cancer at the cost of high rate of unnecessary endometrial biopsy and even hysterectomy [56, 57]. This group of population must be informed in written to report to the physician in case of any change in the vaginal bleeding patterns for further evaluation.

2.6 Novel Tests as Screening Tools for Endometrial Cancer

2.6.1 Liquid-Based Endometrial Cytology

Endometrial cytology has been used in Japan as a routine initial screening method for endometrial cancer since 1987. Its use has not been widely accepted due to low diagnostic accuracy owing to presence of excessive blood and overlapping cells in the cytology samples. Due to the recent development of liquid-based cytology technique, mainly used for cervical cancer screening, endometrial cytology has now been reevaluated as a screening tool for symptomatic women with suspicious endometrial pathology. A total of 1672 women were included in a Chinese study, which aimed to investigate the diagnostic accuracy of liquid-based endometrial cytology, in comparison with histology [58]. All women underwent endometrial cytology using the SAP-1 device, hysteroscopy, and D&C. SAP-1 device (Saipujiuzhou, Beijing, China) (Fig. 2.3) is patented and can be used in China. The SAP-1 sampler measures 3 mm in diameter and 250 mm in

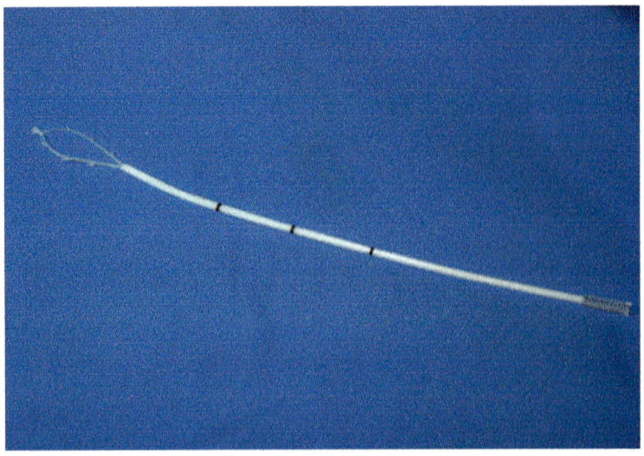

Fig. 2.3 The SAP-1 device (Saipujiuzhou, Beijing, China). Reprinted from Yang X, Ma K, Chen R, Zhao J, Wu C, Zhang N, et al. Liquid-based endometrial cytology associated with curettage in the investigation of endometrial carcinoma in a population of 1987 women. Arch Gynecol Obstet 2017; 296(1): 99–105. With permission from Springer from McCluggage WG (50)

length. It has a flexible soft latex loop with spines to get cytology samples that can be plunged out of outer protective tube to prevent contamination from cervical and vaginal cells when releasing out of the uterine cavity. The cytology samples were immersed in the SurePath vial (BD Diagnostic, Burlington, NC, USA) and processed using AutoCyte PREP automated slide processor (Tri-Path Corporation, USA). In postmenopausal women, 96% ($n = 758/790$) had adequate cytologies as compared to 74.2% ($n = 586$ of 790) adequacy of histologic samples. SAP-1 device provided more adequate samples than D&C ($p < 0.001$). Diagnosing atypical hyperplasia or worse as a positive result, the diagnostic accuracy of liquid-based endometrial cytology was 86.1% with sensitivity, specificity, positive predictive value, and negative predictive value of 70.3%, 88.5%, 48.0%, and 95.2%, respectively. Taking endometrial carcinoma as the positive result, the diagnostic accuracy of liquid-based endometrial cytology was increased to 94.4%, with sensitivity of 53.2%, specificity of 98.6%, positive predictive value at 79.8%, and negative predictive value of 95.3%. The study showed that liquid-based endometrial cytology is a useful method in as a first-line approach in detecting endometrial malignancy. This result shows promising future for endometrial cytology as a screening tool for endometrial cancer, but more robust evidences are needed to support its use.

2.6.2 Multiplex PCR-Based Tests: PapSEEK

The routine screening by Pap smear has improved the diagnosis and thereby treatment of patients with cervical cancer. No such test has been devised for both endometrial and ovarian cancer. Wang et al. [59] performed genetic analysis of fluid obtained through routine Papanicolaou testing (PapSEEK), along with the analysis of tumor DNA circulating in the blood. They also performed intrauterine sampling with Tao brush/Pap brush to increase the sensitivity of detection for the less accessible tumors. Tao brush was used to sample the endometrial cavity, while Pap brush sampled the endocervical canal. The basis of this study was a recent study by Kinde et al. [60], which stated that both the endometrial and ovarian cancer cells shed and get collected at the cervix. These can provide sample for testing the tumor DNA from the fluid collected during cervical Pap screening.

This is a minimally invasive procedure and samples can be conveniently obtained during routine office cervical cancer screening visit. The somatic mutation testing was performed for 18 genes after amplifying the DNA sample obtained for the fluid obtained with Tao brush/Pap brush by using multiplex PCR. The results of this study showed that with PapSEEK, 93% of endometrial cancers were detected with Tao Brush and 81% with Pap brush. The detection rate for ovarian cancers with PapSEEK was 45% with Tao Brush and 33% with Pap brush. The advantage of this method was the high specificity with only 0 and 1.4% of women without cancer testing positive with Tao and Pap brush samples, respectively. The assays for ctDNA in plasma could be used in conjunction with PapSEEK on Pap brush samples, increasing the sensitivity of detecting ovarian cancer to 63%. The combined ctDNA analysis with PapSEEK analysis of Tao brush was not tested in the study.

Table 2.1 Recommendation for endometrial cancer screening

Low-risk and Moderate-risk women [61]	At menopausal age, women should be informed of the risks and symptoms of endometrial cancer Any unexpected bleeding or spotting warrants reporting and evaluation
High-risk women [61]	Annual testing by endometrial biopsy should be considered starting age 35 years
Endometrial sampling technique [7]	Office endometrial biopsy with disposable devices is reliable and accurate for the detection of disease in most cases of endometrial cancer and has become the method of choice for histologic evaluation of the endometrium
Premenopausal women [61]	Evidences on the use of imaging tools to evaluate premenopausal women with abnormal uterine bleeding are not clear Ultrasound measurement of endometrial thickness should not be performed due to poor of diagnostic value
Postmenopausal women [26]	Asymptomatic women: • 14 mm or above endometrial thickness warrants endometrial sampling Symptomatic women: • Initial evaluation by EITHER transvaginal ultrasound or emdometrial sampling • >4 mm endometrial thickness warrants endometrial sampling
Tamoxifen user [56, 57]	Asymptomatic: no routine screening method Symptomatic women: evaluation with TVU and endometrial biopsy

A very important and encouraging finding of this study was the pickup of high-grade endometrial cancer (85% detection rate by Pap brush and 89% detection rate by Tao brush) which is not at all identified by the routine transvaginal ultrasound. Though these high-grade (type II) endometrial cancers contribute very less to the overall incidence of this cancer, the mortality with this type is high and they are picked up at late stage. With this screening modality, we can pick up these high-grade tumors at an early stage, thus contributing to the increased survival rate.

The limitations of the study were that it was a retrospective study rather than prospective. Also, the samples were obtained from the diagnosed endometrial and ovarian cancer patients, though a substantial number of samples were obtained from the early-stage lesions. We need further studies to prove the role of PapSEEK as a screening tool for the endometrial and ovarian cancer.

The summary of endometrial cancer screening is in Table 2.1.

2.7 Conclusion

Since, at present, a good screening method is not available for endometrial cancer and it presents early in the course of progression, routine screening is not advised by different oncology societies. The exception to this is women with high risk, i.e., Lynch syndrome, for which screening is recommended. Emphasis should be given on providing adequate information with respect to abnormal uterine bleeding to women in the perimenopausal age group. For menopausal group, any amount of bleeding should be advised to be reported.

Key Points

- Endometrial carcinoma is the most common gynecological cancer in the developed world and is the second most common in the developing world.
- The available screening modalities for endometrial cancer are transvaginal ultrasound and endometrial sampling.
- TVUS is a good first line of investigation for women presenting with abnormal uterine bleeding, though more beneficial in symptomatic postmenopausal women.
- Postmenopausal women with ET on TVUS measuring more than 4 mm need further evaluation. No specific ET cutoff has been laid down for premenopausal women.
- Endometrial sampling remains the gold standard for diagnosis of endometrial pathology.
- Office endometrial biopsy has considerably replaced the traditional D&C for the screening

and diagnosis of endometrial hyperplasia and neoplasia. The use of pipelle for office procedure has been evaluated as sensitive, specific, and less painful in many studies.
- Screening for endometrial carcinoma is not recommended due to its early symptomatic presentation and good survival rates in early stages.
- The exception to this is the high-risk group, i.e., women with Lynch syndrome who require screening by endometrial sampling.

References

1. Torre LA, Bray F, Siegel RL, Ferlay J, Lortet-Tieulent J, Jemal A. Global cancer statistics, 2012. CA Cancer J Clin. 2015;65(2):87–108.
2. Howlader N, Noone AM, Krapcho M, Miller D, Bishop K, Altekruse SF, et al. SEER cancer statistics review, 1975–2014. Bethesda: National Cancer Institute; 2017.
3. Lortet-Tieulent J, Ferlay J, Bray F, Jemal A. International patterns and trends in endometrial cancer incidence, 1978–2013. J Natl Cancer Inst. 2018;110(4):354–61. https://doi.org/10.1093/jnci/djx214.
4. Jiang X, Tang H. Epidemiology of gynecologic cancers in China. J Gynecol Oncol. 2018;29(1):e7.
5. http://seer.cancer.gov/statfacts/html/corp.html. Accessed 06 June 2016.
6. Galczynski K, Nowakowski L, Rechberger T, Semczuk A. Should we be more aware of endometrial cancer in adolescents? Dev Period Med. 2016;20(3):169–73.
7. Practice Bulletin No. 149: Endometrial cancer. Obstet Gynecol. 2015;125(4):1006–1026.
8. Creasman WT, Odicino F, Maisonneuve P, Quinn MA, Beller U, Benedet JL, et al. Carcinoma of the corpus uteri. FIGO 26th annual report on the results of treatment in gynecological cancer. Int J Gynaecol Obstet. 2006;95(suppl 1):S105–43. (Level III)
9. Siegel R, Ma J, Zou Z, Jemal A. Cancer statistics, 2014. CA Cancer J Clin. 2014;64(1):9–29.
10. Yamagami W, Nagase S, Takahashi F. Clinical statistics of gynecologic cancers in Japan. J Gynecol Oncol. 2017;28(2):e32.
11. Bokhman JV. Two pathogenetic types of endometrial carcinoma. Gynecol Oncol. 1983;15:10.
12. Emons G, Beckmann MW, Schmidt D, et al. New WHO classification of endometrial hyperplasias. Geburtshilfe Frauenheilkd. 2015;75:135.
13. Scully RE, Bonfiglio TA, Kurman RJ, et al. Uterine corpus. In: Histological typing of female genital tract tumours. 2nd ed. New York: Springer; 1994. p. 13.
14. Kim YB, Ghosh K, Ainbinder S, Berek JS. Diagnostic and therapeutic advances in gynecologic oncology: screening for gynecologic cancer. Cancer Treat Res. 1998;95:253–76.
15. Zanotti KM, Kennedy AW. Screening for gynecologic cancer. Med Clin North Am. 1999;83(6):1467–87.
16. Smith RA, von Eschenbach AC, Wender R, Levin B, Byers T, Rothenberger D, et al. American Cancer Society guidelines for the early detection of cancer: update of early detection guidelines for prostate, colorectal, and endometrial cancers. Also: update 2001—testing for early lung cancer detection. CA Cancer J Clin. 2001;51(1):38–75; quiz 7-80
17. Dillon JL, Gonzalez JL, DeMars L, Bloch KJ, Tafe LJ. Universal screening for Lynch syndrome in endometrial cancers: frequency of germline mutations and identification of patients with Lynch-like syndrome. Hum Pathol. 2017;70:121–8.
18. Lancaster JM, Powell CB, Chen LM, et al. Society of Gynecologic Oncology statement on risk assessment for inherited gynecologic cancer predispositions. Gynecol Oncol. 2015;136:3.
19. Tzur T, Kessous R, Weintraub AY. Current strategies in the diagnosis of endometrial cancer. Arch Gynecol Obstet. 2017;296(1):5–14.
20. Goldstein SR, Nachtigall M, Snyder JR, Nachtigall L. Endometrial assessment by vaginal ultrasonography before endometrial sampling in patients with postmenopausal bleeding. Am J Obstet Gynecol. 1990;163:119.
21. Karlsson B, Granberg S, Wikland M, Ylöstalo P, Torvid K, Marsal K, et al. Transvaginal ultrasonography of the endometrium in women with postmenopausal bleeding—a Nordic multicenter study. Am J Obstet Gynecol. 1995;172:1488.
22. Timmermans A, Opmeer BC, Khan KS, Bachmann LM, Epstein E, Clark TJ, et al. Endometrial thickness measurement for detecting endometrial cancer in women with postmenopausal bleeding: a systematic review and meta-analysis. Obstet Gynecol. 2010;116(1):160–7.
23. American College of Obstetricians and Gynecologists. ACOG committee opinion no. 440. The role of transvaginal ultrasonography in the evaluation of postmenopausal bleeding. Obstet Gynecol. 2009;114:409.
24. Goldstein RB, Bree RL, Benson CB, Benacerraf BR, Bloss JD, Carlos R, et al. Evaluation of the woman with postmenopausal bleeding: society of radiologists in ultrasound-sponsored consensus conference statement. J Ultrasound Med. 2001;20:1025.
25. Yasa C, Dural O, Bastu E, Ugurlucan FG, Nehir A, Iyibozkurt AC. Evaluation of the diagnostic role of transvaginal ultrasound measurements of endometrial thickness to detect endometrial malignancy in asymptomatic postmenopausal women. Arch Gynecol Obstet. 2016;294(2):311–6.
26. Louie M, Canavan TP, Mansuria S. Threshold for endometrial sampling among postmenopausal patients without vaginal bleeding. Int J Gynaecol Obstet. 2016;132(3):314–7.

27. Debby A, Malinger G, Glezerman M, Golan A. Intrauterine fluid collection in postmenopuasal women with cervical stenosis. Maturitas. 2006;55:334.
28. Schmidt T, Nawroth F, Breidenbach M, Hoopmann M, Mallmann P, Valter MM. Differential indication for histological evaluation of endometrial fluid in postmenopause. Maturitas. 2005;50:177.
29. Vuento MH, Pirhonen JP, Mäkinen JI, Tyrkkö JE, Laippala PJ, Grönroos M, et al. Endometrial fluid accumulation in asymptomatic postmenopausal women. Ultrasound Obstet Gynecol. 1996;8:37.
30. Breitkopf DM, Frederickson RA, Snyder RR. Detection of benign endometrial masses by endometrial stripe measurement in premenopausal women. Obstet Gynecol. 2004;104:120.
31. Goldstein SR, Zeltser I, Horan CK, Snyder JR, Schwartz LB. Ultrasonography-based triage for perimenopausal patients with abnormal uterine bleeding. Am J Obstet Gynecol. 1997;177:102.
32. Holbert TR. Transvaginal ultrasonographic measurement of endometrial thickness in postmenopausal women receiving estrogen replacement therapy. Am J Obstet Gynecol. 1997;176:1334.
33. Meuwissen JH, Oddens BJ, Klinkhamer PJ. Endometrial thickness assessed by transvaginal ultrasound insufficiently predicts occurrence of hyperplasia during unopposed oestrogen use. Maturitas. 1996;24:21.
34. Torres ML, Weaver AL, Kumar S, Uccella S, Famuyide AO, Cliby WA, et al. Risk factors for developing endometrial cancer after benign endometrial sampling. Obstet Gynecol. 2012;120:998.
35. Kaunitz AM, Masciello A, Ostrowski M, Rovira EZ. Comparison of endometrial biopsy with the endometrial Pipelle and vabra aspirator. J Reprod Med. 1988;33(5):427–31.
36. Wu HH, Harshbarger KE, Berner HW, Elsheikh TM. Endometrial brush biopsy (Tao brush). Histologic diagnosis of 200 cases with complementary cytology: an accurate sampling technique for the detection of endometrial abnormalities. Am J Clin Pathol. 2000;114(3):412–8.
37. Abdelazim IA, Aboelezz A, Abdulkareem AF. Pipelle endometrial sampling versus conventional dilatation & curettage in patients with abnormal uterine bleeding. J Turk Ger Gynecol Assoc. 2013;14(1):1–5.
38. Leng X, Wang M, Zhang SL, Wang D, Cao W, Yang XH. Different methods for the diagnosis of endometrial histological comparative study. Zhonghua Fu Chan Ke Za Zhi. 2013;48(12):891–5.
39. Fakhar S, Saeed G, Khan AH, Alam AY. Validity of Pipelle endometrial sampling in patients with abnormal uterine bleeding. Ann Saudi Med. 2008;28(3):188–91.
40. Machado F, Moreno J, Carazo M, Leon J, Fiol G, Serna R. Accuracy of endometrial biopsy with the Cornier pipelle for diagnosis of endometrial cancer and atypical hyperplasia. Eur J Gynaecol Oncol. 2003;24(3–4):279–81.
41. Zorlu CG, Cobanoglu O, Isik AZ, Kutluay L, Kuscu E. Accuracy of pipelle endometrial sampling in endometrial carcinoma. Gynecol Obstet Investig. 1994;38(4):272–5.
42. Sanam M, Majid MM. Comparison the diagnostic value of dilatation and curettage versus endometrial biopsy by Pipelle—a clinical trial. Asian Pac J Cancer Prev. 2015;16(12):4971–5.
43. Rauf R, Shaheen A, Sadia S, Waqar F, Zafar S, Sultana S, et al. Outpatient endometrial biopsy with Pipelle versus diagnostic dilatation and curettage. J Ayub Med Coll Abbottabad. 2014;26(2):145–8.
44. Gungorduk K, Asicioglu O, Ertas IE, Ozdemir IA, Ulker MM, Yildirim G, et al. Comparison of the histopathological diagnoses of preoperative dilatation and curettage and Pipelle biopsy. Eur J Gynaecol Oncol. 2014;35(5):539–43.
45. Kazandi M, Okmen F, Ergenoglu AM, Yeniel AO, Zeybek B, Zekioglu O, et al. Comparison of the success of histopathological diagnosis with dilatation-curettage and Pipelle endometrial sampling. J Obstet Gynaecol. 2012;32(8):790–4.
46. Guido RS, Kanbour-Shakir A, Rulin MC, Christopherson WA. Pipelle endometrial sampling. Sensitivity in the detection of endometrial cancer. J Reprod Med. 1995;40(8):553–5.
47. Ben-baruch G, Seidman DS, Schiff E, Moran O, Menczer J. Outpatient endometrial sampling with the Pipelle curette. Gynecol Obstet Investig. 1994;37(4):260–2.
48. Du J, Li Y, Lv S, Wang Q, Sun C, Dong X, He M, Ulain Q, Yuan Y, et al. Endometrial sampling devices for early diagnosis of endometrial lesions. J Cancer Res Clin Oncol. 2016;142:2515–22.
49. Visser NCM, Reijnen C, Massuger L, Nagtegaal ID, Bulten J, Pijnenborg JMA. Accuracy of endometrial sampling in endometrial carcinoma: a systematic review and meta-analysis. Acta Chir Belg. 2017;130(4):803–13.
50. McCluggage WG. My approach to the interpretation of endometrial biopsies and curettings. J Clin Pathol. 2006;59(8):801–12.
51. Guidos BJ, Selvaggi SM. Detection of endometrial adenocarcinoma with the ThinPrep Pap test. Diagn Cytopathol. 2000;23:260.
52. Schorge JO, Hossein Saboorian M, Hynan L, Ashfaq R. ThinPrep detection of cervical and endometrial adenocarcinoma: a retrospective cohort study. Cancer. 2002;96:338.
53. Lindor NM, Petersen GM, Hadley DW, Kinney AY, Miesfeldt S, Lu KH, et al. Recommendations for the care of individuals with an inherited predisposition to Lynch syndrome: a systematic review. JAMA. 2006;296:1507.
54. Pilarski R, Stephens JA, Noss R, Fisher JL, Prior TW. Predicting PTEN mutations: an evaluation of Cowden syndrome and Bannayan-Riley-Ruvalcaba syndrome clinical features. J Med Genet. 2011;48:505.

55. Tan MH, Mester JL, Ngeow J, Rybicki LA, Orloff MS, Eng C. Lifetime cancer risks in individuals with germline PTEN mutations. Clin Cancer Res. 2012;18:400.
56. Barakat RR, Gilewski TA, Almadrones L, Saigo PE, Venkatraman E, Hudis C, et al. Effect of adjuvant tamoxifen on the endometrium in women with breast cancer: a prospective study using office endometrial biopsy. J Clin Oncol. 2000;18(20):3459–63.
57. Gerber B, Krause A, Muller H, Reimer T, Kulz T, Makovitzky J, et al. Effects of adjuvant tamoxifen on the endometrium in postmenopausal women with breast cancer: a prospective long-term study using transvaginal ultrasound. J Clin Oncol. 2000;18(20):3464–70.
58. Yang X, Ma K, Chen R, Zhao J, Wu C, Zhang N, et al. Liquid-based endometrial cytology associated with curettage in the investigation of endometrial carcinoma in a population of 1987 women. Arch Gynecol Obstet. 2017;296(1):99–105.
59. Wang Y, Li L, Douville C, Cohen JD, Yen TT, Kinde I, Sundfelt K, et al. Evaluation of liquid from the Papanicolaou test and other liquid biopsies for the detection of endometrial and ovarian cancers. Sci Transl Med. 2018;10(433):eaap8793.
60. Kinde I, Bettegowda C, Wang Y, Wu J, Agrawal N, Shih MI, et al. Evaluation of DNA from the Papanicolaou test to detect ovarian and endometrial cancers. Sci Transl Med. 2013;5:167ra4.
61. Smith RA, Andrews KS, Brooks D, Fedewa SA, Manassaram-Baptiste D, Saslow D, et al. Cancer screening in the United States, 2017: a review of current American Cancer Society guidelines and current issues in cancer screening. CA Cancer J Clin. 2017;67(2):100–21.

Endometrial Hyperplasia: Diagnosis and Management

3

Bijal M. Patel

Abbreviations

AUB	Abnormal uterine bleeding
BMI	Body mass index
BSO	Bilateral salpingo-oophorectomy
CT	Computerized tomography
D&C	Dilatation and curettage
DMPA	Depot medroxyprogesterone acetate
EB	Endometrial biopsy
EC	Endometrial carcinoma
EGF	Epithelial growth factor
EH	Endometrial hyperplasia
EIN	Endometrial intraepithelial neoplasia
ER	Estrogen receptors
ERT	Estrogen replacement therapy
ET	Endometrial thickness
GnRH	Gonadotropin-releasing hormone
H&E	Hematoxylin and eosin
HRT	Hormone replacement therapy
IGF-1	Insulin-like growth factor-1
IL-1β	Interleukin-1β
IUD	Intrauterine device
LNG	Levonorgestrel
MA	Megestrol acetate
MPA	Medroxyprogesterone acetate
MRI	Magnetic resonance imaging
MSI	Microsatellite instability
NETA	Norethisterone acetate
OCs	Oral contraceptives
PCNA	Proliferating cell nuclear antigen
PCOS	Polycystic ovarian syndrome
PMB	Postmenopausal bleeding
PR	Progesterone receptor
RCOG	Royal College of Obstetricians and Gynaecologists
SERM	Selective estrogen receptor modulator
SNPs	Single nucleotide polymorphisms
TAH	Total abdominal hysterectomy
TNF R1	Tumor necrosis factor receptor 1
TNF-α	Tumor necrosis factor-α
TVS	Transvaginal sonography
USG	Ultrasonography
WHO	World Health Organization

3.1 Introduction

Endometrial hyperplasia (EH) is a spectrum of morphological changes ranging from a slightly disordered pattern seen in the late proliferative phase of the menstrual cycle to the irregular proliferation of the endometrial glands with an increase in gland-to-stroma ratio leading to thickening of the endometrium [1]. It is further classified on the basis of the complexity of endometrial glands and any cytological atypia [2]. In fact, EH is the only known direct precursor of endometrial carcinoma (EC). These lesions range from anovulatory endometrium to monoclonal

B. M. Patel (✉)
Department of Gynecologic Oncology,
Gujarat Cancer and Research Institute, Ahmedabad,
Gujarat, India

S. Mehta, A. Singla (eds.), *Preventive Oncology for the Gynecologist*,
https://doi.org/10.1007/978-981-13-3438-2_3

precancers. Menstrual cycle involves a complex interaction of estrogen and progesterone hormones which affects the endometrial lining. Factors like hormonal balance, molecular mechanisms, age, environment, and so forth maintain the fine equilibrium of the endometrium, and any disturbance leading to chronic estrogen stimulation may lead to several endometrial abnormalities [1, 3, 4]. In 1900, Cullen described an etiologic correlation between EH and EC. In 1932, Taylor and also in 1936, Novak and Yui supported this observation. In 1947, Gusberg focused his attention on the role of estrogenic stimulation as a factor that caused EH and EC [5]. Speert (1952) introduced the term "adenomatous atypical hyperplasia" for the premalignant hyperplasias. EH has been classified by various systems over the last 50 years. In 1982, Kurman and Norris first published the study describing reproducible criteria for differentiating EH from well-differentiated EC [6]. The estimated incidence of EH in developed countries is 200,000 new cases per year [1, 7]. EH incidence without atypia and with atypia peaks in the early postmenopausal years and early 60s, respectively [8].

Prospective studies are difficult to conduct to determine the malignant potential of these lesions for several reasons. The obstacle to long-term surveillance is that the condition is usually detected in symptomatic women who therefore require treatment so that follow-up to determine the natural history of the various histological subtypes is difficult. There is also difficulty in accurately differentiating between the atypical hyperplasia and well-differentiated EC [9].

Diagnosis of EH is important because it may cause abnormal uterine bleeding (AUB), indicative of anovulation and infertility, associated with estrogen-producing ovarian tumors, and precede or occur simultaneously with EC [10]. Sensitive and accurate diagnosis can reduce the likelihood of development of invasive EC [11]. Regression of hyperplasia to normal endometrium represents the key to conservative treatment for prevention of the development of EC [1].

A brief overview of the development of a current understanding of EH will serve to understand their diagnosis and management.

3.2 Etiology and Risk Factors

A relative excess of estrogen, unopposed by progesterone, whether it is exogenous or endogenous is thought to be one of the primary etiological factors in both EH and EC. Estrogen stimulates endometrial proliferation by binding to estrogen receptors (ER) in the nuclei of endometrial cells. Known risk factors for EH reflect this etiology [1, 2, 7, 12–14] (Table 3.1).

Hormone replacement therapy (HRT) and obesity are considered as reversible risk factors. Postmenopausal women treated with estrogen replacement therapy (ERT) without progestins are at increased risk of EH. The risk of EH increases by tenfold with each decade of use of ERT [1, 2, 15]. Obese women (body mass index [BMI] > 30 kg/m^2) have a nearly fourfold increase in the incidence of atypical EH due to excessive peripheral conversion of androgens in adipose tissue to estrogen coupled with erratic anovulatory cycles [16, 17].

Table 3.1 Risk factors responsible for development of EH [1, 2, 7, 12–14]

Category of risk factor	Risk factor
Nonmodifiable	Increasing age (age >35 years) Caucasian Family history of endometrium, ovarian, breast, or colon cancer
Lifestyle	Smoking
Menstrual status	Early menarche and/or late menopause, postmenopausal
Reproductive events	Nulliparity, infertility
Comorbidity	Obesity, DM (type II), metabolic syndrome, insulin resistance, HT, PCOS (anovulation), Lynch syndrome (HNPCC), estrogen-secreting ovarian tumors (e.g., ovarian granulosa cell tumors), androgen-secreting tumors of the adrenal cortex
Drug-induced	Unopposed ERT/prolonged HRT, long-term tamoxifen therapy
Others	Immunosuppression, infection
Genetic mutations	MSI, PTEN, K-ras, β-catenin, PIK3CA, SNPs
Cytokine system	TNF-α, PCNA, EGF, Fas, TNF-R1, IGF-1, NF-κB, IL-22

Tamoxifen, which is a selective estrogen receptor modulator (SERM), is used to treat ERα-positive primary and advanced breast cancers. It leads to EH, development of endometrial polyps, abnormal vaginal bleeding, and EC due to its estrogenic effect on the endometrium [1, 17].

In addition to estrogenic stimulation of the endometrium, other elements such as immunosuppression and infection may also be involved in the development of EH [13].

Genetic alterations like microsatellite instability (MSI), PTEN mutations, K-ras mutation, beta-catenin mutation, PIK3CA mutation, functional single nucleotide polymorphisms (SNPs), and so forth are observed in endometrial lesions [1, 14].

Inflammation in the endometrium disturbs the balanced cytokine system which leads to most cases of EH. Inflammation causes decrease in tumor necrosis factor-α (TNF-α), proliferating cell nuclear antigen (PCNA), and epithelial growth factor (EGF) mRNA and increased production of Fas mRNA and IGF-1 receptor (IGF-1R). In glandular cystic hyperplasia, decreased expression of tumor necrosis factor receptor 1 (TNF R1), interleukin-1β (IL-1β), and IL-12 genes is found. The expression of the insulin-like growth factor-1 (IGF-1) gene is reduced only in adenomatous hyperplasia [1].

Risk factors for EH and EC differ in relation to reproductive factors. Parity is found to be protective for EC but not for EH [14]. Long duration of oral contraceptive use has some protective effect [14, 15].

3.3 Risk of Endometrial Carcinoma

EH is a pathologically diversified lesion which encompasses histological subtle and spontaneously reversible proliferative lesions to emerging EC. Women with atypical hyperplasia may have coexistent EC or may progress to carcinoma [18].

3.3.1 Coexistent Carcinoma

EC is found more frequently in women with cytological atypia. Recent studies have shown EC in hysterectomy specimens of up to 50% of women with atypia [2, 5]. Dilatation and curettage (D&C) or hysteroscopy-guided biopsy may not always be completely representative of the entire endometrium. Small foci of malignancy left in situ at the first biopsy might have already been present in the endometrium. In this situation, the term "progression to carcinoma" is less appropriate than "association with cancer/coexistent carcinoma" [19].

EC with concomitant EH are thought to be associated with less aggressive disease, associated with lower grade and stage, significantly lower recurrence risk, and higher 5-year survival rates [2]. The strongest predictors of concurrent EC among women with EH are older age, obesity, diabetes mellitus, and complex hyperplasia [4]. Immunohistochemical staining of complex atypical hyperplasia for PTEN, MIB-1, and *p53* improves the prediction of coexistent EC [10, 20].

3.3.2 Progression to Carcinoma

The natural history of EH is difficult to define, but key factors defining the risk for progression to carcinoma are the presence and severity of cytological atypia and architectural crowding [1, 18, 21, 22]. Simple hyperplasia represents the lowest risk of cancer progression, and the majority spontaneously regress [1]. Among 18% of persistent lesions, there are 8% and 3%, rates of progression to simple atypical hyperplasia and complex atypical hyperplasia and only 1% progress to EC. Complex hyperplasia is reported to have an intermediate risk of progression with 22% persistent and 4% progression to EC, with a mean duration to progression of approximately 10 years. Therefore, both simple hyperplasia and complex hyperplasia are not recognized as preneoplastic forms [2].

Another study reported progression to EC in 1%, 3%, 8%, and 29% of patients with simple hyperplasia, complex hyperplasia, simple atypical hyperplasia, and complex atypical hyperplasia, respectively [23].

The lower risks of progression to EC in women with EH without atypia can help in decision-making for conservative management, whereas the higher risks of atypical hyperplasia progressing to EC required consideration of aggressive approaches [19]. Meticulous knowledge of rates of progression risks for EH to EC encourages better clinical management of EH [18, 21–24].

Thresholds for distinguishing precursors (e.g., atypical hyperplasia or EIN) from carcinoma in biopsies vary among pathologists and by the classification system, but all of these lesions warrant close follow-up. A bigger challenge may be how to evaluate and manage the larger group of women with less severe abnormalities [22].

3.4 Classification

Among several histological classification systems proposed for EH since 1963, two prominent classifications are commonly used for EH at present: the World Health Organization (WHO) classification and the endometrial intraepithelial neoplasia (EIN) classification (Fig. 3.1).

WHO Classification: It was established in 1994 and classified EH in four categories, simple hyperplasia without atypia, complex hyperplasia without atypia, simple atypical hyperplasia, and complex atypical hyperplasia. The latest and fourth classification published in 2014 is the most commonly recognized system with the reduction to two categories only, and it reflects a new concept of molecular genetic changes. Hyperplasia without atypia (Figs. 3.2 and 3.3) expresses no associated genetic changes. They represent benign changes and disappear after the endocrine background returns to normal. Conversely, in atypical hyperplasia (Figs. 3.4 and 3.5), expressions of cellular and genetic changes typical of EC (Figs. 3.6 and 3.7) are found. The diagnosis of EIN in the WHO 2014 classification is interchangeable with atypical hyperplasia [5]. This new classification constitutes an important simplification for clinical practice particularly with concern to management options: hyperplasia without atypia can be treated usually conservatively, while treatment of atypical hyperplasia/EIN is usually total abdominal hysterectomy (TAH) [1, 7, 25].

Gross manifestations of EH are highly different. Changes in endometrium range from diffusely thickened (5–10 mm or greater) to vaguely nodular, tan, and soft without hemorrhage or necrosis. EH may be focal or multifocal in relation to cycling endometrium and polyp or on the diffusely thin endometrium [1, 26–28].

1994 WHO classification	2014 WHO classification		EIN classification
Category	Category	Histopathological features	Category
Simple hyperplasia without atypia	Hyperplasia without atypia	● Variability in gland size and shape ● Cystic glands ● Increased gland to stroma ratio	Endometrial hyperplasia
Complex hyperplasia without atypia			
Simple atypical hyperplasia	Atypical hyperplasia / EIN	● Architectural irregularity of gland ● Glandular crowding with little intervening stroma ● Nuclear atypia	Endometrial intraepithelial neoplasia
Complex atypical hyperplasia			

Fig. 3.1 Schematic representation of 1994 WHO classification, 2014 WHO classification, and EIN classification [7]

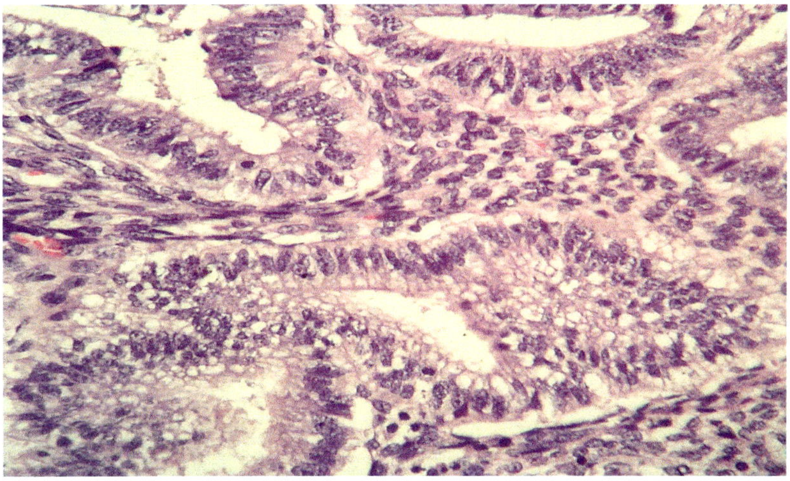

Fig. 3.2 Hyperplasia without atypia (low power 10×): Increased gland-to-stroma ratio is evident. Glands are mildly crowded and dilated

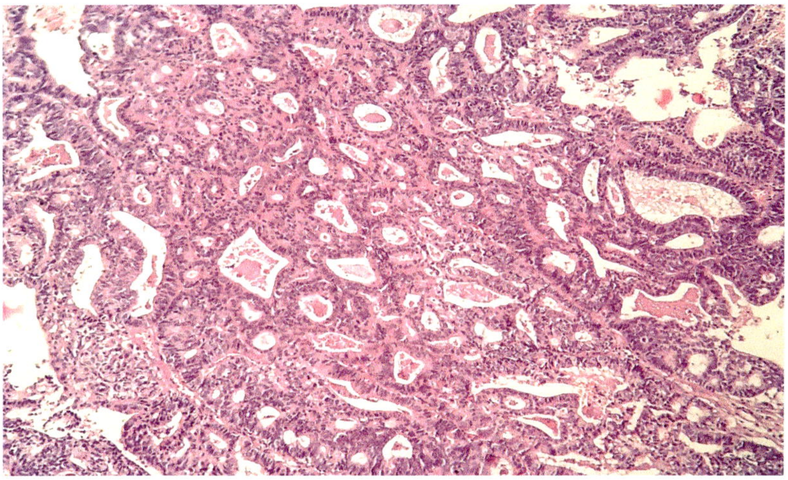

Fig. 3.3 Hyperplasia without atypia (high power 40×): Glands are lined by columnar epithelium and do not show any atypia

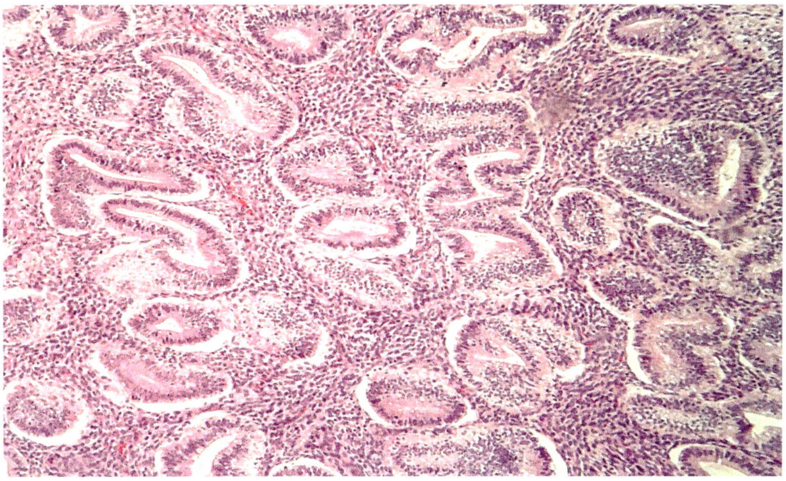

Fig. 3.4 Hyperplasia with atypia (low power 10×): Crowded back to back glands are evident with little intervening stroma

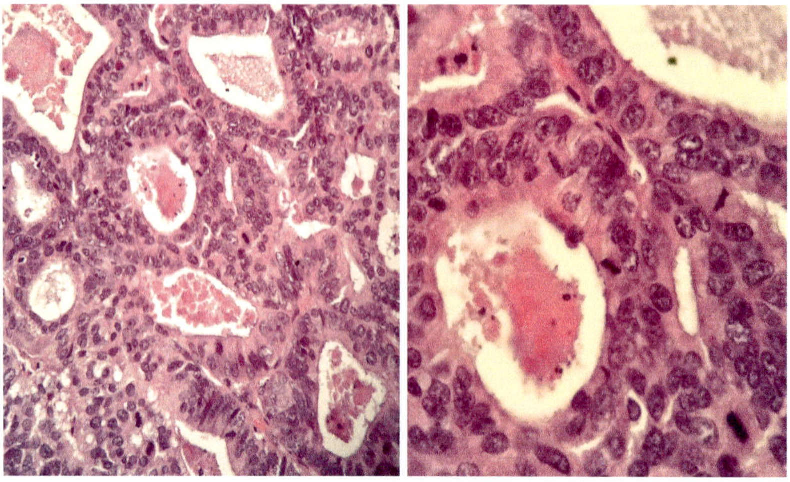

Fig. 3.5 Hyperplasia with atypia (high power). Cells show loss of polarity. Nuclei are enlarged with irregular nuclear membrane, coarse chromatin, and prominent nucleoli. Atypical mitoses are evident

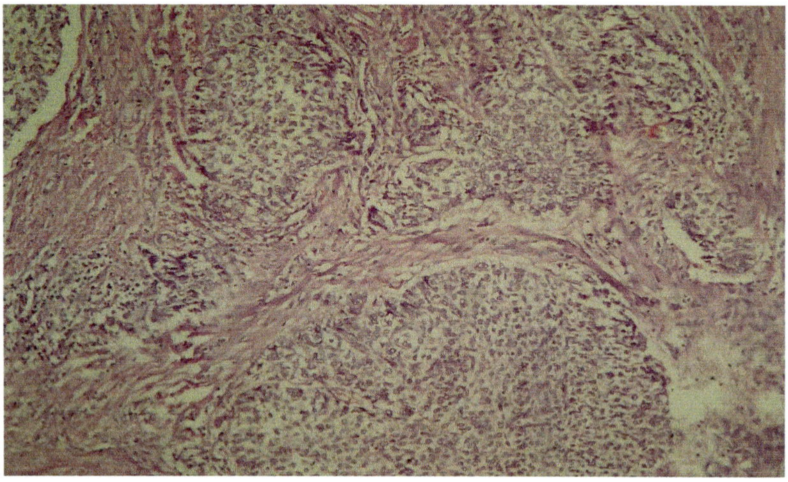

Fig. 3.6 Endometrial carcinoma (low power 10×): Tumor nests invade the myometrium

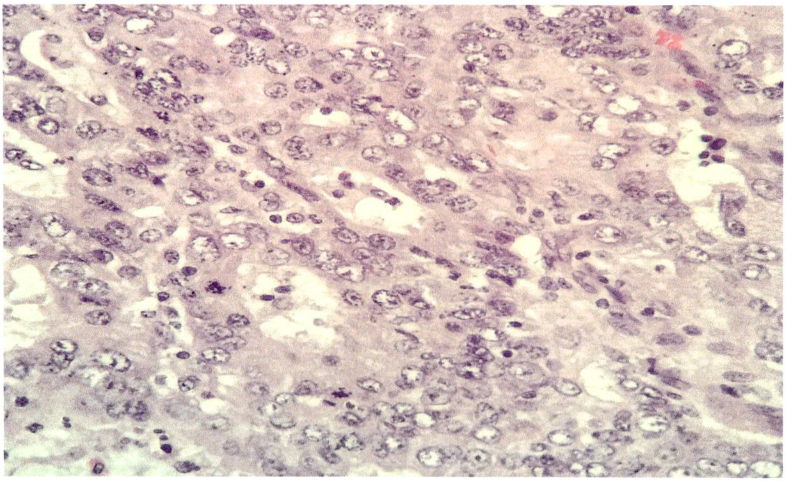

Fig. 3.7 Endometrial carcinoma (high power 40×): Tumor cells with glandular confluence, complex architecture, and lack of intervening stroma. Individual cells show high N/C ratio, pleomorphism, prominent nucleoli, and atypical mitosis

EIN Classification It is an alternative classification which is based on molecular, morphometric, and morphologic data and has been proposed by the International Endometrial Collaborative Group in 2000. It is developed to improve prediction of clinical outcome, improve inter-observer reproducibility, and reduce subjective bias inherent to 1994 WHO classification [7, 13, 29]. In this, nonatypical anovulatory or prolonged estrogen-exposed endometrium is classified as EH. The criteria for diagnosis of EIN are as follows [11, 22, 27, 30].

1. Size of the lesion is at least 1 mm
2. Glandular volume is more than the stromal volume
3. Changes in cytology in relation to background
4. Exclusion of benign mimics like endometrium in secretory phase, effect of exogenous estrogen and polyps and malignancy

The EIN classification can be assigned using computer-assisted morphometric analysis, which provides a D-score or diagnostic criteria that can be applied to standard hematoxylin and eosin (H&E) stained slides subjectively by pathologist [22, 27, 28]. Prior to the formation of EIN classification, it was believed that unopposed estrogenic stimulation will lead to EH. The EIN classification suggests that the initial event in EH is a genetic alteration, and eventually it separates two events: mutational activation and estrogenic stimulation [7]. The EIN system has not gained widespread acceptance, most likely due to cost and/or lack of experience with the computerized D-scoring component [3, 4].

Comparison Between WHO and EIN Classification: Although EIN classification categories do not correspond directly to particular categories in the WHO 1994 classification, there is some distinguishable overlap [7, 25]. The EIN classification may better arrange the distorted cellular architecture and nuclear characteristics, but adequate comparative studies are lacking. The WHO classification is more widely used. The risk of progression to endometrial carcinoma using the WHO and EIN classification was found to be similar [4, 11, 22]. Lesions that cause glandular overactivity (such as decidua basalis or polyps) can be confused with both the WHO (i.e., as EH) and EIN (i.e., as EIN) classifications. Due to sampling errors with endometrial biopsy (EB) specimens and the uncertain natural history of endometrial precursors, it is difficult for any classification to have both high sensitivity and specificity [22].

3.5 Clinical Presentation

Women with EH are diagnosed by EB performed for AUB including menorrhagia, intermenstrual bleeding, irregular bleeding on HRT or tamoxifen, and postmenopausal bleeding (PMB). Consequently, it is the most common symptom for EH. It is common in perimenopausal, in early postmenopausal, or with increasing age in premenopausal women. EH accounts for approximately 15% of women with PMB [2, 12]. In asymptomatic women, EH is detected accidentally, when workup is done for prolonged HRT use or cervical cytology demonstrating endometrial/abnormal glandular cells. The age at presentation relies on the source of excess estrogen. EH secondary to anovulation at menarche is uncommon and easily reversible [3, 4].

3.6 Diagnostic and Surveillance Methods

Management of EIN requires its accurate diagnosis and exclusion of coexistent carcinoma [11]. Women with symptoms suspicious for EH are evaluated at first with physical examination. Diagnosis of EH by cytology is generally unsatisfactory [10].

Histopathological Diagnosis: Diagnosis of EH needs histological confirmation of the endometrial tissue obtained by different techniques which include office EB, D&C, and directed EB by hysteroscopy. Other investigations include transvaginal sonography (TVS) and saline infusion sonography [2, 31]. Apart from diagnosis, endometrial sampling is also required in monitoring regression, persistence, or progression [13].

Office EB technique is usually performed using the several commercially available devices (e.g., Pipelle, Vabra aspirator, Gyno Sampler) and is convenient and safe and has high accuracy for diagnosing EH or EC. It has replaced the procedure of D&C for the diagnosis of EH or EC [3, 32]. Despite a negative biopsy result, 2% of women will still have EH [2, 3, 13]. Mass lesions that encroach on the uterine cavity, for example, polyps or uterine fibroids, may divert Pipelle, which is flexible, preventing sufficient evaluation of the endometrial cavity. In this situation, EB may be performed by a rigid curette during D&C [11]. Office EB can cause some discomfort, and in approximately 8% of patients, it is not possible to perform due to stenotic cervical os [20]. Both Pipelle and D&C are blind sampling techniques and are not representative of the entire endometrial cavity [2]. If hysterectomy is planned for the woman for any reason, then the method of sampling is less important. The accuracy of D&C compared with Pipelle EB in diagnosing a EH, and excluding concurrent EC, is not clear. Both have been reported to have equal rates of cancer detection in patients with AUB [2, 11]. In one meta-analysis, EB with Pipelle was found to be superior to other sampling techniques in the detection of EC and atypical hyperplasia [32].

Diagnostic hysteroscopy is used to examine the entire surface of the endometrium and biopsy suspicious or focal lesions under direct visualization (Figs. 3.8, 3.9, and 3.10). It is especially important when an outpatient sampling fails or is inconclusive, if abnormal bleeding persists or if intrauterine structural abnormalities such as polyps or other discrete focal lesions are suspected on TVS [2, 13, 33]. Office hysteroscopy is conducted in the outpatient setting using miniature hysteroscope and without the requirement of anesthesia or vaginal

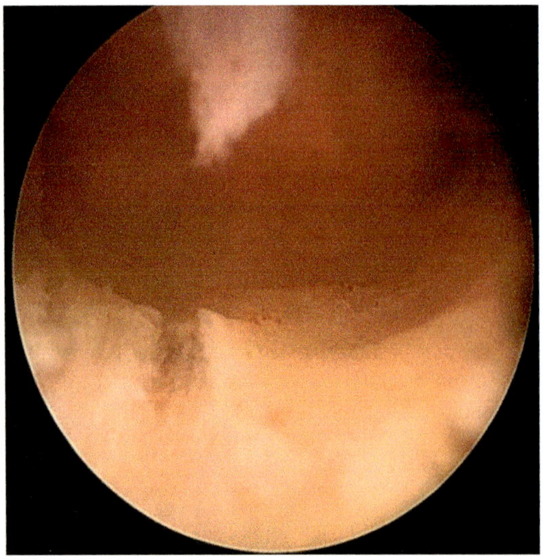

Fig. 3.8 Normal endometrium on hysteroscopy

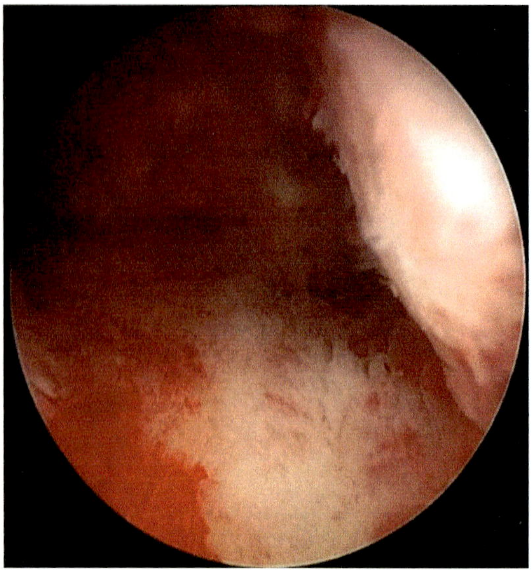

Fig. 3.9 Endometrial hyperplasia on hysteroscopy

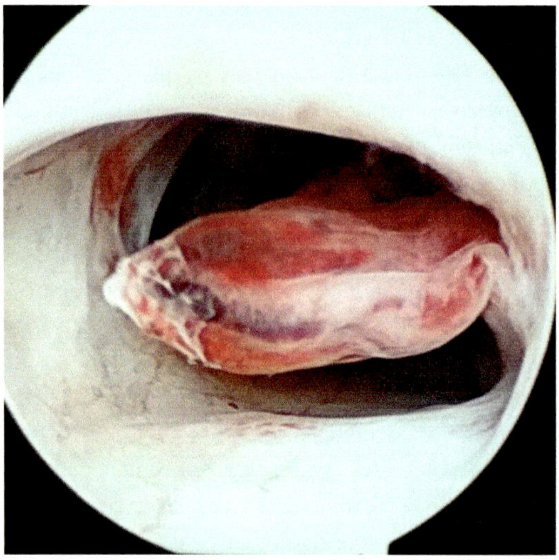

Fig. 3.10 Hysteroscopy demonstrating endometrial polyp in the background of atrophic endometrium in woman on tamoxifen

instrumentation. Hysteroscopy is more precise in detecting than excluding endometrial lesions and has a higher precision for EC than EH [13].

Hysteroscopy with targeted biopsy or D&C compared to hysteroscopy performed alone has very good sensitivity and specificity for detecting EH. The combination of hysteroscopy with D&C or EB is considered to be a superior diagnostic tool compared with hysteroscopy, D&C, or EB performed alone [2].

Practical aspects of diagnosis: Problem in reproducibility of detection of atypical hyperplasia: Diagnostic reproducibility is limited by the size of the lesion, inadequate sample, poor quality of fixation, processing, and staining of tissues [5, 6]. Current diagnostic strategy should include evaluation of sample adequacy, as is recommended for evaluating cervical cytology [5, 9, 11]. There is need to apply multiple diagnostic criteria, and due to imperfect sampling, only few of them may be present in a given specimen. In short, sample or lesion size may be a factor responsible for inaccurate assessment of risk [11]. It is important to remember that atypical hyperplasia is frequently associated with concomitant adenocarcinoma and low level of reproducibility associated with the diagnosis of atypical hyperplasia in EB [6].

Awareness of the artefactual changes generated by EB is necessary to ensure that EH is not overdiagnosed [15]. When the woman is on exogenous progestin, it is better to perform EB after withdrawal of hormones. If EB specimen is compromised by sampling errors or regenerative epithelial changes, either instant additional EB is done or regular follow-up with repeat EB is done after 6 months to detect the presence of pathology in the endometrium. Pathologists must develop their own approach to differentiate between proliferative endometrium and EH especially in women with anovulation or unopposed estrogen exposure [29].

An important issue is the availability of a pathologist experienced in gynecological pathology. As mentioned, there are a range of abnormalities seen in hyperplastic endometrium, and differentiation between them can be quite difficult. Only those with frequent exposure to such specimens are likely to be skilled in interpreting these lesions [9].

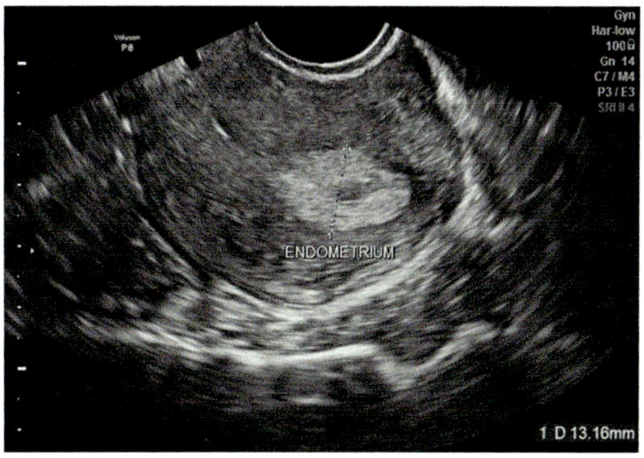

Fig. 3.11 Endometrial hyperplasia as imaged by transvaginal sonography in postmenopausal woman. Endometrial thickness 13.6 mm

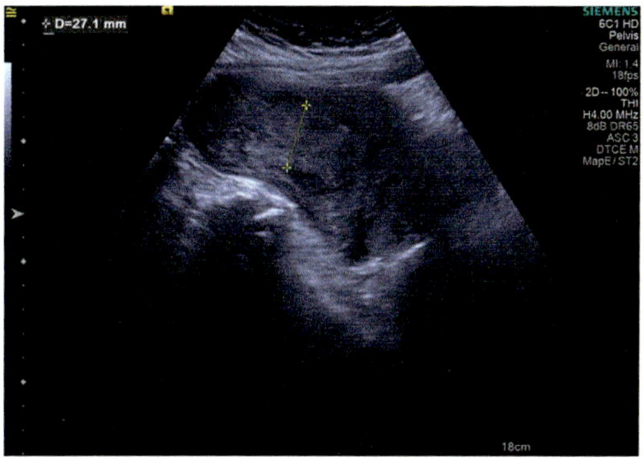

Fig. 3.12 Thickened endometrium as imaged by transabdominal sonography in unmarried patient on tamoxifen (longitudinal view). Endometrial thickness 27 mm

Ultrasonography: TVS, a noninvasive diagnostic method, is of proven value for evaluation of endometrial thickness (ET) and contour as a part of investigation for PMB [2, 34] (Figs. 3.11 and 3.12). It can detect an irregularity of the endometrium or an abnormal double-layer ET measurement. These findings will guide the clinician to determine which women should undergo EB with PMB [13, 33]. Meta-analysis of 5892 symptomatic women with PMB in 35 published studies demonstrated that an ET of 5 mm or more identified 95% of those with EH and EC. In contrast, among them, a woman with an ET of less than 4 mm only had a 1% probability of EC. This cutoff did not differ remarkably between women with and without HRT [2, 9, 11, 34]. However, other systematic reviews have recommended a cutoff of 3 mm or 4 mm to rule out EC. By using this cutoff value, the probability of diagnosis of EC is reduced to less than 1%. A larger cutoff value has been recommended for women on HRT or tamoxifen presenting with AUB or asymptomatic woman with thickened endometrium on TVS [13]. ET more than 1 cm on TVS in postmenopausal women is associated with an increased risk of EC [34]. Overall, assessment of endometrial thickness on TVS is of value in mainly postmenopausal women as there are no cutoff values for endometrial thickness in premenopausal women in whom normal ET can be similar to that with EC [11]. The role of ultrasonography (USG) in premenopausal women is restricted to identifying structural abnormalities, as there appears to be an overlap between normal ET and that caused by endometrial disease. Royal College of Obstetricians and Gynaecologists (RCOG) guidance recommends TVS for women with polycystic ovarian syndrome (PCOS) or AUB. In a woman with PCOS, possibility of EH is less likely if ET is less than 7 mm [13]. It is recommended that both TVS and saline infusion sonography should be performed simultaneously with EB [2]. Occasionally a palpable adnexal mass with solid features on USG should raise the possibility of a coexistent granulosa cell tumor. It is responsible for EH in 40% of cases due to excessive estrogen production [12, 13].

To summarize, a woman with risk factors for EC and with ET more than 5 mm after menopause should undergo EB. However, routine screening for women at high risk of EH has not proven successful or cost-effective except for all Lynch syndrome mutation carriers where annual EB is recommended by National Comprehensive Cancer Network (NCCN) guidelines. An inadequate EB is an indication for further investigation. Even if an office EB is adequate and reported as negative, additional evaluation with TVS and/or D&C/hysteroscopy should be done if symptoms persist or recur [2, 13].

Computerized tomography (CT) and diffusion-weighted magnetic resonance imaging (MRI) in the diagnosis and management of EH are not commonly used. There are no studies evaluating use of CT scan for follow-up of a woman with EH treated conservatively. CT scan is an expensive test and is not routinely advocated because of the radiation exposure associated with it. Diffusion-weighted MRI has the future potential to diagnose EH and other endometrial lesions. It may be a useful imaging for follow-up of a woman with atypical hyperplasia as a predictor for malignant change, but more evidence is needed [13].

Immunohistochemical Biomarkers: Prediction of cases which will progress to EC can increase with the use of several immunohistochemical biomarkers. In some instances, such as for women with hereditary nonpolyposis colon cancer, biomarker may have a role in diagnosis. To date, not a single biomarker is found to merit its clinical utility [2, 11, 13].

3.7 Differential Diagnosis

The differential diagnosis of EH includes other conditions that present with AUB. Confirmation of the source of bleeding is the most important step in evaluation of women with AUB, and bleeding from any other part of the genital tract, anus, or rectum should be excluded. In women with abnormal cervical cytology, the differential diagnosis includes benign endometrial and cervical neoplasia [4].

Even at the level of histopathology, it has to be differentiated from atrophic or weakly proliferative endometrium with the architecture of hyperplasia, endometrial metaplasia, and EH with superimposed secretory changes well-differentiated adenocarcinoma [15, 20, 35].

3.8 Management Options

The choice of management for the woman with EH is determined mainly by woman's age, health, desire for fertility, as well as the risk factor for progression to EC and the type of EH [1, 9, 33, 36]. Nuclear atypia is the main factor, and older age, obesity, and ovulatory dysfunction are additional risk factors in determining the risk for coexistent or progression to EC [4, 37]. EH without atypia is usually treated with hormone therapy. Younger women who desire fertility can be treated by medical management, regardless of the type of EH [1]. However, perimenopausal and postmenopausal women having EH with atypia or symptomatic women having EH without atypia are treated by surgical management unless contraindicated. Regardless of the type of EH, the woman with risk factors for recurrence or progression to EC requires active management and surveillance [1, 9, 30].

All management options should be accompanied by removal of the exogenous or endogenous source of estrogen exposure as it is the main factor contributing to EH. This may be done by discontinuation of ERT without progestin, treatment of ovulatory dysfunction (e.g., PCOS or hyperprolactinemia), weight loss in obese women, or even by removal of estrogen-producing tumor (e.g., granulosa cell tumor) [37].

3.8.1 Observation

In the woman with EH without atypia, spontaneous regression usually occurs during follow-up, and the risk of progression to EC is less than 5% over 20 years [1]. Observation alone can be considered if the risk for coexistent or progression to EC is low and reversible risk factors are identified and treated. The slow progression of EH without atypia to EC offers a window of opportunity to manage these reversible risk factors [1, 12].

Anovulatory cycles can lead to EH especially in a woman with PCOS or in a premenopausal woman. Once a woman with PCOS resumes ovulation or perimenopausal woman reaches menopause, regression of EH occurs. A detailed history regarding the use of exogenous hormones (e.g., long-term use of HRT, unopposed ERT without progestin) should be elicited. The indication and type of HRT should be reviewed especially in relation to dose and mode of administration. Change in the dosage of HRT or discontinuation is often sufficient to induce regression of EH without atypia. The woman on tamoxifen treatment, who developed EH, should be reviewed regarding continuation or change of medicine in conjunction with her treating oncologist. A baseline USG is indicated which also helps to rule out estrogen-secreting granulosa cell tumor of the ovary [1, 37].

However, the woman should be informed that the treatment with progestogen has higher rates of regression of EH compared with observation alone. When a woman with EH fails to regress following observation alone for 12 months, progestogen treatment is required. Observation alone in the symptomatic woman with AUB is rarely advised [1, 12, 13]. In view of a high spontaneous regression rate and a very low rate of progression to more severe disease, it is uncertain whether medical management is appropriate for all women with EH without atypia [1].

3.8.2 Medical Management

Hormonal therapy used in the management of EH includes progestins, selective estrogen receptor modulators, aromatase inhibitors, sulfatase inhibitors, gonadotropin-releasing hormone (GnRH) antagonists, synthetic androgen (danazol), metformin, and protein-tyrosine kinases inhibitor (genistein) [1, 11] (Table 3.2).

3.8.2.1 Progestin Therapy

Progestins, which are synthetic progestogens mimicking natural progesterone, are used most frequently to induce regression of endometrial hyperplasia in women with EH without atypia, those who desire fertility, those who refuse surgery, or those who have contraindications to surgery due to significant medical comorbidities [1, 11, 19]. Therapeutic aims of progestin therapy are complete regression of EH, return to normal endometrial function, and the prevention of EC [11].

Progesterone brings about secretory changes in the normal endometrium. It produces these effects by increasing the catabolism of estrogen receptors and increasing the activity of enzymes 17-b-hydroxysteroid dehydrogenase and sulfotransferase thereby decreasing estrogen levels [1, 19]. It causes apoptosis leading to decreased

Table 3.2 Drugs used in medical management of endometrial hyperplasia

Type of therapy	Routes of administration
Progestin therapy	
Megestrol acetate	Oral
Medroxyprogesterone acetate	Oral/injection
Norethisterone acetate	Oral
Micronized progesterone	Oral/vaginal pessary
Levonorgestrel	Oral/implant/intrauterine insert (IUD)
Therapy other than progestin	
Aromatase inhibitor	Oral
Metformin	Oral
GnRH therapy	Injection/implant/nasal spray
Danazol	Oral
Genistein	Oral
Combination therapy	
Megestrol acetate + metformin	Oral
LNG-IUD + metformin	IUD + oral
LNG-IUD + GnRh agonist	IUD + injection/implant/nasal spray

glandularity and inhibits angiogenesis in the myometrium. Eventually, this causes sloughing and thinning of the endometrium [1, 11].

Contraindications to progestin therapy include current or past history of thromboembolic disorders/stroke, severe liver dysfunction, known or suspected malignancy of progesterone receptor (PR)-positive breast cancer, vaginal bleeding of unknown etiology, pregnancy, and known allergic reaction to progestins [37]. Various routes of administration can be used – oral, intramuscular, and vaginal routes or through intrauterine devices [1].

Unfortunately, optimal progestin regimen and duration have not been investigated, and posttreatment long-term follow-up has not been reported adequately [20, 38]. Sixty-one percent of women on estrogen-only replacement therapy and atypical hyperplasia responded to progestin therapy and were cured [1]. The response to progestin therapy usually begins at 10 weeks and is complete by 6 months. Cyclic progestin has a low regression rate for EH, compared to continuous oral progestin or LNG-IUD [12, 13, 39]. Prognostic factors include low gland-to-stroma ratio, low mitotic activity, loss of cytologic atypia and other changes in histology, cytoplasm or architecture [11]. Progestins used and their dosages are shown in Table 3.3.

Table 3.3 Different types of progestin therapy for treatment of endometrial hyperplasia [1, 11, 37]

Type of progestin	Dose
Megestrol acetate	40–200 mg daily in divided doses or 10 mg × 14 days/month
Medroxyprogesterone acetate	10–20 mg daily or 10–20 mg × 14 days/month
Depot medroxyprogesterone acetate	150 mg intramuscularly every 3 months
Micronized vaginal progesterone	100–200 mg daily or 100–200 mg × 14 days/month
Levonorgestrel IUD	20 μg/day × 1–5 years
Norethisterone acetate	15 mg daily

a. Megestrol acetate (MA)—It is a steroidal progestin and is effective in EH because of its progesterone-like and antigonadotropic effects [1]. It is considered a "chemotherapeutic agent" but best classified as a strong progestin. Dosages vary between 160 and 320 mg/day. At these doses, the beneficial effects on endometrium are maximum with minimal effects on blood glucose levels or lipid profile [1].
b. Medroxyprogesterone acetate (MPA)—It is a synthetic steroidal progestin commonly used in hormone replacement therapy in postmenopausal women in whom its use helps in prevention of EH. The dose commonly given

is 10 mg/day continuously for 6 weeks or 2 weeks/month for 3 months (safer and more acceptable than continuous therapy). If the response is not complete, the therapy can be continued for the next 3 months [1].

c. Norethindrone acetate/norethisterone acetate (NETA)—It is a synthetic, orally active steroidal progestin with antiandrogenic and antiestrogenic effects. It has been shown to reduce EH in postmenopausal women on HRT [1, 37]. The recommended dosage is 15 mg/day.

d. Micronized progesterone—It is a relatively weak progesterone and usually not recommended for first-line treatment of EH. In doses of 200–300 mg daily, it is reserved only for women who are at low risk for progression and cannot tolerate stronger synthetic progestins or refuse levonorgestrel intrauterine device (LNG-IUD). Till date, there are no studies on the use of vaginal micronized progesterone for the treatment of EH. Theoretically, it can be used as maintenance treatment, as high endometrial concentrations may be gained due to local effects [37].

e. Levonorgestrel (LNG)—It is a second-generation progestin (synthetic progestogen) and the intrauterine device containing LNG is an attractive option for managing EH. It releases a constant amount of LNG inside the uterus and effectively opposes the estrogenic effect [1, 11, 40]. The LNG 52/5 starts with an initial dose of 20 mcg/day, and by 5 years the daily dose is approximately 10 mcg/day [37]. The LNG-IUD initially results in irregular bleeding as with other progestin-only therapy, but eventually, most women become amenorrheic or have light tolerable bleeding. For the best outcomes, medical treatment of EH should require LNG-IUD use for up to 5 years [12, 13, 39]. LNG-IUD is also available in lower daily doses (13.5, 17.5, and 18.6 mcg/day) and varies from 3- to 5-year formulations, but these have not been studied in women with EH to determine whether the lower progestin dose is as effective as the LNg 52/5 [37].

Comparison of oral progestins with LNG-IUD—LNG-IUD has high intrauterine but low systemic levels of progestin. Therefore, it has an effect on the endometrium several times stronger without causing side effects such as breast tenderness, mood changes, and weight gain. In addition to higher efficacy, it offers long-acting contraception, does not require daily dosing, and is better tolerated when compared to oral progestins [11, 39, 41]. Other limitations of LNG-IUD are a 1 in 1000 uterine perforation risk and invasive placement in the uterus [39]. There is no significant difference in rates of irregular vaginal bleeding with the LNg 52/5 compared with oral progestins [37].

Oral progestins are preferred over LNG-IUD in women who refuse or cannot tolerate an IUD because of side effects (e.g., dysmenorrhea), women with uterine factors that make placement or retention of an IUD difficult (e.g., severe distortion of the uterine cavity due to fibroids or congenital anomaly), and women who plan to conceive as soon as a complete therapeutic response is achieved. Progestins are contraindicated in pregnancy, and the patient can stop an oral medication without requiring a clinician to remove the device, as with an IUD [37].

f. Progestin injections and implants—Depot medroxyprogesterone acetate (DMPA) is a long-acting progestin, provides contraception, and requires only four injections per year. It has not been well studied for the treatment of EH. In one study, the intramuscular DMPA (150 mg every 3 months) was found to be more successful than NETA (15 mg daily for 14 days/cycle) in the treatment of nonatypical EH. Regarding side effects, nausea and breast discomfort were more with NETA, while amenorrhea was more with DMPA [37].

Common side effects of progestins include weight gain, headache, nausea, vomiting, menstrual irregularities, and sometimes hypertension and depression. The incidence of venous thrombosis and embolism may also be slightly increased [1, 9, 20]. In addition to systemic side effects, oral progestins are associated with poor compliance that may limit its overall efficacy [41]. Bothersome side effects may require an adjustment in dose or a switch to a different progestin therapy. For women on systemic progestins, change over to the LNG-IUD can be considered [37].

Almost 12–53% women with EH fail to respond to progestin therapy [1, 11]. Response to progestins depends not only on patient's age and the type and grade of hyperplasia but also the number of PR and activity of co-activators and co-repressors, insulin resistance, and altered activity of TGF-α and EGFR in endometrial glandular cells [1]. Rarely, resistance to progestin therapy could be a result of paracrine effects. The histologic response of the glands of atypical EH/EIN is strongly coupled to the decidual response in the stroma, so the possibility of a paracrine effect is convincing [11]. Hence, regular follow-up and EB are recommended for patients while on progestin therapy [1]. Recently, the role of HE4 as a novel tissue marker for predicting therapy response and progestin resistance in EH has been studied and proved to be effective in it [42].

3.8.2.2 Therapy Other than Progestins

a. Ovulation induction—In the reproductive-age group, ovulation induction done with clomiphene or aromatase inhibitors will lead to corpus luteum formation, exposure to endogenous progesterone, and resolution of EH in some women. Pregnancy is highly unexpected in the setting of ongoing EH. Careful surveillance is needed to confirm EH regression. This approach is recommended for women with EH without atypia who desire pregnancy [37].
b. Metformin—EH is associated with obesity, metabolic syndrome, PCOS, insulin resistance, and type II diabetes which directly have a mitogen effect on the endometrium. Metformin (*N,N*-dimethylbiguanide) is a biguanide and decreases gluconeogenesis in the liver which in turn decreases insulin resistance [41]. Long-term progestin therapy causes decreased level of progesterone receptors. Metformin induces PR expression in endometrial cells which helps to overcome resistance to progestin therapy [1]. Metformin is also especially helpful in obese women in whom it helps to decrease weight and thereby causes decrease in peripheral conversion of androgen to estrogen and better response to progestins [1, 38, 41]. Metformin is now being studied in combination with LNG-IUD and MA [1, 39].
c. GnRH therapy—GnRH agonists inhibit estrogen by inhibiting the hypothalamic pituitary ovarian axis thereby exerting antiproliferative effect on the endometrial cells. Women with EH, both with and without atypia, can be given GnRH at a dose of 1 ampule/3.75 mg intramuscularly monthly for 6 months [1, 9]. In a study using GnRH and tibolone (a synthetic steroid with both estrogenic and progestagenic effects) for treatment of EH, it was seen that though a complete response was seen in all patients, recurrence occurred within 2 years in 19% after cessation of therapy [1]. In another study, GnRH agonists and LNG-IUD were used in combination with a release rate of 19.5 mcg/day for 5 years (Mirena; LNg52/5) to successfully treat 24 premenopausal women with either atypical EH or early-stage EC [37].
d. Danazol—It is a synthetic androgen which causes atrophy of the endometrium through its ability to produce a hypoestrogenic and hypoandrogenic state [1, 9, 36]. It has been proven to be effective in treatment of EH with a relapse rate of approximately 8 to 9% [1, 9]. The side effects of oral danazol (weight gain, acne, hirsutism, and muscle cramps) are the limiting factors in its use for EH which can be curtailed to some extent by using danazol-containing IUD [1, 37].
e. Genistein—It is an isoflavonoid extracted from soy products. It decreases estrogen level by inhibiting protein-tyrosine kinases and topoisomerase-II. It has still not been established for management of EH till the time more clinical trials are conducted [1].

3.8.3 Surgical Management

Currently, surgical options include hysterectomy with or without bilateral salpingo-oophorectomy

(BSO) by abdominal, vaginal, and minimally invasive procedures (such as laparoscopic or robotic approach). Total extrafascial hysterectomy is the procedure of choice providing a definitive assessment of a coexistent EC and effectively treating EH. Supracervical hysterectomy is unacceptable due the potential for local extension of endometrial neoplasia into the cervix and hence risk of leaving behind residual disease [11, 13]. Morcellation of the uterus should be avoided due to risk of dissemination of coexistent EC [13]. Disadvantages of vaginal hysterectomy include technical difficulty in removing the ovaries and comprehensive surgical staging, if required, is not feasible [11]. During the hysterectomy, gross inspection in routine and frozen section especially in high-risk cases should be performed to evaluate for EC [37]. Discrepancy between the frozen-section interpretation of endometrial tissue and the final diagnosis based on permanent section is problematic. Despite preoperative endometrial sampling and intraoperative evaluation, some women with atypical EH will have EC detected only on final pathology evaluation [13, 37]. Regardless of surgical approach, women with high-risk factors should be explained regarding the need for additional staging surgery if an EC is identified. Following a total hysterectomy, if there is no EC in the specimen, no further surveillance for EH is necessary [11].

For women undergoing hysterectomy as treatment for atypical EH, the choice of bilateral BSO should be decided after weighing the risk of premature menopause and potential risks of oophorectomy versus the risk of a second surgery if EC is found postoperatively. Some women may prefer to undergo bilateral salpingectomy alone instead of oophorectomy, for possible prevention of ovarian, fallopian tubal, or peritoneal cancer (level 3 or 4 evidence) [11, 13]. Endometrial ablation using thermal or electric cautery device is not recommended for the treatment of atypical EH/EIN. No methods are available to confirm the completeness of ablation. Moreover, because of subsequent adhesions, the cavity may be partly inaccessible for surveillance after ablation [11, 13].

3.9 Management Algorithm According to the Type of Endometrial Hyperplasia (Fig. 3.13)

3.9.1 Woman with EH Without Atypia

Premenopausal women—The initial step in the management of EH is the identification of risk factors and removal of the exogenous and endogenous source of unopposed estrogen. The premenopausal woman with EH without atypia can be managed with observation or low-dose progestins for 3–6 months. Hysterectomy can be considered in women aged >40 years [1, 37].

Options for progestin therapy are oral progestins, LNG-IUD, or combined estrogen and progestin oral contraceptives (OCs). Choice of therapy is also according to the need for contraception of patient since many oral progestins do not provide it [37].

If there is a good response after progestin therapy, i.e., menstrual pattern has normalized, annual EB is advised [1, 17]. EB can be performed even with IUD in place [1, 33]. Some authors prefer waiting for a withdrawal bleed before EB, while others perform EB while the patient is on progestin therapy. The rationale behind this dilemma is the decidual reaction that occurs with progestin therapy making it more difficult to interpret pathologic findings [29, 37]. If the bleeding pattern does not normalize, high dose of progestins can be considered after performing repeat EB. If office EB demonstrates abnormal report, D&C or hysteroscopy-directed biopsy is mandatory to rule out coexistent EC or more severe EH. It was reported that the median time to complete response of EH to progestin was 6 months [1]. The best plan for follow-up is undetermined. Follow-up schedules should be individualized. In women with high risk for EH relapse, persistence, or progression, long-term annual follow-up is recommended [12, 13]. If repeat EB shows atypical EH or persistent EH without atypia despite high progestins or if symptoms persist, hysterectomy can be considered [1, 13].

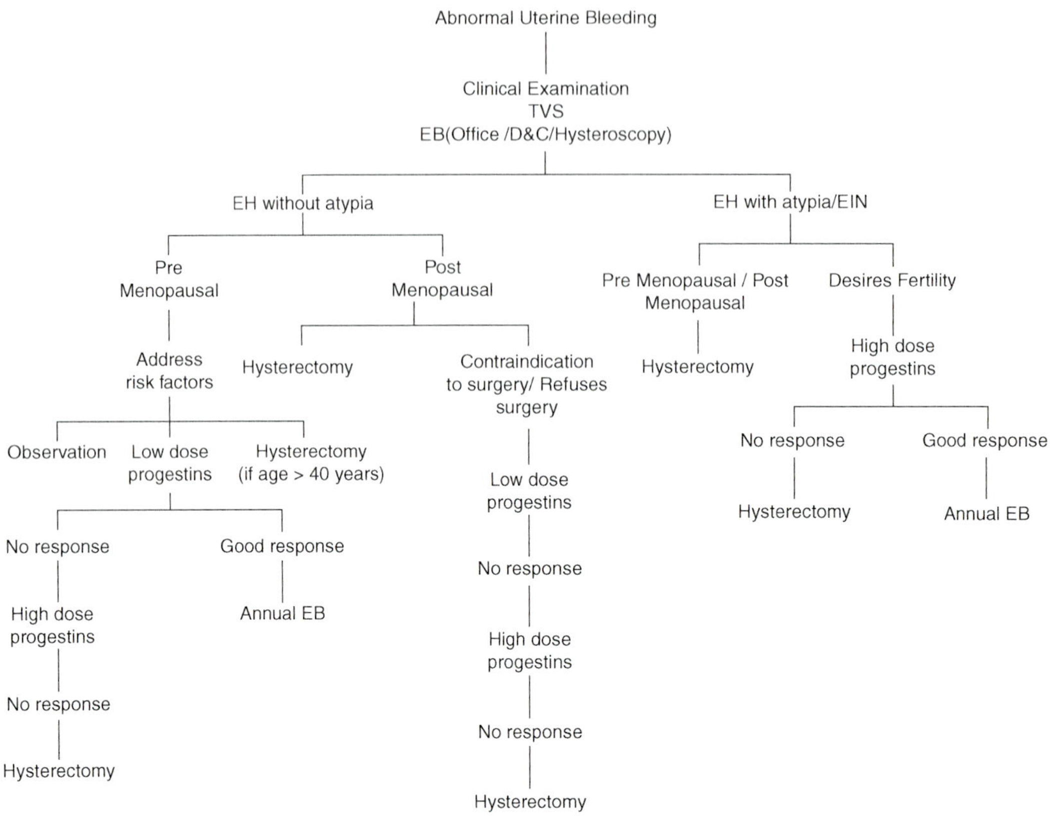

Fig. 3.13 Management algorithm for endometrial hyperplasia

Postmenopausal women—Hysterectomy is usually recommended in the postmenopausal woman with EH without atypia, especially with risk factors for EC or with contraindications to progestin therapy. If there are contraindications to surgery or patient refuses surgery, progestin alone is recommended. OCs are not preferable as these women do not need contraception and also to avoid unnecessary exposure to estrogen [1, 37]. If regression to normal endometrium does not occur after 6 months of progestin therapy, the patient may be treated with higher dose of oral progestin or combination of LNG-IUD and oral progestin after excluding atypical EH or coexistent EC by EB (D&C/hysteroscopy). In the setting of persistent EH, hysterectomy is the standard treatment approach [1, 37].

3.9.2 Women with Atypical Hyperplasia/EIN

Women with atypical hyperplasia have a high risk of coexistent EC or progression to EC. Hysterectomy is curative and the treatment of choice in majority of women who have completed childbearing, do not desire preservation of their fertility, or do not respond to hormone therapy [11, 13]. If diagnosis of atypical EH is made by office EB, further evaluation with D&C/hysteroscopy is recommended to exclude coexistent EC [37].

Women who desire fertility or have contraindication to surgery—Women with atypical EH who desire fertility or have contraindication to surgery can be treated with progestin therapy.

Women should be extensively counseled regarding the risks including a lack of response or even progression or coexistent EC during hormonal therapy. These discussions and patient understanding should be reflected in informed consent. Compliance with medical therapy and adequate and regular follow-up with EB are a prerequisite for medical management [13, 33]. Management is planned after reviewing clinical evaluation, histology, and imaging in multidisciplinary meeting. LNG-IUD is preferred, as it is easy to comply with, is well tolerated, and has a regression rate to normal endometrium in about 90% of cases. Among oral progestins, megestrol acetate is preferred for management of atypical EH in dose of 80 to 160 mg twice per day. It is more potent than MPA. Median time for regression of atypical EH to normal endometrium on progestin therapy is usually 6 to 9 months. If no EH is detected on subsequent EB, a woman can be allowed to consider for natural conception. A decision for assisted reproduction immediately after stopping of progestogen treatment should be made with consultation of a multidisciplinary team weighing between risks of disease progression and fertility prospects. In women with atypical EH, hysterectomy should be recommended once fertility is no longer required because of the high rates of EH recurrence and the potential for EH progression [13]. If there is persistent atypical EH or coexistent EC on subsequent EB, hysterectomy is recommended regardless of fertility issue [13, 36].

3.9.3 Special Issues

Use of HRT in women with endometrial hyperplasia: In women with EH on a sequential HRT, change to continuous combined HRT or LNG-IUD is recommended. In women with EH on continuous combined HRT, review of need of HRT or replacement with LNG-IUD is recommended [13].

Management of endometrial hyperplasia with ongoing tamoxifen use for breast cancer treatment: Women should be informed about increased risk of EH and EC with tamoxifen use and counseled for prompt reporting of AUB. In the presence of EH, use of tamoxifen is reassessed in consultation with medical oncologist and alternative drug is sought. Aromatase inhibitors are studied as an alternative treatment option without increasing the risk of EH and EC. Prophylactic progestin therapy is not recommended in women on tamoxifen [13].

3.10 Prevention of Endometrial Hyperplasia

In women with AUB, it is appropriate to evaluate woman past their fourth decade of life. Women with an intact uterus should never be prescribed ERT as this increases the risk of EC. For women on exogenous estrogens, addition of progestin may prevent EH. Another preventive measure is periodic treatment with a progestin to produce scheduled withdrawal bleeding in the amenorrhoeic or hypermenorrheic perimenopausal women with fluctuating levels of estrogen [27].

Key Points

- A thorough history (age at menarche and menopause, parity, history of infertility, history of dose and duration of HRT and tamoxifen therapy, and family history of uterine or colon cancer) and complete pelvic examination are the key aspects for evaluation of EH.
- The classifications commonly used for endometrial hyperplasia are WHO and EIN classification.
- In the woman with EH without atypia, spontaneous regression usually occurs during follow-up and the risk of progression to EC is less than 5% over 20 years.
- The presence of cellular atypia carries highest chance of persistence, recurrence, and progression to EC or coexistent EC.

- Routine screening for women at high risk of EH has not proven to be successful or cost-effective except for Lynch syndrome mutation carriers.
- Histological examination by an experienced gynecological pathologist is essential to distinguish between different types of EH that are managed differently.
- In younger women with a desire to retain fertility, medical treatment with progestins is appropriate, while in older women especially with atypical hyperplasia, hysterectomy is the treatment of choice.

References

1. Chandra V, Kim JJ, Benbrook DM, Dwivedi A, Rai R. Therapeutic options for management of endometrial hyperplasia. J Gynecol Oncol. 2016;27(1):1–25.
2. Palmer JE, Perunovic B, Tidy JA. Review endometrial hyperplasia. Obstet Gynecol. 2008;10:211–6.
3. Landrum LM, Zuna RE, Walker JL. Endometrial hyperplasia, estrogen therapy, and the prevention of endometrial cancer. In: DiSaia PJ, Creasman WT, editors. Clinical gynecologic oncology. Philadelphia: Mosby Elsevier; 2007. p. 121–8.
4. Classification and diagnosis of endometrial hyperplasia [Internet]. Uptodate.com. 2017. https://www.uptodate.com/contents/classification-and-diagnosis-of-endometrial-hyperplasia?search=reed%20sd,urban%20r.%20r.%20classification%20and%20diagnosis%20of%20endometrial%20-hyperplasia&source=search_result&selectedTitle=1~150&usage_type=default&display_rank=1. Cited19 Dec 2017
5. Trimble CL, Kauderer J, Zaino R, Silverberg S, Lim PC, Burke JJ II, et al. Concurrent endometrial carcinoma in women with a biopsy diagnosis of atypical endometrial hyperplasia. Cancer. 2006;106(4):812–9.
6. Zaino RJ, Kauderer J, Trimble CL, Silverberg SG, Curtin JP, Lim PC, Gallup DG. Reproducibility of the diagnosis of atypical endometrial hyperplasia. Cancer. 2006;106(4):804–11.
7. Sanderson PA, Critchley HOD, Williams ARW, Arends MJ, Saunders PTK. New concepts for an old problem: the diagnosis of endometrial hyperplasia. Hum Reprod Update. 2017;23(2):1–23.
8. Reed SD, Newton KM, Clinton WL, Epplein M, Garcia R, Allison K, et al. Incidence of endometrial hyperplasia. Am J Obstet Gynecol. 2009;200:678.e1–6.
9. Marsden DE, Hacker NF. Optimal management of endometrial hyperplasia. Best Pract Res Clin Obstet Gynaecol. 2001;15(3):393–405.
10. Townsend DE, Marrow CP. Tumors of the endometrium. In: Paul Morrow C, Curtin JP, editors. Synopsis of gynecologic oncology. New York: Churchill Livingstone; 1975. p. 151–5.
11. Trimble CL, Method M, Leitao M, Lu K, Ioffe O, Hampton M, et al. Management of endometrial precancers. Obstet Gynecol. 2012;120(5):1160–75.
12. Naeem S, Duncan T. Management of endometrial hyperplasia. Norfolk and Norwich University Hospitals 2016. 1–7. http://www.nnuh.nhs.uk/publication/download/endometrial-hyperplasia-management_g40_v2/&ved=0ahUKEwijtcjpzLHYAhWMQo8KHQwuDbMQFgg2MAA&usg=AOvVaw2hjRYNHoS-4cGpZG1Xajmv
13. Royal College of Obstetricians and Gynaecologists (RCOG) with the British Society for Gynaecological Endoscopy (BSGE). Management of Endometrial Hyperplasia. Green-top Guideline No. 67. RCOG/BSGE joint guideline. London; 2016. Cited 29 Mar 2016.
14. Ricci E, Moroni S, Parazzini F, Surace M, Benzi G, Salerio B, et al. Risk factors for endometrial hyperplasia: results from a case-control study. Int J Gynecol Cancer. 2002;12:257–60.
15. Wells M. Hyperplasias of the endometrium. In: Gershenson DM, McGuire WP, Gore M, Quinn MA, Gillian T, editors. Gynecologic cancer: controversies in management. Missouri: Elsevier Churchill Livingstone; 2004. p. 249–57.
16. Wise MR, Jordan V, Lagas A, Showell M, Wong N, Lensen S, et al. Obesity and endometrial hyperplasia and cancer in premenopausal women: a systematic review. Am J Obstet Gynecol. 2016;214:689.e1–689.e17.
17. van der Meer ACL, Hanna LS. Development of endometrioid adenocarcinoma despite Levonorgestrel-releasing intrauterine system: a case report with discussion and review of the RCOG/BSGE guideline on the management of endometrial hyperplasia. Clin Obes. 2017;7:54–7.
18. Lacey JV Jr, Ioffe OB, Ronnett BM, Rush BB, Richesson DA, Chatterjee N, et al. Endometrial carcinoma risk among women diagnosed with endometrial hyperplasia: the 34-year experience in a large health plan. Br J Cancer. 2008;98:45–53.
19. Horn LC, Schnurrbusch U, Bilek K, Hentschel B, Einenkel J. Risk of progression in complex and atypical endometrial hyperplasia: clinicopathologic analysis in cases with and without progestogen treatment. Int J Gynecol Cancer. 2004;14:348–53.
20. Hacker NF, Friedlander ML. Uterine cancer. In: Berek JS, Hacker NF, editors. Berek & Hacker's gynecologic oncology. Philadelphia: Wolters Kluwer; 2015. p. 390–434.
21. Lacey JV Jr, Sherman ME, Rush BB, Ronnett BM, Ioffe OB, Duggan MA, Glass AG, Richesson DA, Chatterjee N, Langholz B. Absolute risk of endometrial carcinoma during 20-year follow-up among women with endometrial hyperplasia. J Clin Oncol. 2010;28(5):788–92.
22. Lacey JV Jr, Mutter GL, Nucci MR, Ronnett BM, Ioffe OB, Rush BB, et al. Risk of subsequent endo-

metrial carcinoma associated with endometrial intraepithelial neoplasia classification of endometrial biopsies. Cancer. 2008;113(8):2073–81.
23. Kurman RJ, Kaminski PF, Norris HJ. The behavior of endometrial hyperplasia: a long-term study of "untreated" hyperplasia in 170 patients. Cancer. 1985;56:403–12.
24. Kurman RJ, Norris HJ. Evaluation of criteria for distinguishing atypical endometrial hyperplasia from well-differentiated carcinoma. Cancer. 1982;49:2547–59.
25. Emons G, Beckmann M, Schmidt D, Mallmann P. New WHO classification of endometrial hyperplasias. Geburtshilfe Frauenheilkunde. 2015;75(2):135–6.
26. Rao S, Sundaram S, Narasimhan R. Biological behaviour of preneoplastic conditions of the endometrium: a retrospective 16-year study in South India. Indian J Med Paediatr Oncol. 2009;30(4):131–5.
27. Trope C, Alektiar K, Sabbatini P, Zaino R. Corpus: epithelial tumor. In: William JH, Carlos AP, Robert CY, Richard B, Maurie M, Marcus R, editors. Principles and practice of gynecologic oncology. Philadelphia: Lippincott Williams & Wilkins; 2005. p. 823–72.
28. McMeekin DS, Yashar C, Campos S, Zaino RJ. Corpus: epithelial tumors. In: Barakat R, Berchuck A, Markman M, Randal ME, editors. Principles and practice of gynecologic oncology. Philadelphia: Wolters Kluwer; 2013. p. 661–714.
29. Mutter GL, The Endometrial Collaborative Group. Endometrial Intraepithelial Neoplasia (EIN): will it bring order to chaos? Gynecol Oncol. 2000;76:287–90.
30. Raychaudhuri G, Bandyopadhyay A, Sarkar D, Mandal S, Mondal S, Mitra PK. Endometrial hyperplasia: a clinicopathological study in a Tertiary Care Hospital. J Obstet Gynecol India. 2013;63(6):394–8.
31. Memon MJ, Gupta Y. Endometrial Hyperplasia: a 3—years study at a rural based hospital. Schol J App Med Sci. 2016;4(10B):3707–10.
32. Dijkhuizen FPHLJ, Mol BWJ, Brolmann HAM, Heintz APM. The accuracy of endometrial sampling in the diagnosis of patients with endometrial carcinoma and hyperplasia. Cancer. 2000;89(8):1765–72.
33. Iglesias DA, Huang M, Soliman PT, Djordjevic B, Lu KH. Endometrial hyperplasia and cancer. In: Karlan BY, Bristow RE, Andrew LJ, editors. Gynecologic oncology clinical practice & surgical atlas. New York: McGraw Hill; 2012. p. 250–326.
34. Karlsson B, Gransberg S, Wiklan M, Pekka Y, Torvid K, Marsal K, et al. Transvaginal ultrasonography of the endometrium in women with postmenopausal bleeding-A Nordic multicenter study. Am J Obset Gynecol. 1995;172(5):1488–94.
35. Christopherson WM, Gray LA. Premalignant lesions of the endometrium: endometrial hyperplasia and adenocarcinoma in situ. In: Coppelson M, Monaghan JM, Morrow CP, Tattersall MHN, editors. Gynecologic oncology: fundamental principles and clinical practice (Vol 1 & 2). New York: Churchill Livingstone; 1992. p. 731–45.
36. Trope C, Lindahl B. Premalignant lesions of the endometrium: clinical features and management. In: Coppelson M, Monaghan JM, Morrow CP, Tattersall MHN, editors. Gynecologic oncology: fundamental principles and clinical practice (Vol 1 & 2). New York: Churchill Livingstone; 1992. p. 747–51.
37. Management of endometrial hyperplasia [Internet]. Uptodate.com. 2017. https://www.uptodate.com/contents/management-of-endometrial-hyperplasia?search=reed%20sd,urban%20r.%20r.%20classification%20and%20diagnosis%20of%20endometrial%20hyperplasia&source=search_result&selectedTitle=2~150&usage_type=default&display_rank=2. Cited 19 Dec 2017.
38. Gunderson CC, Fader AN, Carson KA, Bristow RE. Oncologic and reproductive outcomes with progestin therapy in women with endometrial hyperplasia and grade 1 adenocarcinoma: a systematic review. Gynecol Oncol. 2012;125:477–82.
39. Nwanodi O. Progestin intrauterine devices and metformin: endometrial hyperplasia and early stage endometrial cancer medical management. Healthcare. 2017;5(30):1–10.
40. Wildemeersch D, Dhont M. Treatment of nonatypical and atypical endometrial hyperplasia with a levonorgestrel-releasing intrauterine system. Am J Obstet Gynecol. 2003;188:1297–8.
41. Kim MK, Seong SJ. Conservative treatment for atypical endometrial hyperplasia: what is the most effective therapeutic method? J Gynecol Oncol. 2014;25(3):164–5.
42. Orbo A, Arnes M, Lysa LM, Borgfelt C, Straume B. HE4 is a novel tissue marker for therapy response and progestin resistance in medium- and low-risk endometrial hyperplasia. Br J Cancer. 2016;115:725–30.

Hereditary Endometrial and Ovarian Cancers

4

Garima Yadav and Anshuja Singla

4.1 Introduction

The most common cancers affecting women all over the world are breast cancers, epithelial ovarian cancers, and endometrial cancers, with large number of new cases being diagnosed every year. Ovarian cancer alone accounts for about 2.25 lac new cases diagnosed worldwide and around 1.54 lac deaths every year mainly because ovarian cancers are diagnosed in advanced stages secondary to subtle or absent symptoms [1]. The origin and progression of cancer cells are secondary to genetic alterations resulting from either accumulation of multiple somatic mutations or inheritance of one or more germline mutations in various genes controlling cell growth, proliferation, and apoptosis. About 12% of all ovarian cancers and 5% of endometrial cancers are considered to be hereditary [2, 3]. Germline mutations require multiple mutations at various gene loci for tumor genesis to occur. Hence, by identifying the specific germline mutations associated with particular hereditary cancer syndromes, targeted genetic diagnosis and therapies can be used to reduce morbidity and mortality associated with these malignancies.

Hereditary cancers are usually suspected in women who present with gynecological malignancies at a relatively young age or with a family history of cancer, usually of a specific cancer syndrome, in two or more relatives. The presence of ovarian cancer in a single first-degree relative increases a woman's chances of developing this disease by three- to fourfold [4]. Various studies have documented a relative risk of 1.2–2.8 for developing endometrial cancer, if it ever affected any first-degree relative [5–7]. The familial aggregation of cancers can be attributed to both genetic and environmental factors common within families, but genetic factors are thought to be more important [8].

4.2 Cancer Genetics

Two types of genes determine the origin and proliferation of cancer cells. The first ones are the "gatekeeper genes" which control cellular proliferation like various oncogenes and tumor suppressor genes. The second ones are the "caretaker genes" which are mainly involved in DNA repair. On the genomic level, the pro-oncogenes may get converted to oncogenes following gain of functional gene mutation; similarly, loss of functional gene mutations can inactivate tumor suppressor genes and hence can favor unchecked growth of

G. Yadav (✉)
Department of Obstetrics and Gynaecology, All India Institute of Medical Sciences, Jodhpur, Rajasthan, India

A. Singla
Department of Obstetrics and Gynaecology, University College of Medical Sciences and Guru Teg Bahadur Hospital, New Delhi, India

S. Mehta, A. Singla (eds.), *Preventive Oncology for the Gynecologist*, https://doi.org/10.1007/978-981-13-3438-2_4

tumor cells. Various genetic and epigenetic changes can also cause activation of oncogenes or deactivation of tumor suppressor genes allowing the cells to invade and metastasize, grow independently of growth factor support, and escape from antitumor immune responses. In all the developmental stages of genital malignancies, genomic alterations like point mutations, gene amplification, gene deletions, and rearrangements have been identified [9].

4.2.1 Types of Genomic Alterations in Hereditary Ovarian and Endometrial Cancers

Amplification It refers to an increase in the number of copies of a gene resulting in increased amount of template DNA undergoing transcription, thus leading to an overall increase in gene expression. Pro-oncogene overexpression following amplification is a relatively common event in various malignancies affecting women, e.g., overexpression of *HER2/neu* was demonstrated in about 30% of breast cancers, 20% of advanced ovarian cancers, and as many as 50% of endometrial cancers [10].

Point Mutation It refers to an alteration of a codon sequence and subsequent disruption of the normal function of a gene product. The most common genetic mutations described in solid tumors is the p53 point mutation. The nonfunctional normal *p53* within a cancer cell results in uninhibited cell proliferation where the DNA damage repair mechanism is not effective leading to genetic instability. *P53* gene has been found to be affected in approximately 50% of advanced ovarian cancers and 30–40% of endometrial cancers [11, 12]. Similarly, point mutations in the *BRCA1* and *BRCA2* genes, which mainly function as DNA repair genes, can cause accumulation of genetically instable cells and predispose to genesis of breast and ovarian cancers [13]. Table 4.1 provides the list of various hereditary cancer syndromes associated with gynecological tumors.

Table 4.1 Hereditary cancer syndromes associated with gynecological tumors

Hereditary syndrome	Gene mutation	Tumor phenotype
Li-Fraumeni syndrome	TP53, CHEK2	Breast cancer, soft tissue sarcoma, adrenal cortical carcinoma, brain tumors
Cowden syndrome, Bannayan-Zonana syndrome	PTEN	Breast cancer, hamartoma, glioma, endometrial cancer
Hereditary breast and ovarian cancer	BRCA1, BRCA2	Cancer of the breast, ovary, fallopian tube
Hereditary nonpolyposis colorectal cancer (HNPCC)	MLH1, MSH2, MSH3, MSH6, PMS2	Cancer of the colon, endometrium, ovary, stomach, small bowel, urinary tract
Multiple endocrine neoplasia type 1	Menin	Cancer of the thyroid, pancreas, and pituitary, ovarian carcinoid
Multiple endocrine neoplasia type 2	RET	Cancer of the thyroid and parathyroid, pheochromocytoma, ovarian carcinoid
Peutz-Jeghers syndrome	STK11	Gastrointestinal hamartomatous polyps; tumors of the stomach, duodenum, and colon; ovarian sex cord tumor with annular tubules (SCTAT)

4.3 Hereditary Endometrial Cancers

4.3.1 Hereditary Nonpolyposis Colorectal Cancer (HNPCC) Syndrome or Lynch Syndrome

Lynch syndrome has autosomal dominant transmission and can lead to both ovarian and endometrial cancer in the affected individual. It is caused by the germline mutation in one of the DNA mismatch repair (MMR) genes like MSH2, MSH3, MSH6, MLH1, and PMS2. This syndrome is associated with multiple malignancies, most common being colorectal cancers and endometrial cancer followed by ovarian, renal,

Table 4.2 Lifetime cumulative risk of endometrial cancer in women with Lynch syndrome

Study	Gene defect	Cumulative lifetime risk (%)
Dunlop et al. [18]	*hMLM* and *hMSH2*	42
Aarnio et al. [15]	*hMLH1* and *hMSH2*	60
Vasen et al. [19]	*hMLH1* and *hMSH2*	42 (*hMLH1*); 61 (*hMSH2*)
Hendriks et al. [20]	*hMLH1* *hMSH2* *hMSH6*	27 40 71
Hampel et al. [21]	*hMLH1* and *hMSH2*	54
Baglietto et al. [22]	*hMSH6*	44

stomach, pancreas, small bowel, and brain cancers [14]. Although colorectal cancer is considered as a primary cancer in Lynch syndrome, more than 50% of women in Lynch syndrome families present with malignancy of either the endometrium or ovaries [15–17]. The lifetime cumulative risk of endometrial cancers as discovered by various authors in women with MMR gene mutations is listed in Table 4.2.

The lifetime risk of developing ovarian cancer in women with a germline MMR mutations is around 6.7% as estimated in European and American population [23], and the cumulative lifetime risk of ovarian cancer increases to 10% by the age of 70 in *hMLH1 or hMSH2 mutation carriers* [24]. *In the general population, MMR gene mutations are present in 2% of ovarian cancer irrespective of age* [25, 26] *and in 9% of endometrial cancer cases under 50 years of age* [27, 28]. *If a woman is diagnosed with endometrial cancer at <50 years of age along with a positive family history of Lynch syndrome-related cancers in the first-degree relative, the chances of her being a carrier for MMR mutation is around 45%. In the presence of two or more first-degree relatives with endometrial cancer, MMR gene mutations can be present in 10% of women with such families* [29]. *Ovarian and endometrial cancers in Lynch syndrome are mostly endometrioid or clear cell type, which present at an early stage and have relatively better prognosis in terms of stage-specific survival.*

4.3.1.1 Screening Recommendations for Mutation Positive

Women with proven HNPCC genetic mutations are at high risk for developing endometrial cancer and must undergo genetic counseling in order to explain the associated risk, need for genetic testing in other family members (cascade testing), and options for preventive surgeries. Evaluation of the endometrium by transvaginal sonography and endometrial sampling may be offered, starting from age 35 to 40 years for early detection [30]. Lynch syndrome is usually associated with endometrioid-type pathology, which has a relatively better prognosis, and presents at an early stage; thus, it has been argued that screening would not result in a survival advantage for mutation-positive women. With respect to the prophylactic risk-reducing surgery in women with Lynch syndrome, proper recommendations are missing, but in light of the associated high risk, total laparoscopic hysterectomy and bilateral salpingo-oophorectomy (TLH-BSO) may be planned in these women once they have completed their families [31].

For patients with HNPCC syndrome, who choose against risk-reducing surgery, the National Comprehensive Care Network (NCCN) recommends follow-up starting from the age of 35 years, using transvaginal sonography and CA 125 measurement every 6 months during the proliferative phase of menstrual cycle. Screening for endometrial and ovarian cancer can also begin 5–10 years earlier than the earliest age of diagnosis of genital cancer in the family.

4.3.1.2 Cowden Syndrome

Cowden syndrome is a rare disorder with autosomal dominant transmission. This syndrome results secondary to the germline mutations in the PTEN tumor suppressor gene leading to the development of hamartomas and an increased risk of breast and non-medullary thyroid cancers. Cowden syndrome is found to be associated with increased chances of endometrial cancers (up to 30% of affected women); thus, the revised criteria for Cowden syndrome also include endometrial cancer as an important component cancer and were supported by NCCN panel for research purpose and clinical practice until robust data is available to disapprove this association [32].

4.3.2 Hereditary Ovarian Cancers

4.3.2.1 Hereditary Breast and Ovarian Cancer (HBOC) Syndrome

BRCA1 and/or BRCA2 gene mutations are detected in a majority of families with history of four or more members affected by either breast or ovarian cancer as components of HBOC syndrome [33, 34]. Around 65–85% of hereditary ovarian tumors are because of germline mutations in BRCA1/BRCA2 genes, which mainly function as DNA repair genes. The cumulative risk of ovarian cancer by age 70 is found to be 44–63% in BRCA1 carriers and 27–31% in BRCA2 carriers as suggested by case-based studies, although a relatively lower risk was estimated in population-based studies (39% for BRCA1 and 11% for BRCA2) which may be explained by the various lifestyle and environmental genetic modifiers that segregate the families (Table 4.3) [35, 36].

The ovarian tumors associated with BRCA1/2 mutations are found to be either serous, mixed malignant mesodermal tumors or undifferentiated type with high genomic instability. A novel hypothesis proposes that these tumors mostly arise in the tubal fimbria from intraepithelial lesions also known as serous tubal intraepithelial carcinoma (STIC). These abnormal cells may implant on the ovarian surface and the peritoneum. These hereditary ovarian cancers are usually high-grade pelvic serous tumors, which are aggressive in nature and present at advanced stages [37, 38]. Another theory proposed by Kurman and Sama et al. suggests that normal epithelium from the fimbria implants onto the ovarian surface during the process of ovulation and forms a cortical inclusion cyst (CIC) where malignant transformation of ovarian epithelium occurs [37, 39].

Table 4.3 Prevalence of BRCA1 and BRCA2 genes in women with family history of breast and ovarian cancers

Family history of breast and/or ovarian cancer	Prevalence of BRCA1 and/or BRCA2
Two or more first-degree relatives with ovarian cancer	37% and 9%
Three cases only of ovarian cancers	54% for BRCA1/2
Three or more cases of ovarian cancer and at least one case of breast cancer	81% for BRCA1/BRCA2

4.3.2.2 Ovarian Cancers Associated with Mutations Other than BRCA1/2

Majority of the hereditary ovarian cancers are found to be associated with BRCA1 or BRCA2 mutations, but more than 15% of these cancers are found to be secondary to genetic mutations other than BRCA genes, several of which still remain unknown [40]. Interestingly the clinicopathological features and behavior of non-BRCA-related tumors are also different from those associated with BRCA genes and TP53 gene (Table 4.4).

Screening Recommendations

The United States Preventive Service Task Force (USPSTF) recommends genetic counseling and

Table 4.4 Types of hereditary ovarian cancers and their clinicopathological features

	Type 1	Type 2
Prevalence	30%	70%
Histology	Serous, endometrioid, mucinous, and clear cell tumors	Serous, mixed malignant mesodermal tumors, carcinosarcomas, and undifferentiated tumors
Grade	Low and borderline	High
Mutations	PTEN, KRAS, BRAF, PIK3CA, ERBB2, CTNNB1, ARID1A, PPPR2R1A, and microsatellite instability	TP53 BRCA1/2
Clinical behavior	Large cystic masses confined to the ovary with a relatively indolent course	Diagnosed at advanced stages and have aggressive behavior

Table 4.5 Family history associated with hereditary breast and ovarian cancer syndrome

Ethnicity	Family history of malignancy
Ashkenazi Jewish women	One first-degree relative with breast or ovarian cancer Two second-degree relatives on the same side of the family with breast or ovarian cancer
All other women	Two first-degree relatives with breast cancer, one of whom was diagnosed by 50 years of age Three or more first- or second-degree relatives with breast cancers A combination of breast and ovarian cancers among first- and second-degree relatives One first-degree relative with bilateral breast cancer Two or more first- or second-degree relatives with ovarian cancer One first- or second-degree relative with a combination of breast and ovarian cancers Breast cancer in a male relative

offering BRCA testing in women who have a family history suggestive of cancers associated with BRCA1 or BRCA2 gene mutations as elaborated in Table 4.5.

Evidence supports that BRCA1 and BRCA2 mutation testing should be offered to every woman diagnosed with high-grade pelvic serous tumors (epithelial ovarian, fallopian tube, and primary peritoneal carcinoma), regardless of age and family history. This approach could be useful in offering cascade testing in close blood relatives in whom there is a role of routine screening and risk-reducing surgeries [41].

Next-generation sequencing with multigene panels: It is important to identify these cancer susceptibility genes not only to prevent ovarian cancers in high-risk population but also to guide treatment. In women already affected with ovarian cancer, genetic evaluation might help in identifying potential targets for emerging therapies like PARP (poly (ADP-ribose) polymerase) inhibitors in selected pathologies. Next-generation sequencing (NSG) offers a higher sensitivity and specificity in analyzing multiple cancer susceptibility genes in a single setting. Various panels of multiple genes including known ovarian cancer-associated loci have been introduced to screen germline mutations, thus reducing the cost and delay and optimizing the molecular diagnosis of hereditary ovarian cancers [42–44]. Despite the abovementioned advantages, geneticists and clinicians face challenges while interpreting and managing the results of these multigene panels secondary to identification of various mutations which are variants of unknown significance (VUS). Therefore, the clinician has uncertainties about interpreting the results and counseling the affected individual about future course of management. Hence, genetic screening and counseling using NSG technology should only be carried out at specialized family cancer clinics wherein a multidisciplinary expert can manage these families over an extended period of time.

Management Options for BRCA1/2 Mutation Positive

- Prophylactic risk-reducing bilateral salpingo-oophorectomy (RRBSO) is the main risk-reducing approach for preventing ovarian malignancies in women who are carriers of *BRCA1* or *BRCA2* mutation. Breast surgery like bilateral mastectomy or routine screening using modalities like self-breast examination, clinical breast examination, and breast imaging can be offered, in order to reduce the risk of breast cancer in BRCA mutation carriers [45]. It has been observed that removal of bilateral tubes and ovaries can decrease ovarian cancer risk largely (80–96%) [46–49]. Hence, all the women with BRCA gene mutations must be counseled for risk-reducing bilateral salpingo-oophorectomy (RRBSO), once their families are complete. The proposed age for undergoing RRBSO is between 35 and 40 years, as there is significant increase in the risk of developing ovarian cancer after the fourth decade. Upcoming evidence supports the role of RRBSO in reducing the risk of breast cancer by 56% in BRCA1 mutation carriers and 46% in BRCA2 mutation carriers, although more robust evidence is needed, before the information about this additional benefit becomes a standard part of counseling

[50, 51]. However, in BRCA mutation carriers, the need for routine breast screening continues even after RRBSO.

- In BRCA gene mutation carriers, who chose against RRBSO and need lifetime screening, the role of transvaginal scan or CA 125 is still not established but can be offered after the age of 30–35 years at clinician's discretion.
- Role of poly (ADP-ribose) polymerase (PARP) inhibitors in hereditary ovarian cancers: PARP1 and PARP2 help in DNA repair and are active components of repair of single-strand breaks (SSBs) and base excision repair (BER). These enzymes are activated by DNA damage and help in subsequent survival of tumor cells by helping in DNA repair of these cells. Brief suppression of PARP enzymes using PARP inhibitors will lead to the accumulation of unrepaired SSBs causing accumulation of double-strand breaks (DSBs) which are toxic for the survival of tumor cells. Notably, BRCA1- and BRCA2-mutated cells are highly dependent on PARP enzymes for DNA repair and hence are potential targets for PARP inhibitors.
- The most recent phase III trials of several PARP inhibitors like talazoparib, niraparib, olaparib, and veliparib have shown promise in terms of clinical use, efficacy, and safety profile. Olaparib has been granted accelerated approval to be used only in life-threatening disease, with or without platinum-based chemotherapy although more evidence is needed to understand the whole biological spectrum of PARP inhibitors in terms of their target tumors and safety index [52].

4.3.2.3 Li-Fraumeni Syndrome (LFS)

Li-Fraumeni syndrome is caused by mutations in the tumor suppressor gene TP53 and has autosomal dominant transmission. The cardinal cancers in this syndrome are early-onset sarcomas, breast cancers, and adrenocortical carcinomas, which account for 77–80% of LFS-associated tumors. Other tumors, leukemia, and lung, skin, gastrointestinal, and epithelial ovarian malignancies account for the remaining LFS-associated cancers [53]. The median age for ovarian cancers secondary to TP53 gene mutation is 40 years as against 64.3 years for sporadic cases [54]. Looking at the rarity of gynecological malignancies in this syndrome, there are no available guidelines for routine screening.

4.3.3 Peutz-Jeghers Syndrome

Peutz-Jeghers syndrome (PJS) is caused by the germline mutations in the *STK11* gene and has autosomal dominant transmission. It is typically a gastrointestinal polyposis disorder, which is also associated with increased risk of gynecological and breast tumors. The presence of pigmented lesions on the lips and buccal mucosa is a typical sign, which can indicate toward the diagnosis of PJS. The characteristic female malignancies are sex cord stromal tumor of the ovary and minimal deviation adenocarcinoma of the cervix, previously known as "adenoma malignum." Hence, annual screening with cervical cytology from the age of 18 years and transvaginal ultrasound along with CA 125 measurement starting from 25 years have been suggested in known mutation carriers [55] although a definitive advantage and guidelines for screening are not available.

4.3.4 Multiple Endocrine Neoplasia (MEN) Syndrome

Multiple endocrine neoplasia is a cancer syndrome that typically affects various organs of the endocrine system. The major forms of MEN syndrome are type 1, type 2, and type 4, and the associated tumors can be either benign or malignant. MEN type 1 has an autosomal dominant inheritance caused by mutations in the MEN1 gene and comprises of tumors of the pituitary gland, parathyroid gland, and pancreas along with several other benign tumors like lipomas, angiomyofibromas, and uterine fibroids, along with malignant carcinoid tumors of the lungs, thymus, and colon. MEN2 syndrome is caused by RET gene mutations and includes tumors like medullary thyroid cancer, pheochromocytoma, and hyperparathyroidism. MEN syndrome is reported to be associated with ovarian carcinoids and granulosa cell tumors of the ovary [56]. Carney complex is the most recent addition to MEN syndrome, and it refers to tumors of the gonads, thyroid gland, adrenal cortex, and pituitary gland. This complex occurs secondary to the mutations in the gene that codes for regulatory subunit type 1A of protein kinase A (PKA) (*PRKAR1A*) [57].

4.3.5 Muir-Torre Syndrome

Muir-Torre syndrome is a subtype of Lynch syndrome (HNPCC) most commonly associated with MSH2 gene mutation and has autosomal dominant transmission like HNPCC. The syndrome is characterized by rare skin lesions like adenoma, epithelioma, and carcinomas of the sebaceous glands along with visceral malignancies in more than 50% of affected patients. Various visceral malignancies in Muir-Torre syndrome are cancers of the gastrointestinal tract, followed by genitourinary cancers (endometrial and ovarian), parotid gland cancers, lung and breast cancers, and hematological malignancies [58]. Diagnosis of sebaceous tumor can point toward Muir-Torre syndrome, and affected individuals should undergo screening for associated malignancies. Individuals with proven mutation and their first-degree relatives are offered a yearly breast examination, CA 125 levels, pelvic examination along with a transvaginal scan, and annual endometrial biopsy [59].

4.3.5.1 Small Cell Carcinoma of the Ovary-Hypercalcemic Type (SCCOHT)

Small cell carcinoma of the ovary is an extremely rare and highly aggressive cancer affecting women of younger age group, with hypercalcemia occurring in around 65% of cases. The diagnosis is based on histopathological evidence of small cells with hyperchromasia, scanty cytoplasm, and high mitosis along with necrosis. Immunohistochemically, these tumors are positive for vimentin, along with focal expression of epithelial markers. In 75% of cases, the affected gene identified is SMARCA4; leading to nonproduction of BRG1 protein which is a product of the SMARCA4 gene. This genetic mutation involving SMARCA4 is also found in malignant rhabdoid tumors which are also found to be hereditary on occasions and are frequently associated with hypercalcemia; thus, SCCOHT tumors can also be termed as "malignant rhabdoid tumors of the ovary" [60]. In early stages, radical surgery including panhysterectomy, omentectomy, and pelvic and para-aortic lymphadenectomy followed by adjuvant chemotherapy with cisplatin and etoposide is recommended. Since SCCOHT affects young women, fertility preservation surgery, which involves proper staging and removal of the affected ovary only, followed by chemotherapy, must be considered. For advanced stages, neoadjuvant chemotherapy should be the first-line treatment, followed by debulking surgery [61]. The long-term, disease-free survival is very poor in these patients even in patients with an early-stage disease.

4.4 Conclusion

It is estimated that around 5% of endometrial and 20% of ovarian cancers are hereditary. Hereditary gynecological cancers are usually suspected when these tumors arise in young females with family history of these cancers. The most common syndrome associated with hereditary endometrial cancers is the Lynch syndrome (HNPCC) and that with ovarian cancers is hereditary breast and ovarian cancer syndrome. Several genetic mutation loci have been identified for diagnosing the susceptibility of an individual to develop these cancers. It is important to confirm these genetic mutations in potentially susceptible women with a strong family history, not only to prevent the development of cancers by advising them risk reduction procedures but also to offer them targeted therapies against the identified genetic mutations.

For the prevention of hereditary gynecological cancers in individuals with confirmed genetic mutations, proper screening must be done according to the above laid guidelines after proper genetic counseling. These patients must be managed by multi-speciality teams at dedicated family cancer clinics. After the identification of multiple genetic mutations in hereditary gynecological cancers, the use of next-generation sequencing (NSG) has provided the opportunity to analyze even non-BRCA gene-related mutations in the same reaction. The clinicians must understand the importance of taking family history in detail in endometrial and ovarian cancers in order to offer genetic counseling and testing in the index patient and also in the unaffected individuals of the family. If a genetic mutation is present in the affected women, other family members can undergo targeted testing also known as "cascade testing," thus saving resources. Prophylactic risk reduction surgeries can be offered, once the genetic mutation has been identified and risk assessment has been done. There is an emerging evidence in support of the chemoprotective therapies besides the time-tested platinum-based chemotherapy, which indicates that PARP inhibitors can be proven to be effective in managing BRCA-related ovarian malignancies.

Key Points

- Approximately 5% of endometrial carcinomas and 20% of epithelial ovarian carcinomas are hereditary.
- Majority of these hereditary cancers have autosomal dominant inheritance, and the commonest disorders are hereditary breast and ovarian cancer (HBOC) syndrome and Lynch syndrome.
- The family history of single first-degree relative affected with ovarian cancer increases a woman's chances of developing this disease by three- to fourfold.
- For endometrial cancer, having an affected first-degree relative increases the chances of a woman with a relative risk of 1.2–2.8.
- More than 50% of women in Lynch syndrome families present with malignancy of either the endometrium or ovaries as their first malignancy.
- Screening of high-risk women, i.e., women with proven MMR pathway mutations or women with family history of Lynch syndrome, must begin by the age of 35–40 years using transvaginal ultrasound and aspiration biopsy.
- *Around 65–85% of hereditary ovarian tumors are because of* BRCA1/BRCA2 gene mutations.
- Every woman with high-grade pelvic serous tumors should be offered *BRCA1* and *BRCA2* gene testing, regardless of the family history.
- Women who carry *BRCA1* or *BRCA2* mutation must be offered risk-reducing bilateral salpingo-oophorectomy (RRBSO) and risk-reducing breast surgery or breast screening.
- Various other genes, besides BRCA genes, have now been identified using massive gene sequencing, and targeted therapies against these mutations are being evaluated.

References

1. Ferlay J, Shin HR, Bray F, Forman D, Mathers C, Parkin DM. Estimates of worldwide burden of cancer in 2008. Int J Cancer. 2010;127(12):2893–917.
2. Berends MJ, Wu Y, Sijmons RH, et al. Toward new strategies to select young endometrial cancer patients for mismatch repair gene mutation analysis. J Clin Oncol. 2003;21:4364–70.
3. King MC, Marks JH, Mandell JB. Breast and ovarian cancer risks due to inherited mutations in BRCA1 and BRCA2. Science. 2003;302:643–6.
4. Stratton JF, Pharoah PDP, Smith SK, Easton DF, Ponder BAJ. A systematic review an metaanalysis of family history an risk of ovarian cancer. Br J Obstet Gynaecol. 1998;105:493–9.
5. Gruber SB, Thompson WD. A population base study of endometrial cancer and familial risk in younger women. Cancer and Steroid Hormone Study Group. Cancer Epidemiol Biomark Prev. 1996;5(6):411–7.
6. Lucenteforte E, Talamini R, Montella M, Dal Maso L, Pelucchi C, Franceschi S, La Vecchia C, Negri E. Family history of cancer and risk of endometrial cancer. Eur J Cancer Prev. 2009;18(2):95–9.
7. Parazzini F, Negri E, La Vecchia C, Restelli C, Francesci S. Family history of reproductive cancers and ovarian cancer risk: an Italian case control study. Am J Epidemiol. 1992;135(1):35–40.
8. Lichtenstein P, Holm NV, Verkasalo PK, Iliadou A, Kaprio J, Koskenvuo M, Pukkala E, Skytthe A, Hemminki K. Environmental and heritable factors in the causation of cancer- analyses of cohorts of twins from Sweden, Denmark, Finland. N Engl J Med. 2000;343(2):78–85.

9. Baker VV. Update on the molecular carcinogenesis of cervix cancer. Clin Consult Obstet Gynecol. 1995;7:86–93.
10. Hogdall EV, Christensen L, Kjaer SK, et al. Distribution of HER-2 overexpression in ovarian carcinoma tissue and its prognostic value in patients with ovarian carcinoma: from the Danish MALOVA Ovarian Cancer Study. Cancer. 2003;98:66–73.
11. Kastan MB, Onyekwere O, Sidransky D, et al. Participation of p53 protein in the cellular response to DNA damage. Cancer Res. 1991;51:6304–11.
12. Kuerbitz SJ, Plunkett BS, Walsh WV, et al. Wild type p53 is a cell cycle checkpoint determinant following irradiation. Proc Natl Acad Sci U S A. 1992;89:7491–5.
13. Bacolod MD, Schemmann GS, Giardina SF, et al. Emerging paradigms in cancer genetics: some important findings from high-density single nucleotide polymorphism array studies. Cancer Res. 2009;69:723–7.
14. Meyer LA, Broadus RR, Lu KH. Endometrial cancer and Lynch syndrome: clinical and pathologic considerations. Cancer Control. 2009;16(1):14–22.
15. Aarnio M, Sankila R, Pukkala E, Salovaara R, Aaltonen LA, de la Chapelle A, Peltomaki P, Mecklin JP, Jarvinen HJ. Cancer risk in mutation carriers of DNA-mismatch-repair genes. Int J Cancer. 1999;81(2):214–8.
16. Vasen HF, Watson P, Mecklin JP, Lynch HT. New clinical criteria for hereditary non polyposis colorectal cancer (HNPCC,Lynch syndrome) proposed by the international collaborative group on HNPCC. Gastroenterology. 1999;116(6):1453–6.
17. Watson P, Lynch HT. Cancer risk in mismatch repair genes mutation carriers. Familial Cancer. 2001;1:57–60.
18. Dunlop MG, Farrington SM, Carothers AD, Wyllie AH, Sharp L, Burn J, Liu B, Kinzler KW, Vogelstein B. Cancer risk associated with germline DNA mismatch repair gene mutations. Hum Mol Genet. 1997;6(1):105–10.
19. Vasen HF, Wijnen JT, Menko FH, Kleibeuker JH, Taaal BG, Griffioen G, Nagengast FM, Meijers-Heijboer EH, Bertario L, Varesco L, et al. Cancer risk in families with hereditary nonpolyposis colorectal cancer diagnosed by mutation analysis. Gastroenterology. 1996;110(4):1020–7.
20. Hendriks YM, Wagner A, Morreau H, Menko F, Stormorken A, Quehenberger F, Sandkuijl L, Moller P, Genuardi M, van Houwelingen H, et al. Cancer risk in hereditary nonpolyposis colorectal cancer ue to MSH6 mutations: impact on counseling and surveillance. Gastroenterology. 2004;127(1):17–25.
21. Hampel H, Stephens JA, Pukkala E, Sankila R, Aoltonen LA, Mecklin JP, de la Chapelle A. Cancer risk in hereditary nonpolyposis colorectal cancer syndrome: later age of onset. Gastroenterology. 2005;129(20):415–21.
22. Baglietto L, Lindor NM, Dowty JG, White DM, Wagner A, Gomez Garcia EB, Vriends AH, Dutch Lynch Syndrome Study Group, Cartwright NR, Barnetson RA. Risk of LYNCH syndrome cancers in MSH6 mutation carriers. J Natl Cancer Inst. 2010;102(3):193–201.
23. Watson P, Vasen HF, Mecklin JP, Bernstein I, Aarnio M, Jarvinen HJ, Myrhoj T, Sunde L, Wijnen JT, Lynch HT. The risk of extra-colonic, extra-endometrial cancer in the Lynch syndrome. Int J Cancer. 2008;123(2):444–9.
24. Vasen HF, Stormorken A, Menko FH, Nageggast FM, Kleibeuker JH, Griffioen G, Taal BG, Moller P, Wijnen JT. MSH2 mutation carriers are at higher risk of cancer than MLH1 mutation carriers: a study of hereditary non polyposis colorectal cancer families. J Clin Oncol. 2001;19:4074–80.
25. Malander S, Rambech E, Kristoffersson U, Halvarsson B, Ridderheim M, Borg A, Nilbert M. The contribution of the hereditary non polyposis colorectal cancer syndrome to the development of ovarian cancer. Gynecol Oncol. 2006;101:238–43.
26. Rubin SC, Blackwood MA, Bandera C, Behbakht K, Benjamin I, Rebbeck TR, Boyd J. BRCA1, BRCA 2, and hereditary nonpolyposis colorectal cancer gene mutations in an unselected ovarian cancer population: relationship to family history and implications for genetic testing. Am J Obstet Gynecol. 1998;178:670–7.
27. Lu KH, Schorge JO, Roabaugh KJ, Daniels MS, Sun CC, Soliman PT, White KG, Luthra R, Gershenson DM, Broaddus RR. Prospective determination of prevalence of Lynch syndrome in young women with endometrial cancer. J Clin Oncol. 2007;25:5158–64.
28. Berends MJ, Wu Y, Sijmons RH, van der Sluis T, Ek WB, Ligtenberg MJ, Arts NJ, ten Hoor KA, Kleibeuker JH, de Vries EG, et al. Toward new strategies to select endometrial cancer patients for mismatch repair gene mutation analysis. J Clin Oncol. 2003;21:4364–70.
29. Ollikainen M, Abdel-Rehman WM, M oisio AL, Lindroos A, Kariola R, Jarvela I, Poyhonen M, Butzow R, Peltomaki P. Molecular analysis of familial endometrial carcinoma: a manifestation of hereditary nonpolyposis colorectal cancer or a separate syndrome? J Clin Oncol. 2005;23:4609–16.
30. Vasen HF, Blanco I, Aktan-Collan K, Gopie JP, Alonso A, Aretz S, et al. Revised guidelines for the clinical management of Lynch syndrome (HNPCC): recommendations by a group of European experts. Gut. 2013;62:812–23.
31. Schmeler KM, Lynch HT, Chen LM, Munsell MF, Soliman PT, Clark MB, et al. Prophylactic surgery to reduce the risk of gynecologic cancers in the Lynch syndrome. N Engl J Med. 2006;354:261–9.
32. Eng C. Will the real cowden syndrome please stand up: revised diagnostic criteria. J Med Genet. 2000;37:828–30.
33. Gayther SA, Russell P, Harrington P, Antoniou A, Easton DF, Ponder BAJ. The contribution of germline BRCA1 and BRCA2 mutations to familial ovarian cancer: no evience for other ovarian cancer susceptibility genes. Am J Hum Genet. 1999;65:1021–9.

34. Ramus SJ, Harrington PA, Pye C, Dicioccio RA, Cox MJ, Garlinghouse-Jones K, Oakley-Girvan I, Jacobs IJ, Hardy RM, Whittemore AS, et al. Contribution of BRCA1 and BRCA2 mutations to inherited ovarian cancer. Hum Mutat. 2007;28(12):1207–15.
35. Antoniou AC, Sinilnikova OM, Simard J, Leone M, Dumont M, Neuhausen SL, Struewing JP, Stoppa-Lyonnet DD, Barjhoux L, Hughes DJ, et al. RAD51 135G>C modifies breast cancer risk among BRCA2 mutation carriers: results from a combined analysis of 19 studies. Am J Hum Genet. 2007;81(6):1186–200.
36. Antoniou AC, Spurdle AB, Sinilnikova OM, Healey S, Pooley KA, Schmutzler RK, Versmold B, Engel C, Meindl A, Arnold N, et al. Common breast cancer predisposition alleles are associated with breast cancer risk in BRCA1 and BRCA2 mutation carriers. Am J Hum Genet. 2008;82(4):937–48.
37. Kurman RJ. Origin and molecular pathogenesis of ovarian high grade serous carcinoma. Ann Oncol. 2013;10:1016–21.
38. Kurman RJ, Shih IM. Pathogenesis of ovarian cancer: lessons from morphology and molecular biology and their clinical implications. Int J Gynecol Pathol. 2008;27(2):151–60.
39. Sama AR, Schilder RJ. Refractory fallopian tube carcinoma—current perspectives in pathogenesis and management. Int J Women's Health. 2013;6(1):149–57.
40. Walsh T, Casadie S, Lee MK, Penil CC, Nord AS, Thornton AM, et al. Mutations in 12 genes for inherited ovarian, fallopian tube, and peritoneal carcinoma identified by massive parallel sequencing. Proc Natl Acad Sci U S A. 2011;108(44):18032.
41. Trainer AH, Meiser B, Watts K, Mitchell G, Tucker K, Friedlander M. Moving toward personalized medicine: treatment-focused genetic testing of women newly diagnosed with ovarian cancer. Int J Gynecol Cancer. 2010;20:704–16.
42. Castéra L, Krieger S, Rousselin A, Legros A, Baumann JJ, Bruet O, et al. Next-generation sequencing for the diagnosis of hereditary breast and ovarian cancer using genomic capture targeting multiple candidate genes. Eur J Hum Genet. 2014;22(11):1305–13.
43. Tung N, Battelli C, Allen B, Kaldate R, Bhatnagar S, Bowles K, et al. Frequency of mutations in individuals with breast cancer referred for BRCA1 and BRCA2 testing using next-generation sequencing with a 25-gene panel. Cancer. 2015;121(1):25–33.
44. Ruiz A, Llort G, Yagüe C, Baena N, Viñas M, Torra M, et al. Genetic testing in hereditary breast and ovarian Cancer using massive parallel sequencing. Biomed Res Int. 2014;2014:542541, 8 p
45. Manchanda R, Abdelraheim A, Johnson M, Rosenthal AN, Benjamin E, Brunell C, et al. Outcome of risk-reducing salpingo-oophorectomy in BRCA carriers and women of unknown mutation status. BJOG. 2011;118:814–24.
46. Kauff ND, Satagopan JM, Robson ME, Scheuer L, Hensley M, Hudis CA, et al. Risk- reducing salpingo-oophorectomy in women with a BRCA1 or BRCA2 mutation. N Engl J Med. 2002;346:1609–15.
47. Rebbeck TR, Lynch HT, Neuhausen SL, Narod SA, van't Veer L, Garber JE, et al. Prophylactic oophorectomy in carriers of BRCA1 or BRCA2 mutations. N Engl J Med. 2002;346:1616–22.
48. Kauff ND, Domchek SM, Friebel TM, Robson ME, Lee J, Garber JE, et al. Risk-reducing salpingo-oophorectomy for the prevention of BRCA1- and BRCA2-associated breast and gynecologic cancer: a multicenter, prospective study. J Clin Oncol. 2008;26:1331–7.
49. Finch A, Beiner M, Lubinski J, Lynch HT, Moller P, Rosen B, et al. Salpingo-oophorectomy and the risk of ovarian, fallopian tube, and peritoneal cancers in women with a BRCA1 or BRCA2 mutation. JAMA. 2006;296:185.
50. Ford D, Easton DF, Stratton M, Narod S, Goldgar D, Devilee P, et al. Genetic heterogeneity and penetrance analysis of the BRCA1 and BRCA2 genes in breast cancer families. Am J Hum Genet. 1998;62:676–89.
51. Rosenthal AN, Fraser L, Manchanda R, Badman P, Philpott S, Mozersky J, Hadwin R, Cafferty FH, Benjamin E, Singh N, Evans DG, Eccles DM, Skates SJ, Mackay J, Menon U, Jacobs IJ. Results of annual screening in phase I of the United Kingdom familial ovarian cancer screening study highlight the need for strict adherence to screening schedule. J Clin Oncol. 2013;31(1):49–57.
52. Dziadkowiec KN, Gąsiorowska E, Markwitz EN, Jankowska A. PARP inhibitors: review of mechanisms of action and BRCA1/2 mutation targeting. Prz Menopauzalny. 2016;15(4):215–9.
53. Sorrell AD, Espenschied CR, Culver JO, Weitzel JN. Tumor protein p53 (TP 53) testing and li-fraumeni syndrome: current status of clinical applications and future directions. Mol Diagn Ther. 2013;17(1):31–47.
54. Olivier M, Goldgar DE, Sodha N, et al. Li-Fraumeni and related syndromes: correlation between tumor type, family structure, and TP53 genotype. Cancer Res. 2003;63(20):6643–50.
55. Giardiello FM, Trimbath JD. Peutz-Jeghers syndrome and management recommendations. Clin Gastroenterol Hepatol. 2006;4:408–15.
56. Hall MJ, Innocent J, Rybak C, Veloski C, Scott WJ, Wu H, et al. Bilateral granulosa cell tumors: a novel malignant manifestation of multiple endocrine neoplasia 1 syndrome found in a patient with a rare menin in-frame deletion. Appl Clin Genet. 2015;8:69–73.
57. Stratakis CA. Clinical genetics of multiple endocrine neoplasias, carney complex and related syndromes. J Endocrinol Investig. 2001;24:370–83.

58. Jones B, Oh C, Mangold E, Egan CA. Muir–Torre syndrome: diagnostic and screening guidelines. Aust J Dermatol. 2006;47:266–9.
59. Pancholi A, Collins D, Lindley R, Gandhi P. Muir–Torre syndrome: a case report and screening recommendations. Ann R Coll Surg Engl. 2008;90(8):W9–1.
60. Karanian-Philippe M, Velasco V, Longy M, Floquet A, Arnould L, Coindre JM, et al. SMARCA4 (BRG1) loss of expression is a useful marker for the diagnosis of ovarian small cell carcinoma of the hypercalcemic type (ovarian rhabdoid tumor): a comprehensive analysis of 116 rare gynecologic tumors, 9 soft tissue tumors, and 9 melanomas. Am J Surg Pathol. 2015;39:1197–205.
61. Harrison ML, Hoskins P, du Bois A, Quinn M, Rustin GJ, Ledermann JA, Baron-Hay S, Friedlander ML. Small cell of the ovary, hypercalcemic type—analysis of combined experience and recommendation for management. A GCIG study. Gynecol Oncol. 2006;100:233–8.

5 Chemoprevention for Endometrial Cancers

Monisha Gupta

5.1 Introduction

Endometrial cancer (EC) is the sixth leading cause of cancer-related death in women worldwide, with the majority of cases arising in postmenopausal women. Endometrial adenocarcinoma originates in the inner lining of the uterus, and it accounts for about 90% of uterine cancers, while uterine sarcoma originates in the myometrium and accounts for less than 10% of the cases [1, 2]. Endometrioid adenocarcinoma is the most common histology (90% cases of EC) and has a good prognosis in early stage (5-year survival rate >90%) [2].

5.2 Why Chemoprevention for Endometrial Cancer?

Chemoprevention for cancer means ingestion of any drug (allopathic, homeopathic, or ayurvedic) to prevent, suppress, or reverse the pathogenesis of cancer in an individual with no signs and symptoms. To identify individuals/patients who may require chemoprevention, it is advisable that their chances of developing cancer must be weighed against toxic effects of such drugs. Thus, an ideal chemoprevention study should recruit individuals from a high-risk population and should involve the drug/chemical agent with minimal side effects.

Cancer chemoprevention for certain high-risk population as well as for certain cancers is the current topic of interest. For instance, in the case of hormone-dependent cancers like breast cancer, hormone modulators such as tamoxifen, raloxifene, and aromatase inhibitors have shown to significantly decrease the risk of breast cancer [3]. Likewise, the use of oral contraceptive pills has already been documented to reduce the risk of ovarian cancer in women with BRCA 1 and BRCA 2 germline mutations, thus an alternative to prophylactic oophorectomy in young premenopausal women [4].

Recent literature indicates toward increasing interest for chemoprevention of EC. Its occurrence is related to both endogenous and exogenous hormone exposures and that too in a dose-response relationship. Combination oral contraceptives (COC) and menopausal hormone therapy are the most common forms of exogenous hormones. Other risk factors that lead to excess hormonal levels and, thus, increase the risk of EC are increasing age, obesity, low parity, late menopause, HRT, polycystic ovarian disease (PCOD), and certain estrogen-secreting ovarian tumors.

Also, family history (having close relatives with EC and/or colorectal cancer) pointing toward Lynch syndrome or self-history of ovarian

M. Gupta (✉)
Department of Surgical Oncology, Max Super Speciality Hospital, Shalimar Bagh, New Delhi, India

Department of Surgical Oncology, Max Super Speciality Hospital, Pitampura, New Delhi, India

S. Mehta, A. Singla (eds.), *Preventive Oncology for the Gynecologist*,
https://doi.org/10.1007/978-981-13-3438-2_5

or breast cancer significantly increases the risk for EC. Thus, EC is among certain cancers that have a well-defined risk factor profile and, thus, gives an easy access to identify women at high risk of developing EC.

Currently, various studies on a variety of hormonal and non-hormonal agents for chemoprevention of EC are being conducted. In the chapter, we will discuss the rationale of their use, their side effects, and their effect on EC risk reduction.

5.3 Chemoprevention of Endometrial Cancer

5.3.1 Hormonal Contraception and Endometrial Cancer Risk Reduction

In the early 1980s, hormonal chemoprevention of endometrial cancer with OCs was first demonstrated, and it was shown that the protection was clinically highly significant and dependent on the duration of use: 5 years of OC use provides 46%, and 10 years of use gives 71% reduction in risk of cancer [5]. Thus, irrespective of type and dose of progestins, longer duration of COC use provides significant reduction in risk of EC [6, 7]. Moreover, this reduction persists for about 20 years even after stopping COC [8].

Majority of risk factors for EC are explained by the mitogenic action of estrogen in the absence of progestin (so-called unopposed estrogen) in stimulating endometrial cell division. The age-incidence curve of cancer of the endometrium shows a distinct decrease at the age of menopause as the concentration of unopposed estrogen reduces to very low level at menopause (Fig. 5.1). Thus, early menopause reduces the risk of EC to a very low level. Progesterone effectively reduces the effect of unopposed estrogen throughout pregnancy; thus increasing parity also decreases endometrial cancer risk. Obesity significantly increases the serum estradiol levels in both premenopausal (increased anovulation) and postmenopausal women (also decreases sex hormone-binding globulin) and, thus, significantly increases the risk for EC. Estrogen replacement therapy in postmenopausal women significantly increases endometrial cancer risk.

A dose-response relationship between unopposed estrogen and EC has also been suggested in literature (5–50 pg/ml) [5].

The high dose of progestins in OCs protects endometrial cells from unopposed estrogen for about 21 days in 28 day cycle; thus, only during 7 days (when OCs are not taken), the endometrial cells are exposed to unopposed estrogen. In this way, various epidemiological studies show an 11.7% reduction in EC risk per year of OC use [5].

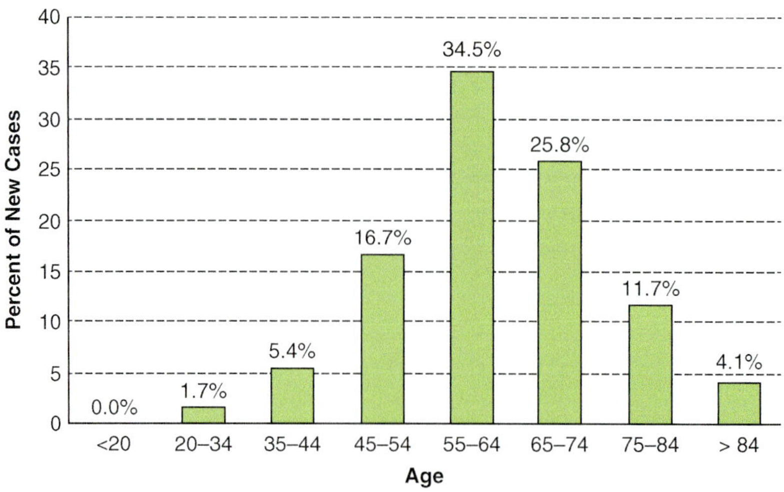

Fig. 5.1 SEER data 18 2010–2014, all races, females

Since the most immediate effect of COC use on risk of EC is well documented, how COC use results in long-term protective effects remains largely unknown. It has been hypothesized that progestin antagonizes the estrogens' proliferative effect on endometrial cells and that is exactly how COC provides risk reduction for EC [9]. A randomized trial by Lu et al. has also shown the same results [10]. Various studies have shown a variety of molecular effects of progestins, i.e., it promotes cell cycle arrest, induces apoptosis, and also regulates expression of multiple signaling pathways involved in oncogenesis [11]. Another study has suggested that COC use has a long-term effect on various hormone levels, estradiol, estrone, androstenedione, testosterone, and sex hormone-binding globulin in our body [12], and also, age at menopause is also older in COC users as compared to nonusers [13]. The exact mechanism of action behind all these effects of progestins is largely unknown; however, enduring epigenetic changes, progestin-mediated decrease in receptor expression and long-term effects on hormone metabolism are speculated to be the prime reasons [13, 14].

To have a minimal effect on breast tissue, progestins need to be delivered to the endometrium in such a manner so as to have minimal serum concentration such as vaginal route or direct endometrial route. The vaginal route provides a high endometrial progestin level with very low serum levels [15]. The direct endometrial route of administration with an intrauterine device has even lower serum progestin levels [1].

5.3.1.1 Chemoprevention for Lynch Syndrome-Related Endometrial Cancer

Lynch syndrome (LS) is an autosomal dominant cancer syndrome carrying a high risk of colorectal cancer (CRC) as well as non-colonic cancers such as endometrial cancer (second most common), ovarian cancer, gastric cancer, intestinal cancer, etc. LS has been reported to affect as many as 1 in 370 individuals [16]. The increase risk of cancer is due to inherited mutations in MSH2, MLH1, MSH6, and PMS2 genes that impair DNA mismatch repair mechanism. The cumulative risk of endometrial cancer is 54% for MLH1, 21% for MSH2, and 16% for MSH6 carriers with syndrome-related EC manifesting 10 years earlier than their sporadic counterpart [17]. For many women with LS, the risk of EC is comparable or even exceeds their risk of CRC [18]. However, studies regarding the efficacy of chemopreventive agents in LS-associated EC are few.

Women with LS are at high risk for endometrial cancer and are ideal candidate for prophylactic surgery. However, most women are eager for alternatives to surgery (as are relatively young at age) and, thus, should be offered chemoprevention because the risk-benefit profile of potential chemopreventive agents for EC is favorable.

Lu and colleagues [19] have demonstrated that oral contraceptive pills (OCPs) and depoMPA induce an expected physiologic endometrial response when administered to premenopausal women with Lynch Syndrome. With each woman as her own control, after 3 months of treatment, there was a significant decrease in endometrial epithelial cell proliferation (Ki-67) in both dMPA and OCP arms. Also on histology, 20 of the 23 women in depoMPA arm and 21 of 22 women in the OCP arm demonstrated the presence of secretory type glands. This suggests that both depoMPA and OCPs can be used as chemopreventive agents in women with LS. However, right now, it will be premature to conclude that this effect of hormonal agent will decrease the incidence of EC in this high-risk population. Thus, further large studies are needed to clearly delineate the molecular mechanism of development of EC in women with LS and whether that mechanism can be prevented or reversed with hormonal agents.

5.3.2 Effect of Metformin on Obesity-Related Endometrial Proliferation and Cancer

It is a well-known fact that being overweight and obese are significant risk factors for cardiovascular diseases and type II DM as well as for many cancer types [20, 21]. In females, increased BMI associated very strongly with risk of EC with

>50% of all EC attributed to obesity [22]. In obese female, fat cells are prime site for conversion of estrogen to estradiol: an active form of female hormone that leads to endometrial cell proliferation. Moreover, other factors including hyperinsulinemia also contribute to cancer pathogenesis as well as progression. It has been suggested in a study that an obese female is at 2.5 times higher risk of death due to EC as compared to nonobese counterpart [22].

Metformin which is an antidiabetic drug from biguanide class commonly used to treat type II diabetes has recently been demonstrated to exert chemopreventive and antiproliferative effects for a variety of cancers in diabetic patients, including those with endometrial cancer [23–25]. Metformin inhibits cell growth both by insulin- and non-insulin-dependent mechanisms. Metformin increases insulin receptor sensitivity and increases insulin uptake, thereby reducing systemic insulin levels. It also inhibits cell proliferation by activating the growth inhibitory AMPK, which counteracts signaling through both the PI3K/AKT and MAPK pathways downstream of the insulin and IGF1 receptors (Fig. 5.2) [26]. Metformin further downregulated signaling through the MAPK pathway, as demonstrated by a decrease in phospho-ERK1/2 in estrogen-treated obese rat endometrium. Finally, metformin effectively hindered induction of the estrogen-responsive, pro-proliferative transcription factors c-myc and c-fos [27].

Metformin induces changes in signaling both upstream and downstream of insulin and IGF1 receptors [27, 28]. Also, it has direct growth-inhibitory effects on cells via activation of the AMPK pathway [29]. Thus, metformin controls cell division as it increases AMP relative to ATP levels inside the cells, thus regulating the ATP consuming pathways [27].

Regarding non-endometrioid endometrial cancer, diabetic endometrial cancer patients with non-endometrioid tumors who were taking metformin (dose is gradually increased from 500 mg/day to 2 gm/day over 1 month) were demonstrated to have a lower risk of mortality than that of patients with endometrial cancer who did not use metformin [29]. Metformin may therefore function as an adjuvant therapy for the treatment of non-endometrioid endometrial cancer.

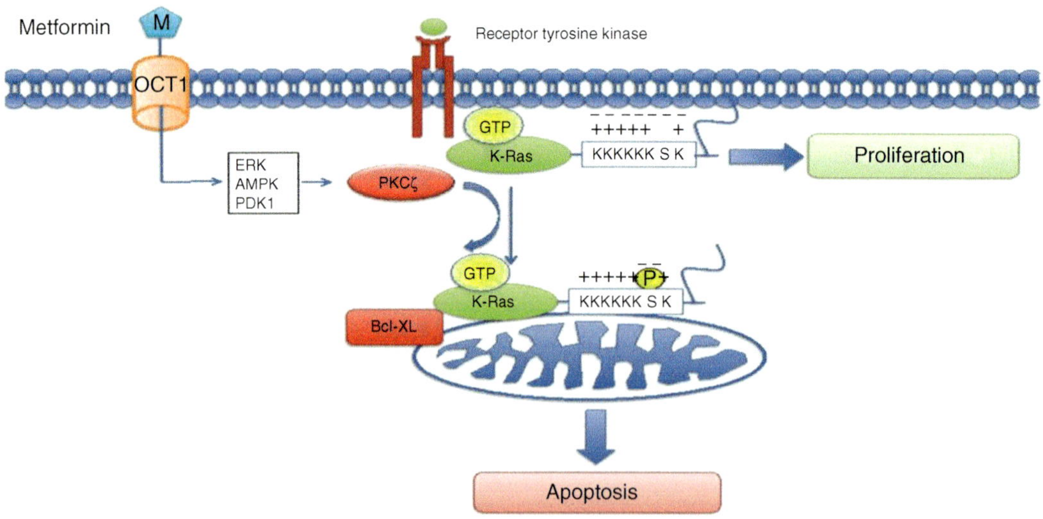

Fig. 5.2 Proposed mechanism by which metformin causes translocation of activated K-Ras from the plasma membrane and promotes cell death. Previous studies have shown that metformin activates atypical PKC (PKCζ) through an AMPK-, ERK-, and PDK1-dependent mechanism. PKCζ then phosphorylates the lysine-rich tail of activated K-Ras, acting as an electrostatic switch that causes K-Ras to be repelled from the membrane. This phosphorylation also promotes association between oncogenic K-Ras and Bcl-XL on the mitochondrial outer membrane, inducing apoptosis

Thus, there is enough epidemiological evidence that metformin exerts chemopreventive and antiproliferative effects for a variety of cancers by modulating insulin receptor and IGF1R autophosphorylation and also by attenuating the proliferative pathways of the endometrium in response to estrogen in the context of obesity.

5.3.3 COX-2 Inhibitors as Chemopreventive Agents

Molecular targets identified as a result of increasing knowledge of the molecular biological structure and genetic defects have been useful in designing new antineoplastic agents that can halt the progression of human malignancies with minimal systemic damage [30], and cyclooxygenase-2 (COX-2) is emerging as one of the major players among them [30, 31]. Both cyclooxygenase-1 (COX-1) and COX-2 are catalytic enzymes involved in prostaglandin synthesis. Prostaglandin E2 (PGE2) functions to promote the primary process of carcinogenesis and its further consolidation and progression via increased cell proliferation, decreased natural killer cell activity, in situ immune down-modulation, induction of neoangiogenesis, and the elevated expression of antiapoptotic protein Bcl-2 [32]. COX enzyme overexpression has been associated with neoplasms at various sites, including the gastrointestinal tract, lung, and skin.

COX-2 is the form of the enzyme cyclooxygenase that is inducible by cytokines, mitogens, and growth factors [30] and has emerged as one of the principal targets of the current antineoplastic chemotherapy regimens. In fact, COX-2 inhibitors that have been employed in cancer chemoprevention are now under active investigation for systemic cancer therapy.

During the last few years, there has been an emerging interest in the study of COX-2 in human gynecological neoplasms, and the clinical role of COX-2 inhibitors in this area is currently a subject of investigation [33, 34]. While COX-2 overexpression generally localizes to the adenocarcinoma cells [33], some authors have identified increasing COX-2 presence in the neoplastic cells with increasing FIGO grades of endometrioid adenocarcinoma (EACAs) [35] and have shown an association between COX-2 positivity and shorter disease-free survival [35].

5.3.3.1 How is the COX-2 Expression Tested on Samples in Various Studies?

The immunohistochemical antigen detection was performed using a DAKO autostainer employing 3-micron-thick paraffin sections from each of the representative tumor blocks selected [36]. The sections were deparaffinized, rehydrated, and subjected to antigen retrieval by using EDTA/Tris buffer at pH 8.0 for 10 min in a microwave oven. Endogenous peroxidase was blocked with 3% H2O2. The sections were then incubated overnight with a 1:100 dilution of the primary antibody, human monoclonal anti-COX-2 (Cayman Chemical, Ann Arbor, MI, USA), according to the COX-2 staining protocol optimized in our laboratory. The sections were then washed in TBS/Tween, and the COX-2 immunoreactivity was detected using a LSAB staining kit and DAB (diaminobenzidine) liquid chromogen (DAKO, Carpenteria, CA, USA). After light counterstaining with modified Mayer's hematoxylin, the sections were cleared, mounted in Permount, and examined under a light microscope (Fig. 5.3a and b).

In a study by Nasir et al. [36], the overall frequency of COX-2 expression increases from precursor lesions to EACAs, i.e., 1 out of 5 (20%) of the cases with foci of atypical complex hyperplasia (ACH) and 1 out of 9 (11%) cases with foci of endometrial hyperplasia (EH) showed moderate expression of COX-2 protein, while 17 of 22 (77%) EACAs showed moderate to strong COX-2 expression. These findings seem to be of potential clinical relevance in supporting the role of COX-2 inhibition in designing chemoprevention strategies for patients with precursor lesions of endometrial adenocarcinoma. Also, since COX-2 is one of the principal targets of COX-2 inhibitor therapy, identifying COX-2-positive EACAs may provide an objective tool to identify a subset of EACAs that may receive a potential therapeutic benefit from COX-2 inhibitor therapy.

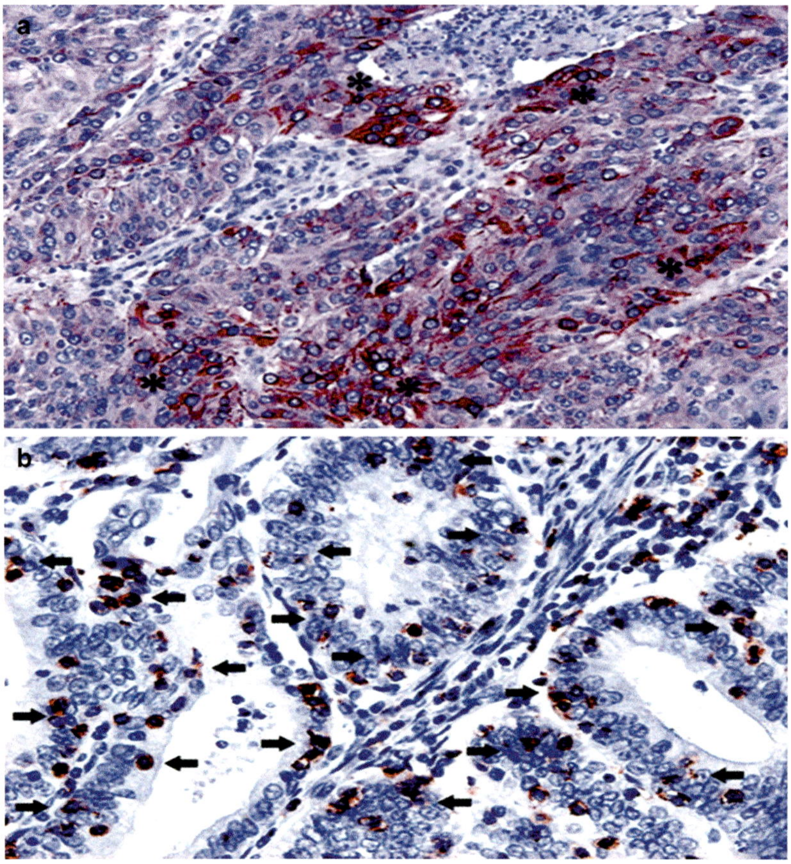

Fig. 5.3 Representative sections of endometrial cancer with strong cytoplasmic staining of COX-2 in tumor cells presented by the asterisks (**a**) endometrioid adenocarcinoma with grade 3 and enriched infiltration of CD8+ T cells presented by the arrow (**b**) endometrioid adenocarcinoma with grade 1 are shown

Also, in the same study, Nasir and colleagues [36] observed that the degree of expression of COX-2 in ACH (mean COX-2 IHC score 70) is comparable to EACAs (mean COX-2 IHC score 76) rather than EH (mean COX-2 IHC score 22), and it suggested that higher expression of COX-2 may be an early event in the neoplastic progression of EH to ACH and EACA. Similar observations have been reported in another study [32], in which the expression of COX-2 was found to be higher in cases with atypical endometrial proliferations as compared to normal endometrium and cases with endometritis [37]. However, more evidence in the form of studies on a larger series of cases are warranted to study the expression of COX-2 in EACA and precursor lesions. If the trend toward increasing COX-2 expression from precursor lesions to invasive EACA remains evident in such studies, COX-2 inhibitors (celecoxib 50 ppm in diet or exemestane 50 mg/kg weekly) may be considered as potentially useful chemopreventive agents to slow down the progression of EH toward ACH and EACA.

Knowledge about COX-2 staining in various FIGO grades of endometrial cancer will also have clinical utility. In a study by Cao et al. [38], well-differentiated EACAs showed minimal COX-2 staining, while moderately and poorly differentiated EACAs demonstrated the strongest COX-2 expression (Fig. 5.3) making a case for a possible role of COX-2 in tumor progression rather than tumor initiation. Similar observations were reported by Ferrandina et al. [38].

COX-2 inhibitors may play an important role in the clinical management of endometrial cancer and may also have a potential chemopreventive role in inhibiting the progression of precursor lesions into invasive endometrial adenocarcinoma. Inhibitors of COX-2 represent another component to be considered when developing the "cocktail" that will lead to the most efficacious treatment of neoplastic disease.

Thus, routine evaluation of COX-2 status of formalin-fixed, paraffin-embedded human endometrial cancer tissues and precursor lesions may be of potential clinical utility in the effective control of human endometrial cancer and precursor lesions. However, more evidence in the form of larger case-controlled studies is needed.

5.3.4 Chemopreventive Effect of Statins

As already stated, obesity (and increased BMI) is a well-known risk factor for EC. However, the relation between other comorbid conditions like dyslipidemia, HT, and EC is less clear.

Statins or 3-hydroxy-3-methylglutaryl-coenzyme A (HMG-CoA) reductase inhibitors are the drug of choice to reduce plasma cholesterol levels and prevent cardiovascular diseases. Statins block the HMG-CoA reductase, the enzyme required for conversion of HMGCoA to the cholesterol precursor mevalonic acid. Thus, statins are thought to lead critical changes at molecular level through inhibition of the mevalonic acid pathway. Also, it has been postulated that statins have antiproliferative and anti-metastatic effects in endometrial cancer cells, possibly through regulation of the MAPK and AKT/mTOR pathways [39].

Recently, relationship between statin use and endometrial cancer risk has been evaluated in a number of studies [39, 40]. However, the findings from these studies are controversial, with no beneficial effect in the majority of studies [40], whereas others supported a reduced risk.

To date, most of the available results of statin use and endometrial cancer risk are from observational studies; only two RCTs reported endometrial cancer risk as a secondary end point.

5.3.5 Progestin Therapy for Chemoprevention of Endometrial Cancer

EC is a disease of postmenopausal women. However, 5% of EC and endometrial hyperplasia commonly presents in premenopausal younger age group, where fertility and hormonal function preservation usually remain desirous. Thus, these women are ideal candidate for conservative management with progestins that usually has 70% success rates. Thirty percent of women may fail to respond [41], and currently, there is no way to identify this subgroup of women.

In the last two decades, significant research work has been done to understand the mechanism of progestin resistance as it will help immensely to choose the suitable candidates for progestin therapy as well as to counsel them about the success rate, so that they can make their own decision [42, 43]. One of the postulated theories for such progestin resistance is downregulation of progestin receptors (PR) due to continuous progestin administration leading to desensitization of receptors [44]. On the other hand, intermittent progestin therapy has shown to significantly increase the apoptotic rate of EC cells [45]. In another study, other molecular pathways including EGF/EGFR and insulin hormones have been speculated to be involved in progestin resistance [46].

NF-E2-related factor 2 (Nrf2), a transcription factor, has a critical role in cancer development as well as its recurrence and resistance to adjuvant chemotherapy and radiation therapy [47, 48]. It has been shown that both Nrf 2 and AKR1C1 are overexpressed in both partially responding and nonresponding endometrial cancer and endometrial hyperplasia. On the other hand, for women who respond completely to progestin therapy, their endometrial sampling shows either normal or no expression of Nrf-2 and AKR1C1. Thus it can be concluded that normal or reduced Nrf-2-AKR1C1 function may indicate good response to progestin therapy [48].

5.3.6 Rosiglitazone: Peroxisome Proliferator-Activated Receptor Gamma Agonist

For development of endometrial cancer, loss of PTEN (phosphatase and tension homolog) function plays an important role. The *PTEN* gene is located at chromosome 10q23.31. The PTEN protein plays a crucial role in the control of the PI3K-AKT pathway through dephosphorylation of PIP3 at the cell membrane. The absence of functional PTEN protein leads to unopposed action of PI3K with resultant uncontrolled PIP3 production. One major effector of the PI3K-AKT pathway is mTOR, which stimulates protein synthesis, initiates entry into G1 phase of the cell cycle, and interacts with proteins that regulate apoptosis. PTEN mutations have been found in 55% of precancerous endometrial lesions and in up to 83% of endometrioid endometrial cancer [49].

Peroxisome proliferator-activated receptor gamma (PPAR-y) is a member of the nuclear hormone receptor superfamily of transcription factors [50]. Upon ligand binding, PPAR-y forms heterodimers with the retinoid X receptor (RXR) and modulates gene expression via binding to a specific DNA regulatory element [51]. It has been shown that PPAR-y ligands exert chemopreventive effects through both PPAR-y-dependent and PPAR-y-independent pathways [52]. In a recent study, PPAR-y agonists have been shown to have an inhibitory effect on mammary and gastric carcinogenesis in different animal models [53]. Although the exact mechanism is not clear, various possible pathways of PPAR-y agonist (thiazolidinediones) induced anti-tumorigenic effects, cell cycle arrest, induction of apoptosis, inhibition of angiogenesis, modulation of differentiation, and stemness processes, and cross talk with other signaling pathways has been suggested and also speculated to be involved in proliferation and survival [53]. All of these events may be exerted by PPAR-γ genomic or non-genomic actions (Fig. 5.4) [54]. Another study has suggested that the tumor suppressor actions of PPAR-y agonists are also mediated via upregulation of PTEN [55].

Recently, in a study by Celestino and colleagues [56], it has been shown that PPAR-y agonist rosiglitazone inhibits the proliferation and induces apoptosis in both PTEN wild-type and PTEN-null cancer cell lines and that too in a dose-dependent manner. Both a low dose (4 mg/

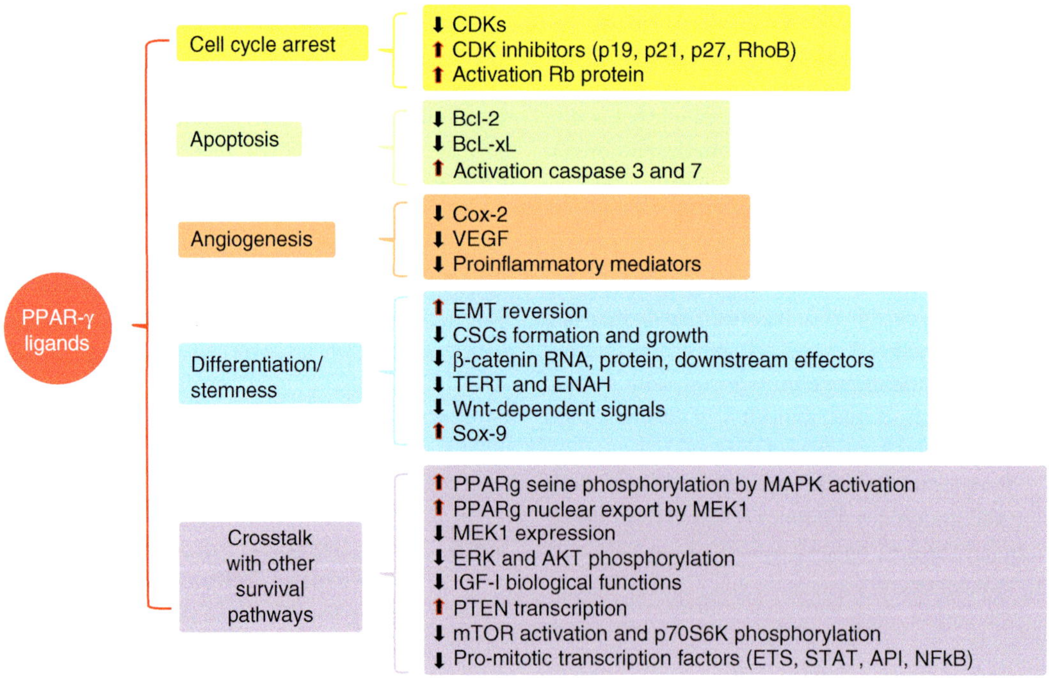

Fig. 5.4 Mechanisms underlying anti-tumorigenic actions of peroxisome proliferator-activated receptor (PPAR)-γ agonists. *CDKs* cyclin-dependent kinases, *RhoB* rho-related GTP-binding protein, *Rb protein* retinoblastoma-associated protein, *Bcl-2* B-cell lymphoma 2, *Bcl-xL* B-cell lymphoma-extra large, *Cox-2* cyclooxygenase-2, *VEGF* vascular endothelial growth factor, *EMT* epithelial to mesenchymal transition, *CSCs* cancer stem cells, *TERT* telomerase reverse transcriptase, *ENAH* enabled homolog, *ETS* E26-transformation-specific family, *STAT* signal transducer and activator of transcription, *AP1* activator protein-1

kg) and a high dose (8 mg/kg) of rosiglitazone showed similar results. Similar results are also shown in relation to endometrial hyperplasia.

PPAR-γ agonist is currently used clinically as an insulin sensitizer in patients with type II diabetes to control high blood glucose. Because obesity and diabetes are high-risk factors for the development of endometrial cancer, further studies are necessary to determine whether PPAR-γ agonists may be useful in both insulin sensitization and chemoprevention.

Thus, rosiglitazone may be a reasonable primary chemopreventive agent against the development of PTEN-mediated endometrial hyperplasia and subsequent cancer.

5.4 Summary

1. Endometrioid adenocarcinoma is the most common histology (90% cases of EC) and has a good prognosis in early stage (5-year survival rate >90%).
2. Endometrial cancer, like breast cancer, is presumed to be an estrogen-driven malignancy. EC is among certain cancers that has a well-defined risk factor profile and, thus, gives an easy access to identify women at high risk of developing EC.
3. Hormonal chemoprevention of endometrial cancer is seen with OCPs: 5 years of use provides a long-term reduction in risk of about 46%, and 10 years of use causes a reduction of about 71%. In addition, studies report that after cessation of COC use, a reduction in risk persists for 20 years or more.
4. Women with LS are at high risk for endometrial cancer and thus represent an ideal population for chemoprevention. OCPs and depoMPA induce an expected physiologic endometrial response when administered to premenopausal women with Lynch syndrome.
5. Metformin exerts chemopreventive and antiproliferative effects by modulating insulin receptor and IGF1R autophosphorylation and also attenuates the proliferative pathways of the endometrium in response to estrogen in the context of obesity.
6. COX-2 inhibitors may play an important role in the clinical management of endometrial cancer and may also have a potential chemopreventive role in inhibiting the progression of precursor lesions into invasive endometrial adenocarcinoma.
7. PPAR-γ agonist rosiglitazone may be a reasonable primary chemopreventive agent against the development of PTEN-mediated endometrial hyperplasia and subsequent cancer.
8. Progestin resistance may be related to the intrinsic overexpression of Nrf2-AKR1C1 signal transduction pathway, while normal or decreased Nrf2AKR1C1 function may be indicative of good response to progestin treatment.

References

1. MayoClinic.com. Endometrial cancer. http://www.mayoclinic.com/health/endometrial-cancer/DS00306. Updated 7 Dec 2004.
2. The American Cancer Society. Cancer facts and figures, 1998. Atlanta: The American Cancer Society; 1998.
3. Goss PE, Ingle JN, Alés-Martinez JE, Cheung AM, Chlebowski RT, Wactawski-Wende J, et al. Exemestane for breast-cancer prevention in postmenopausal women. N Engl J Med. 2011;364:2381–91.
4. Narod SA, Risch H, Moslehi R, Dorum A, Neuhausen S, Olsson H, et al. Oral contraceptives and the risk of hereditary ovarian cancer. Hereditary Ovarian Cancer Clinical Study Group. N Engl J Med. 1998;339:424–8.
5. Pike MC, Spicer DV. Oral contraceptives and cancer. In: Shoupe D, Haseltine F, editors. Contraception. New York: Springer; 1993. p. 67–84.
6. Mueck AO, Seeger H, Rabe T. Hormonal contraception and risk of endometrial cancer: a systematic review. Endocr Relat Cancer. 2010;17:R263–71.
7. Hannaford PC, Selvaraj S, Elliott AM, Angus V, Iversen L, Lee AJ. Cancer risk among users of oral contraceptives: cohort data from the Royal College of General Practitioner's oral contraception study. BMJ. 2007;335:651.
8. Maxwell GL, Schildkraut JM, Calingaert B, Risinger JI, Dainty L, Marchbanks PA, et al. Progestin and estrogen potency of combination oral contraceptives and endometrial cancer risk. Gynecol Oncol. 2006;103:535–40.
9. Key TJ, Pike MC. The dose-effect relationship between 'unopposed' oestrogens and endometrial mitotic rate: its central role in explaining and predicting endometrial cancer risk. Br J Cancer. 1988;57:205–12.

10. Lu KH, Loose DS, Yates MS, Nogueras-Gonzalez GM, Munsell MF, Chen LM, et al. Prospective Multicenter randomized intermediate biomarker study of oral contraceptive versus depo-provera for prevention of endometrial cancer in women with lynch syndrome. Cancer Prev Res. 2013;6:774–81.
11. Rodriguez GC, Rimel BJ, Watkin W, Turbov JM, Barry C, Du H, et al. Progestin treatment induces apoptosis and modulates transforming growth factor-beta in the uterine endometrium. Cancer Epidemiol Biomark Prev. 2008;17:578–84.
12. Chan M-F, Dowsett M, Folkerd E, Wareham N, Luben R, Welch A, et al. Past oral contraceptive and hormone therapy use and endogenous hormone concentrations in postmenopausal women. Menopause. 2007;15:332–9.
13. Gold EB, Crawford SL, Avis NE, Crandall CJ, Matthews KA, Waetjen LE, et al. Factors related to age at natural menopause: longitudinal analyses from SWAN. Am J Epidemiol. 2013;178:70–83.
14. Zhou X, Dowdy S, Podratz K, Jiang S. Epigenetic considerations for endometrial cancer prevention, diagnosis and treatment. Gynecol Oncol. 2007;107:143–53.
15. Miles RA, Paulson RJ, Lobo RA, Press MF, Dahmoush L, Sauer MV. Pharmacokinetics and endometrial tissue levels of progesterone after administration by intramuscular and vaginal routes: a comparative study. Fertil Steril. 1994;62:485–90.
16. Hampel H, de la Chapelle A. The search for unaffected individuals with Lynch syndrome: do the ends justify the means? Cancer Prev Res. 2011;4:1–5.
17. Bonadona V, Bonaïti B, Olschwang S, Grandjouan S, Huiart L, Longy M, et al. Cancer risks associated with germline mutations in MLH1, MSH2, and MSH6 genes in Lynch syndrome. JAMA. 2011;305:2304–10.
18. Stoffel E, Mukherjee B, Raymond VM, Tayob N, Kastrinos F, Sparr J, et al. Calculation of risk of colorectal and endometrial cancer among patients with Lynch syndrome. Gastroenterology. 2009;137:1621–7.
19. Lu KH, Loose DS, Yates MS, Nogueras-Gonzalez GM, Munsell MF, Chen LM, et al. Prospective, multicenter randomized intermediate biomarker study of oral contraceptive vs. Depo-Provera for prevention of endometrial cancer in women with Lynch syndrome. Cancer Prev Res. 2013;6:774–81.
20. Haslam DW, James WP. Obesity. Lancet. 2005;366:1197–209.
21. Yach D, Stuckler D, Brownell KD. Epidemiologic and economic consequences of the global epidemics of obesity and diabetes. Nat Med. 2006;12:62–6.
22. Calle EE, Kaaks R. Overweight, obesity and cancer: epidemiological evidence and proposed mechanisms. Nat Rev Cancer. 2004;4:579–91.
23. Zhang Q, Shen Q, Celestino J, et al. Enhanced estrogen-induced proliferation in obese rat endometrium. Am J Obstet Gynecol. 2009;200:186 e1–8.
24. Del Barco S, Vazquez-Martin A, Cufi S, et al. Metformin: multi-faceted protection against cancer. Oncotarget. 2011;2:896–917.
25. Dowling RJ, Goodwin PJ, Stambolic V. Understanding the benefit of metformin use in cancer treatment. BMC Med. 2011;9:33.
26. Cantrell LA, Zhou C, Mendivil A, Malloy KM, Gehrig PA, Bae-Jump VL. Metformin is a potent inhibitor of endometrial cancer cell proliferation--implications for a novel treatment strategy. Gynecol Oncol. 2010;116:92–8.
27. Zhang Q, Celestino J, Schmandt R, et al. Chemopreventive effects of metformin on obesity-associated endometrial proliferation. Am J Obstet Gynecol. 2013;209(1):24.e1–24.e12.
28. Zakikhani M, Dowling R, Fantus IG, Sonenberg N, Pollak M. Metformin is an AMP kinase-dependent growth inhibitor for breast cancer cells. Cancer Res. 2006;66:10269–73.
29. Hardie DG, Ross FA, Hawley SA. AMPK: a nutrient and energy sensor that maintains energy homeostasis. Nat Rev Mol Cell Biol. 2012;13:251–62.
30. Bodey B. Genetically engineered antibodies for direct antineoplastic treatment and systematic delivery of various therapeutic agents to cancer cells. Expert Opin Biol Ther. 2001;1:603–17.
31. Hawk ET, Viner JL, Dannenberg A, DuBois RN. COX-2 in cancer–a player that's defining the rules. J Natl Cancer Inst. 2002;94:545–6.
32. Tuynman JB, Hulscher JB, Steller EP, van Lanschot JJ, Richel DJ. Cyclooxygenase (COX)-2-inhibition in the prevention and treatment of colorectal carcinoma. Ned Tijdschr Geneeskd. 2003;147:2207–12.
33. Landen CN Jr, Mathur SP, Richardson MS, Creasman WT. Expression of cyclooxygenase-2 in cervical, endometrial, and ovarian malignancies. Am J Obstet Gynecol. 2003;188:1174–6.
34. Hayes EC, Rock JA. COX-2 inhibitors and their role in gynecology. Obstet Gynecol Surv. 2002;57:768–80.
35. Ferrandina G, Legge F, Ranelletti FO, Zannoni GF, Maggiano N, Evangelisti A, Mancuso S, Scambia G, Lauriola L. Cyclooxygenase-2 expression in endometrial carcinoma: correlation with clinicopathologic parameters and clinical outcome. Cancer. 2002;95:801–7.
36. Nasir A, Boulware D. Cyclooxygenase-2 (COX-2) expression in human endometrial carcinoma and precursor lesions and its possible use in cancer chemoprevention and therapy. In Vivo. 2007;21:35–44.
37. Li J, Lu Y, Ma D. Cyclooxygenase-2 expression in endometrium carcinoma. Zhonghua Fu Chan Ke Za Zhi. 2002;37:408–10.
38. Cao QJ, Einstein MH, Anderson PS, Runowicz CD, Balan R, Jones JG. Expression of COX-2, Ki-67, Cyclin D1, and P21 in endometrial endometrioid carcinomas. Int J Gynecol Pathol. 2002;21:147–54.
39. Lavie O, Pinchev M, Rennert HS, Segev Y, Rennert G. The effect of statins on risk and survival of gynecological malignancies. Gynecol Oncol. 2013;130:615–9.

40. Sperling CD, Verdoodt F, Friis S, Dehlendorff C, Kjaer SK. Statin use and risk of endometrial cancer: a nationwide registry-based case-control study. Acta Obstet Gynecol Scand. 2017;96:144–9. https://doi.org/10.1111/aogs.13069.
41. Perez-Medina T, Bajo J, Folgueira G, Haya J, Ortega P. Atypical endometrial hyperplasia treatment with progestogens and gonadotropin-releasing hormone analogues: long-term follow-up. Gynecol Oncol. 1999;73:299–304.
42. Zhang Z, Dong L, Sui L, Yang Y, Liu X, Yu Y, Zhu Y, Feng Y. Metformin reverses progestin resistance in endometrial cancer cells by downregulating GloI expression. Int J Gynecol Cancer. 2011;21:213–21.
43. Zhao S, Chen X, Lu X, Yu Y, Feng Y. Epidermal growth factor receptor signaling enhanced by long-term medroxyprogesterone acetate treatment in endometrial carcinoma. Gynecol Oncol. 2007;105:45–54.
44. Satyaswaroop PG, Clarke CL, Zaino RJ, Mortel R. Apparent resistance in human endometrial carcinoma during combination treatment with tamoxifen and progestin may result from desensitization following downregulation of tumor progesterone receptor. Cancer Lett. 1992;62:107–14.
45. Zheng W, Baker HE, Mutter GL. Involution of PTEN-null endometrial glands with progestin therapy. Gynecol Oncol. 2004;92:1008–13.
46. Shen ZQ, Zhu HT, Lin JF. Reverse of progestin-resistant atypical endometrial hyperplasia by metformin and oral contraceptives. Obstet Gynecol. 2008;112:465–7.
47. Shibata T, Kokubu A, Saito S, Narisawa-Saito M, Sasaki H, Aoyagi K, Yoshimatsu Y, Tachimori Y, Kushima R, Kiyono T, Yamamoto M. NRF2 mutation confers malignant potential and resistance to chemoradiation therapy in advanced esophageal squamous cancer. Neoplasia. 2011;13:864–73.
48. Jiang T, Chen N, Zhao F, Wang XJ, Kong B, Zheng W, Zhang DD. High levels of Nrf2 determine chemoresistance in type II endometrial cancer. Cancer Res. 2010;70:5486–96.
49. Mutter GL, Ince TA, Baak JP, et al. Molecular identification of latent precancers in histologically normal endometrium. Cancer Res. 2001;61:4311–4.
50. Issemann I, Green S. Activation of a member of the steroid hormone receptor superfamily by peroxisome proliferators. Nature. 1990;347:645–50.
51. Kliewer SA, Umesono K, Noonan DJ, et al. Convergence of 9-cis retinoic acid and peroxisome proliferator signalling pathways through heterodimer formation of their receptors. Nature. 1992;358:771–4.
52. Clay CE, Monjazeb A, Thorburn J, et al. 15-Deoxy-delta12, 14-prostaglandin J2-induced apoptosis does not require PPAR-gamma in breast cancer cells. J Lipid Res. 2002;43:1818–28.
53. Lu J, Imamura K, Nomura S, et al. Chemopreventive effect of peroxisome proliferator-activated receptor gamma on gastric carcinogenesis in mice. Cancer Res. 2005;65:4769–74.
54. Grommes C, Landreth GE, Heneka MT. Antineoplastic effects of peroxisome proliferator-activated receptor gamma agonists. Lancet Oncol. 2004;5:419–29.
55. Teresi RE, Shaiu CW, Chen CS, et al. Increased PTEN expression due to transcriptional activation of PPAR-gamma by Lovastatin and Rosiglitazone. Int J Cancer. 2006;118:2390–8.
56. Celestino J, Milam MR, et al. Primary chemoprevention of endometrial hyperplasia with the peroxisome proliferator-activated receptor gamma agonist rosiglitazone in the PTEN heterozygote murine model. Int J Gynecol Cancer. 2008;18:329–38.

Part II

Cervix

Cervical Squamous Intraepithelial Lesions: A Pathologist's Perspective

6

Charanjeet Singh and Grace N. Kim

6.1 Introduction

The histologically well-defined precursor squamous lesions and their temporal relationship with invasive squamous carcinoma were recognized more than a century ago; however, their association with human papillomavirus (HPV) is relatively recent (1970s). The evolution from precursor to cervical cancer is not only temporal; the lesion also has a spatial preference. Anatomically, the squamocolumnar junction of the cervix is a sharp border between the stratified squamous epithelium of ectocervix and the mucin-producing columnar epithelium of endocervix. However, puberty and menarche-associated physiological changes result in a more gradual and functional border characterized by metaplastic squamous epithelium, the so-called "transformation zone" mucosa. HPV infection and, therefore, virtually all cervical neoplasms and their precursors have a predilection for this transformation zone.

The clinical ease of recognition of this colposcopically visible transformation zone perhaps underlies the success of cervical cancer screening and that of the management of the precursor squamous lesions of cervix.

6.2 Evolution of the Terminology of Cervical Squamous Precursor Lesions

The terminology for histopathological classification of cervical squamous precursor lesions has evolved over the last century, driven primarily by the understanding of the natural history of HPV infection and secondarily by evolution of the management options. Historically, the terms surface carcinoma, intraepithelial carcinoma, and carcinoma in situ (CIS) were used to describe the precursor lesions in which the cells looked malignant but did not invade into the stroma. The two-tiered CIS and non-CIS terminology meant hysterectomy for women with CIS and no treatment for the latter group. Studies by Reagan, Hicks [1], Seidemann [2], and other investigators showed that some of these surface lesions of the cervix, despite having abnormal looking cells, were not as aggressive as CIS and had lower risk for progressing to invasive cancer. These lesions were termed variously as anaplasia, basal cell

C. Singh
Department of Pathology, Florida Hospital, Orlando, FL, USA

Department of Pathology, University of Central Florida, Orlando, FL, USA

G. N. Kim (✉)
Department of Pathology, LAC+USC Medical Center, Los Angeles, CA, USA

Department of Pathology, Keck Hospital of USC, Los Angeles, CA, USA
e-mail: gkim4@dhs.lacounty.gov; grace.kim2@med.usc.edu

S. Mehta, A. Singla (eds.), *Preventive Oncology for the Gynecologist*,
https://doi.org/10.1007/978-981-13-3438-2_6

hyperplasia, and atypical hyperplasia. Reagan et al. proposed the term "dysplasia" in 1953 [2] and graded it as mild, moderate, or severe based on the degree of squamous epithelial differentiation with respect to CIS, giving rise to a four-tiered system of precursor lesions. Based on this system, the women with CIS underwent hysterectomy, while the patients with "severe dysplasia" were subjected to cold knife conization.

The seminal investigation from Richart in 1969 [3] established that morphologic changes in the form of mild dysplasia to cervical cancer represented a disease continuum and that there was an absence of objective evidence to separate severe dysplasia from CIS. This led to the proposal of cervical intraepithelial neoplasia (CIN) terminology as follows: CIN1 for mild dysplasia, CIN2 for moderate dysplasia, and CIN3 for severe dysplasia. Due to proposed disease continuum of all lesions, CIN1 and CIN2 were treated with ablation (such as laser, CO_2, etc.), and CIN3 was treated with hysterectomy.

The work by zur Hausen [4] and colleagues in 1976 hypothesized the role of HPV in cervical cancer with identification of types HPV16 and HPV18 in cervical cancers in 1983–1984. Further understanding of the HPV biology led to increasing recognition that CIN1 was a more indolent lesion, while CIN2 was at the action threshold with CIN3. Based on this, the lesions were biologically regarded as "low-grade squamous intraepithelial lesion" (LSIL, which included CIN1/mild dysplasia) and "high-grade squamous intraepithelial lesion" (HSIL, which included CIN2/moderate and CIN3/severe dysplasia). The discovery of two-tiered biological significance of the cervical lesions coincided with the US Congress passing the Clinical Laboratory Improvement Amendments (CLIA) in 1988. The Bethesda system (TBS) [5] for reporting of cervical cytology was a by-product of CLIA 1988 amendment. TBS adopted the terminology of "LSIL" and "HSIL" for reporting cervical precursor lesions, along with the use of terms "negative for squamous intraepithelial lesion and malignancy (NILM)" and its most controversial term "atypical squamous cells of undetermined significance (ASCUS)," for lesions that were indeterminate morphologically (Fig. 6.1).

In the 1990s and early 2000s, despite the usage of LSIL and HSIL terminology for reporting cervical cytology, the three-tiered system of CIN1, CIN2, and CIN3 remained in use for cervical biopsy, cone, and LEEP reporting.

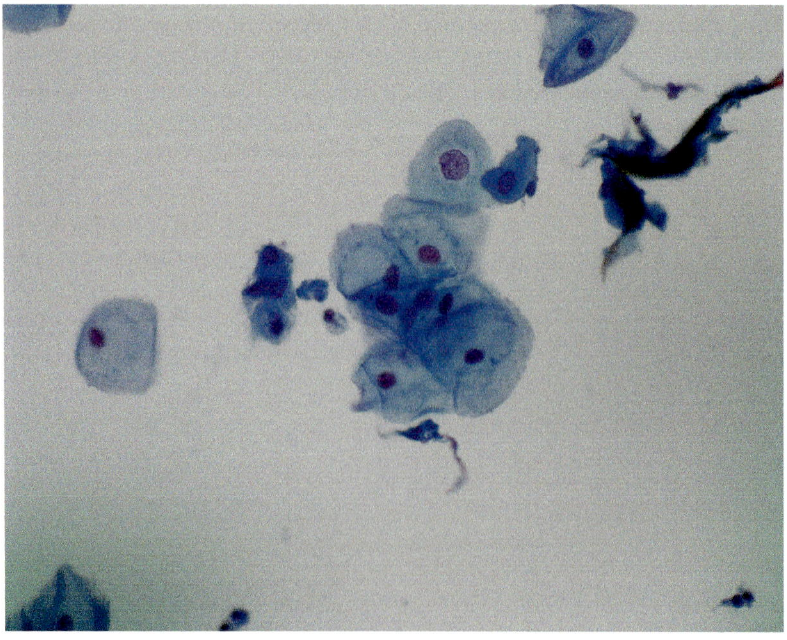

Fig. 6.1 Note a single cell in the group shows slight nuclear enlargement and irregularity, along with cytoplasmic clearing, consistent with atypical squamous cell of undetermined significance. This cell, by itself, is not diagnostic of an HPV infection-related lesion (Pap stain, ThinPrep smear, 600× magnification)

This discrepant use of terminology by pathologists was a result of utilization of three-tiered terminology for clinical management by the American Society for Colposcopy and Cervical Pathology (ASCCP) Consensus Guidelines: expectant management was advocated for CIN1, and in-office excision using cold knife cone or LEEP was advised for CIN2 and CIN3.

As is now well-recognized that HPV is associated with intraepithelial lesions and invasive cancers in the entire anogenital region and in both genders, a task force called the Lower Anogenital Squamous Terminology (LAST) Project was co-sponsored by the College of American Pathologists (CAP) and the ASCCP in order to unify the terminology between cytology and histology. The LAST terminology recommendations of 2012 [6] unified the terminology across all lower anogenital sites and created a nomenclature system that reflected the current knowledge of HPV biology and current use of HPV biomarkers, in order to facilitate clear communication for management of these lesions, across different medical specialties. As per the LAST recommendations:

- A two-tiered nomenclature is recommended for noninvasive HPV-associated squamous proliferations of the lower anogenital tract.
- The recommended terminology for HPV-associated squamous lesions is LSIL and HSIL, which may be optionally classified by the –IN subcategorization.
- The –IN refers to intraepithelial neoplasia. For a specific location, the appropriate complete term such as CIN (cervix), VaIN (vagina), and VIN (vulva) should be used.

6.3 Morphology of Squamous Intraepithelial Lesions

Cytological examination of Pap smears is the primary method of recognition of SIL lesions, followed subsequently by histopathological examination of tissue based on the ASCCP guidelines. Herein, we are using the two-tiered system and the most current LSIL and HSIL terminology to describe the morphological changes associated with these lesions. The cytological appearances of these lesions are discussed first, followed by their histological counterparts.

6.3.1 Cytological Diagnosis of LSIL and HSIL

The Bethesda system of cervical cytology provides criteria for diagnosing various categories, beginning at NILM, ASCUS, LSIL, HSIL, and cancer, for liquid-based cytology (such as ThinPrep and SurePath) and conventional cytology.

The cytological criteria used for the diagnosis of LSIL (Fig. 6.2) include:

- Enlarged superficial cells with distinct borders; cells present singly or in groups.
- Enlarged nuclei of the squamous cells with at least 3× nuclear enlargement compared to the background intermediate cell nuclei; nuclear-to-cytoplasmic ratio is only slightly increased.
- Perinuclear cytoplasmic vacuolation (the so-called koilocytic change), which has sharp delineation from dense, peripheral orangeophilic cytoplasm, in the presence of appropriate nuclear changes.
- The nuclei tend to show hyperchromasia and slight irregularity (raisinoid appearance) and often show binucleation.
- The chromatin is coarsely granular to dense opaque, and nucleoli are either absent or small and inconspicuous.

As opposed to LSIL, the cytological changes of HSIL are seen more so in the intermediate and basal-like cells, which have cytoplasmic appearance like that of "metaplastic" squamous cells. The criteria diagnostic of HSIL (Fig. 6.3) are:

- Affected cells are present singly more often than in LSIL, and when present in clusters, the cells tend to have syncytial appearance with ill-defined borders.
- Nuclear hyperchromasia with variation in nuclear size and shape, marked nuclear

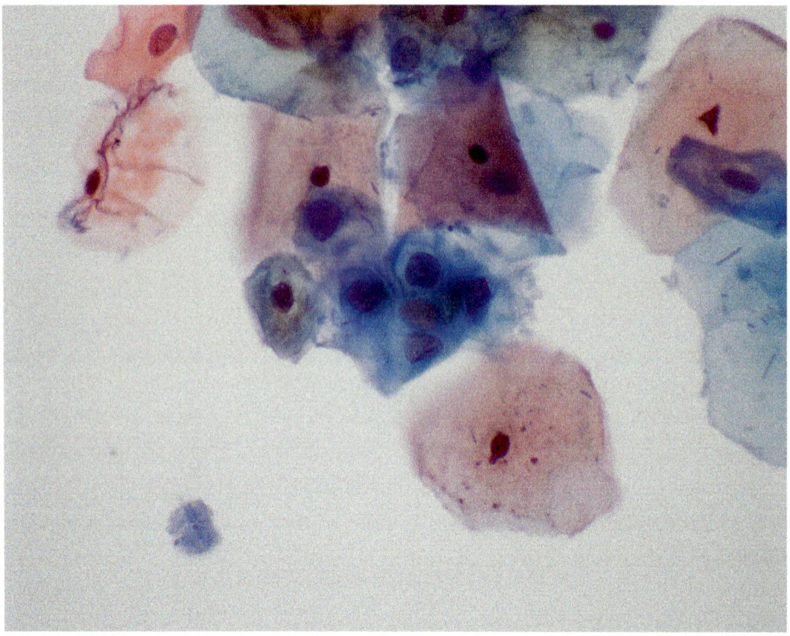

Fig. 6.2 Classic example of "koilocytic change" diagnostic of low-grade squamous intraepithelial lesion. The superficial cells show nuclear hyperchromasia, irregularity, and enlargement. The cytoplasm shows a clearly demarcated perinuclear halo (Pap stain, ThinPrep smear, 600× magnification)

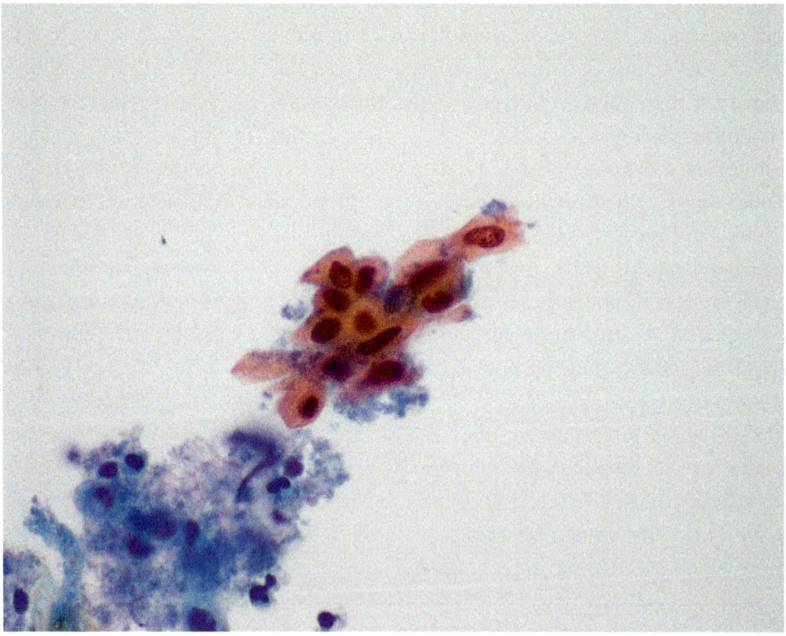

Fig. 6.3 Compared to the cells of LSIL (see Fig. 6.2), note the HSIL cells have marked variation in sizes of individual nuclei and thickened nuclear membranes (Pap stain, ThinPrep smear, 600× magnification)

enlargement, and high nuclear-to-cytoplasmic ratios.

- Nuclear irregularities are marked and grooves are common. The nuclear membranes are thicker and pronounced.
- The chromatin is finer and evenly distributed. Similar to LSIL, the nucleoli are still uncommon.
- Also uncommon is keratinized cytoplasm in HSIL lesions; and when present, differential diagnostic consideration is with squamous carcinoma especially together with necrosis.

6.3.2 Histological Findings of Squamous Intraepithelial Lesions

As discussed in detail elsewhere in this book, patients with cytological diagnosis of LSIL, depending on the age, may undergo co-testing for HPV and/or colposcopy-guided biopsy of the cervix and/or endocervical curettage. Usually, on the other hand, patients with HSIL on cytology almost always have colposcopy followed by a biopsy or LEEP or cold knife cone. The purpose of the biopsy is either to confirm the cytological diagnosis or find a more worrisome component so that definitive management can be performed timely. As previously alluded to, the changes are usually first and often best seen at the functional border of endocervical and squamous epithelium, the so-called "transformation zone" mucosa. The normal transformation zone cells show proliferation of immature/basal layer and early squamous differentiation, but not keratinization/epidermidalization.

The LSIL (CIN1) lesions are generally flat; however, less commonly they may be exophytic (condyloma) or papillary. The major histologic criteria for diagnosis are prominent nuclear enlargement in superficial cells, at least three times the normal nuclear size. The transition from normal epithelium to LSIL is generally discrete. As previously noted, the cells may show binucleation and/or multinucleation, and at least two such cells [7] are needed for a convincing diagnosis. Parakeratosis may be present, but is not required for the diagnosis. The basal layers are normal and do not show dysplastic features in LSIL. When the surface epithelial features of LSIL coexist with loss of polarity, the presence of abnormal mitoses or a high mitotic rate, and atypia beyond the parabasal layers, it should invoke the diagnosis of HSIL and more particularly CIN2.

The cells in CIN2 show surface epithelial koilocytosis or abnormal keratinization and/or bizarre nuclei; on the contrary, a complete lack of maturity characterizes CIN3 (HSIL). In the CIN3 lesions, nuclear hyperchromasia involves full thickness of epithelium, with minimal to no surface maturation and with irregularly spaced nuclei. The mitoses, both typical and atypical, can be seen in any layer of the squamous epithelium.

6.4 Morphology of Glandular Intraepithelial Lesions

Endocervical adenocarcinoma in situ (AIS) is a premalignant, high-risk HPV-related glandular counterpart of HSIL. Most cases of AIS are associated with HPV18 followed by HPV16. Despite the continuity of glandular epithelium of endocervix with squamous epithelium of ectocervix, at the transformation zone, AIS is less frequent than HSIL. However, most cases of AIS tend to have coexistent SIL.

Cytological criteria for diagnosis of AIS (Fig. 6.4), as detailed in the Bethesda system for reporting of cervical cytology, include:

- Sheets, clusters, or strips of glandular cells with nuclear crowding and overlap
- Nuclear elongation, stratification, and variation in size
- Hyperchromatic nuclei with coarsely granular to evenly distributed chromatin
- Presence of mitoses and/or apoptosis
- Inconspicuous to absent nucleoli
- Absence of tumor diathesis (tumor necrosis)

It is noteworthy that in glandular lesions, on cytological examination, the presence of prominent nucleoli (Fig. 6.5) and/or diathesis should invoke the consideration for an invasive adenocarcinoma. A well-differentiated invasive adenocarcinoma can lack both the nucleoli and diathesis and is a challenging differential of AIS on cytology and histology.

Histologically, AIS can involve the epithelium of a group of glands or a single gland, either in entirety or in patches. Paramount to its diagnosis are preserved glandular architecture and enlarged, hyperchromatic, stratified nuclei with high mitotic and apoptotic rate. The cytoplasm can be muco-depleted to abundant and basophilic or

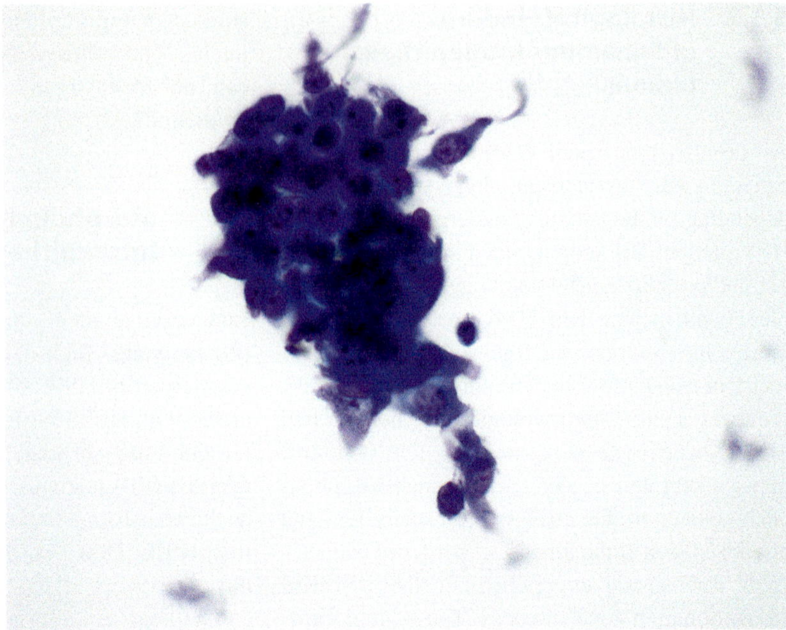

Fig. 6.4 Endocervical adenocarcinoma in situ with a hyperchromatic cell group that shows nuclear crowding. Noted at the periphery of the clusters are individual cells with "feathering" and high nuclear-to-cytoplasmic ratios (Pap stain, ThinPrep smear, 600× magnification)

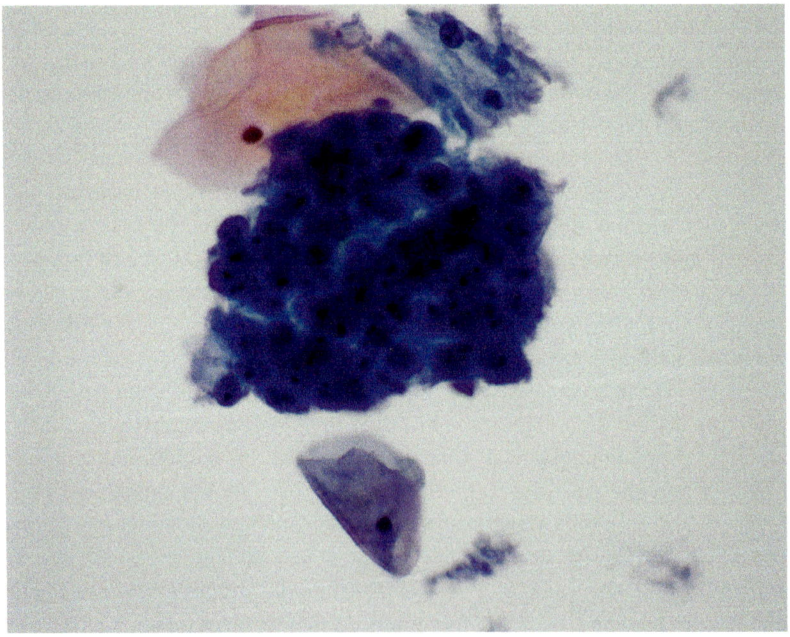

Fig. 6.5 In this group, compared to that in Fig. 6.4, the nuclei have prominent nucleoli, and there is a variation in nucleolar size. Some cells have more than one nucleoli. These features are more suggestive of an invasive adenocarcinoma, compared to AIS (Pap stain, ThinPrep smear, 600× magnification)

eosinophilic. Presence of glandular complexity and/or desmoplasia, AIS-like features in deeper glands and/or marked nuclear atypia even in superficial glands, should invoke the consideration for invasive adenocarcinoma. This is an important distinction to make, and in difficult cases, review by multiple pathologists and/or consultation with an expert gynecologic pathologist should be considered. Compared to the risk of squamous carcinoma in HSIL, AIS has a higher risk to transform to invasive adenocarcinoma, which when stage-matched with squamous carcinoma has higher risk of nodal involvement.

6.5 Stratified Mucin-Producing Intraepithelial Lesion (SMILE)

These are uncommon lesions which are thought to arise from the reserve cells at the transformation zone. The current Bethesda terminology for cytologic reporting does not recognize SMILE as a diagnostic category, given that it would be a challenging lesion to diagnose on cytology and that its histologic features are like that of HSIL. SMILE have stratified immature cells that display intracytoplasmic mucin or cytoplasmic vacuoles. These mucinous cells are typically seen in the mid to lower layers of the epithelium. AIS-like gland formation is not identified in SMILE. Most of the cases with SMILE-like lesions have coexistent HSIL or AIS or both.

6.6 Morphologic Evaluation of Cone and LEEP Excision Biopsies

Both cone and LEEP biopsies are procured once the diagnosis of cervical squamous or glandular intraepithelial lesions has been established. The role of the pathologist in LEEP and cone biopsies includes:

- To estimate the burden of intraepithelial lesion or adenocarcinoma in situ (i.e., the number of quadrants involved)
- To identify if there is a potential more worrisome component (e.g., invasive carcinoma in the setting of a previous CIN-3)
- To establish if the dysplasia extends higher into the endocervical canal

As such, during the evaluation of these specimens, the endocervical margins of the cone and endocervical curetting specimen (which may be separately submitted depending on the local practice) must be evaluated carefully. Due to the location at the transformation zone, it is not uncommon for CIN3 to involve and extend into the endocervical glands; this phenomenon should be carefully distinguished from stromal invasion. In such cases, evaluation of the deep margin of cone or LEEP is equally important.

6.7 Differential Diagnoses

Apart from extension of the CIN into endocervical glands, and mimicking invasion, the other significant differential diagnoses of cervical squamous intraepithelial lesions include radiation atypia, immature repair, atrophy, immature metaplasia, polyp-associated atypia, and pregnancy implantation-associated atypia. The differential diagnoses for AIS include tubal or endometrioid metaplasia, reactive endocervical gland atypia, Arias-Stella-like reactions, etc.

While LSIL, HSIL, and AIS can be distinguished from each other and from reactive atypia in most cases, ancillary studies are both useful and required in others. Studies [8] have also shown that routine use of ancillary studies lowers the rate of major cytohistologic discrepancies and is associated with a higher rate of HSIL (CIN2+) diagnoses and lower CIN1/CIN2+ ratios. To understand HPV ancillary testing, an understanding of the HPV types and life cycle is critical.

6.8 The Human Papillomavirus

HPV, for which more than 200 different types have been studied thus far, is a circular, double-stranded DNA virus. It has strains that range from innocuous, nearly commensal to pathologic and infectious. While HPV infections are commonplace, and most infections are cleared by the host's robust immune system, a persistent HPV infection can lead to stepwise and temporal progression from preneoplastic lesions to neoplasia [6]. Within the lower anogenital tract, HPV viruses are recognized as part of the alpha genus and are generally divided into two broad, mutually exclusive families: "low-risk" HPV and "high-risk" HPV. The most common types of "low-risk" HPV include HPV 6 and 11, while "high-risk" types include 16, 18, 31, 33, 35, 39, 45, 51, 52, 56, 58, and 59, to name a few. Viral oncogenic potential is the main distinguishing characteristic between the "low-risk" and "high-risk" groups, in that "low-risk" HPV types contribute to the pathogenesis of benign mucosal lesions without potential for significant clinical progression, while the "high-risk" HPV types carry notable malignant potential, not only as mucosal carcinomas but also as precursor mucosal lesions [4–6, 9].

High-risk HPV types distinguish themselves from low-risk types by their ability to integrate the viral genome into the host DNA. However, depending on the specific high-risk HPV type, a viral genome may or may not be integrated within the affected tumor cells of cervical carcinoma. In particular, the most common high-risk HPV strain that occurs in cervical carcinoma, HPV 16, exhibits integration of viral genome into the host's DNA in approximately 70% of cervical cancer cases. Similarly, nearly 100% of HPV 18-infected carcinomas have integration of viral sequences [10]. The remainder of the cases demonstrates viral episomes within the affected cell without integration.

6.8.1 Life Cycle of the Human Papillomavirus

Despite the significant differences between low-risk and high-risk HPV types, the broad principles of the HPV life cycle are comparable. The episomal genome of the HPV virus has three distinct sets of encoding regions: (a) the early genes (E1, E2, E4, E5, E6, E7, E8), (b) the late region (proteins L1 and L2 coding the viral capsid), and (c) the long control region (LCR) or the upstream regulatory region (URR) [9]. The first inciting event in the HPV life cycle is infection, which introduces virions into the nucleus of the squamous epithelial basal cells secondary to surface epithelial trauma. At this point in the life cycle, the viral episome remains extrachromosomal and undergoes viral genome replication, with copy numbers ranging from 50 to 200 copies per infected cell. Once a constant copy number is reached, the life cycle enters a maintenance phase [10]. The vital players in the steps of replication and maintenance are the E1 and E2 genes which regulate transcription and replication.

After replication, a daughter cell of the infected undifferentiated basal cell travels away from the basal layers and into the superficial layers where it enters a period of squamous differentiation. Differentiation normally halts replication within suprabasal cells; however, in infected cells, replication is maintained. This process is called "cell cycle reentry," signifying aberrant reentry of superficial cells into S-phase of the cell cycle to allow for viral amplification. Of note, in some scenarios of high-risk HPV infection, the infection may remain dormant in the basal cells without further propagation into the upper squamous layers and without clinical evidence of an HPV-driven lesion. As such, the detection of high-risk HPV by ancillary testing does not necessarily equate to the presence of a dysplastic lesion [11]. In such cases of dormancy, as well as in low-risk HPV infections, the significance of the two proteins vital for neoplastic cellular proliferation, E6 and E7, is not well known. On the contrary, the role of E6 and E7 protein in high-risk HPV types is critical for neoplastic growth [10].

E6 and E7 are proteins transcribed from early viral genes, which are critical in high-risk HPV types as oncogenic drivers. E6 binds and targets tumor suppressor protein p53 for inactivation, which renders p53 incapable of its normal function of pausing cell cycle progression and signaling cell death when cell cycling is overstimulated. Only in high-risk HPV types is p53 marked for ubiquitination and degradation [10]. E7, on the other hand, binds with retinoblastoma (Rb) protein, also signaling this protein for degradation. The absence of Rb protein function prevents the proper functioning of proteins that usually regulate S-phase entry [4]. Interestingly, a critical difference in low-risk and high-risk HPV types is the affinity of E7 protein to Rb. The binding affinity of E7 to Rb in low-risk HPV is ten times weaker when compared to that of high-risk HPV types. Low-risk HPV also lacks affinity to the entire family of Rb proteins, while high-risk HPV can target all members. In addition, integration of the viral genome into the host's DNA is not a calculated event but rather one of chance, often occurring at weak points in the host's genome [10]. During integration, the E2 locus, which is responsible for keeping E6 and E7 gene products at lower levels, is often damaged allowing for uncontrolled E6 and E7 production [6].

One of the late events during the HPV life cycle is the assembly of virions that solely occurs in the superficial squamous cells. L1 and L2 are late gene products for major and minor capsid proteins. A single viral genome is packaged in the capsid, and this virion is then released during natural cell shedding of terminally differentiated keratinocytes [4, 6, 12].

6.8.2 Laboratory Testing for HPV

The confirmation of HPV in tissue samples has become an adjunctive test in the diagnosis and management of dysplastic lesions and, more recently, the prognosis of malignant tumors. For instance, the finding of high-risk HPV in a head and neck squamous cell carcinoma has been shown to have improved therapy response and disease-free survival compared to HPV-unrelated carcinomas [13]. HPV detection methods are of two types, indirect methods and direct methods. The indirect methods rely on the life cycle of HPV, and since HPV virus cannot be cultured in-vitro, the direct methods of detection are predominantly molecular-based [14].

Various tests for HPV detection and their clinical implications are discussed in Chap. 9, and the reader can refer to that chapter for details. Only a brief mention of the tests will be done here.

6.8.2.1 Indirect Methods

The indirect methods use surrogate markers of HPV infection, such as p16 immunostaining and Pro-Ex C.

P16 Immunostaining

Immunostaining for p16 exhibits block positivity (strong nuclear and cytoplasmic reactivity) in high-grade lesions (CIN-2 and CIN-3, and AIS). This relies on the principle that the p16 protein is upregulated with disruption of Rb protein function by E7 in high-risk HPV-associated lesions. Consequently, it is more so a surrogate marker of high-risk HPV type. The staining in reactive atypia and in low-risk HPV-associated lesions tends to be patchy and weak. The advantage in using p16 immunostain is the ease and objectivity in interpretation by pathologists on routine tissue biopsies, obtained for follow-up after Pap smear or a previous diagnosis of dysplasia. The published literature shows large inter-observer variability found by multiple studies in the diagnosis and grading of CIN by pathologists. This has been attributed variously to:

- Technical factors: Small biopsy, poor processing, incomplete representation, thermal crush, and other artifacts.
- Patient-related factors: Pregnancy, menopause, exogenous hormone, coexistent infections, and prior radiation.
- Pathologist-related factors: These are mainly seen in grading, especially when the epithelium is thin, metaplastic, or denuded.

Study by Singh et al. [8] has shown that the more frequent use of an objective marker such as p16, alone or together with Ki-67 (which is a marker of proliferation), in difficult cases, allows pathologists to modify their diagnostic thresholds and render a more objective diagnosis between low-grade (CIN-1) and high-grade (CIN-2 +) lesions. The LAST working group advocates the use of p16 in the following situations:

- To differentiate HSIL from benign mimics (such as immature metaplasia or atrophy)
- To classify indeterminate lesions (essentially CIN 2 in the old terminology) as either LSIL or HSIL
- To reach a consensus on possible cases of HSIL with differing pathologists' interpretation

Pro-Ex C Assay

Pro-Ex C is another immune-cytochemical assay, which is an S-phase proliferation marker with a specific pattern of staining. TOP2A and MCM2 are S-phase proteins, which are induced upon integration of HPV viral DNA into the host genome, leading to increased levels of E6 and E7 proteins. This leads to aberrant S-phase induction and at the morphological level correlates with high-grade dysplasia. In cervical biopsies, positive staining for Pro-Ex C is defined by staining of nuclei of more than half of the mucosal thickness. While Pro-Ex C has been shown to be a more specific marker than Ki-67, its specificity and sensitivity are lower compared to p16. For this reason and due to difficulties in laboratory validation and standardization of Pro-Ex C stain, p16 immunostaining continues to be the preferred marker for indirect testing of high-risk HPV in dysplastic lesions.

6.8.2.2 Direct Methods

The predominance of innovation in HPV detection has been in the arena of direct methodology. The most frequently used assays currently are signal amplification assays and nucleic acid target amplification assays, five of which are FDA-approved in the United States. The majority of these tests detect HPV genomic DNA. The first to be FDA-approved was the Digene Hybrid Capture 2 in 2003, followed by Hologic's Cervista HPV HR and Cervista HPV 16/18 in 2009. The Roche Cobas HPV test was more recently approved for testing in 2011.

1. Signal Amplification Tests
   - The Digene Hybrid Capture 2 High-Risk HPV DNA Test: RNA probes are utilized directly against HPV DNA of 13 high-risk HPV types (HPV 16, 18, 31, 33, 35, 39, 45, 51, 52, 56, 58, 59, and 68). If these viral genotypes are present, a DNA-probe hybrid is formed in a solution of isolated DNA from the patient's sample and recognized by a chemiluminescent compound. The intensity of the emitted light is proportional to high-risk HPV DNA content, and a semiquantitative value beyond a designated cutoff determines reporting of the specimen as positive or negative for HPV. This assay can be automated on the Qiagen Rapid Capture System resulting in high-throughput processing [14].
   - The Cervista HPV HR Test: This test by Hologic utilizes a specific proprietary method called Invader. A cocktail of oligonucleotide probes targeting 14 high-risk HPV genotypes (16, 18, 31, 33, 35, 39, 45, 51, 52, 56, 58, 59, 66, 68) and the Invader probes are added to the isolated specimen DNA, which ultimately results in a conformational change at the target. The Cervista assay is automated, and the presence of an internal control is beneficial in that it accounts for specimen cellularity. Cervista HPV 16/18 is a reflex test similar to the Cervista HPV HR and also uses the same Invader chemistry technology; however, the probes are specific to HPV strains 16 and 18 only [14].
   - Cobas 4800 HPV Test: It is the newest edition of a real-time PCR assay that is specific to 14 high-risk HPV types and also HPV16/18 as a distinct duo. Hence, the Cobas test is unique in that it can simultaneously report a pooled result on 12 high-risk HPV types and also individual HPV 16 and 18 genotype results without extra cost. In contrast, all prior PCR-based assays target a combination of both low- and high-risk HPV types. The Cobas 4800 HPV test is the only FDA-approved test that can be used singularly without an adjunctive Pap test for cervical cancer screening in women over the age of 25 years. Additionally, all the aforementioned FDA-approved HPV tests are approved only for ThinPrep cervical specimens and not SurePath, with the exception of the Cobas HPV test, which was approved for use on SurePath-collected cells on July 7, 2016 [14].
   - Aptima HPV Assay: A FDA-approved HPV assay which utilizes the fully automated GenProbe TIGRIS DTS System. It is the only assay which detects E6 and E7 mRNA via transcription-mediated amplification. Detection of viral oncogenes E6 and E7 serves as direct evidence of HPV transcriptional activity, and this is regarded as the gold standard in confirmation of clinically relevant HPV infection [13]. E6 and E7 mRNA transcripts are highly specific to HPV genotypes, and as such, the Aptima assay can detect mRNA of 14 high-risk HPV genotypes. Unlike the Cobas system, the Aptima assay cannot differentiate between the 14 genotypes nor specify the presence of HPV 16/18. In women in which

the Aptima HPV assay is positive, the specimen can be further tested by the Aptima HPV 16 18/45 genotype assay [14].

2. Nucleic Acid Hybridization Assays
   - Historically, the Southern blot and dot blot hybridizations have been available; however, due to their labor-intensive techniques, high DNA content requirements, and low overall sensitivity, these methods are not being used [15].
   - HPV DNA in situ hybridization (ISH) test: This test is no longer commercially available, though laboratory-validated editions do still exist. It targets 21 HPV genotypes inclusive of the most common high-risk HPV genotypes and few low-risk genotypes [16]. In situ hybridization is performed on a tissue section similar to immunohistochemistry, and thus, advantageously, the morphologic context of the lesion in question remains intact during the evaluation process, though the sensitivity of the DNA ISH test is low.
   - RNA in situ hybridization tests: These tests use a similar technique, and only one, the Ventana Inform HPV III, is currently commercially available for clinical use [17]. The Inform HPV III ISH test targets E6 and E7 mRNA of either a pooled high-risk HPV panel of 18 subtypes (16, 18, 26, 31, 33, 35, 39, 45, 51, 52, 53, 56, 58, 59, 66, 68, 73, and 82), a pooled low-risk HPV panel of 10 subtypes (6, 11, 40, 43, 44, 54, 69, 70, 71, and 74), or a focused detection of HPV 16/18. The Ventana Inform HPV III demonstrates different patterns of staining that can detect either episomal or integrated HPV genetic material; however, the test has been plagued by interlaboratory variability, with complications of background staining and low sensitivity [17].
   - RNA ISH test: The latest addition to the armamentarium of HPV tests is developed by Advanced Cell Diagnostics. It has been studied to have superior sensitivity and specificity compared to p16 immunohistochemistry, DNA ISH, and DNA PCR [11, 13, 18, 19], along with a high concordance rate with p16 immunostaining. Mills et al. [14] recently in mid-2017 demonstrated its usage on the clinically available Leica Bond III. Compared to DNA-based detection systems and particularly PCR assays, RNA ISH testing is promising in that it is not overly sensitive in detecting HPV DNA in samples without cytologic or histologic changes of viral infection but also direct detection of E6 and E7 mRNA viral oncogenes may be more clinically relevant since E6 and E7 mRNA detection correlates with active HPV transcription and proliferation of lesions [11, 18].

The choice between the abovementioned direct methods of HPV testing is largely based on extraneous factors such as the size of the laboratory, the test volume, the available infrastructure, and the preference of the clinicians between HPV testing and cytology for primary screening of cervical lesions. It is noteworthy though that in April of 2014, the FDA approved the use of the Roche Cobas HPV assay for primary cervical cancer screening in women over the age of 25 years, without the concomitant Pap test. This approval recommended either colposcopy or a Pap cytology for patients with specific high-risk HPV types detected by the HPV test.

6.9 Conclusion

In conclusion, this chapter highlights the different aspects of life cycle of HPV and upregulation of p16 due to integration of genome of hrHPV in the host DNA. In the biopsy specimens, p16 immunostain can serve as a surrogate marker for hrHPV detection and in differentiating low-grade squamous intraepithelial lesions from high-grade squamous intraepithelial lesions. Alternatively, in cellular material obtained for Pap smear, molecular methodologies detailed in this chapter may be used to detect and sub-type HPV into high-risk and low-risk groups. Detection of hrHPV and/or a HSIL lesion is the action threshold for a more frequent follow-up and/or a cone/LEEP procedure, based on the current ASCCP guidelines.

Key Points

- The cytological criteria used for the diagnosis of LSIL include enlarged superficial cells with nuclear enlargement to at least three times the reference intermediate cell and perinuclear cytoplasmic vacuolation.
- The important cytological features of HSIL include nuclear hyperchromasia with very high nuclear-to-cytoplasmic ratio, marked nuclear irregularities with grooves, and thick nuclear membranes.
- The cytological features of glandular intraepithelial lesions include sheets, clusters, or strips of glandular cells with nuclear crowding and overlap, nuclear elongation, stratification and variation in size, presence of mitoses and/or apoptosis, and inconspicuous to absent nucleoli.
- SMILE are uncommon lesions which are thought to arise from the reserve cells at the transformation zone; Bethesda terminology does not recognize SMILE as a diagnostic category, given that it would be a challenging lesion to diagnose on cytology and that its histologic features are like that of HSIL.
- Tests for HPV detection include indirect methods (p16 immunostaining and Pro-Ex C) and direct methods (signal amplification tests and nucleic acid hybridization assays).

References

1. Reagan JW, Hicks DJ, Scott RB. A study of in-situ and squamous cell cancer of the uterine cervix. Cancer. 1953;6(6):1200–14.
2. Reagan JW, Seidemann IL, Saracusa Y. The cellular morphology of carcinoma in situ and dysplasia or atypical hyperplasia of the uterine cervix. Cancer. 1953;6(2):224–34.
3. Richart RM. A theory of cervical carcinogenesis. Obstet Gynecol Surv. 1969;24(7 Pt 2):874–9.
4. zur Hausen H. Papillomaviruses in the causation of human cancers—a brief historical account. Virology. 2009;384(2):260–5.
5. National Cancer Institute Workshop. The 1988 Bethesda system for reporting cervical/vaginal cytologic diagnoses. JAMA. 1989;262:931–4.
6. Darragh TM, Colgan TJ, Cox JT, Heller DS, Henry MR, Luff RD, et al. The Lower Anogenital Squamous Terminology Standardization Project for HPV-associated lesions: background and consensus recommendations from the College of American Pathologists and the American Society for Colposcopy and Cervical Pathology. J Low Genit Tract Dis. 2012;16:205–42.
7. Kurman RJ, Ellenson H, Ronnett BM. Blaustein's pathology of the female genital tract. 6th ed. New York: Springer; 2011.
8. Singh C, Manivel JC, Truskinovsky AM, Savik K, Amirouche S, Holler J, et al. Variability of pathologists' utilization of p16 and ki-67 immunostaining in the diagnosis of cervical biopsies in routine pathology practice and its impact on the frequencies of cervical intraepithelial neoplasia diagnoses and cytohistologic correlations. Arch Pathol Lab Med. 2014;138(1):76–87.
9. Lee C, Laimins LA, editors. The differentiation-dependent life cycle of human papillomaviruses in keratinocytes. Boston: Springer; 2007.
10. Graham SV. Keratinocyte differentiation-dependent human papillomavirus gene regulation. Viruses. 2017;9(9). https://doi.org/10.3390/v9090245.
11. Steinback A, Riemer AB. Immune evasion mechanisms of human papillomavirus: an update. Int J Cancer. 2018;142(2):224–29.
12. Graham SV. The human papillomavirus replication cycle, and its links to cancer progression: a comprehensive review. Clin Sci (Lond). 2017;131(17):2201–21.
13. Doorbar J, Egawa N, Griffin H, Kranjec C, Murakami I. Human papillomavirus molecular biology and disease association. Rev Med Virol. 2015;25(Suppl 1):2–23.
14. Mills AM, Dirks DC, Poulter MD, Mills SE, Stoler MH. HR-HPV E6/E7 mRNA in situ hybridization: validation against PCR, DNA in situ hybridization, and p16 immunohistochemistry in 102 samples of cervical, vulvar, anal, and head and neck neoplasia. Am J Surg Pathol. 2017;41(5):607–15.
15. Thomas JT, Oh ST, Terhune SS, Laimins LA. Cellular changes induced by low-risk human papillomavirus type 11 in keratinocytes that stably maintain viral episomes. J Virol. 2001;75(16):7564–71.
16. Bishop JA, Ma XJ, Wang H, Luo Y, Illei PB, Begum S, et al. Detection of transcriptionally active high-risk HPV in patients with head and neck squamous cell carcinoma as visualized by a novel E6/E7 mRNA in situ hybridization method. Am J Surg Pathol. 2012;36(12):1874–82.
17. Guo M, Gong Y, Deavers M, Silva EG, Jan YJ, Cogdell DE, et al. Evaluation of a commercialized in situ hybridization assay for detecting human papillomavirus DNA in tissue specimens from patients with cervical intraepithelial neoplasia and cervical carcinoma. J Clin Microbiol. 2008;46(1):274–80.
18. Nishino HT, Tambouret RH, Wilbur DC. Testing for human papillomavirus in cervical cancer screening: a review of indications and methodology. Cancer Cytopathol. 2011;119(4):219–27.
19. Abreu AL, Souza RP, Gimenes F, Consolaro ME. A review of methods for detect human papillomavirus infection. Virol J. 2012;9:262.

Cytology and HPV Testing in Primary Cervical Cancer Screening

7

Satinder Kaur and Shilpa Jamwal

7.1 Introduction

Cervical cancer is the only female genital tract cancer which can be diagnosed and treated in precancerous state by simple screening techniques. The incidence of the disease has come down drastically in countries which have successfully implemented the screening programmes. Cytology, visual inspection with acetic acid, visual inspection with Lugol's iodine and various HPV diagnostic tests have been used alone or in sequencing for screening. With the advent of newer diagnostics tests with better sensitivity and specificity, it has been possible to triage patients more effectively. This has also helped in increasing the screening interval leading to better compliance. Cytology and HPV testing are the two main methods which are universally adopted for primary screening of cervical cancer.

7.2 Cytology

Cervical cytology involves evaluation of exfoliated cervical cells. The cells from the cervix are collected with the help of cytobrush and spatula and examined microscopically for any abnormality. The concept of cytology was introduced by George Papanicolaou in 1920 and is named after him as Pap smear. There have been many modifications in the reporting system since then [1]. He originally classified findings of cervical cytology into five major categories (classes I–V) depending upon their resemblance to malignant cells (Table 7.1).

The concept of dysplasia was then introduced by Reagen et al. [3] in the 1950s and cervical intraepithelial neoplasia by Richart et al. [4] in the 1960s leading to modification of classification by the World Health Organization. In 1988, The Bethesda system (TBS) was devised to standardize cervical cytology nomenclature [5]. It broadly categorized clinically similar intraepithelial lesions into low-grade squamous intraepithelial lesion (LSIL) and high-grade squamous intraepithelial lesion (HSIL). Koilocytic changes in the smear and early precancerous lesions, i.e. cervical intraepithelial neoplasia I (CIN I), were clubbed as LSIL. Higher-grade lesions like CIN II and III were labelled as HSIL. TBS is now

Table 7.1 Classification of cervical cytology [2]

Class	Description
I	Absence of atypical or abnormal cells
II	Atypical cytology, but no evidence for malignancy
III	Cytology suggestive of, but not conclusive for, malignancy
IV	Cytology strongly suggestive of malignancy
V	Cytology conclusive for malignancy

S. Kaur (✉) · S. Jamwal
Department of Gynae-Oncology, Dharamshila Narayana Superspeciality Hospital, New Delhi, India

S. Mehta, A. Singla (eds.), *Preventive Oncology for the Gynecologist*,
https://doi.org/10.1007/978-981-13-3438-2_7

internally accepted as a standardized method of reporting cervical cytology. The reporting system was re-revised in 2006 in the Bethesda Workshop and is being followed all over the world.

Decrease in incidence of cervical cancer with the use of conventional Pap smear in primary cervical cancer screening itself strongly supported the efficacy of the method. However, the accuracy of technique was questioned on critical evaluation of the results. Meta-analysis of 62 studies by Fahey et al. compared Pap tests with histology and found sensitivity of cytology ranging 11–99% and specificity ranging 14–97%. Pap test was unable to achieve both high sensitivity and specificity, concurrently [6]. False negative rate of Pap test was about 14–33% and usually occurred due to sampling or slide preparation limitations [7]. As only a small part of the sample is taken and smeared on the Pap slide and most of the sample is discarded with the collecting device, using this method leads to inaccuracies and equivocal diagnosis.

To overcome these limitations, in the mid-1990s, liquid-based cytology (LBC) was introduced. The first LBC approved by US Food and Drug Administration (FDA) was ThinPrep^{R} Pap test (Hologic, Inc., Marlborough, MA) followed by the SurePath^{TM} Pap test (Becton, Dickinson and Company, Franklin Lakes, NJ) in 1999. In this method a spatula with sample was immersed directly into the preservative solution rather than being spread on a slide. An automated process is used to process the sample, so that the impurities and dead cells are filtered out. The processed sample is then used to form a monolayer on the slide which is first analysed by a computer-based imager and then reviewed by a pathologist and/or cytotechnologist. With the change in sample collection technique and betterment of sample quality, the clinical sensitivity of single LBC test in detection of high-grade lesions is reported from 88% to 93% which is much better than conventional Pap smear [8, 9]. Hence, the advantage of LBC over conventional Pap test became obvious not only in advancement in technology but also in detecting precancerous lesions or cervical cancer.

The advantage of ThinPrep Pap test was emphasized in the pivotal trial where it was shown that ThinPrep test provides a 65% increase ($P < 0.001$) in diagnosis of LSIL or greater cytology and better specimen quality compared with conventional Pap test ($P < 0.001$) [10]. Similarly, the SurePath Pap test showed increased detection rate of LSIL by 47% ($P = 0.0011$) and high-grade squamous intraepithelial lesions by 116% ($P = 0.0002$), respectively, as compared with the conventional Pap test [11]. After these results in early 2000, there was a drastic increase in lab offering only liquid-based cytology (9.3% vs. 25.5%) as compared to only conventional Pap testing (24.4% vs. 13.7%) [12].

Contrasting results were however shown in a meta-analysis of 109 studies by Arbyn et al. that compared test adequacy and results of conventional Pap with LBC. In only six studies, cytology tests were verified with histopathology. Pooled sensitivity and specificity in these studies with gold standard verification for HSIL were 57% and 97%, respectively, for LBC and 55.2% and 96.7% for conventional Pap smear. When atypical squamous cells of undetermined significance (ASCUS) were taken as cut-off, the pooled sensitivities and specificities were 90.4% and 64.6% for LBC and 88.2% and 71.3% for conventional Pap, respectively. Hence, it was concluded that for detection of HSIL, LBC and conventional cytology have equal sensitivity and specificity [13].

Despite liquid-based cytology showing controversial data in some studies, it is being widely adopted all over the world, including cancer screening programmes in developed countries. To add to it, many high-income countries are investigating molecular testing as a complementary screening test to cytology. Being objective in nature, molecular-based HPV testing has been shown to be of importance in identifying women at risk for developing preinvasive lesions of the cervix and later invasive cancer, decreasing subjective errors in cervical cytology reporting [14].

7.3 HPV DNA Testing

Human papillomavirus (HPV) has around 40 genotypes which can affect the genital mucosa of which around 13 are high-risk type. Infection and persistence of these high-risk types lead to the development of precancerous conditions of the cervix, which can further progress to invasive cancer. Ninety-nine percent of cervical cancers are caused by HPV infection. Genotype 16, 18, 31 and 33 are responsible for 80% of the cervical cancers [15]. So, HPV molecular-based detection and genotyping technologies may have an added advantage when used for screening cervical cancer.

HPV DNA is presently detected by three principal methods: (1) direct probe methods (e.g. Southern transfer hybridization and in situ hybridization [ISH]); (2) signal amplification (e.g. hybrid capture second-generation [HC2] assay); and (3) target amplification (polymerase chain reaction [PCR] variants).

7.3.1 Direct Probe Method

This method involves direct hybridization with DNA probes like in situ hybridization or Southern blotting. In 1980, in situ hybridization using cloned or synthetic oligonucleotide probes was first used for HPV detection. This clinically applicable method had the benefit of retaining the cellular structure and localization [16, 17]. However, Southern blot test used initially for hybridization technique showed variable results. Hence, clinical utility of this test was questionable and not recommended for routine practice.

7.3.2 Signal Amplification

Signal amplification, as the name suggests, amplified the detection signals without causing any modification in initial amount of nucleic acids in the sample. Hence, as compared from direct methods, lower amount of DNA could be detected with this method. It includes the second-generation hybrid capture assays [18].

7.3.2.1 Hybrid Capture HPV DNA Assay (Digene, Gaithersburg, MD)

This technique utilizes two non-isotopic single-stranded long RNA probes. Five low-risk types (6, 11, 42, 43 and 44) are detected by probe A, and 13 high-risk types (16, 18, 31, 33, 35, 39, 45, 51, 52, 56, 58, 59 and 68) are detected by probe B mixture. Each probe is separately used for hybridization with patient's sample which contains whole HPV DNA. The specific HPV DNA -RNA hybrids thus formed are added to antibodies specific to RNA-DNA hybrids coated microtiter plate leading to capture or immobilization of previously formed HPV DNA-RNA hybrids on the plate. The captured hybrids are bound to antibodies conjugated to alkaline phosphatase. Chemiluminescent substrate is added to it after removing the excess antibodies and non-hybridized probes. Viral load is calculated by using a luminometer (detects remaining immobilized hybrids) in which the intensity of light emitted by the sample is divided by the light emitted by a positive control which corresponds to the quantity of target DNA in the patient's specimen. However, this is an expensive and time-consuming test. To reduce the expenses, only high-risk probes are mostly used, and the result is interpreted as positive or negative for a high-risk group.

7.3.2.2 Care HPV (Qiagen, Gaithersburg, MD)

The major limitation with all the above tests is the high cost and time taken for the results. Care HPV is a rapid test broadly based on the principle of HC assay. It takes less than 2.5 h in contrast to 6 h with HC2 and requires minimum infrastructure. The contributing factor to this advantage is the unique reagents used in patient collection device which does not need prolonged mechanical agitation. The surfactant in it is nontoxic and quickly solubilizes cervical specimens. Also, magnetic beads are used in place of microtiter plates, and temperature requirements are varied in some steps as compared to HC2. Care HPV efficacy was first evaluated in a comprehensive study done in Shanxi province of rural China, where screening tests Care HPV, HC2 and simple visual inspection with acetic acid (VIA) were compared with gold standard colposcopy with biopsy. With Care HPV, the sensitivity and specificity to detect high-grade CIN (CIN 2 and higher) were 90% and 84% as compared to HC2 (97% and 86%) and VIA (41% and 95%) [19]. This test is ideal for developing countries as it is a rapid test, does not require much expertise and can be performed under limitation of space and temperature.

7.3.2.3 Target Amplification

Nucleic acid amplification techniques have brought into light the natural history of HPV infection. PCR has high sensitivity in detecting most genital HPV types and in variant analysis of HPV types. Type-specific PCR and consensus PCR are the two principle techniques in detecting HPV. Type-specific PCR test targets a sequence of viral genes leading to amplification of single HPV genotype. Practical feasibility of type-specific PCR is however questionable due to a large number of HPV in genital infections. Consensus PCR assay amplifies the majority of anogenital HPV genotypes in one reaction. Amplified genes are then typed using filters by hybridization with type-specific oligonucleotide probes [18].

7.3.2.4 Line Blot HPV Test

It is a L1 consensus primer-based PCR assay which uses PGMY09/11 following which line blot assay is done. In this test multiple probes are fixed as lines on a membrane strip. Twenty-seven HPV genotypes (6, 11, 16, 18, 26, 31, 33, 35, 39, 40, 42, 45, 51–59, 66, 68, 73, 82, 83, 84) are detected using reverse line blot hybridization. Additional 11 non-oncogenic types (61, 62, 64, 67, 69–72, 81, 82, 89) can also be detected by an extended version of this test. This test has been used in multiple past studies in research settings to examine the molecular epidemiology of HPV. Commercial version of this test, LINEAR ARRAY test, is widely used in research settings but is not US FDA cleared. This qualitative test detects 37 high- and low-risk HPV genotypes. Comparison between linear assay and HC2 test was evaluated in a study on 3,488 women with ASCUS on Pap testing at baseline. The sensitivity (93% vs. 93%), specificity (48% vs. 51%), negative predictive value (99% vs. 99%) and positive predictive value (15% vs. 15%) of the baseline detection of high-risk HPV types (HPV types 16, 18, 31, 33, 35, 39, 45, 51, 52) to predict biopsy-proven cervical intraepithelial neoplasia (CIN) grade 3 at 2 years were similar when comparing both tests, respectively [20].

7.3.2.5 AMPLICOR HPV Test

This test involves amplification of target DNA by polymerase chain reaction followed by nucleic acid hybridization to various HPV types. The 13 high-risk HPV types detected by HC2 are also detected by AMPLICOR utilizing the amplification of beta-globin gene which is essential for sample integrity and adequacy. AMPLICOR test is like HC2 in terms of performance characteristics to determine the presence or absence of any high-risk HPV type (except the specific HPV genotype). 23 AMPLICOR is not clinically approved by the US FDA but has Europe approval for clinical use.

7.3.2.6 The Cobas HPV Test

The US FDA has approved Cobas^R 4800 HPV test, a qualitative in vitro test, for the detection of HPV in specimens of patients. This test is efficient enough for detection of 14 high-risk HPV types in single analysis by amplification of target DNA by the polymerase chain reaction (PCR) followed by nucleic acid hybridization. This test specifically detects HPV 16 and 18 types with concurrent detection of rest of high-risk types (31, 33, 35, 39, 45, 51, 52, 56, 58, 59, 66 and 68). The test was validated on CIN 2+ lesions in ATHENA trial [21].

7.4 HPV Viral Load Evaluation by Real-Time PCR

The real-time PCR evaluates the viral load (amount of HPV DNA) in a cervical sample. Utility of HPV detection methods is improved by real-time PCR. Real-time PCR assay by measuring the increase of fluorescence released during the amplification reaction gives accurate measurements of the initial copy number of target DNA present in samples. This advantage cannot be gained with conventional PCR. Real-time PCR incorporates amplification by rapid thermocycling with fluorescence detection. For each specimen from patient, a human gene (such as beta-globin) and HPV DNA can be amplified.

The signal hence obtained is then compared with concentration reactivity from a titration curve of HPV and cellular DNA. The signal obtained for HPV DNA is then adjusted with the amount of cellular DNA deduced from the signal obtained with beta-globin amplification [22].

Despite the limitation of this method in sequencing multiple HPV genotypes, it is a useful method to identify specific HPV types [23].

7.5 HPV mRNA Testing

Overexpression of the viral oncogenes E6 and E7 is the real causative factor for cervical cancer and not HPV infection per se as earlier thought. Too many 'false positives' are identified with DNA assays as episomal HPV DNA may be present, but the infection regresses and there is no clinical disease. However, when HPV persists and integrates, overexpression of E6/E7 mRNA occurs; there is less probability of infection to regress. APTIMA test for detection of E6/E7 mRNA is more specific for detecting the progression of disease. Seeing the fact that specificity of HPV DNA tests for CIN 3+ is low and the positive predictive value is low in groups with low incidence, it implies that test for detection of overexpression of E6 and E7 messenger RNA is more specific than a test that detects the presence of viral DNA. E6/E7 mRNA of five main high-risk HPV types (16, 18, 31, 33 and 45) which are responsible for 86% of cervical cancers is detected by HPV mRNA test PreTect HPV-Proofer [24].

7.6 HPV and Cytology Co-testing

In 2012 the American Cancer Society (ACS) updated the guideline on screening for early detection of cervical precancerous lesions and cancer by including HPV DNA testing in screening [25]. FDA has approved HPV DNA testing as a primary screening test only in conjunction with cervical cytology and only in women aged 30 years and older. The 2012 screening guidelines for cervical cancer are stated in Table 7.2.

Table 7.2 ACS-ASCCP-ASCP 2012 screening guidelines

Population	Recommended screening method	Comments
Age <21 years	No screening	Irrespective of onset of sexual activity
Age 21–29 years	Cytology alone every 3 years	No role of HPV testing No role of yearly testing
Age 30–65 years	HPV and cytology co-testing every 5 years (preferred) Cytology alone every 3 years (acceptable)	
Age >65 years	No screening following adequate negative prior screening	Women with history of CIN 2 or higher should continue screening for 20 years
After hysterectomy	No screening	No history of CIN 2 or more for the past 20 years or cervical cancer ever

Women who are negative for both cytology and HPV test should be screened less frequently as they are at very low risk for CIN 3+. This fact was evaluated in a prospective cohort study carried out on 332,000 US women of age 30 years and older who underwent co-testing with cervical cytology and HPV DNA every 3 years. Incidence of CIN 3+ in women negative for both tests was 0.047% at 3 years and 0.16% at 5 years [26]. In another study involving 43,000 women aged 29–61 years, co-testing was carried out every 5 years for 15 years in one half of the patients. Incidence of CIN 3+ in those negative for both tests was 0.01% (95% confidence interval [CI], 0.00–0.05%) at 9 years and 0.07% (95% CI, 0.03–0.17%) at 14 years of follow-up [27]. Hence, it was concluded that screening more frequently than every 3 years is not very fruitful as it would only increase the cost and lead to over-treatment, causing no improvement in sensitivity [28, 29].

It has been shown in many studies that women with CIN 2 positivity are better identified by

HPV DNA testing than with cytology (range of sensitivities 84–97%). In a randomized trial in women aged 30–69 years, where both Pap and HPV testing were used, sensitivity of HPV was found to be 95% as compared to Pap cytology where it was 55%. The combined use of HPV and cytology had a sensitivity of 100% and referral rate of 7.9% [30].

Although HPV DNA has better sensitivity than cytology, it lacks in specificity. It has been found that cytology has a specificity of 97% compared with 94% for HPV testing in women older than 30 years [30]. Women younger than 30 years who have transient HPV infection have even lower specificity of HPV DNA testing. So, efforts in detecting such women would add to unnecessary follow-up workload and expenses. However, few reports have found that though sensitivity increases with co-testing, this strategy adds a little when compared with primary HPV screening alone.

7.7 HPV as a Primary Screening Tool

ACS-ASCCP-ASCP 2012 guidelines discussed the application of HR-HPV testing alone as a primary screening tool, but there was no official recommendation for its regular use in screening. At present many studies carried out on women over 30 years of age support efficacy of HPV testing as a primary screening modality alone. Accuracy of HPV testing in screening helps in increasing the screening interval leading to more comfort for the patients, more compliance and better cost-benefit ratio. Meta-analysis by Arbyn et al. including 49 studies (with eight randomized controlled trials) strongly proved HPV test to be more sensitive as compared to cytology for CIN 2+ and CIN 3+ detection. Also, in the second round of screening, HPV-negative women had lower incidence of CIN 3+ as compared to cytology-negative women [31].

In the ARTISTIC screening trial, HPV and cytology testing were compared in terms of efficacy in detecting CIN 2 or worse (CIN 2+) and CIN 3 or worse (CIN 3+). HPV testing is done using the HC2 (Qiagen) assay for high-risk types and genotyped by linear array (Roche) and PapilloCheck (Greiner) assays. ThinPrep was used for liquid-based cytology. The data has indicated that the protective value of single negative HPV test is more than three rounds of cytology testing. It suggested that if HPV testing is incorporated as a primary screening modality in place of cytology for women over 30 years of age, the screening interval can be increased to 6 years [32].

In 2014, seeing the growing evidence in support of use of HPV testing as a primary screening tool, 13 experts including representatives from the Society for Colposcopy and Cervical Pathology, Society of Gynaecologic Oncology, American Society of Obstetricians and Gynaecologists, American Cancer Society, American Society of Cytopathology, College of American Pathologists and American Society for Clinical Pathology came together to discuss the role of HR-HPV testing as a primary screening approach. Data based on literature review and from the FDA registration study was discussed and guidelines formulated incorporating expert's opinion. These guidelines stated that primary HR-HPV screening can be considered as an alternative to current US cytology-based cervical cancer screening approaches including cytology alone and co-testing [33].

Incorporating HPV as a primary screening test is a challenge due to technicality attached to the procedure, increasing the workload and the logistics. In low-income countries, using HPV as a primary screening modality is impracticable considering the high cost of the kit. Care HPV test has shown some ray of hope in this respect. Further studies need to be done for evaluating its applicability [19].

Another area of debate and research is the management of women tested positive for HPV, if incorporated as a primary screening modality. Castle et al. carried out a study on a sub-cohort of women enrolled in population-based cohort in Guanacaste, Costa Rica. They found that testing for short-term persistence of HPV infection helps in assessing the risk of CIN 2+. Twenty percent of women with HPV persistence and 40% with HPV 16 persistence had a higher probability of high-grade CIN in the following 3–5 years. These patients were advised repeat HPV testing after 1 year [34]. Carozzi et al. showed p16 testing had higher sensitivity for detection of CIN 3+ than that of conventional cytology (77.8% at all ages) at a 3-year follow-up [35].

Primary HPV testing in women less than 30 years of age has a limited clinical efficacy in view of high positive rates [35]. Thus, recommending primary HPV screening is a challenging issue. This problem is more cumbersome in countries who are organizing regular screening programmes such as the USA, where high coverage is achieved as compared to countries where women are less screened. Countries which start screening at 30 years of age are facing fewer challenges than countries where screening age is less than 30 years of age. It is also important to give clear and adequate information once there is a proposal for change of screening modality from present cytology screening to 'HPV-first' approach.

7.8 HPV as a Triage Test

Since many years, HPV testing has been used for triaging low-grade abnormalities in different countries. It has been found that the sensitivity of this approach in order to detect CIN 2+ is more than repeat cytology especially when using a test which has efficacy comparable to HC2. Marc Arbyn et al. recently proved in a recent meta-analysis that HPV triage with HC2 assay test has higher sensitivity and similar specificity than repeat cytology and APTIMA test (mRNA testing) being similarly sensitive but more specific as compared to HC2 [31].

In young women who have rampant transient HPV infection, the sensitivity of HPV test for triage purpose for detection of low-grade abnormalities (LSIL) or mild dyskaryosis is unquestionable, but as far as its specificity is concerned, its role is disputed. RNA-based tests have the potential to improve specificity as compared to DNA tests as found in APTIMA assay in a recent meta-analysis where the sensitivity was shown equivalent to HC2 test but with a higher specificity [36]. Women who have undergone treatment for CIN 2 or CIN 3 positivity have a high risk of recurrence or even progression to invasive cancer following treatment [37]. If HPV testing is added in post-treatment follow-up protocol than due to its high sensitivity and negative predictive value, the number of follow-ups can fall drastically. In a recent analysis by Rebolj et al. on Dutch women post-treatment for any preinvasive lesion, who had three subsequent normal smears as part of standard follow-up, approximately fourfold risk of cancer was identified [38]. This has often led to prolonged post-treatment follow-ups and inconvenience to women undergoing these follow-ups. So, incorporating HPV testing in these post-treatment follow-up protocols will be a good idea. In a Dutch study from Kocken et al., one HPV-negative test at 6 months post-treatment had a 10-year risk of CIN 3+ of 2.1%. However, with negative co-testing, the risk reduced to 1.4%. Conversely, if a woman was found to be HPV positive at 6 months post-treatment, the risk of CIN 3 over a 10-year period was 9.2%. Hence, a test with higher sensitivity is required in post-treatment follow-ups [39].

Higher efficacy of HPV test in detecting residual and recurrent high-grade CIN than follow-up cytology has also been shown in a meta-analysis of Arbyn et al. [40] and in study by Chan et al. [41]. These analyses have drawn conclusions predominantly on the performance of HC2 assay. These studies are in fact one of the initial studies done comparing various HPV assays.

Despite the need for high sensitivity, attaining a perfect investigation is challenging. Real challenge is patient who are referred for colposcopy due to their HPV positive status, but clinically have a no evidence of disease. Hence, more studies are required for appropriate and safe direction for the treatment of such women.

7.9 Conclusion

Screening is essential to bring down the incidence of cervical cancer and subsequently morbidity and mortality associated with it. Cytology-based screening has traditionally been used for cervical cancer. Knowing the etiological relationship with the disease, HPV testing has been suggested as an alternate test for screening. Although HPV test has low sensitivity in detecting CIN 2+and CIN 3+ and leads to unrequired referrals, this test is more reassuring than a negative conventional cytology test. Cytological tests have greater probability of being falsely negative, which leads to the delay in receiving appropriate treatment. Further prospective longitudinal studies are required to establish the relative clinical implications.

Key Points

- Cytology and HPV testing are the main methods that are universally adopted for primary cervical cancer screening.
- Liquid-based cytology has been shown beneficial over conventional cytology in improvements in technology; however, advantage in clinical utility for detecting precancerous lesions or cervical cancer is still questionable.
- Human papillomavirus (HPV) has around 40 genotypes which can affect the genital mucosa of which around 13 are high-risk type and are the precursors of cervical cancer development. Therefore, HPV molecular-based detection and genotyping technologies are beneficial clinically in screening for cervical cancer.
- HPV DNA testing has been FDA approved only in combination with cervical cytology as a primary screening test and that also in women 30 years and older.
- Many studies at present support efficacy of HPV testing as a primary screening modality alone in women above 30 years of age.
- HPV as primary test is a challenge due to technicality attached to the procedure, increasing the workload and the logistics.
- Appropriate information needs to be provided to women when moving on from cervical cytology screening to 'HPV-first' approach, as appropriate management of these patients is important.
- Incorporation of HPV testing in post-treatment follow-up provides high sensitivity and negative predictive value, decreasing follow-up significantly.

References

1. Papanicolaou GN. New cancer diagnosis. In: Proceedings third race betterment conference. Battle Creek, MI: Race Betterment Foundation; 1928. p. 528–34.
2. Papanicolaou GN. Atlas of exfoliative cytology. Boston: Commonwealth Fund University Press; 1954.
3. Reagan JW, Seidemann IL, Sarcusa Y. Cellular morphology of carcinoma in situ and dysplasia or atypical hyperplasia of uterine cervix. Cancer. 1953;6:224–35.
4. Richart RM. Natural history of cervical intraepithelial neoplasia. Clin Obstet Gynecol. 1968;10:748–84.
5. National Cancer Workshop. The 1988 Bethesda system for reporting cervical/vaginal cytologic diagnosis. JAMA. 1989;262:931–4.
6. Fahey MT, Irwig L, Macaskill P. Meta-analysis of Pap test accuracy. Am J Epidemiol. 1995;14:680–9.
7. Hartmann K, Hall SA, Nanda K, et al. Systematic evidence review number 25: screening for cervical cancer. Rockville: US Department of Health and Human Services; 2002.
8. Clavel C, Masure M, Bory JP, et al. Human papillomavirus testing in primary screening for the detection of high-grade cervical lesions: a study of 7932 women. Br J Cancer. 2001;84:1616–23.
9. Hutchinson ML, Zahniser DJ, Sherman ME, et al. Utility of liquid-based cytology for cervical carcinoma screening: results of a population-based study conducted in a region of Costa Rica with a high incidence of cervical carcinoma. Cancer. 1999;87:48–55.
10. Lee KR, Ashfaq R, Birdson GG, et al. Comparison of conventional Papanicolaou smears and a fluid-based, thin-layer system for cervical cancer screening. Obstet Gynecol. 1997;90:278–84.
11. Marino JF, Fremont-Smith M. Direct-to-vial experience with Auto Cyte PREP in a small New England regional cytology practice. J Reprod Med. 2001;46:353–8.
12. Eversole GM, Moriarty AT, Schwartz MR, et al. Practices of participants in the College of American Pathologists interlaboratory comparison program in cervicovaginal cytology, 2006. Arch Pathol Lab Med. 2010;134:331–5.
13. Arbyn M, Bergeron C, Klinkhamer P, et al. Liquid compared with conventional cervical cytology: a systemic review and meta-analysis. Obstet Gynecol. 2008;111:167–77.
14. Boulet GA, Horvath CA, Berghmans S, Bogers J. Human papillomavirus in cervical cancer screening: important role as biomarker. Cancer Epidemiol Biomarkers Prev. 2008;17:810–7.
15. Wheeler CM, Hunt WC, Schiffman M, Castle PE, Atypical Squamous Cells of Undetermined Significance/Low-Grade Squamous Intraepithelial Lesions Triage Study Group. Human papillomavirus genotypes and the cumulative 2-year risk of cervical precancer. J Infect Dis. 2006;194:1291–9.

16. Ungar E, Budgeon LR, Myerson D, et al. Viral diagnosis by in situ hybridization. Am J Surg Pathol. 1986;10:1–8.
17. Cubie HA, Norval M. Detection of human papillomaviruses in paraffin wax sections with biotinylated synthetic oligonucleotide probes and immunogold staining. J Clin Pathol. 1989;42:988–91.
18. Coutlée F, Mayrand MH, Provencher D, Franco E. The future of HPV testing in clinical laboratories and applied virology research. Clin Diagn Virol. 1997;8:123–41.
19. Qiao YL, Sellors JW, Eder PS, et al. A new HPV-DNA test for cervical-cancer screening in developing regions: a cross-sectional study of clinical accuracy in rural China. Lancet Oncol. 2008;9(10):929–36.
20. Gravitt PE, Schiffman M, Solomon D, Wheeler CM, Castle PE. A comparison of linear array and hybrid capture 2 for detection of carcinogenic human papillomavirus and cervical precancer in ASCUS-LSIL triage study. Cancer Epidemiol Biomarkers Prev. 2008;17:1248–54.
21. Heideman DA, Hesselink AT, Berkhof J, et al. Clinical validation of the cobas® 4800 HPV Test for cervical screening purposes. J Clin Microbiol. 2011;49(11):3983–5.
22. Swan DC, Tucker RA, Tortolero-Luna G, et al. Human papillomavirus (HPV) DNA copy number is dependent on grade of cervical disease and HPV type. J Clin Microbiol. 1999;37:1030–4.
23. Mayrand MH, Coutlee F, Hankins C, et al. Detection of human papillomavirus type 16 DNA in consecutive genital samples does not always represent persistent infection as determined by molecular variant analysis. J Clin Microbiol. 2000;38:3388–9.
24. Molden T, Kraus I, Skomedal H, Nordstrøm T, Karlsen F. PreTect HPV-Proofer: real-time detection and typing of E6/E7 mRNA from carcinogenic human papillomaviruses. J Virol Methods. 2007;142(1-2):204–12.
25. Saslow D, Solomon D, Lawson HW, Killackey M, Kulasingam SL, Cain J, et al. American Cancer Society, American Society for Colposcopy and Cervical Pathology, and American Society for Clinical Pathology screening guidelines for the prevention and early detection of cervical cancer. CA Cancer J Clin. 2012;62:147–72.
26. Katki HA, Kinney WK, Fetterman B, et al. Cervical cancer risk for women undergoing concurrent testing for human papillomavirus and cervical cytology: a population-based study in routine clinical practice. Lancet Oncol. 2011;12(7):663–72.
27. Dijkstra MG, van Zummeren M, Rozendaal L, et al. Safety of extending screening intervals beyond five years in cervical screening programmed with testing for high risk human papillomavirus: 14-year follow-up of population based randomized cohort in the Netherlands. BMJ. 2016;355:i4924.
28. Saslow D, Runowicz CD, Solomon D, et al. American Cancer Society guideline for the early detection of cervical neoplasia and cancer. CA Cancer J Clin. 2002;52(6):342–62.
29. Goldie SJ, Kim JJ, Wright TC. Cost-effectiveness of human papillomavirus DNA testing for cervical cancer screening in women aged 30 years or more. Obstet Gynecol. 2004;103(4):619–31.
30. Mayrand MH, Duarte-Franco E, Rodrigues I, et al. Human papillomavirus DNA versus papanicolaou screening tests for cervical cancer. N Engl J Med. 2007;357(16):1579–88.
31. Arbyn M, Ronco G, Anttila A, et al. Evidence regarding human papillomavirus testing in secondary prevention of cervical cancer. Vaccine. 2012;30(Suppl 5):F88–99.
32. Kitchener HC, Gilham C, Sargent A, et al. A comparison of HPV DNA testing and liquid based cytology over three rounds of primary cervical screening: extended follow up in the ARTISTIC trial. Eur J Cancer. 2011;47:864–71.
33. Huh WK, Ault KA, Chelmow D, et al. Use of primary high-risk human papillomavirus testing for cervical cancer screening: interim clinical guidance. Gynecol Oncol. 2015;125(2):330–7.
34. Castle PE, Rodriguez AC, Burk RD, et al. Short-term persistence and risk of cervical precancer and cancer: population-based cohort study. BMJ. 2009;339:b2569.
35. Carozzi F, Gillio-Tos A, Confortini M, et al. Risk of high-grade cervical intraepithelial neoplasia during follow-up in HPV-positive women according to baseline p16-INK4A results: a prospective analysis of a nested sub study of the NTCC randomized controlled trial. Lancet Oncol. 2013;14:168–76.
36. Arbyn M, Roelens J, Cuschieri K, et al. The APTIMA HPV assay versus the hybrid capture 2 test in triage of women with ASC-US or LSIL cervical cytology: a meta-analysis of the diagnostic accuracy. Int J Cancer. 2013;132:101–8.
37. Strander B, Andersson-Ellstrom A, Milsom I, et al. Long-term risk of invasive cancer after treatment for cervical intraepithelial neoplasia grade 3: population-based cohort study. BMJ. 2007;335:1077.
38. Rebolj M, Helmerhorst T, Habbema D, et al. Risk of cervical cancer after completed post-treatment follow-up of cervical intraepithelial neoplasia: population-based cohort study. BMJ. 2012;345:e6855.
39. Kocken M, Helmerhorst TJM, Berkhof J, Louwers JA, Nobbenhuis MAE, Bais AG, et al. Risk of recurrent high-grade cervical intraepithelial neoplasia after successful treatment: a long-term multi-cohort study. Lancet Oncol. 2011;12(5):441–50.
40. Arbyn M, Paraskevaidis E, Martin-Hirsche P, et al. Clinical utility of HPV–DNA detection: triage of minor cervical lesions, follow-up of women treated for high-grade CIN: an update of pooled evidence. Gynecol Oncol. 2005;99:S7–11.
41. Chan BKS, Melnikow J, Slee CA, et al. Posttreatment human papillomavirus testing for recurrent cervical intraepithelial neoplasia: a systematic review. Am J Obstet Gynecol. 2009;200:422.e1–9.

Management of Abnormal Cytology

8

Fredric Willmott, Samuel George Oxley, and Tony Hollingworth

8.1 Introduction

Cervical cytology is a routine screening test for cervical preinvasive conditions. Other conditions might also be seen, i.e. infective or malignant diseases. It is a technique that involves microscopic examination of individual cells or cell clusters. The collection of the cells (the test) is performed by fully visualising the patient's cervix and then either scraping, brushing or washing the cells from the surface of the cervix. These cells are then stained with Papanicolaou stain to aid cytological examination [1]. The degrees of cervical abnormality are diagnosed by the nuclear characteristics and nuclear-cytoplasmic ratio, shown in Fig. 8.1 [2].

Abnormal cervical cytology or a positive result for high-risk human papillomavirus (hr-HPV) indicates the presence of an abnormality within the cervix. Cytology reports provide clear and consistent communication to clinicians, to enable triage of high-risk patients to colposcopy and reassure the majority of low-risk patients who may continue with routine screening. This chapter will discuss the degrees of cytological abnormality and their initial management.

8.2 Main Article

Dyskaryosis or dysplasia seen on cervical cytology refers to the disproportionate nuclear enlargement in relation to the surrounding cytoplasm. Dyskaryotic cells have abnormal chromatin and distribution leading to possible abnormal shapes of the nucleus [3]. Additional "reflex" testing of samples for hr-HPV enables further refinement in risk assessment, and this is mainly used as an adjunct to triage those with borderline and low-grade dyskaryosis, although primary HPV screening is becoming more popular, with cytology as the adjunct. In some systems hr-HPV testing is not yet routinely performed. Other programmes adjust hr-HPV testing with age. The Canadian system recommends women less than 30 years old should not have hr-HPV testing done as a screen with cytology [4]. This is based on the relative high rate of women below the age of 35 years who will test positive for hr-HPV. The information below relates primarily to cytology with reflex HPV testing, but management plans without a hr-HPV result are mentioned.

F. Willmott (✉) · S. G. Oxley
Department of Women's Health, Whipps Cross University Hospital, London, UK
e-mail: fredric.willmott@bartshealth.nhs.uk

T. Hollingworth
Department of Women's Health, Whipps Cross University Hospital, London, UK

Department of Gynaecology, Barts Health NHS Trust, London, UK

Centre for Cancer Prevention, Wolfson Institute for Preventive Medicine, QMUL, London, UK

S. Mehta, A. Singla (eds.), *Preventive Oncology for the Gynecologist*, https://doi.org/10.1007/978-981-13-3438-2_8

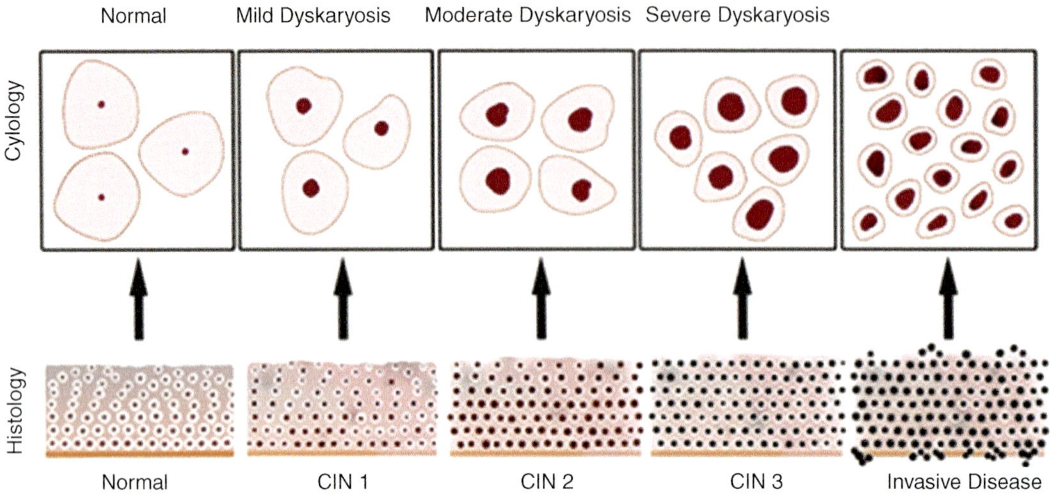

Fig. 8.1 Cytological and histological appearance of cervical abnormalities

There are harms and benefits with any screening programme and this is true with prevention of cervical cancer. Risk can never be reduced to zero as this would result in overtreatment and the problems that come with removing part of the cervix. It was noted in a consensus conference on cervical screening which took place in 2011 that optimal prevention strategies should identify those HPV-related abnormalities likely to progress to invasive cancers [5]. These strategies should also avoid non-excision treatment of abnormalities not destined to become cancerous.

Strategies should incorporate HPV testing and this recommendation is based on studies that have used validated HPV assays. Therefore management should completely avoid HPV tests that have not been validated as the outcomes may be unpredictable and run the risk of harm to the patient [5]. Testing should be restricted to high-risk (oncogenic) HPV types (mainly 16, 18, 31, 33, 35, 39, 45, 51, 52, 56, 58 and 59). There is no role for testing of low-risk (non-oncogenic) HPV types in the evaluation of women with abnormal cervical cytology results [5].

In selecting appropriate patients for onward referral, a balance must be struck between sensitivity in detection of preinvasive or invasive disease and the avoidance of unnecessary assessment which may provide a burden on patients in the form of anxiety, overtreatment and inconvenience, as well as on colposcopy services. The overall incidence of high-grade disease is low. As the natural course of the condition is known, there is a long time to cancer development. Therefore, repeated smears in routine or earlier screening intervals can be used rather than colposcopy in certain cases to monitor progression and HPV clearance. There is no international consensus, and some guidelines may adopt a more risk-averse strategy depending on local availability of robust screening programmes and colposcopists; however, the same principles of safe management apply.

Commonly infective organisms are seen in conjunction with cervical cytology. These include trichomonas vaginalis, fungal organisms morphologically consistent with a *Candida* species, shifts in vaginal flora suggestive of bacterial vaginosis, actinomyces, cellular changes consistent with herpes simplex virus and reactive cellular changes consistent with inflammation [1]. If found, treatment and possible further sexual health screening should be discussed with the patient. In the UK, it is becoming routine to offer HIV testing to all women attending for their first colposcopy clinic visit. This is due to the fact that the immunocompromised state of untreated HIV patients can make managing cervical pathology very difficult. This improves with effective antiretroviral medication.

Cytology will be reported as inadequate, negative, borderline, low-grade or high-grade (moderate

Table 8.1 Terminological changes to cervical cytology reporting [1, 6]

Previous terminology (BSCC 1986)	2001 Bethesda System (Abridged)	New terminology (NHS England)
Borderline change	Atypical squamous cells (ASC)	Borderline changes in squamous cells Borderline changes in endocervical cells
Mild dyskaryosis Borderline change with koilocytosis	Low-grade squamous intraepithelial lesion (LSIL)	Low-grade dyskaryosis
Moderate dyskaryosis	High-grade squamous intraepithelial lesion (HSIL)	High-grade dyskaryosis (moderate)
Severe dyskaryosis		High-grade dyskaryosis (severe)
Severe dyskaryosis? Invasive	Squamous cell carcinoma	High-grade dyskaryosis? Invasive squamous carcinoma
Glandular neoplasia	Atypical glandular cells (AGC)	Glandular neoplasia of endocervical type
	Atypical glandular cells, favour neoplastic Endocervical adenocarcinoma in situ (AIS) Adenocarcinoma	Glandular neoplasia (non-cervical)

or severe), and occasionally invasive squamous carcinoma, glandular neoplasia and benign endometrial cells may be seen (Table 8.1). The significance of these may vary depending on clinical circumstances.

Within the UK screening programme, there are target timelines for colposcopic assessment following detection of an abnormal smear. These standards are [6]:

1. Three consecutive inadequate samples: appointment within 6 weeks
2. Borderline change/hr-HPV positive: appointment within 6 weeks
3. Low-grade/hr-HPV positive: appointment within 6 weeks
4. High-grade (moderate): appointment within 2 weeks
5. High-grade (severe): appointment within 2 weeks
6. Invasive squamous carcinoma/Invasive glandular neoplasia: appointment within 2 weeks

8.2.1 Inadequate Samples

If a liquid-based cytology (LBS) sample is reported as inadequate, the test should be repeated. This repeat should be deferred for 2–4 months [5] to allow the surface layer of squamous cells to regenerate, giving a representative sample. The time frame is 3 months within the NHS screening programme. A sample will also be classed as inadequate if the sample taker has not confirmed seeing the entire cervix, as this could lead to false-negative results. Despite this, if borderline or dyskaryotic cells are seen in a sample, the test cannot be called inadequate [6].

If there are repeated inadequate LBC samples, three in the NHS screening programme [6], then a referral should be made to colposcopy. Inadequate samples account for less than 1% of cytology results and are caused mainly by insufficient squamous cells [5]. Reflex HPV testing is not usually possible due to the concern that the cervix has not been adequately sampled.

In the postmenopausal population, the rate of inadequate samples can be greater due to atrophic changes and the transformation zone inverting into the cervical canal. The inadequate cytology rate can be decreased by applying a vaginal oestrogen preparation for a time prior to screening. The use of an endocervical brush can also help obtain an adequate sample.

8.2.2 Negative Result

Negative cytology is highly reassuring, and patients can be returned to routine recall. Following a negative result, there is a 61–84% risk reduction in developing cervical cancer over the following 3–5 years [6]. In the UK, reflex

HPV testing is not required for these patients. Where HPV testing is performed and found to be positive, repeat cytology should be performed within a year [6]. This is due to the known risk of developing high-grade lesions or malignancy in these patients. If HPV has been cleared, then these patients can safely be returned to the routine national screening recall system; however, if HPV persists, then a referral for colposcopy should be made. The presence of high-risk subtypes 16 or 18 justifies referral for colposcopy, particularly as subtype 18 is associated with adenocarcinomas, the detection of which is problematic with cytological screening alone. In up to 10–20% of cytological samples, there will be scanty endocervical/transformation zone (EC/TZ) sampling, suggesting insufficient cells from the squamocolumnar junction. This has previously raised concerns over the possibility of falsely negative results. However, it appears that such women, many of whom are older with lower baseline rates of CIN 3+, do not have increased risk of high-grade disease [7]. As such, negative cytology has good specificity despite insufficient EC/TZ sampling, and women can safely be returned to routine screening, although high-risk HPV testing can be considered for such women aged 30–64 years with management as detailed above, which adds a further element of safety.

8.2.3 Borderline Change in Squamous or Endocervical Cells (Atypical Squamous Cells of Undetermined Significance (ASCUS))

In the UK, the detection of borderline cells prompts reflex hr-HPV testing. If the hr-HPV test is positive, then it is recommended that women warrant referral to a colposcopy clinic. If negative the patient returns to routine recall, 3 or 5 years depending on their age. This corresponds with 2011 screening guidelines from the USA recommending women "with HPV-negative ASC-US co-testing results be managed with routine follow-up" [5].

Where the HPV result is unreliable due to insufficient cellularity, then a repeat cytology sample should be taken between 6 months [6] and 1 year [5]. A negative HPV result at this time is reassuring, and patients can be returned to routine recall. If the result is positive for hr-HPV, then that woman should be referred to colposcopy [6].

8.2.4 Low-Grade (LG) Dyskaryosis

The detection of LG dyskaryosis triggers reflex hr-HPV testing. If positive the patient is referred to colposcopy. A positive hr-HPV result is found in 77% of cases with LG dyskaryosis [5]. If hr-HPV negative, the woman can be returned to the national recall system for her next routine smear at the designated interval. If LG dyskaryosis is confirmed but the hr-HPV testing is inadequate or unreliable, a referral should be made to colposcopy [6].

Once at colposcopy the patient should be assessed. To prevent overtreatment, it is not recommended to manage women with LG dyskaryosis with immediate treatment, i.e. "see and treat" [6]. Representative biopsies should be the first line of management.

8.2.5 High-Grade Dyskaryosis (Moderate or Severe)/High-Grade Squamous Intraepithelial Lesion (HSIL)

High-grade (HG) dyskaryosis or greater should prompt urgent referral to colposcopy, without the need for high-risk HPV testing. Moderate dyskaryosis is associated with a 74% likelihood of CIN 2 or 3 and severe dyskaryosis with an 80–90% risk [6]. This strong correlation helps justify a "see and treat" approach with immediate excision of the transformation zone for many women [5]. The decision for "see and treat" depends on the clinical suspicion, patient's consent, patient's fertility wishes and the ability to follow patients up following diagnostic biopsies. Patients at risk from loss to follow-up, for example, geographical proximity concerns, may be more suited to immediate treatment and are more likely to benefit from immediate treatment.

Cervical cancer is diagnosed at colposcopy in approximately 2% of women with high-grade lesions [5]. However, risk also rises with age. With regard to hr-HPV status, HPV-negative HG cytology is rare. Some guidelines state it still carries a 5-year risk for CIN 3+ of 29% and 7% will develop cancer. Therefore, it is not currently suggested reflex hr-HPV is performed on HG cytology. In HPV-positive HG dyskaryosis, the 5-year risk of CIN 3+ was 50%, whilst the 5-year cancer risk was 7% [5]. The current role for HPV testing in this group of women could be to guide the clinician towards immediate treatment versus close monitoring.

8.2.6 Invasive Squamous Cell Carcinoma

These patients are referred urgently for colposcopy. The concern for a malignant process is very high as the correlation between this result and the histological diagnosis of invasive cancer is high. One case series suggested that invasive cytology has a 56% positive predictive value [8].

8.2.7 Glandular Neoplasia

Glandular neoplasia may be seen, and such cells may originate from the endocervix or another gynaecological site such as the endometrium. It can be associated with polyps and metaplasia but also with neoplasia, including adenocarcinomas of the endometrium, cervix, ovary, fallopian tube and other sites [5]. Urgent colposcopy is required for visualisation of the endocervix where the former is suspected, as glandular neoplasia is strongly associated with invasive (40–43%) as well as preinvasive disease (20–28%) [6]. Where cells from a non-cervical location are seen, an urgent referral to a gynaecology clinic is appropriate, alongside consideration of further investigations such as transvaginal ultrasound and endometrial biopsy. It is important to ensure communication is appropriate, as such results will be outside routine screening programmes. The Canadian guidelines recommend all women with glandular cytology should have an endocervical curettage [4].

In one cohort, CIN 3+ was found in 9% of patients 30 years and older with glandular cytology, with cancer in 3% [5]. Although the cytological description of this group regards glandular abnormalities, the most common findings are squamous lesions. Nevertheless, squamous and glandular lesions often coexist, with CIN found in approximately half of women with glandular invasion cytology. Therefore, identification of CIN does not preclude the presence of preexisting CGIN or adenocarcinoma [5].

Fortunately, cervical adenocarcinoma is HPV associated and therefore can be detected with HPV testing. However, endometrial cancer is not HPV related; consequently reflex HPV testing does not identify a subgroup of women who need less invasive assessment [5]. If cytology showed glandular cells and the sample was hr-HPV negative, then one would be concerned about excluding the possibility of an endometrial cancer.

8.2.8 Benign Endometrial Cells

Benign endometrial cells may be reported in up to 9.8% of cytology samples [5], and the interpretation of this varies with the patient's age and other clinical details, which is usually for the referring clinician to assess. Most endometrial pathology is symptomatic and occurs in postmenopausal women. For patients under 40 years, benign endometrial cells are unlikely to reflect pathology, and this does not need to be reported. The presence of benign endometrial cells in the cytology of women over the age of 40 years should be reported as the likelihood of endometrial pathology increases, reaching a 20.7% incidence of adenocarcinoma in those over 59 years in one study [5]. These cells are more likely to be present in the follicular phase of the menstrual cycle, but if present during the luteal phase are more concerning. However, patients on hormone replacement therapy, oral contraceptives, tamoxifen, or with intrauterine contraceptive devices can shed normal endometrial cells throughout the cycle, and this has not been shown to be associated with any increase in the risk for malignancy if visualised on cytology [6].

Occasionally, cytologists may have difficulty interpreting cytological samples, and such women should be referred for colposcopy. If colposcopy is similarly non-specific, or there is significant difference in colposcopic impression versus cytology, then cases should be discussed in the multidisciplinary meeting with a cytologist, colposcopist and histopathologist where appropriate [7].

8.2.9 Abnormal Cytology and Pregnancy

It is not uncommon that an abnormal cytological result is identified in conjunction with the patient detecting a pregnancy. Ideally, routine cervical screening should not be done in pregnancy and be deferred until the pregnancy is over. Nevertheless, if a patient has been previously poorly compliant in having routine cytology then one could make an argument for opportunistic screening for that particular woman [6]. Colposcopy is possible whilst pregnant, but becomes more difficult in late pregnancy. Also with the increased blood flow to the gravid uterus, caution must be taken when treatments are planned.

If a low-grade lesion (borderline or low-grade dyskaryosis) is found during pregnancy, even with hr-HPV, cytology should be repeated 3 months postpartum [4, 6]. This practice is safe as the rate of cancer in this group of women is very low. If high-grade dyskaryosis is found, prompt evaluation with colposcopy is essential and the same timelines should be followed as the non-pregnant patient. If colposcopy is unsatisfactory in the first trimester, it should be repeated after 20 weeks' gestation when, because of the physiological changes, the cervix everts itself and the squamocolumnar junction may become easier to visualise [4]. Caution with biopsies should be taken due to the risk of excessive bleeding in pregnancy. The gravid state is an exception for biopsying lesions not thought to be invasive [6], although close follow-up is required. If CIN 3 or carcinoma is suspected, biopsy is recommended. There is no evidence that taking a biopsy of the cervix during pregnancy will jeopardise it in any way [4]. There is a theoretical risk that abnormalities may worsen during pregnancy due to the woman's altered immune status. This emphasises the need for close follow-up and senior input for pregnant patients. Women with high-grade dysplasia in pregnancy should be seen by an experienced colposcopist.

Follow-up appointments for low-grade lesions can be delayed until after pregnancy. However, it is advisable that assessment should not be delayed if the first appointment for follow-up cytology or colposcopy is following treatment for CGIN. The "test of cure" appointment should not be delayed after treatment for CIN 2 or CIN 3 with involved or uncertain margin status [6]. On a practical note, colposcopy whilst a woman is breast-feeding can be unsatisfactory due to the relative hypo-oestrogenic state of the vaginal epithelium.

8.2.10 HPV Primary Screening

HPV testing as a primary method of screening is expected to be more sensitive than cytology, resulting in an increased detection of CIN 2+ lesions. It may also allow the screening interval to be extended for HPV-negative women [9]. Initial evidence led to a pilot of HPV testing as primary screening in six sites across England that previously acted as pilot and sentinel sites for HPV triage.

These studies found the total referral rates were significantly higher for HPV primary screening than for primary cytology for all ages combined. This was especially evident in the younger age group (25–49), but slightly lower in the age group 50–64 [9].

The planned triaging flow will depend on the hr-HPV result. If the result is negative, then the patient can be returned to routine screening. However, if the result proves positive, then a cytological examination will be performed. A referral to colposcopy will be arranged if there is any degree of cytological abnormality. If the cytology is negative, HPV testing will be repeated in 1 year. If again positive and the cytology is negative, the test will be repeated in 1 year. If after the third test the cytology is still negative despite a positive HPV result, a referral to colposcopy will be arranged [10]. Within the study 8.6% of women tested were HPV positive/cytology negative and scheduled for recall at 12 months. After retesting, 40% had become HPV negative, 21% were referred (either due to abnormal cytology or persistent HPV 16 or 18) and 38% remain on nonroutine recall. The study suggested the detection rate of CIN 2+ for all ages is significantly higher with HPV primary screening (1.25 vs 1.09, $p < 0.001$), as is the detection rate of CIN 3+ (0.82% vs 0.72%, $p < 0.01$) [9].

Therefore, the evidence for screening by HPV primary testing achieves a higher detection rate of CIN 2 or worse, with a small increase also in the number of referrals to colposcopy. The NHS screening programme is planning to convert to this protocol in 2019.

Primary HPV testing might also be beneficial outside of a screening programme in patients who fail to attend for their cervical cytology screening. One randomised trial investigated whether women who do not attend for cervical screening are more likely to respond to the opportunity to collect a self-sample for HPV. Three thousand women from London were randomly selected if they had missed two or more invitations for cervical screening. The women were randomised to either receive another invitation for cervical cytology or an HPV self-sampling kit. There was a 10.2% response rate in those offered self-sampling compared to 4.5% in the group invited for conventional cytology sampling. This was shown to be statistically significant ($P < 0.0001$). In the self-sampling group, eight tested positive for HPV; seven attended for a cervical smear and at the same time had a colposcopic assessment. Three of these cases (43%) had CIN 2+, and one case was diagnosed with invasive cancer (stage 1b) and one CIN 3 [11]. This study suggested self-sampling could have a role in patients who are otherwise missing cytological screening.

8.2.11 Cytology in Adolescents and Young Women

As stated above, a balance must be struck between sensitivity in detection of preinvasive or invasive disease and the avoidance of unnecessary assessment which may provide a burden on patients in the form of anxiety or overtreatment. Cytological examination is not a diagnostic test, and clinical concerns of cervical pathology should be referred to colposcopy for a diagnostic procedure. Therefore, cytology will be applied to an asymptomatic population. There is a concern regarding the timing a screening programme should start, as the prevalence of HPV infection is high but the rate of high-grade preinvasive lesions is low. It is very rare for women under 25 years to develop cervical cancer. In 2007, 56 cases of cervical cancer were registered among women aged 15–24 in England and Wales [13]. There were three reported deaths in the same period.

The problem is that the prevalence of transient HPV infection after coitarche is high. Almost one in six cervical cytology samples obtained in this age group is abnormal. However, much of this disease is likely to be low grade and consequently will resolve spontaneously [13]. Screening this age group thus leads to unnecessary attendances at colposcopy. This is associated with increased anxiety, overtreatment and potentially negative consequences for future pregnancies. Furthermore, screening has not been shown to be effective at reducing the incidence of invasive cancer in women under the age of 25 [6].

The association between surgical treatment of CIN and subsequent preterm birth has been a topic of great interest recently. Meta-analysis suggested that women post LLETZ (large loop excision of transformation zone) are at approximately twice the risk of a preterm birth than pregnant women in general [12]. A study from England, and a recent meta-analysis, found a lower relative risk and no association after adjusting for confounding factors. Further recent research suggests that the increased risk of late miscarriage/premature labour might be associated with large loop excisions alone (10–14 mm and particularly >15 mm) and that the reason for the lack of association in some studies was that the majority of women treated had small excisions performed.

Therefore, data suggests that abnormal cytology in the younger age group, i.e. <25 years old, does not correlate well with invasive disease. Also, the impact of treatment on subsequent pregnancies needs to be considered. For these reasons routine screening is not recommended, but if a clinical suspicion arises, a referral for diagnostic tests should be considered [6].

8.3 Summary

Cervical cytology has proved to be a very successful method for screening for cervical abnormalities. It not only alerts the clinician to the presence of premalignant conditions which are not routinely visible without colposcopy but also helps guide management. This is done by triaging how rapidly a patient should be seen and guiding whether aggressive treatment is indicated. Terminologies differ throughout the world, e.g. the UK vs the USA, but principles are very similar. The information in this chapter is designed to be an overall review for management of abnormal cervical cytology, but in practice local or national guidelines should be the reference guide for clinical practice.

Key Points

- Cervical cytology is a screening test for cervical preinvasive conditions.
- Colposcopy and histopathology are the diagnostic tests.
- hr-HPV-positive tests allow triaging of the higher-risk groups to colposcopy.
- hr-HPV-negative tests are reassuring in low-risk groups.
- During colposcopic examination, cytology can help in the detection of CIN2+ disease. This can target management towards diagnostic biopsies or immediate treatment, i.e. "see and treat".
- Screening programmes around the world differ in certain points, and local or national guidelines should be consulted for management.
- Other pathologies might be suggested on cervical cytology which might need investigation or treatment, e.g. infections or non-cervical malignancies.
- Pregnancy can prove a challenge to managing abnormal cytology. If low risk of invasive disease, a conservative approach should be taken.
- Primary HPV screening detects more high-grade lesions than primary cytology screening with a slight increase in colposcopy referrals.

References

1. Jones H, Rock J. Te Linde's operative gynecology. 11th ed. Philadelphia: Wolters Kluwer; 2015.
2. Courtesy of Andreas Wessel-Therhorn.
3. Shafi M, Nazeer S. Colposcopy: a practical guide. 2nd ed. Cambridge: Cambridge University Press; 2012.
4. Bentley J. Colposcopic management of abnormal cervical cytology and histology. J Obstet Gynaecol Can. 2012;34:1188–202.
5. Massad L, Einstein M, Huh W, Katki H, Kinney W, Schiffman M, et al. 2012 update consensus guidelines for the management of abnormal cervical screening tests and cancer precursors. Obstet Gynecol. 2013;121:829–46.
6. Public Health England. NHS cervical screening programme: colposcopy and programme management. London: Public Health England; 2016.
7. Fadare O, Ghofrani M, Chacho M, et al. The significance of benign endometrial cells in cervicovaginal smears. Adv Anat Pathol. 2005;12(5):274–87.
8. Johnson S, Wadehra V. How predictive is a cervical smear suggesting invasive squamous cell carcinoma? Cytopathology. 2001;12:144–50.
9. Moss S, Gibney A. HPV primary screening pilots: evaluation report to the national screening committee. London: Centre for cancer prevention, Wolfson institute, Queen Mary University of London; 2015.
10. Jo's cervical cancer trust. HPV primary screening. 2017. http://www.jostrust.org.uk/about-cervical-cancer/cervical-screening-smear-test-and-abnormal-cells/primary-hpv-testing. Accessed Dec 2017.
11. Szarewski A, Cadman L, Mesher D, Austin J, Ashdown-Barr L, Edwards R, et al. HPV self-sampling as an alternative strategy in non-attenders for cervical screening – a randomised controlled trial. Br J Cancer. 2011;104:915–20.
12. Sasieni P, Castanon A, Landy R, Kyrgiou M, Kitchener H, Quigley M, et al. Risk of preterm birth following surgical treatment for cervical disease: executive summary of a recent symposium. BJOG. 2016;123(9):1426–9.
13. Willmott F, Ritchie S, Chenoy R. Key questions on cervical cancer. Pulse Magazine. 5/11/2014. http://pulse-learning.co.uk/clinical-modules/cancer/key-questions-cervical-cancer.

HPV Infection: Pathogenesis and Detection

9

Pakhee Aggarwal

9.1 Introduction

Human papillomavirus (HPV) infections are one of the most common sexually transmitted infections (STIs) across the world. There are more than 150 types of HPV, of which about 40 are known to affect humans [1]. HPV can be subgrouped into cutaneous types and mucosal types based on the tissue tropism. Cutaneous types infect keratinizing epithelium, e.g., skin of hands/feet, and are linked to warts (plantar warts, flat warts, common warts) on the hands, face, and feet. The mucosal types infect nonkeratinizing epithelium, e.g., mucosa of anogenital tract, oral mucosa, conjunctiva, and respiratory tract [2]. The mucosal HPV types are further classified into high-risk and low-risk types, based on whether they cause cancerous or benign changes in the tissues affected [3].

The high-risk oncogenic types are linked to cervical, vaginal, vulvar, and anal cancer in women and penile, anal, and oropharyngeal cancer in men [4]. The low-risk non-oncogenic types are responsible for warts and other benign pathologies in both sexes (Table 9.1).

Although HPV infection is easily acquired, most infections are subclinical and transient [5]. Detection of HPV infection in the asymptomatic population is by screening or when persistent HPV infection causes clinical manifestations like warts or cancer. Since HPV infection is not a notifiable infection (unlike HIV or certain other STDs), its true incidence is difficult to estimate, but the prevalence of asymptomatic infection varies from 2 to 44%, depending on the population and region [6].

Table 9.1 Mucosal HPV types

Mucosal HPV	HPV types	Associated diseases
Low-risk	6, 11	Low-grade cellular changes; genital warts (condylomata acuminata, smooth papules, flat papules, keratotic warts); lesions on oral, upper respiratory, upper gastrointestinal, and ocular sites; recurrent respiratory papillomatosis
High-risk	16, 18, 31, 33, 45, 52, 58	High-grade cellular changes, anogenital (i.e., cervical, vulvar, vaginal, anal) and oropharyngeal cancer

HPV infection is common in the general population and also found in immune-compromised people. The virus is transmitted by direct contact with an infected tissue or through fomites. In general, the infection resolves spontaneously within 1–5 years. This chapter is focused on the pathogenesis of HPV infection and how it can be detected in the asymptomatic population.

To better understand the pathogenesis of HPV infection, one needs to be familiar with the structure and life cycle of the virus. This is also important so that we may know how and when to detect HPV.

P. Aggarwal (✉)
Department of Obstetrics and Gynaecology, Fortis Memorial Research Institute, Gurugram, Haryana, India

S. Mehta, A. Singla (eds.), *Preventive Oncology for the Gynecologist*, https://doi.org/10.1007/978-981-13-3438-2_9

9.2 HPV: Structure and Life Cycle

9.2.1 Structure of Human Papillomavirus

It is a non-enveloped DNA virus, having an icosahedral outer shell composed of L1 and L2 capsid proteins and a single molecule of double-stranded, circular DNA as its genome. The HPV genome is functionally divided into three regions [7]:

1. A noncoding upstream regulatory region (URR) or long control region (LCR). This regulates DNA replication by controlling the transcription of the "early" and "late" regions through enhancer and silencer sequences.
2. An "early" region which includes the genes E1, E2, E3, E4, E5, E6, E7, and E8. The expression of these is important for determining whether an HPV infection would be active or latent or would undergo malignant transformation. The early region is involved in viral replication and oncogenesis.
3. A "late" region, which encodes the L1 and L2 structural proteins for the viral capsid.

The vital functions of these genes in the early and late regions in the HPV genome are outlined in Table 9.2.

Table 9.2 Functions of the HPV genome

Gene	Function
E1	Viral DNA replication
E2	Modulation of viral transcription, DNA replication, and segregation of viral genomes
E3, E8	Unknown
E4	Controlling virus maturation and release of virions (productive viral infections)
E5	Enhances transforming activity of E6/E7
E6	Oncoprotein; interaction with p53 protein
E7	Oncoprotein; interaction with pRB protein
L1	Major capsid protein
L2	Minor capsid protein

9.2.2 Life Cycle of HPV

HPV infection in humans has a predilection for the mucosa, e.g., genital HPV has a predilection for the genital mucosa and skin, and its replication is closely linked to the replication and differentiation process of the host cell. There is some evidence to indicate that due to the anatomical, histological, physiological, and immunological features of the transformation zone, this is a vulnerable site of entry of the HPV infection [8].

The life cycle of HPV can be divided into two phases [9]:

1. Maintenance phase: infection enters the body through sexual intercourse and begins as an infliction of the basal layer of the stratified squamous epithelium. It is presumed that the infection requires microtrauma or abrasion of the epithelium to enter. The basal layer of the stratified squamous epithelium contains stem cells, which divide periodically, with one daughter cell migrating upward to undergo terminal differentiation and the other remaining in the basal layer as a slow-cycling, self-renewing population [10]. Once the infection gains access to the basal layer, a productive infection begins, wherein the viral genome is maintained in the basal cells at a stable level with a low copy number. This is also the reservoir to develop a viral wart [11]. Viral DNA replication is supported by early HPV genes, and the cells infected with HPV can be sustained in the lesion for a long period. These infected daughter cells migrate upward to the surface, and viral late gene products (L1 and L2) are produced, which causes the viral DNA to be packaged into capsids, and progeny virions are released to reinitiate infection in sexual contacts. In benign lesions caused by HPV, viral DNA is located extrachromosomally (episomal DNA) in the nucleus.

   At this stage, though there is amplification of the viral genome, the viral DNA is yet to integrate in the host genome, and the infection

Table 9.3 HPV infection and its clinical correlates

Variables	hr HPV infection	hr HPV persistence	hr HPV persistence	hr HPV persistence
Type of HPV infection	Transient/latent hr HPV infection	Productive hr HPV infection	Transforming hr HPV infection	Transforming hr HPV infection
CIN (Richart)	Normal	CIN1	CIN2/CIN3	Invasive carcinoma
Dysplasia (WHO)	Normal	Mild-moderate dysplasia	Moderate-severe dysplasia, CIS	Invasive carcinoma
Cytology (Bethesda)	NILM	ASCUS-LSIL	HSIL	Invasive carcinoma

is a "productive infection," which cytologically and histologically corresponds to LSIL and CIN1, respectively [12]. As there is no cellular transformation in this vegetative phase of the HPV life cycle, the body can still clear this infection. This is outlined in Table 9.3.

2. Differentiation-dependent phase: in a small percentage of women with persistent HPV infection, the virus integrates with the host genome, leading to what is called a "transforming infection." Once the integration of HPV DNA is complete, it results in deletion and loss of expression of E2 region [13]. This interferes with the function of E2, which in the normal course of events is to downregulate the transcription of the E6 and E7 genes. This leads to an increased expression of E6 and E7 genes. The overexpression of early genes results in increased production of the E6 and E7 proteins. This results in increased proliferation of the squamous epithelium. This cytologically and histologically corresponds to HSIL and CIN2/3, respectively. This is depicted in Table 9.3. At a molecular level, the host cell machinery is used by the HPV to encode for viral proteins. Overexpression of viral early genes E6 and E7 in proliferating cells alters the viral life cycle [14]. The suprabasal differentiated cells reenter into S-phase of the cell cycle caused by the early proteins E6 and E7. This activates the host replication machinery needed for amplification of viral genomes for virion synthesis. There is a continuous mode of DNA replication, DNA amplification to high copy number, capsid synthesis, and viral assembly. The virus copy number increases from 50 to 200 copies to several thousands of copies per cell [9].

9.3 Pathogenesis of HPV Infection

Most sexually active men and women will acquire the infection at some point in their lives, but majority of them will clear the infection without manifesting any symptoms. At 12 months, 66% of all infections and at 24 months 90% of all infections are cleared by immune-competent individuals [15, 16]. This also means that 10% of the women will have a persistent infection that can predispose to cancer.

The incubation period of the infection, i.e., time from acquiring the infection to the development of clinical manifestations, can be anywhere from weeks to months for genital warts, months to years for cervical abnormalities, and years to decades for cervical cancer. This is a variable process continuing back and forth from clearance of HPV infection, persistence of HPV infection, progression to precancer, regression of precancer, and progression to invasive cancer based on the immune status and other risk factors of the patient (Fig. 9.1). Certain conditions like immunosuppression, older age, and multiple partners increase the risk of persistent infections. It is difficult to distinguish persistent HPV infection from clearance followed by reinfection, although reinfection with the same HPV type appears to be uncommon [9]. Also, when the levels

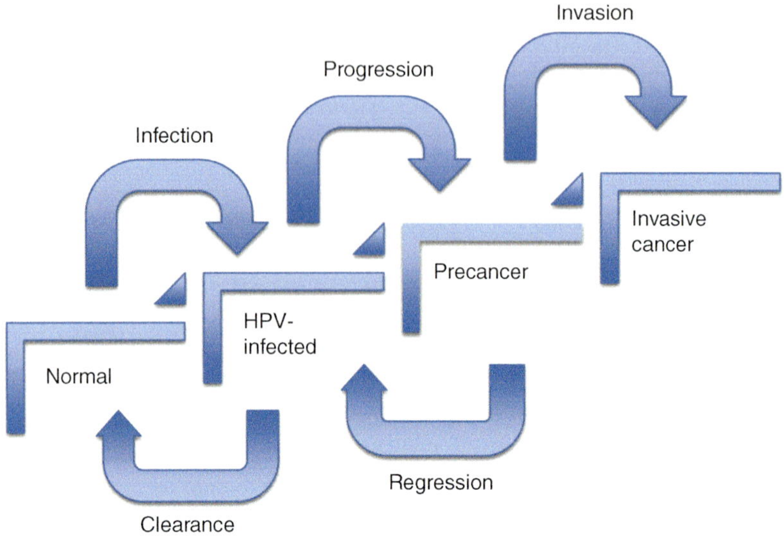

Fig. 9.1 HPV infection cycle

are below the threshold of detection of assays due to viral latency, the HPV infection may go undetected [17].

In precancerous changes due to persistent HPV infection, CIN1 and some CIN2 lesions show relatively low levels of E6 and E7 expression (in which the viral genome replicates episomally), whereas invasive cancer, CIN3, and some CIN2 lesions have high levels of E6 and E7 expression (due to integration of viral DNA into the host cell genome) [18].

The frequency of integration varies between the high-risk HPV types. For example, HPV 16, 18, and 45 are found more often in the integrated state compared to HPV 31 and 33. Because of this, precancers induced by the former HPV types progress to invasive cervical cancer much faster compared to the latter [19].

In addition, two features in the HPV life cycle indirectly contribute to carcinogenesis. First, replicative phase of HPV occurs in differentiated epithelial cells, which are not usually involved in DNA synthesis as they have exited the cell cycle [20]. This means that the viral DNA replication and assembly occur in a cell that will be terminally differentiated and die by natural causes. As a result, the virus lies dormant for many months to years, during which time, host defense mechanisms apparently remain unaware of the pathogen and the immune response generated is insufficient to eliminate the virus, thus developing persistent infection. As the terminal keratinocyte is already programmed to die, HPV replication and release do not cause cell death and inflammation and thus escape recognition. Also, due to the absence of viremia, cell lysis, necrosis, or any other inflammatory signals, there is an inadequate humoral immune response [21]. The viral infectious cycle is confined to the intraepithelial compartment, thus there is no viremia or spread through blood and lymphatics, and thus cellular immunity is not activated. But since they require the host machinery and cellular enzymes to replicate while at the same time maintaining differentiation, they require the help of E6 and E7 proteins. However, any disruption in this process can lead to immortalization of cells. Even so, integration is not a normal part of the HPV life cycle. Integration of high-risk HPV genomes represents a noteworthy event associated with progression from preneoplastic lesions to invasive cancer [22].

Second, the site of DNA replication within the epithelium in high- and low-risk HPV types differs. In low-risk HPV, DNA replication is initiated in the less differentiated cell population where elements of the cellular DNA replication machinery are still present. In high-risk HPV, this replication occurs in more differentiated cells and thus requires more forceful priming of the cell division machinery [20].

Thus, in a transforming infection, protein products of viral genes result in altered expression of cell cycle and DNA repair regulators, enhancing the oncogenic potential of the infection by immortalization, genomic instability, and malignant transformation. Essential to the pathogenesis of HPV is the role of oncoproteins E6 and E7 which are described below.

Role of E6 The E6 protein binds and degrades p53, which is a tumor-suppressor gene product, thus resulting in inhibition of apoptosis [23]. This anti-apoptotic activity of E6 is of critical significance in the development of cervical cancer, as this compromise in the process cellular DNA damage repair allows the accumulation of secondary mutations to go unchecked and predisposes to cancer [24]. The degradation of p53 or blocking of its function by E6 consequently inhibits the apoptotic signaling that would destroy the HPV-infected cell in the usual course of events. The E6 protein is able to disrupt both extrinsic and intrinsic pathways to facilitate a protective environment and prevent cell death.

Low-risk HPV E6 proteins do not bind p53 at detectable levels and have no effect on p53 stability in vitro. The high-risk HPV E6 in addition to binding p53 has another function that is important for immortalization. This is the ability to activate the expression of the catalytic subunit of telomerase (hTERT). Thus, the E6 protein is able to promote the maintenance of the telomere, through the action of telomerase [25].

Role of E7 The E7 protein drives cells into S-phase as it binds and inactivates the retinoblastoma protein (pRB), which is a tumor-suppressor protein, thus resulting in progression of the cell cycle [26]. This results in increased cellular DNA synthesis and cell proliferation. The E7 protein from low-risk HPV types has lower affinity to pRB. It also results in upregulation of p16 expression. These lead to uncontrolled cellular proliferation which is no longer controlled at G1/S transition.

Malignant progression occurs when additional mutations are accumulated over time, e.g., ras or fos genes. This is also why cervical cancer occurs many years after the initial HPV infection, indicating that although HPV infection is essential for initiation of the process, the culmination to cancer occurs only when host genome mutations accumulate over time [27].

Infection with HPV causes cellular growth, thereby increasing the demand for nutrients and oxygen. To overcome this, angiogenesis is induced by increased activity of hypoxia-inducible factor-1 (HIF-1) and its target genes. It is this activity which is responsible for persistence of infection with HPV [28].

The increase in cellular proliferation and genomic instability leads to increased amount of damaged DNA which cannot be repaired, thus transforming cells into malignancy. Supplementary to this chromosome instability, other potential mechanisms for carcinogenesis are methylation of viral and cellular DNA, telomerase activation, and immunogenetic factors. Both humoral and cellular responses can be elicited by oncoproteins E6 and E7, and so they can play an important role in therapeutics [29].

Supplementary Role of E5 HPV infection also leads to formation of tetraploid cells by inducing cell fusion and failure of cytokinesis, thus causing aneuploidy [15]. Tetraploid cells formed by accident cannot undergo normal mitosis and thus are unresponsive to p53-induced apoptosis. This chromosomal instability favors integration of HPV genomes, further leading to generation of viral-cellular fusion transcripts and expression of the E6-E7 genes. Thus, the role of E5-induced cell fusion is in the early stage of development of HPV-associated cervical cancer, rather than tumor maintenance [30].

The endogenous interferon response, which is important in activating the innate immunity, is inhibited by infection with high-risk HPV. In the absence of this, the adaptive immunity is also not activated, effectively creating an HPV antigen-tolerant milieu. There is decreased expression of pro-inflammatory cytokines (IL-1, IL-6, TNF-α, and TGF-β) and increased expression of anti-inflammatory cytokine (IL-10) [31]. Development of HPV-specific T-cell response is also suppressed due to the downregulation of major histocompatibility complex (MHC) I expression [32].

9.4 Detection of HPV Infection

After acquiring the infection, it can be detected by the commercially available tests for a period of up to 1 year [33]. More than 90% of cervical and anal cancers are caused by HPV. Approximately 70% of vulvar, vaginal, and oropharyngeal cancers are also linked to infection with HPV [34].

HPV infection is diagnosed using clinical (warts) and molecular evidence of infection. Immunological evidence of HPV infection is difficult due to the innate life cycle of HPV wherein late (capsid) proteins are only expressed in productive infections and early proteins are expressed in low amounts in infected tissues and lack of a robust antibody response to the viral infection.

Since the HPV cannot be grown in tissue culture, its detection is dependent on the detection of viral nucleic acids (DNA or RNA) using molecular techniques like nucleic acid probe technology and DNA sequencing. In addition to knowing whether high-risk HPV (hr HPV) infection is present, there is also an increasing need to know the type of hr HPV infection (genotyping). The potential advantages of genotyping are:

1. Certain HPV types are more linked to certain cancers, e.g., HPV 18 to adenocarcinoma (AC) and adenocarcinoma in situ (AIS) and HPV 16 to both squamous cell carcinoma (SCC) and AC [35].
2. Some infections have multiple HPV genotypes, and knowing the proportion of each is sometimes relevant.
3. Genotyping is crucial after rolling out a vaccination program to know the efficacy of prophylactic vaccines in reducing the prevalence of infection types covered by the vaccine.
4. In the clinical scenario, HPV genotyping may have prognostic significance in monitoring the response to treatment (LEEP/cryotherapy). The same strain of HPV in the posttreatment follow-up smear as in the pretreatment sample may indicate inadequate removal or inability of the body to clear the infection (more severe consequences), while a different strain may indicate reinfection (less severe consequences).
5. Multiple HPV genotypes are found in about a third of the HPV-infected patients and in half of those with HIV positivity [36]. Multiple genotypes are less common in those with carcinoma.

There are three main types of detection methods currently in use—non-amplified hybridization assays, signal-amplification techniques, and target amplification techniques [37]. These are discussed in detail below and outlined in Table 9.4.

I. Non-Amplified Hybridization Assays These include Southern blot for DNA, Northern blot for RNA, dot blot hybridization, and in situ hybridization (ISH). There are some disadvantages with the first three of these methods that is why they are not commonly used. Mainly, it is the requirement of large amounts of purified DNA to perform analysis, labor-intensive process, poorly reproducible and having only moderate sensitivity [38]. They cannot be run on fixed tissues where the DNA has degraded. ISH, on the other hand, can be run on processed and fixed tissues. It identifies specific

Table 9.4 Types of HPV tests

Technique of HPV testing	Commercially available tests
Non-amplified hybridization assay	Southern blot, Northern blot, Dot blot, In situ hybridization
Signal-amplification assay	HC2 (and care HPV), Cervista HPV
Nucleic acid amplification assay	Amplicor, PapilloCheck microarray, Clinical arrays HPV test, INNO-LiPA, Linear Array HPV genotyping, Luminex microarray (MCHA), real-time PCR (Abbott RT-PCR, Cobas 4800, GenoID), genome sequencing, CLART HPV 2, HPV E6/E7 mRNA (PreTect Proofer, NucliSENS EasyQ HPV, APTIMA HPV)

nucleotide sequences with conserved morphology in cell or tissue sections, thereby determining the spatial location of target genomes in the specimen [39]. The sensitivity of ISH can be improved by combining it with PCR (known as in situ PCR) [40]. ISH can be used to detect mRNA as a marker of gene expression [41].

II. Signal-Amplification Techniques These can be liquid phase or morphological techniques and are based on the technique of amplification of signals generated by DNA/RNA hybrids and DNA in situ hybridization, respectively. These are non-PCR-based tests. Two commonly used tests are HC2 and Cervista HPV.

a. Hybrid Capture (HC2®) (Qiagen, USA, *formerly Digene Co.*): It is FDA approved and detects DNA from 13 hr HPV to 5 lr HPV types at sensitivity of 5000 copies of HPV genome per reaction well using the technique of chemiluminescence to detect RNA/DNA hybrids [42]. It uses RNA probes complimentary to the genomic sequence of 13 hr HPV and 5 lr HPV types, which are used to prepare high- and low-probe cocktails. DNA present in the specimen is hybridized with each of the probe cocktails leading to the formation of RNA/DNA hybrids. These bind to the antibodies in the reaction well that are programmed to bind the RNA/DNA hybrids. The final detection is using a luminometer to detect the intensity of emitted light by the hybrid product. The amount of light (in relative light units—RLU) gives an indirect/semiquantitative measurement of the amount of hr HPV DNA present in the specimen. Usually only the high-probe mix is used (as it more clinically relevant) which reduces the cost of the test. More than or equal to 1 RLU (which equals 1 pg of DNA per ml of buffer) is considered a positive test. It is performed in a 96-well microtiter plate, which can run many automated samples in one go. Another advantage is that it is not susceptible to cross-contamination, as it does not use PCR to amplify the DNA [43]. This assay distinguishes between hr HPV and lr HPV but is not able to tell the specific type of HPV (genotyping). Genotyping is important, as the risk of high-grade changes is 10–15% with HPV 16/18 and less than 3% for all other hr HPV types combined [44].

   A recently developed low-cost assay, for use in low-resource countries (*careHPV*®, Qiagen NV), uses RNA probes (like HC2) to detect 14 hr HPV types. It is a rapid point-of-care test that takes about 2.5 h to perform and does not require specialized laboratory or staff. It was clinically validated in a large study in rural China and found to have an accuracy of 90% in detecting premalignant lesions [45].

   To reduce cross-reactivity, an automated third-generation Hybrid Capture assay has been introduced recently. It is based on biotin-labeled oligonucleotide sequences for capture of target regions [46].
b. Cervista® HPV (Hologic Inc., Marlborough, USA) detects the presence of 14 hr HPV types (Cervista® HPV HR and Genfind® DNA Extraction) with or without individual genotyping for HPV 16/18 (Cervista® HPV 16/18). It is more sensitive than HC2 and has a lesser false-positive rate [47]. It is also FDA approved.

III. Target Amplification Techniques These are PCR-based assays that amplify the target segments of HPV DNA and aid detection of hr HPV types and specific genotypes. This assay relies on a thermostable DNA polymerase, type-specific or general/consensus primers, which bind to and replicate the area of interest. After several cycles of replication, the viral DNA is amplified sufficiently in vitro to allow it to be visualized. This amplification can be real time (which can help to quantify viral load) using reverse hybridization techniques. Theoretically, PCR can detect a single copy of the target sequence in the reaction tube as it is highly sensitive and specific. In practice, the sensitivity is 100–1000 genome equivalents per reaction tube (i.e., 10–100 HPV genomes in a background of 100 ng of cellular DNA). Due to this PCR can be performed even in specimens that have a low DNA content. PCR has the advantage of generating one billion copies after just 30 cycles of replication, from a single double-stranded DNA molecule [38]. Detection of HPV using PCR can be done using primers. Primers can be of three types:

1. Type-specific primers (which will amplify specific HPV genotypes): they are more expensive and time-consuming than using consensus primers.
2. General/consensus primers: these are based on the conserved regions common to all HPV genotypes, generally the long control region L1 or E6/E7 regions [48, 49]. Commonly used consensus primers are GP5/6 pair, and its extended set GP5+/6+ pair aimed at L1 region and MY09/11 degenerate primers and its modified version, PGMY09/11 [50]. The disadvantage of using degenerate primers like MY09/11 is a large batch-to-batch variation and poor reproducibility [51]. The modified primers, PGMY09/11, have more consistency and better sensitivity for a large number of HPV genotypes [46].
3. Combined primers: contain inosine which matches with any nucleotide and can target the location of the viral genome with accuracy and reproducibility.

In any PCR reaction, the efficiency is inversely proportional to the size of the amplicon or PCR product. The smaller the size of amplicon, the more is the efficiency of the PCR, especially when the DNA sample is degraded or low in quantity [52]. In addition, the sensitivity and specificity of the individual PCR-based method depend on the primer set, reaction conditions, function of DNA polymerase, HPV types amplified, and the ability to detect multiple or specific types of HPV. To reduce the false-positive rates from DNA contamination, strict PCR protocols need to be followed. Once the PCR is run and the products are amplified, they can be analyzed by restriction fragment length polymorphism (RFLP) and plated on agarose gel [53]. Another way is to use type-specific probes using enzyme immune assay (EIA). The PCR product is hybridized onto the chip and read using a DNA chip scanner. This has a high sensitivity (more than 90%) and can be used to identify the type of HPV as well as multiple infections [54]. However, the disadvantages are the false-negative results if multiple subtypes of HPV are present in the sample with low copy number. Because multiple infections are common, PCR may not detect all the HPV genotypes [55]. To overcome this problem, a simple technique of PCR-RFLP can allow the HPV to be genotyped, at a lower cost and effort [56]. It can also detect multiple HPV types in the same infection and differentiate them into lr HPV and hr HPV. Amplicor® HPV MWP assay (Roche Molecular Systems) was the first commercially available PCR kit using nondegenerate primers, which detected 13 hr HPV without individual genotyping by amplifying a short fragment (170 bp) of the L1 gene using primers. It is more sensitive than HC2 and amenable to high-throughput testing [57].

In addition to DNA, viral mRNA can also be amplified using reverse transcriptase PCR or nucleic acid sequence-based amplification (NASBA). For example, detection of E6/E7 mRNA from the hr HPV types can indicate high specificity for detection of high-grade lesion. One such commercially available assay is the APTIMA® HPV assay, which identifies mRNA from 14 hr HPV types [58]. The PreTect HPV-Proofer (NorChip AS, Norway) uses NASBA amplification of E6/E7 mRNA prior to type-specific detection of 5 hr HPV types.

Various target amplification techniques are:

a. PapilloCheck® microarray analysis: It uses a DNA chip and allows for parallel analysis of multiple DNA samples. Currently, the main role of microarray analysis is in gene expression profiling and mutation analysis [59]. PapilloCheck® is a commercially available microarray chip which detects 24 genotypes of high- and low-risk HPV using a chip scanner. Its advantage is identification of hr HPV and lr HPV for screening [60]. However, it cannot detect HPV types 35 and 53 and is expensive to run [61].
b. Clinical Array Technology (CLART)® HPV kit (Genomica SAU, Spain): It is a commercially available test kit, which uses the human

cystic fibrosis transmembrane conductance regulator (CFTR) gene plasmids to check the PCR method and DNA integrity, detecting 35 hr HPV types [62].

Both these methods are based on a prior target sequence amplification by PCR followed by hybridization using labeled type-specific oligonucleotide probes fixed on a chip/slide or solid support. After DNA hybridization, an automatic detection system can be used to determine the possible presence of up to 42 different HPV genotypes [46].

c. INNO-LiPA® (LiPA HBV GT; Innogenetics NV, Ghent, Belgium): In this test part of the L1 region of the HPV genome is amplified using SPF10 primers. This short PCR fragment (SPF-PCR) is designed to discriminate between a broad spectrum of HPVs in a reverse line blot hybridization (LiPA) which is interpreted visually. The position of the blot is related to the HPV genotype. The INNO-LiPA HPV Genotyping v2® test detects 11 hr HPV and 5 lr HPV, while Genotyping Extra® can detect 22 hr HPV and 6 lr HPV types [63]. It can be used on cervical swab specimens but is less efficacious than real-time PCR [64].
d. Linear Array® HPV Genotyping (Roche Molecular Diagnostics, Pleasanton, USA): It is a PCR-based assay using PGMY09/11 amplification system coupled with reverse line blot hybridization. It can detect 37 HPV types including the 15 most common hr HPV types. This is done using the Auto-LiPA instrument (Innogenetics, Ghent, Belgium), which uses colored signals on strips than can easily be interpreted as per the Linear Array® reference guide [65].
e. Microplate colorimetric hybridization assay® (MCHA) (Boehringer Mannheim, Germany)/ Luminex microarray technology: It allows high-throughput, simultaneous identification and quantification of 6 hr HPV types using PCR-based technology and colorimetric hybridization with type-specific probes attached to dyed polystyrene beads. These are then passed through a Luminex analyzer in order to determine the spectral signatures indicative of specific HPV genotypes [66]. It has a high analytical sensitivity, specificity, and reproducibility for identifying HPV 16/18 as well as 31/33/45 and somewhat less for HPV 39. Probes for other HPV types can be added [67].
f. Real-time PCR: "In-house" real-time PCR can detect viral load as well as HPV genotypes from a very small concentration of nucleic acids using fluorescence to detect the HPV. It can simultaneously amplify different nucleic acid targets. It can be run on both tissue samples and cellular slides. It is rapid, reliable, sensitive, specific, and validated for use for screening in high-throughput testing [68]. Examples of real-time PCR tests are:
   - Abbott® RT-PCR, which detects HPV 16/18 as well as other 12 high-risk genotypes (pooled) [69]. It serves a dual diagnostic purpose of hr HPV screening and viral genotyping in the same test.
   - Cobas® 4800 (Roche Molecular Systems, Pleasanton, USA) HPV test also uses real-time PCR to detect 14 hr HPV types from a single sample. It detects HPV 16, HPV 18, and HPV 12 pooled hr HPV types [70]. It is easy to use and gives rapid results (within 4 h), making it suitable for screening. It is reliable and clinically validated to detect hr HPV and for ASCUS triage [71]. It is FDA approved.
   - GenoID® real-time PCR assay, which amplifies the L1 region of HPV and detects non-integrated copies of HPV. It detects 15 hr HPV and 6 lr HPV with a sensitivity of 100 infected cells [72].
g. HPV genome sequencing: There are two techniques for this. The first is the traditional Sanger technique [73] and its subsequent modification using fluorescent dyes (both of which have not been clinically validated), and the second is using pyrosequencing. This technique can be applied to any source of DNA or RNA that can be amplified by PCR, be it fresh or formalin-fixed. This latter method has several advantages over the former. It is easy to decipher readout in real time, inexpensive, rapid, and quantitative [74].

h. CLART® Human Papillomavirus 2 (Genomica, Madrid, Spain): It can detect 35 HPV DNA types in a semiquantitative manner using PCR technology. It is a highly sensitive (98%) and specific test (nearly 100%) [75].
i. HPV E6/E7 mRNA: Because of the role of E6/E7 mRNA in cervical carcinogenesis, their detection has a stronger correlation with cervical disease than detection of HPV DNA alone [76]. There are three commercially available assays:
   - PreTect® HPV-Proofer assay (NorChip AS, Norway): It has high sensitivity and specificity and is based on real-time PCR (real-time nucleic acid sequence-based amplification assay (NASBA)) [77]. It detects E6/E7 mRNA from 5 hr HPV types (HPV 16/18/31/33/45).
   - NucliSENS® EasyQ HPV (bioMerieux): It also detects E6/E7 mRNA from 5 hr HPV types (HPV 16/18/31/33/45) [78].
   - APTIMA® HPV assay (Gen-Probe, San Diego, USA) which detects HPV E6/E7 mRNA from 14 hr HPV types. Thus it is more sensitive than PreTect Proofer assay [79]. In addition, it is fully automated, does not cross react with lr HPV, has lower limits of detection, and can predict advancement of disease more accurately. It is FDA approved.

Detecting E6/E7 mRNA has been found to be more specific in detecting individuals that develop high-grade disease rather than HPV DNA detection by PCR with GP5+/6+ consensus primers [80]. There is a significant association between E6/E7 oncogene transcripts and severity of disease on cytology and histology, for both HPV 16 and 18. Also, this identifies persistent hr HPV infections without having to perform repeated testing [81].

In addition, one can determine the HPV DNA viral load and markers for HPV DNA integration as markers for HPV infection.

1. *HPV DNA Viral Load*: It can be determined using quantitative real-time PCR and semi-quantitatively using HC2. It rises as the severity of disease on cytology and histology worsens [82]. The best correlation is seen with HPV 16 infection [83]. There is a positive correlation of HPV 16 and 31 DNA load with severity of disease and a fair to poor correlation of HPV 18 and 33 DNA with severity of disease [84]. Viral load declines with therapy and can guide further management. High viral load production occurs in severe disease but is the effect rather than the cause [85].
2. *HPV DNA Integration*: In the initial phase of infection, HPV DNA lies extrachromosomally in the cell. However, during the process of integration, it becomes intrachromosomal. This causes changes in the expression of several viral genes, all toward one aim of persistence and dissemination of infection [86]. Viral integration occurs earlier than even morphological changes, such that viral integration may not always correspond to high-grade lesion as the molecular events predate clinical events [87]. HPV integration is detected using real-time PCR, which can calculate the ratio of E2 and E6/E7 genes. A 1:1 ratio indicates integration [88]. Other methods are FISH and PCR. In the former fluorescent probes are used for TERC gene and MYC gene loci [89]. One of the key functions of E6 is activating telomerase reverse transcriptase (TERT) gene expression on chromosome 5p. Telomerase is located at the ends of chromosomes. It has a structural RNA component (TERC) that serves as a template during telomere elongation and a catalytic subunit (hTERT) that has reverse transcriptase activity. Its purpose is stabilizing and repairing repeated DNA sequences at telomere end of chromosomes [90]. Telomerase can be detected using quantitative RT-PCR. Increase in the catalytic subunit activity is seen in cervical carcinogenesis [91]. PCR can also be used to detect pure integrated DNA, using type-specific E1 and E2 primers but without the site of integration [92].

A protocol for the amplification of papillomavirus oncogene transcripts (APOT) from cervical specimens can allow differentiation of episomal DNA from integrated DNA. In normal cells and early dysplasia, the HPV genomes are episomal, while in advanced dysplasia and invasive cancer, they are integrated into the host cells. Using APOT, a strong correlation between detection of integrated high-risk HPV transcripts and presence of high-grade disease was seen [93]. However, because this technique tests for RNA, and RNA is more labile than DNA, the time and type of specimen storage also influence the results and amount of RNA available for analysis. Collection media that can preserve both RNA and DNA integrities, such as methanol-based liquid media, are preferred [94].

9.5 Which Test to Choose?

The ideal test should have high sensitivity to detect all infections as well as good specificity to avoid unnecessary anxiety to all women who have screened positive. The first is achieved by having a PCR-based test, which has a high sensitivity, and using amplification primers which can detect all variations and integrations in the hr HPV genome and specifically the E6/E7 region which is the most preserved [95]. Low specificity of such testing is then overcome by using secondary triage with E6/E7 mRNA analysis or HPV viral load quantification. In an epidemiological study to know prevalence of HPV or efficacy of vaccination, tests with high sensitivity are used, as the offset in specificity is not important in these settings.

In general, there is good correlation between HC2 and PCR using consensus primers. While testing for more than one HPV type in the biologic specimen is preferentially done by PCR-based method, HC2 is more accurate in HPV detection as low- or high-risk groups and does not distinguish between individual HPV types. Both are suitable to high-throughput testing and automation.

9.6 Samples for HPV Detection

For target amplification methods, which are PCR based, the specimen needs to be such where the nucleic acids are not degraded or exposed to PCR-inhibiting organic solvents. In the LBC media, preservation of nucleic acids occurs, and media like the Universal Collection Medium (UCM) by Qiagen (Digene) do not contain large amounts of organic solvents. Formalin-fixed and paraffin-embedded specimens may have nuclear degradation but no exposure to PCR-inhibiting substances.

For detecting mRNA, special media that preserve the integrity of mRNA as well as DNA (PreservCyt LBC) are needed so that mRNA can be analyzed through RT-PCR and NASBA. Also, mRNA can be detected on biopsy specimens and extracted through special techniques.

For signal-amplification methods, e.g., HC2, the specimen can be both cervical smears and biopsy specimens transported in Specimen Transport Medium (STM) by Qiagen (Digene). This medium destroys cell morphology and causes release of nucleic acids without the use of additional solvents [96]. Cervical smears can also be collected in ThinPrep Medium by Cytyc. This medium preserves cell integrity and requires additional solvents to cause cell lysis and release of DNA. A middle ground between the two is UCM that has the advantages of both. Leftover fluid after preparing an LBC slide can also be used to detect HPV DNA using HC2.

Although the analytic sensitivity of some HPV detection tests is very high (thus useful to know prevalence of HPV infection), its corresponding clinical significance is not. This is because all HPV infections may not persist or lead to clinically relevant disease [97].

Detection of HPV has certain advantages as compared to other methods of screening. First, its high sensitivity and negative predictive value means that very frequent screening can be avoided. Second, detection of HPV DNA in a woman over the age of 30 years puts her at higher risk of developing CIN, and thus appropriate management can be instituted early. Third, the testing itself is objective and automated [98].

9.7 Conclusion

Thus, a deep understanding of the life cycle of HPV and its role in cervical carcinogenesis is important to understand the advantages and limitations of detection methods for HPV. Despite several tests being available, there is no gold standard molecular test. There is a need for testing to become more rapid, automated, low-cost, and easily accessible in all resource situations.

Key Points

- Human papillomavirus (HPV) is one of the most common sexually transmitted infections with more than 150 subtypes, subdivided into low-risk (non-oncogenic) and high-risk (oncogenic) types.
- Low-risk HPV 6/11 cause majority of genital warts; high-risk HPV 16/18 cause 70% of all HPV-associated cervical cancers, with 31/33/45/52/58 accounting for another 10%.
- Most HPV infections, whether low-risk or high-risk, are asymptomatic and transient and resolve spontaneously without any clinical sequelae.
- In persistent infection, unique characteristics of the HPV genome make it a suitable pathogen to infect and transmit disease.
- E6 and E7 protein expression plays a major role in carcinogenesis induced by persistent HPV infection.
- In early precancer (CIN1), the viral genome is episomal (extrachromosomal), while in late precancer (CIN2/3) and invasive cancer, the viral DNA integrates into the host cell genome.
- HPV cannot be grown in culture; hence detection relies on molecular methods.
- Two basic techniques in use are signal amplification (HC2) and target amplification (PCR based).
- Several tests are available but only five are US FDA approved. These are *Digene Hybrid Capture® 2*, QIAGEN (hr HPV and lr HPV); *Cervista® HPV HR* and Genfind® DNA Extraction Hologic (14 hr HPV types); *Cervista® HPV 16/18 Hologic* (HPV 16/18); *Cobas® 4800*, *Roche* (14 hr HPV, specifically HPV 16/18); and *APTIMA®*, *Gen-Probe*, Hologic (E6/E7 mRNA of 14 hr. HPV types).
- In a clinical setting, tests with high sensitivity and good specificity are preferred, with secondary triage by a test which has high specificity. In a population-based/epidemiological setting, tests with high sensitivity are adequate.

References

1. de Villiers EM, Fauquet C, Broker TR, Bernard HU, zur Hausen H. Classification of papillomaviruses. Virology. 2004;324:17–27.
2. Bonnez W, Reichman RC. In: Mandell GL, Bennett JE, Dolin R, editors. Principles and practice of infectious diseases. Philadelphia: Churchill Livingstone; 2000. p. 1630–44.
3. Zur Hausen H. Papillomavirus infections-a major cause of human cancers. Biochem Biophys Acta. 1996;1288:F55–78.
4. Saraiya M, Unger ER, Thompson TD, Lynch CF, Hernandez BY, Lyu CW, et al. US assessment of HPV types in cancers: implications for current and 9-valent HPV vaccines. J Natl Cancer Inst. 2015;107(6):djv086.
5. Bosch FX, de Sanjosé S. The epidemiology of human papillomavirus infection and cervical cancer. Dis Markers. 2007;23(4):213–27.
6. de Sanjosé S, Diaz M, Castellsagué X, Clifford G, Bruni L, Muñoz N, et al. Worldwide prevalence and genotype distribution of cervical human papillomavirus DNA in women with normal cytology: a meta-analysis. Lancet Infect Dis. 2007;7(7):453–9.
7. Gómez DT, Santos JL. Human papillomavirus infection and cervical cancer: pathogenesis and epidemiology. In: Méndez-Vilas A, editor. Communicating current research and educational topics and trends in applied microbiology: Formatex. p. 660–8.
8. Herfs M, Hubert P, Moutschen M, Delvenne P. Mucosal junctions: open doors to HPV and HIV infections? Trends Microbiol. 2011;19(3):114–20.
9. Fernandes JV, Fernandes TAA. In: Broeck DV, editor. Human papillomavirus: biology and pathogenesis, human papillomavirus and related diseases—from bench to bedside—a clinical perspective. London: Intech; 2012. p. 1–39.
10. Watt FM. Epidermal stem cells: markers, patterning and the control of stem cell fate. Philos Trans R Soc Lond Ser B Biol Sci. 1998;353:831–7.
11. Doorbar J. The papillomavirus life cycle. J Clin Virol. 2005;32(S1):S7–15.
12. Ebisch RM, Siebers AG, Bosgraaf RP, Massuger LF, Bekkers RL, Melchers WJ. Triage of high-risk HPV positive women in cervical cancer screening. Expert Rev Anticancer Ther. 2016;16(10):1073–85.
13. Yoshinouchi M, Hongo A, Nakamura K, Kodoma J, Itoh S, Sakai H, et al. Analysis by multiplex PCR of the physical status of human papillomavirus type 16 DNA in cervical cancers. J Clin Microbiol. 1999;37(11):3514–7.
14. Doorbar J, Egawa N, Griffin H, Kranjec C, Murakami I. Human papillomavirus molecular biology and disease association. Rev Med Virol. 2015;25(Suppl 1):2–23.
15. Ho GY, Bierman R, Beardsley L, Chang CJ, Burk RD. Natural history of cervicovaginal papillomavirus infection in young women. N Engl J Med. 1998;338:423–8.

16. Rodriguez AC, Schiffman M, Herrero R, Wacholder S, Hildesheim A, Castle PE, et al. Rapid clearance of human papillomavirus and implications for clinical focus on persistent infections. J Natl Cancer Inst. 2008;100(7):513–7.
17. Baseman JG, Koutsky LA. The epidemiology of human papillomavirus infections. J Clin Virol. 2005;32(Suppl 1):S16–24.
18. von Knebel Doeberitz M. New markers for cervical dysplasia to visualise the genomic chaos created by aberrant oncogenic papillomavirus infections. Eur J Cancer. 2002;38:2229–42.
19. Vinokurova S, Wentzensen N, Kraus I, Klaes R, Driesch C, Melsheimer P, et al. Type-dependent integration frequency of human papillomavirus genomes in cervical lesions. Cancer Res. 2008;68:307–13.
20. Doorbar J, Foo C, Coleman N, Medcalf L, Hartley O, Prospero T, et al. Characterization of events during the late stages of HPV16 infection in vivo using high-affinity synthetic Fabs to E4. Virology. 1997;238(1):40–52.
21. Stanley MA. Immune responses to human papilloma viruses. Indian J Med Res. 2009;130(3):266–76.
22. Pett M, Coleman N. Integration of high-risk human papillomavirus: a key event in cervical carcinogenesis? J Pathol. 2007;212:356–67.
23. Mantovani F, Banks L. The human papillomavirus E6 protein and its contribution to malignant progression. Oncogene. 2001;20:7874–87.
24. Grm HS, Bergant M, Banks L. Human papillomavirus infection, cancer & therapy. Indian J Med Res. 2009;130(3):277–85.
25. Howie HL, Katzenellenbogen RA, Galloway DA. Papillomavirus E6 proteins. Virology. 2009;384(2):324–34.
26. Pang CL, Thierry F. Human papillomavirus proteins as prospective therapeutic targets. Microb Pathog. 2013;58:55–65.
27. Mitelman F, Johansson B, Mertens F. The impact of translocations and gene fusions on cancer causation. Nat Rev Cancer. 2007;7(4):233–45.
28. Bodily JM, Mehta KP, Laimins LA. Human papillomavirus E7 enhances hypoxia-inducible factor 1-mediated transcription by inhibiting binding of histone deacetylases. Cancer Res. 2011;71(3):1187–95.
29. Arbyn M, Anttila A, Jordan J, Ronco G, Schenck U, Segnan N, et al. European guidelines for quality assurance in cervical cancer screening. Second edition-summary document. Ann Oncol. 2010;21(3):448–58.
30. Gao P, Zheng J. High-risk HPV E5-induced cell fusion: a critical initiating event in the early stage of HPV-associated cervical cancer. Virol J. 2010;7:238.
31. Alcocer-Gonzalez JM, Berumen J, Tamez-Guerra R, Bermudez-Morales V, Peralta-Zaragoza O, Hernandez-Pando R, et al. In vivo expression of immunosuppressive cytokines in human papillomavirus—transformed cervical cancer cells. Viral Immunol. 2006;19(3):481–91.
32. van der Burg SH, Palefsky JM. Human immunodeficiency virus and human papilloma virus—why HPV-induced lesions do not spontaneously resolve and why therapeutic vaccination can be successful. J Transl Med. 2009;7:108.
33. Insinga RP, Perez G, Wheeler CM, Koutsky LA, Garland SM, Leodolter S, et al. Incidence, duration, and reappearance of type-specific cervical human papillomavirus infections in young women. Cancer Epidemiol Biomark Prev. 2010;19(6):1585–94.
34. Muñoz N, Bosch FX, Castellsagué X, Díaz M, de Sanjose S, Hammouda D, et al. Against which human papillomavirus types shall we vaccinate and screen? The international perspective. Int J Cancer. 2004;111(2):278–85.
35. Bulk S, Berkhof J, Bulkmans NW, Zielinski GD, Rozendaal L, van Kemenade FJ, et al. Preferential risk of HPV16 for squamous cell carcinoma and of HPV18 for adenocarcinoma of the cervix compared to women with normal cytology in The Netherlands. Br J Cancer. 2006;94(1):171–5.
36. Levi JE, Kleter B, Quint WG, Fink MC, Canto CL, Matsubara R, et al. High prevalence of human papillomavirus (HPV) infections and high frequency of multiple HPV genotypes in human immunodeficiency virus-infected women in Brazil. J Clin Microbiol. 2002;40(9):3341–5.
37. Brink AATP, Snijders PJF, Meijer CJLM. HPV detection methods. Dis Markers. 2007;23:273–81.
38. Zaravinos A, Mammas IN, Sourvinos G, Spandidos DA. Molecular detection methods of human papillomavirus (HPV). Int J Biol Markers. 2009;24(4):215–22.
39. Villa LL. Human papillomavirus. In: Rosenblatt A, Guidi HGC, editors. Laboratory methods for detection of human papillomavirus infection. Berlin: Springer; 2009. p. 23–30.
40. Nuovo GJ, Moritz J, Walsh LL, MacConnell P, Koulos J. Predictive value of human papillomavirus DNA detection by filter hybridization and polymerase chain reaction in women with negative results of colposcopic examination. Am J Clin Pathol. 1992;98(5):489–92.
41. Stoler MH, Wolinsky SM, Whitbeck A, Broker TR, Chow LT. Differentiation-linked human papillomavirus types 6 and 11 transcription in genital condylomata revealed by in situ hybridization with message-specific RNA probes. Virology. 1989;172(1):331–40.
42. Ylitalo N, Sorensen P, Josefsson AM, Magnusson PK, Andersen PK, Pontén J, et al. Consistent high viral load of human papillomavirus 16 and risk of cervical carcinoma in situ: a nested case-control study. Lancet. 2000;355(9222):2194–8.
43. Lorincz A, Anthony J. Advances in HPV detection by hybrid capture. Papillomavirus Rep. 2001;12:145–54.
44. Abreu AL, Souza RP, Gimenes F, Consolaro ME. A review of methods for detect human papillomavirus infection. Virol J. 2012;9:262.
45. Qiao YL, Sellors JW, Eder PS, Bao YP, Lim JM, Zhao FH, et al. A new HPV-DNA test for cervical cancer screening in developing regions: a cross sectional study of clinical accuracy in rural China. Lancet Oncol. 2008;9(10):926–36.

46. Piana A, Sotgiu G, Castiglia P, Pischedda S, Dettori M, Cocuzza C, et al. Molecular methods for the detection of human papillomavirus infection: new insights into their role in diagnostics and epidemiological surveillance. JPH. 2009;7(6):164–71.
47. Einstein MH, Martens MG, Garcia FA, Ferris DG, Mitchell AL, Day SP, et al. Clinical validation of the Cervista HPV HR and 16/18 genotyping tests for use in women with ASC-US cytology. Gynecol Oncol. 2010;118:116–22.
48. Tieben LM, ter Schegget J, Minnaar RP, Bouwes Bavinck JN, Berkhout RJ, Vermeer BJ, et al. Detection of cutaneous and genital HPV types in clinical samples by PCR using consensus primers. J Virol Methods. 1993;42:265–79.
49. Carvalho NO, del Castillo DM, Perone C, Januário JN, Melo VH, Brasileiro FG. Comparison of HPV genotyping by type-specific PCR and sequencing. Mem Inst Oswaldo Cruz. 2010;105:73–8.
50. Gravitt PE, Peyton CL, Alessi TQ, Wheeler CM, Coutlée F, Hildesheim A, et al. Improved amplification of genital human papillomaviruses. J Clin Microbiol. 2000;38(1):357–61.
51. Peyton CL, Schiffman MA, Lorincz AT, Hunt WC, Mielzynska I, Bratti C, et al. Comparison of PCR and hybrid capture-based human papillomavirus detection system using multiple cervical specimen collection strategies. J Clin Microbiol. 1998;36:3248–54.
52. Kado S, Kawamata Y, Shino Y, Kasai T, Kubota K, Iwasaki H, et al. Detection of human papillomaviruses in cervical neoplasias using multiple sets of generic polymerase chain reaction primers. Gynecol Oncol. 2001;81(1):47–52.
53. Grce M, Husnjak K, Skerlev M, Lipozencić J, Pavelić K. Detection and typing of human papillomaviruses by means of polymerase chain reaction and fragment length polymorphism in male genital lesions. Anticancer Res. 2000;20:2097–102.
54. Kim CJ, Jeong JK, Park M, Park TS, Park TC, Namkoong SE, et al. HPV oligonucleotide microarray-based detection of HPV genotypes in cervical neoplastic lesions. Gynecol Oncol. 2003;89:210–7.
55. Brandstetter T, Böhmer S, Prucker O, Bissé E, zur Hausen A, Alt-Mörbe J, et al. A polymerase based DNA biochip platform for human papillomavirus genotyping. J Virol Methods. 2010;163:40–8.
56. Coser J, Boeira TR, Fonseca AS, Ikuta N, Lunge VR. Human papillomavirus detection and typing using a nested-PCR-RFLP assay. Braz J Infect Dis. 2011;15:467–72.
57. Iftner T, Villa LL. Human papillomavirus technologies. J Natl Cancer Inst Monogr. 2003;31:80–8.
58. Szarewski A, Ambroisine L, Cadman L, Austin J, Ho L, Terry G, et al. Comparison of predictors for high-grade cervical intraepithelial neoplasia in women with abnormal smears. Cancer Epidemiol Biomark Prev. 2008;17:3033–42.
59. Hoheisel JD. Microarray technology: beyond transcript profiling and genotype analysis. Nat Rev Genet. 2006;7:200–10.
60. Didelot MN, Boulle N, Damay A, Costes V, Segondy M. Comparison of the PapilloCheck assay with the digene HC2 HPV DNA assay for the detection of 13 high-risk human papillomaviruses in cervical and anal scrapes. J Med Virol. 2011;83:1377–82.
61. Dalstein V, Merlin S, Bali C, Saunier M, Dachez R, Ronsin C. Analytical evaluation of the PapilloCheck test, a new commercial DNA chip for detection and genotyping of papillomavirus. J Virol Methods. 2009;156:77–83.
62. Otero-Motta AP, Ordóñez JL, González-Celador R, Rivas B, Macías M, Macías MC, et al. Prevalence of human papillomavirus genotypes in cytologic abnormalities from unvaccinated women living in North-Western Spain. APMIS. 2011;119:204–15.
63. Kocjan BJ, Seme K, Poljak M. Comparison of the Abbott real time high risk HPV test and INNO-LiPA HPV genotyping extra test for the detection of human papillomaviruses in formalin-fixed, paraffin- embedded cervical cancer specimens. J Virol Methods. 2011;175:117–9.
64. van Hamont D, van Ham MA, Bakkers JM, Massuger LF, Melchers WJ. Evaluation of the SPF10-Inno LiPA human papillomavirus (HPV) genotyping test and the roche linear array HPV genotyping test. J Clin Microbiol. 2006;44:3122–9.
65. Dobec M, Bannwart F, Kilgus S, Kaeppeli F, Cassinotti P. Human papillomavirus infection among women with cytological abnormalities in Switzerland investigated by an automated linear array genotyping test. J Med Virol. 2011;83:1370–6.
66. Schmitt M, Bravo IG, Snijders PJ, Gissmann L, Pawlita M, Waterboer T. Bead-based multiplex genotyping of human papillomaviruses. J Clin Microbiol. 2006;44:504–12.
67. Barcellos RB, Almeida SE, Sperhacke RD, Verza M, Rosso F, Medeiros RM, et al. Evaluation of a novel microplate colorimetric hybridization genotyping assay for human papillomavirus. J Virol Methods. 2011;177:38–43.
68. Roberts I, Ng G, Foster N, Stanley M, Herdman MT, Pett MR, et al. Critical evaluation of HPV16 gene copy number quantification by SYBR green PCR. BMC Biotechnol. 2008;8:57.
69. Halfon P, Benmoura D, Agostini A, Khiri H, Penaranda G, Martineau A, et al. Evaluation of the clinical performance of the Abbott RealTime high-risk HPV for carcinogenic HPV detection. J Clin Virol. 2010;48(4):246–50.
70. Heideman DA, Hesselink AT, Berkhof J, van Kemenade F, Melchers WJ, Daalmeijer NF, et al. Clinical validation of the Cobas 4800 HPV test for cervical screening purposes. J Clin Microbiol. 2011;49:3983–5.
71. Mateos ML, Rodríguez-Domínguez M, Sanz I, Rubio MD, Antonio J, Chacón D. Evaluation of a prototype real-time PCR assay for the separate detection of human papillomavirus genotypes 16 and 18 and other high risk human papillomavirus in cervical cancer screening. Enferm Infecc Microbiol Clin. 2011;29:411–4.
72. de Araujo MR, De Marco L, Santos CF, Rubira-Bullen IR, Ronco G, Pennini I, et al. GP5+/6+ SYBR green methodology for simultaneous screening and

quantification of human papillomavirus. J Clin Virol. 2009;45:90–5.
73. Sanger F, Nicklen S, Coulson AR. DNA sequencing with chain-terminating inhibitors. Biotechnology. 1992;24:104–8.
74. Novais RC, Thorstenson YR. The evolution of pyrosequencing for microbiology: from genes to genomes. J Microbiol Methods. 2011;86:1–7.
75. Pista A, Verdasca N, Oliveira A. Clinical performance of the CLART human papillomavirus 2 assay compared with the hybrid capture 2 test. J Med Virol. 2011;83:272–6.
76. Wentzensen N, von Knebel DM. Biomarkers in cervical cancer screening. Dis Markers. 2007;23:315–30.
77. Hwang SJ, Shroyer KR. Biomarkers of cervical dysplasia and carcinoma. J Oncol. 2012;2012:507286.
78. Varnai AD, Bollmann M, Bankfalvi A, Speich N, Schmitt C, Griefingholt H, et al. Predictive testing of early cervical pre-cancer by detecting human papillomavirus E6/E7 mRNA in cervical cytologies up to high-grade squamous intraepithelial lesions: diagnostic and prognostic implications. Oncol Rep. 2008;19(2):457–65.
79. Dockter J, Schroder A, Eaton B, Wang A, Sikhamsay N, Morales L, et al. Analytical characterization of the APTIMA HPV assay. J Clin Virol. 2009;45(Suppl 1):39–47.
80. Molden T, Kraus I, Karlsen F, Skomedal H, Nygård JF, Hagmar B. Comparison of human papillomavirus messenger RNA and DNA detection: a cross-sectional study of 4,136 women >30 years of age with a 2-year follow-up of high-grade squamous intraepithelial lesion. Cancer Epidemiol Biomark Prev. 2005;14(2):367–72.
81. Cuschieri KS, Whitley MJ, Cubie H. Human papillomavirus type specific DNA and RNA persistence—implications for cervical disease progression and monitoring. J Med Virol. 2004;73:65–70.
82. Lowe B, O'Neil D, Loeffert D, Nazarenko I. Distribution of human papillomavirus load in clinical specimens. J Virol Methods. 2011;173:150–2.
83. Gravitt PE, Kovacic MB, Herrero R, Schiffman M, Bratti C, Hildesheim A, et al. High load for most high risk human papillomavirus genotypes is associated with prevalent cervical cancer precursors but only HPV16 load predicts development incident disease. Int J Cancer. 2007;21:2787–93.
84. Broccolo F, Chiari S, Piana A, Castiglia P, Dell'Anna T, Garcia-Parra R, et al. Prevalence and viral load of oncogenic human papillomavirus types associated with cervical carcinoma in a population of North Italy. J Med Virol. 2009;81:278–87.
85. Hart KW, Williams OM, Thelwell N, Fiander AN, Brown T, Borysiewicz LK, et al. Novel method for detection, typing, and quantification of human papillomaviruses in clinical samples. J Clin Microbiol. 2001;39:3402–12.
86. Kulmala SM, Syrjänen SM, Gyllensten UB, Shabalova IP, Petrovichev N, Tosi P, et al. Early integration of high copy HPV16 detectable in women with normal and low grade cervical cytology and histology. J Clin Pathol. 2006;59:513–7.
87. Gallo G, Bibbo M, Bagella L, Zamparelli A, Sanseverino F, Giovagnoli MR, et al. Study of viral integration of HPV-16 in young patients with LSIL. J Clin Pathol. 2003;56:532–6.
88. Yoshida T, Sano T, Kanuma T, Owada N, Sakurai S, Fukuda T, et al. Quantitative real-time polymerase chain reaction analysis of the type distribution, viral load, and physical status of human papillomavirus in liquid-based cytology samples from cervical lesions. Int J Gynecol Cancer. 2008;18:121–7.
89. Jin Y, Li JP, He D, Tang LY, Zee CS, Guo SZ, et al. Clinical significance of human telomerase RNA gene (hTERC) amplification in cervical squamous cell lesions detected by fluorescence in situ hybridization. Asian Pac J Cancer Prev. 2011;12:1167–71.
90. Meyerson M, Counter CM, Eaton EN, Ellisen LW, Steiner P, Caddle SD, et al. hEST2, the putative human telomerase catalytic subunit gene, is upregulated in tumor cells and during immortalization. Cell. 1997;90:785–95.
91. Liu X, Yuan H, Fu B, Disbrow GL, Apolinario T, Tomaic V, et al. The E6AP ubiquitin ligase is required for transactivation of the hTERT promoter by the human papillomavirus E6 oncoprotein. J Biol Chem. 2005;280:10807–16.
92. Matovina M, Sabol I, Grubisić G, Gasperov NM, Grce M. Identification of human papillomavirus type 16 integration sites in high-grade precancerous cervical lesions. Gynecol Oncol. 2009;113:120–7.
93. Klaes R, Woerner SM, Ridder R, Wentzensen N, Duerst M, Schneider A, et al. Detection of high-risk cervical intraepithelial neoplasia and cervical cancer by amplification of transcripts derived from integrated papillomavirus oncogenes. Cancer Res. 1999;59(24):6312–6.
94. Nonogaki S, Wakamatsu A, Longatto Filho A, Pereira SM, Utagawa ML, Ferreira Alves VA, et al. Hybrid capture II and polymerase chain reaction for identifying HPV infections in samples collected in a new collection medium. A comparison. Acta Cytol. 2004;48(4):514–20.
95. Choo KB, Pan CC, Han SH. Integration of human papillomavirus type 16 into cellular DNA of cervical carcinoma: preferential deletion of the E2 gene and invariable retention of the long control region and the E6/E7 open reading frames. Virology. 1987;161:259–61.
96. Rabelo-Santos SH, Levi JE, Derchain SF, Sarian LO, Zeferino LC, Messias S, et al. DNA recovery from hybrid capture II samples stored in specimen transport medium with denaturing reagent, for the detection of human papillomavirus by PCR. J Virol Methods. 2005;126(1–2):197–201.
97. Snijders PJ, van den Brule AJ, Meijer CJ. The clinical relevance of human papillomavirus testing: relationship between analytical and clinical sensitivity. J Pathol. 2003;201(1):1–6.
98. Villa LL, Denny L. Methods for detection of HPV infection and its clinical utility. Int J Gynaecol Obstet. 2006;94(Suppl 1):S71–80.

10 Biomarkers for the Early Detection of Cervical Cancer

Md Kausar Neyaz and Saman Ahmad

10.1 Introduction

Cancer is a genetic disease caused by a multistep process involving activation of oncogenes, loss of function of tumor suppressor genes, and alteration of modifier genes, for instance, genes involved in DNA repair and genomic stability. Cervical cancer is the fourth most common cancer affecting women worldwide [1]. India alone accounts for one-quarter of the worldwide cervical cancer burden [2]. In last decade, significant advancement in understanding the causes of cervical cancer and identification of biomarkers have been achieved for its early diagnosis, prevention, and treatment. The human papillomavirus (HPV) is considered as one of the major etiological factors for cervical cancer along with other factors [3]. HPVs are epitheliotropic viruses and possess a small, circular double-stranded DNA. These viruses cause a variety of benign epithelial lesions such as warts or condylomata acuminata and neoplasia of the lower genital tract in humans [4, 5]. Presently, more than 120 HPV types have been described, of which at least 40 are associated with anogenital lesions, 15 of these have been classified as high risk (HR-HPV) (HPV 16, 18, 31, 33, 35, 39, 45, 51, 52, 56, 58, 59, 68, 73, and 82) and 12 as low risk (LR-HPV) (HPV 6, 11, 40, 42, 43, 44, 54, 61, 70, 72, 81, and 89) [6, 7]. Among these, infection of HPV types 16 and 18 [8, 9] is found to be the most oncogenic type that leads to the development of cervical cancer, while the infection of low-risk HPV types 6 and 11 is mainly associated with the development of benign lesions and genital warts. This causal relationship between HR-HPV infection and cervical cancer has been proved from various epidemiological and experimental studies [10, 11]. These HR-HPVs have been detected in almost 100% of cervical squamous cell carcinomas (SCCs) [7, 12] and 94–100% of cervical adenocarcinoma and adeno-squamous carcinoma [13, 14]. In India, cancer of the uterine cervix is the major cancer harboring HPV in almost 98%, and more than 90% of them are infected with specifically HPV type 16 [15].

PCR detection of HPV DNA by L1 consensus primers and typing by HPV type-specific primers should be performed to detect the presence of high-risk HPVs. Most widely used MY9 and MY11 consensus primers are capable of detecting about 27 HPV types which include all 15 high-risk HPVs (HPV 16, 18, 31, 35, 39, 45, etc.) and 6 low-risk HPVs [16].

Cytology-based screening for cervical cancer has shown to reduce the incidence and mortality rate since the last few decades. Addition of HR-HPV DNA screening in cervical cancer

M. K. Neyaz (✉)
Department of Research and Development, DSS Imagetech Pvt. Ltd., New Delhi, India

S. Ahmad
Content Department, Applect Learning Systems Pvt. Ltd., New Delhi, India

S. Mehta, A. Singla (eds.), *Preventive Oncology for the Gynecologist*, https://doi.org/10.1007/978-981-13-3438-2_10

screening has improved the sensitivity, but it is also associated with low specificity. Thus, other markers are needed to triage test for maintaining acceptable sensitivity and specificity. Various protein biomarkers for the detection of cervical cancer have been identified. Most of them are involved in cell cycle regulation, signal transduction, DNA replication, and cellular proliferation [17–19]. The altered expression of these proteins is a consequence of the binding of the high-risk HPV E6 and E7 oncogenes to host regulatory proteins, resulting in the degradation of the p53 tumor suppressor gene product, ultimately leading to dysregulation of the cell cycle. The evidence regarding the use of these biomarkers have shown their ability to triage mildly abnormal and indeterminate cytology cases, with those found to have elevated levels of biomarkers staining more likely to represent cases with true high-grade cervical cancer.

10.2 Biomarker Principles and Cervical Cancer

The biomarkers help in improving the management of cervical cancer at every point from screening and prognosis to assessment of treatment response. A significant advancement in understanding the causes of cervical cancer and identification of many different biomarkers have been achieved for its early diagnosis, prevention, and treatment.

Cytology still forms the mainstay of screening programs in most parts of the world, especially the USA. It is used either as a stand-alone test or as a co-test with HPV testing [20–23]. Presently with evidence building up, some European countries are using HPV as a primary screening modality and triaging positive results with cytology [24].

New biomarkers would be potentially useful in triaging women with primary cytology or HPV testing positive. The hallmark of cervical screening is to identify lesions which are most likely to progress to cancer. The biomarkers have a crucial role to play as they can identify significant changes that occur during any of the important steps of the functional progression model. There are two main groups of markers, viral or cellular markers (Table 10.1). Table 10.2 lists the commercially available viral and cellular biomarkers.

Table 10.1 Markers for cervical cancer screening

Viral markers	Cellular markers
HPV DNA detection	$p16^{ink4a}$
E6/E7 mRNA	Proliferation—Ki67, MCM2, Top2a
Viral integration	Chromosomal instability—3q, 5p
Viral and host methylation	

10.3 Viral Biomarkers

10.3.1 HPV DNA Detection and Genotyping

With time the importance of molecular basis of HPV infection and HPV genotyping has been recognized. Studies have shown that the sensitivity of high-risk HPV DNA testing is more sensitive than cytology [25, 26]. The National Comprehensive Cancer Network (NCCN) recommends co-testing with Pap and HPV every 5 years in women between 30 and 65 years as the preferred option for cervical cancer screening [27].

The ASCUS-LSIL Triage Study (ALTS) trial which was conducted by the National Cancer Institute concluded that doing reflex HPV testing in cytology reports of ASCUS identified 96% of CIN3+ cases, and only 56% of cases were referred for colposcopy [28].

Follow-up is mandatory for women after treatment for CIN, and HPV testing is a good option for doing so due to its high sensitivity in picking up recurrences [29, 30]. The prediction for recurrences can be further improved if genotyping for the type of HV infection is also done [31]. But the specificity for the test is low which can be improved by triaging positive results with cytology or methylation markers [32].

Table 10.2 Commercially available assays targeting viral as well as cellular biomarkers

Available assays approved	Manufacturer	Target	HPV genotypes	Genotyping	FDA
Viral assay HPV DNA					
COBAS 4800	Roche	L1 DNA	13 HR HPV and HPV66	16 and 18	Yes
Cervista	Hologic	L1 DNA	13 HR HPV and HPV66	16 and 18	Yes
Hybrid capture 2	QIAGEN	Full genome	13 HR HPV and HPV66	No	Yes
Amplicor	Roche	L1 DNA	13 HR HPV	No	No
careHPV	QIAGEN	L1 DNA	13 HR HPV and HPV66	No	No
Digene HPV eHC	QIAGEN	Full genome	13 HR HPV, HPV66 and 82	No	No
EIA kit HPV GP HR	Diassay	L1 DNA	13 HR HPV and HPV66	No	No
INFINITI HPV-HR QUAD	AutoGenomics	E1 DNA	13 HR HPV and HPV66	No	No
RT HPV	Abbott	L1 DNA	13 HR HPV and HPV66	16 and 18	No
Digene HPV eHC 16 18/45	QIAGEN	Full genome	13 HR HPV, HPV66 and 82	16, 18, and 45	No
CLART	Genomica	L1 DNA	13 HR HPV and 22 no HR	Yes	No
InfinitiTM	Genomica	L1 DNA	13 HR HPV and 12 no HR	Yes	No
INNO-LiPA	Innogenetics	L1 DNA	13 HR HPV and 15 no HR	Yes	No
Linear array	Roche	L1 DNA	13 HR HPV and 24 no HR	Yes	No
Multiplex HPV genotyping	Multimetrix	L1 DNA	13 HR HPV and 11 no HR	Yes	No
PapilloCheck	Greiner bio-one	E1 DNA	13 HR HPV and 11 no HR	Yes	No
HPV RNA					
Aptima	Gen-probe	E6/E7 mRNA	13 HR HPV and HPV66	No	Yes
NucliSens EasyQ	Biomerieux	E6/E7 mRNA	5 HR HPV	16, 18, 31, 33, and 45	No
OncoTect	IncellDx	E6/E7 mRNA	13 HR HPV	Yes	No
PreTect proofer	Norchip	E6/E7 mRNA	5 HR HPV	16, 18, 31, 33, and 45	No
HPV proteins					
Cytoactiv	Cytoimmun diagnostics	L1	All known HPVs	No	No
OncoE6	Arbor Vita	E6	3 HR HPV	16, 18, and 45	No
Cellular assay					
CINtec	Mtm laboratories	p16ink4a			No
CINtec plus	Mtm laboratories	p16ink4a/K1-67			No
Ki-67 (MIB1)	DakoCytomation	Ki-67			No
ProEx C	Becton Dickinson	TOP2A/MCM2			No

10.3.2 HPV E6/E7 mRNA

As established HPV DNA testing has an important role in cervical cancer prevention, other biomarkers with higher specificity and prognostic value need to be used to identify patients who are at higher risk of this disease. There are evidences which suggest that HPV messenger RNA transcripts' detection proves to be a more specific method for diagnosing clinically important infection than detection of viral DNA. It has been found that HPV E6/E7 mRNA testing for high-risk types correlates better with the severity of the lesions as compared to HPV DNA testing and is considered as a potential marker for the identification of women who are at high risk of contracting cervical cancer [33]. Various studies supported the above finding that the detection of E6/E7 mRNA expression is much helpful in predicting the risk of cervical cancer than HPV DNA testing [34] as mRNA expression profile shows better correlation with the severity of the lesions. The persistent and regressive infections cannot be distinguished by HPV DNA detection methods. Hence, such methods are not specific enough to identify patients at risk of cervical cancer [35].

The oncogenic potential of the HPV early genes E6 and E7 is well known. It is widely accepted that HPV can cause cancer only if there is persistent infection and a cellular environment which allows high-level expression of viral E6 and E7 genes. The E6 and E7 proteins are essential for the replication of the virus and are expressed during the productive normal life cycle, where their regulation is under tight control. When this regulation is disrupted and E6 and E7 are overexpressed, they can evade normal tumor suppressive function and cell cycling [36]. This may lead to a disturbance in cell cycle control and a deficiency in DNA repair, causing genomic instability and an elevated risk of malignant transformation [37]. Thus, targeting E6/E7 mRNA may lead to more trusted outcomes than detecting the presence of viral DNA.

10.3.3 HPV Viral Load and Integration

Several studies suggest that there exists a close link between HPV viral copy number and integration of viral genome into the host cell which increases the risk for progression to invasive cancer [38]. The grade of the lesion is directly linked to the HPV viral, and a much higher number have been found in high-grade lesions. Integration of the viral DNA to host cell genome is yet another biomarker as persistent HPV infection leads to integration of viral DNA into the host cell genome, leading to tumorigenic transformation of cervical epithelium.

The tests for viral DNA detection, E6/E7 mRNA, and viral integration have been discussed in detail in Chap. 9, and out of the viral markers, only DNA methylation will be discussed here.

10.3.4 DNA Methylation as Biomarkers

Tumorigenesis involves modifications in the epigenes within the promoter genes which is crucial for progression to cancer. There are reports showing evidence of hypermethylation of DNA of tumor suppressor gene causing its activity to cease and thereby leading to progression of the lesion [39]. This methylation is nonrandom, with certain genes being methylated in some tumor types and others are not. Also, some reports show contradictory results with DNA hypomethylation of oncogenes in cancers [40–42].

Hypermethylated markers are DNA based as they are inherently more stable than RNA. As gene promoter hypermethylation is common to many cancers, so marker panels can be made which would pick up 70% of all major cancers [43].

Hypermethylated CpG islands are very sensitive tumor markers which utilize methylation-specific polymerase-chain-reaction (MS-PCR) methods to detect methylated DNA sequences [44, 45]. By utilizing these approaches, abnormally methylated gene sequences have been detected in DNA from serum [46, 47].

Host Methylation Methylation of many genes has been studied in cervical cancer, and these are listed in Table 10.3. As these genes are negative regulators of cell growth, they are most probably methylated and silenced in cervical cancer and its precursor lesions. Also, the frequency of DNA methylation increases with increasing severity of precursor lesions. These genes have been studied

Table 10.3 Methylation markers studied in cervical specimens

Gene	Number of studies	Methylation frequency (number positive) NL	HGCIN[a]	Ca	Full name	Biological function
DAPK	22	0.068 (33)	0.296 (158)	0.582 (659)	Death-associated protein kinase-1	Serine-threonine kinase; positive mediator of IFN-γ-induced apoptosis
RASSF1	17	0.031 (10)	0.102 (31)	0.141 (175)	Ras association (RalGDS/AF-6) domain family member-1	Ras effector protein; microtubule regulation, cell migration, proliferation, and apoptosis
CDH1	15	0.159 (37)	0.129 (36)	0.521 (456)	Cadherin 1, E-cadherin	Calcium-dependent cell adhesion glycoprotein
CDKN2A/p16	15	0.049 (17)	0.131 (26)	0.220 (187)	Cyclin-dependent kinase inhibitor 2A	Inhibits CDK4 kinase; regulation of cell cycle control in G1
MGMT	12	0.091 (33)	0.124 (37)	0.183 (124)	0-6-Methylguanine-DNA methyltransferase	DNA repair
RARB	12	0.045 (15)	0.130 (40)	0.343 (169)	Retinoic acid receptor-β	Regulates gene expression in response to thyroid-steroid hormones
CADM1	10	0.256 (43)	0.385 (106)	0.657 (236)	Cell adhesion molecule 1	Intracellular adhesion
FHIT	10	0.072 (21)	0.020 (2)	0.398 (268)	Fragile histidine triad gene	Diadenosine 5′,5‴-P1,P3-triphosphate hydrolase; purine metabolism
TIMP3	9	0 (0)	0.107 (6)	0.189 (82)	TIMP metallopeptidase inhibitor 3	Matrix metalloproteinase; degradation of the extracellular matrix
TERT	7	0.156 (12)	0.388 (73)	0.628 (120)	Telomerase reverse transcriptase	Enzymatic component of telomerase; responsible for the addition of short repeats to the ends of chromosomes or telomeres
CDH13	5	0.177 (25)	0.047 (7)	0.391 (79)	Cadherin 13, H-cadherin	Calcium-dependent cell adhesion glycoprotein
PAX1	4	0 (0)	0.356 (36)	0.917 (33)	Paired box 1	Pattern formation during embryogenesis
TFPI2	4	0.200 (20)	0.342 (13)	0.721 (88)	Tissue factor pathway inhibitor 2	Regulation of plasmin-mediated matrix remodeling
CCNA	3	0.108 (8)	0.387 (24)	0.696 (94)	Cyclin A2	Activates CDK2 kinases; promotes G1/S and G2/M transitions
MAL	3	0.098 (4)	0.577 (71)	0.942 (227)	T-lymphocyte maturation-associated protein	Candidate linker protein in T-cell signaling; implicated in myelin biogenesis and function in the nervous system; formation, stabilization, and maintenance of glycosphingolipid-enriched membrane microdomains
TWIST	3	0.0928 (4)	0.403 (27)	0.362 (68)	Twist homolog 1	Transcription factor; differentiation and cell lineage determination

Inclusion criteria: Genes that have been studied in normal, high-grade, and cancer samples; genes that showed a low level of methylation (<20%) in normal samples that increased in precancerous lesions and/or cancer samples; genes that have been reported in at least three studies; or genes that have been utilized in a marker panel.

Ca cervical cancer, *HGCIN* high-grade cervical intraepithelial neoplasia, *NL* no lesion

[a]Includes CIN2, CIN3, and HSIL in calculations.

as single markers as well as marker panels, but further studies are needed to confirm their role as markers in cervical cancer prevention.

Viral Methylation Detecting methylation of the HPV genome can add to the list of biomarkers for detection of CIN and its progression. E6 and E7 promoter regions get methylated late in the tumor cycle. Also, methylation of CpGs within L1 has been shown to be increased in high-grade lesions. The clinical relevance of these findings is still under research [48, 49].

10.4 Cellular Biomarkers

10.4.1 p16

p16 (also known as p16^{INK4a}), a cyclin-dependent kinase inhibitor, is a cell cycle regulatory protein. This tumor suppressor protein, p16INK4a, plays a critical role in regulation of the cell cycle. It is a cellular correlate of the increased expression of HPV E7 oncoprotein and causes disturbance in the cell cycle regulator pRb. This further leads to compensatory overexpression of p16^{INK4a} through negative feedback. It is clearly identified from the result of several studies that p16^{INK4a} is a useful diagnostic marker for squamous and glandular epithelial dysplasia in the uterine cervix [50, 51] (Fig. 10.1). A recent study showed that a p16^{INK4a} immunocytochemical assay has much better specificity as compared to HPV DNA testing to predict underlying high-grade dysplastic lesions [52]. The sensitivity ranges between 59 and 96% and the specificity between 41 and 96% for the detection of CIN2+ lesions. It has been evaluated as a stand-alone and as an adjunct to cytology and HPV testing. p16 overexpression has been found in majority of the cases of cervical precancers and cancers, while it is rarely expressed in normal tissue [50]. It is commercially available as CINtec (mtm lab) and has been widely validated. It is also available as a dual immunostain with Ki67 as CINtecPlus.

10.4.2 Markers of Abnormal Cell Proliferation

10.4.2.1 Ki-67

Ki-67 is a nuclear protein which is expressed during all active phases of the cell cycle, and its expression is directly linked with cellular proliferation. Increased expression of Ki-67 can be found in superficial layers of the cervical epithelium in CIN [53]. Several studies have concluded that Ki-67 can be used as an independent prognostic marker to identify women who are at high risk for progression and/or recurrence of CIN [54].

10.4.2.2 TOP 2A and MCM2

A combination of antibodies against minichromosome maintenance protein 2 (MCM2) and topoisomerase II alpha (TOP2A) has been studied as a biomarker for detection of CIN [55–58]. Both MCM2 and TOP2A regulate different steps of DNA replication, and their expression is increased in situations of aberrant cell cycle and cellular proliferation including cervical neoplasia related to high-risk HPV. Rather than testing for either one of them, which will leave out some dysplastic lesions, it is generally approved to apply the combination of MCM2 and TOP2A immunostaining (ProExC) for diagnosis of CIN. The sensitivity of the test ranges from 67 to 99% and specificity between 61 and 85% according to the few studies done which had a limited sample size [57, 58].

10.4.3 Chromosomal Aberrations

Cervical cancers and precancers are associated with a high degree of genomic instability in the form of recurrent chromosomal amplifications and deletions. The regions typically lost are 2q, 3p, 4p, 5q, and 18q, while regions amplified are 1q, 3q, 5p, and 8q [59–61].

Gain of 3q is the most consistent abnormality seen in cervical cancer; one gene TERC within this region is of particular importance. According

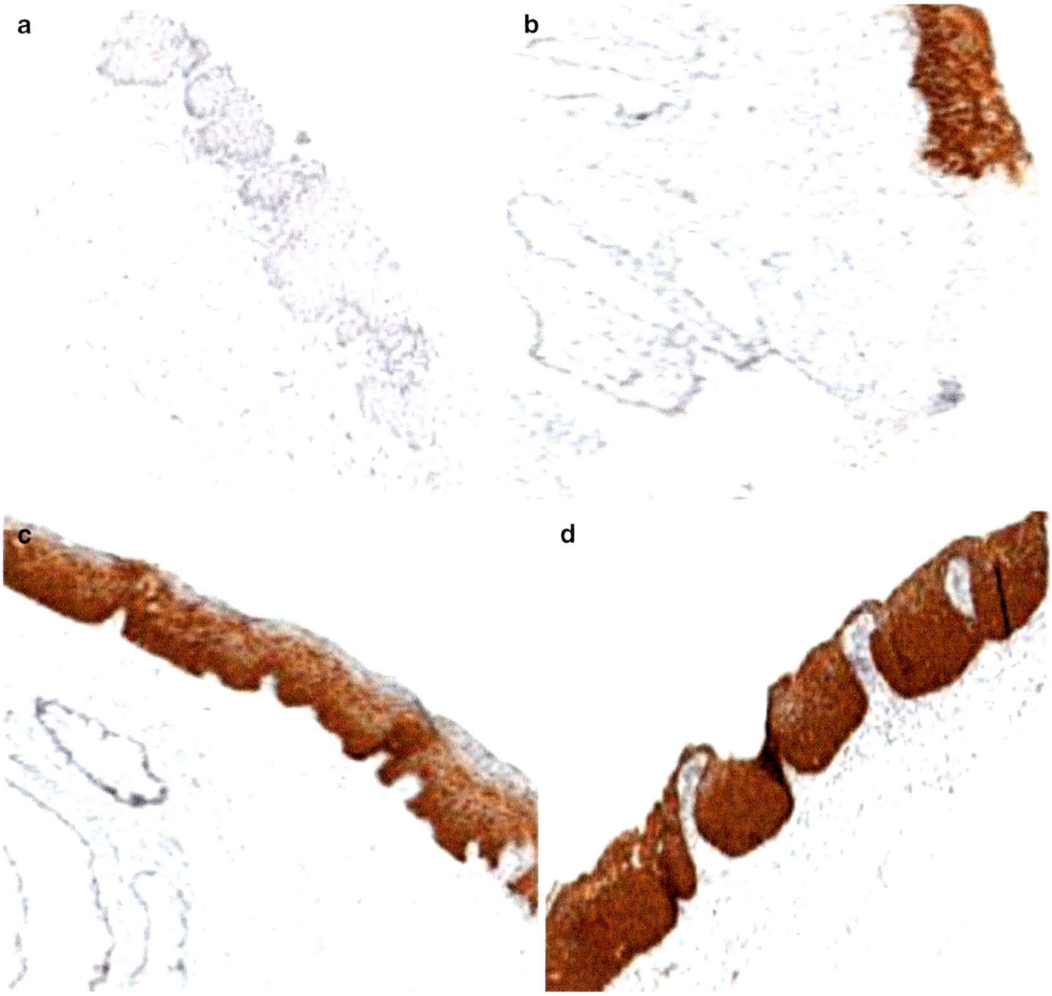

Fig. 10.1 p16 staining: (**a**) normal, (**b**) CIN 1, (**c**) CIN 2, and (**d**) CIN 3. Reprinted with permission from Kaur S. (2017) Pathology of Preinvasive Lesions of the Cervix. In: Mehta S., Sachdeva P. (eds) Colposcopy of Female Genital Tract. Springer, Singapore

to a multicentric study in China, TERC amplification was seen only in women who progressed to high-grade lesions. Another study showed that amplification of 3q had a high negative predictive value for progression of LSIL to CIN2+ [61]. So, TERC amplification could be used to triage HPV-positive women with ASCUS/LSIL cytology. Other chromosomal aberrations still require further research.

10.4.4 Protein Biomarkers

Protein biomarkers help in improving the cervical screening results. Many different protein biomarkers have been identified that are involved in cell cycle regulation, signal transduction, DNA replication, and cellular proliferation. The clinically significant protein markers for the detection of cervical cancer have been summarized in Table 10.4.

Table 10.4 Protein biomarkers

S. No.	Biomarkers	Significance
1.	p53	It is a tumor suppressor protein that prevents the outgrowth of aberrant cells, by inducing cell cycle arrest, DNA repair, or programmed death. The E6 protein of oncogenic HPV types has been shown to complex with p53 and target it for rapid degradation [62]. As a consequence, p53's growth-arrest and apoptosis-inducing activities are abrogated. This suggests the potential importance of E6-p53 interaction for therapeutic intervention
2.	p16	It is considered as a surrogate marker for high-risk HPV infection according to several reports which have mainly examined HPV 16 and 18 subtypes. Its overexpression is well established in CIN and invasive cancer by many studies [50, 63–65]
3.	c-fos	It specifically shows exclusive high expression with the increasing severity of lesion. As a member of transcription factor AP-1, c-Fos has been implicated mainly in signal transduction, cell differentiation, and proliferation [66]. Many studies focused on its oncogenic functions and found that c-Fos-regulated genes are important for tumorigenesis, causing downregulation of tumor suppressor genes [67] and leading to invasive growth of cancer cells [68]
4.	Fra-1	It is normally expressed in cervical tissue, but its expression gets diminished as the lesion progresses from precancer to cancer [69]. It has been found that there is a distinct pattern of gradual increase of c-fos and a concomitant decrease of fra-1 expression that perfectly match the progression of cervical lesions
5.	NF-κB	The NF-κB family consists of transcription factors that play a complex and essential role in innate immunity, inflammation, viral replication, and the initiation and progression of cancer. The classic form of NF-κB is a heterodimer between p65 (RelA) and p50 subunits. p50 subunit of NF-κB shows enhanced expression in high-grade cervical lesions and changes in relation to disease progression [69]
6.	pRB	It is a tumor suppressor protein which plays a pivotal role in the negative control of the cell cycle and in tumor progression. It has been found that pRB is responsible for a major G1 checkpoint, blocking S-phase entry and cell growth. The pRb protein represses gene transcription, required for transition from G1 to S phase, by associating with the E2F family of transcription factors. E7 binding to pRB releases E2F that leads to the expression of proteins necessary for DNA replication [70]
7.	Ki67	It is a marker of cell proliferation. Various studies have shown that an increased expression of Ki67 is correlated with higher cervical CIN grade and is a highly sensitive biomarker for differentiating between CIN1 and CIN2/3 [71, 72]. It can be used as an independent prognostic marker to identify women with high risk for progression and/or recurrence of cervical squamous precancerous lesions
8.	E-cadherin	It is mainly involved in the cell adhesion and is considered as an important biomarker for tumor development [73, 74]. The decrease or loss of expression of these molecules can be correlated with aggressive behavior and progression of cervical cancer. Several recent studies have already focused on changes in intercellular adhesion in different tumors, revealing the pivotal role of E-cadherin during tumor progression and invasion [75, 76]

Few important biomarkers have been discussed in detail.

10.4.4.1 p53

p53 is a tumor suppressor protein which plays an important role in the cells' response to genotoxic stresses like DNA damage, cellular senescence, and apoptosis and helps to maintain genomic stability of the cell. It has been found that disruption of p53 function by the viral E6 protein is one of the major events in cervical carcinogenesis [77]. The E6 protein of oncogenic HPV types makes complex with p53 and targets its rapid degradation [78]. As a consequence, growth-arresting and apoptosis-inducing activities of p53 are abrogated. This makes p53 as a robust prognostic biomarker in cervical cancer.

10.4.4.2 pRB

pRB is a negative regulator of the cell cycle that normally prevents S-phase entry by associating with the E2F family of transcription factors [70].

In case of cervical cancer, HPV infection affects the complex of pRB with E2F and causes its disruption upon binding of oncoprotein E7 that leads to the expression of E2F-responsive genes and degradation of pRB [77, 79]. Various studies have shown the inverse relationship between pRB levels and grade of the lesion with decreasing levels of pRB associated with higher grades of CIN [80, 81].

10.5 Newer Biomarkers

10.5.1 miRNAs

miRNAs are short noncoding RNAs and prevent translation of mRNA by negatively regulating the expression of genes. Abnormalities in their expression patterns are responsible for tumorigenesis as well as prognosis in cervical and other cancers [82]. Expression of some miRNAs (miR-21, miR-127, and miR-199a) is increased in CIN, while miR143, miR214, miR-218, and miR-34a expressions are decreased in cervical cancer compared with normal tissue [83–85]. The changes in miRNA expression is seen in the preinvasive stage of the disease, and so they can contribute as biomarkers for cervical cancer screening [86, 87].

10.5.2 Proteomics

Proteomics is a new emerging field which includes identification of differentially expressed proteins in biospecimens. Studies have shown sensitivity of 87.5% and specificity of 90% for these markers. A serum-based study which included 165 patients was able to mark out three peaks by MALDI-TOF that were different between cancer patients and healthy volunteers [88].

Alternative specimens have also been tried for the study of proteomics including cervicovaginal fluid or cervical mucus [89, 90]. However, the role of proteomics as marker in CIN or cervical cancer still needs to be validated in larger studies.

10.6 Conclusion

In cervical cancer which is associated high morbidity and mortality rates, a better understanding of the molecular mechanisms underlying tumor progression in the disease could reveal the novel pathway of high clinical relevance. Since development of cervical cancer progresses through various stages, it offers a unique opportunity to study the changes occurring at cellular and molecular levels that lead to the development of invasive cancer.

The main causative factor for cervical cancer is persistent HPV infection, but the incidence varies with the genotype of HPV. Tests for HPV genotyping thus help in the development of better screening protocols for prevention of cervical cancer. Currently, a number of molecular markers for cervical cancer screening are commercially available.

The significantly higher HPV load is a possible prognostic marker of high-grade squamous intraepithelial lesions. Integration of the viral DNA to host cell genome is yet another biomarker as persistent HPV infection leads to integration of viral DNA into the host cell genome. It has been found that HPV E6/E7 mRNA testing for high-risk types correlates better with the severity of lesions as compared to HPV DNA testing and is considered as a potential marker for the identification of women who are at high risk of contracting cervical cancer.

Various studies suggest the importance of protein biomarkers like Ki-67, p16, p53, and pRB, for use in cervical cancer screening. They help as predictive markers to identify high-grade lesions which are most likely to progress to cervical cancer.

Cancer of the cervix is the most preventable major form of cancer. The novel biomarkers not only help in screening, detection, and diagnosis of cervical cancer at an appropriate time, but they also help in prognostic evaluation, monitor treatment and predict recurrence, and also play major role in clinical decision-making.

Key Points

- New biomarkers have a potential role to play in primary screening for cervical cancer as well as for triaging primary cytology or HPV screening.
- Viral and cellular biomarkers indicating key steps of the functional progression model (HPV infection, precancer and invasive cancer) are being studied. Of these two main types of biomarkers are viral and cellular.
- The viral biomarkers include HPV DNA testing, HPV E6/E7 mRNA, HPV integration, and methylation; the cellular markers include p16^{INK4a}, chromosomal aberrations, and protein markers.
- Detection of HPV E6/E7 mRNA as well as cellular markers p16^{INK4a}/Ki-67 immunostaining is commercially available mainly as triage markers.
- Cervical cancers and precancers are associated with a high degree of genomic instability with numerous recurrent chromosomal amplifications and deletions; gain of 3q is the most consistent abnormality seen in cervical cancer.
- Role of miRNAs and proteomics is still under research and needs validation.

References

1. International Agency for Research on Cancer (IARC), World Health Organization (WHO). GLOBOCAN 2012: estimated cancer incidence, mortality and prevalence worldwide in 2012: cancer fact sheets: cervical cancer. Lyon: IARC; 2014.
2. Ferlay J, Soerjomataram I, Ervik M, Forman D, Bray F, Dixit R. GLOBOCAN 2012, cancer incidence and mortality worldwide in 2012. Lyon: International Agency for Research on Cancer; 2012.
3. Neyaz MK, Hussain S, Hassan MI, Das BC, Husain SA, Bharadwaj M. Novel missense mutation in FHIT gene: interpreting the effect in HPV-mediated cervical cancer in Indian women. Mol Cell Biochem. 2010;335:53–8.
4. zur Hausen H. Condylomata acuminata and human genital cancer. Cancer Res. 1976;36(2 pt 2):794.
5. zur Hausen H. Papillomavirus infections—a major cause of human cancer. Biochim Biophys Acta. 1996;1288(2):F55–78.
6. zur Hausen H. Papillomaviruses in human cancers. Proc Assoc Am Physicians. 1999;111(6):581–7.
7. Munoz N, Bosch FX, de Sanjose S, Herrero R, Castellasague X, Shah KV, et al. Epidemiologic classification of human papillomavirus types associated with cervical cancer. N Engl J Med. 2003;348:518–27.
8. Durst M, Gissmann L, Ikenberg H, zurHausen H. A papillomavirus DNA from a cervical carcinoma and its prevalence in cancer biopsy samples from different geographic regions. Proc Natl Acad Sci U S A. 1983;80(12):3812–5.
9. zur Hausen H. Papillomaviruses causing cancer: evasion from host-cell control in early events in carcinogenesis. J Natl Cancer Inst. 2000;92(9):690–8.
10. zur Hausen H. Papillomaviruses and cancer: from basic studies to clinical application. Nat Rev Cancer. 2002;2(5):342–50.
11. Bosch FX, de Sanjose S. Chapter 1: human papilloma virus and cervical cancer burden and assessment of casualty. J Natl Cancer Inst Monogr. 2003;31:3–13.
12. Walboomers JMM, Jacobs MV, Manos MM, Bosch FX, Kummer JA, Shah KV, et al. Human papillomavirus is a necessary cause of invasive cervical cancer worldwide. J Pathol. 1999;189:12–9.
13. van Muyden RC, ter Harmsel BW, Smedts FM, Hermans J, Kuijpers JC, Raikhlin NT, et al. Detection and typing of human papillomavirus in cervical carcinomas in Russian women: a prognostic study. Cancer. 1999;85(9):2011–6.
14. Zielinski GD, Snijders PJ, Rozendaal L, Daalmeijer NF, Risse EK, Voorhorst FJ, et al. The presence of high-risk HPV combined with specific p53 and p16INK4a expression patterns points to high-risk HPV as the main causative agent for adenocarcinoma in situ and adenocarcinoma of the cervix. J Pathol. 2003;201(4):535–43.
15. Das BC, Sehgal A, Murthy NS, Gopalkrishna V, Sharma JK, Das DK, et al. Human papillomavirus and cervical cancer in Indian women. Lancet. 1989;2(8674):1271.
16. Gravitt PE, Peyton CL, Apple RJ, Wheeler CM. Genotyping of 27 human papillomavirus types by using Li consensus PCR products by single-hybridization, reverse line blot detection method. J Clin Microbiol. 1998;36:30203027.
17. Malinowski DP. Molecular diagnostic assays for cervical neoplasia: emerging markers for the detection of high-grade cervical disease. BioTechniques. 2005;suppl:17–23.
18. Malinowski DP. Multiple biomarkers in molecular oncology. I. Molecular diagnostics applications in cervical cancer detection. Expert Rev Mol Diagn. 2007;7(2):117–31.
19. Wentzensen N, von Knebel Doeberitz M. Biomarkers in cervical cancer screening. Dis Markers. 2007;23(4):315–30.
20. Jordan J, Arbyn M, Martin-Hirsch P, et al. European guidelines for quality assurance in cervical cancer screening: recommendations for clinical management of abnormal cervical cytology, part 1. Cytopathology. 2008;19(6):342–54.

21. Mitchell H. The price of guidelines: revising the national guidelines for managing Australian women with abnormal pap smears. Sex Health. 2006;3(1):53–5.
22. Barzon L, Giorgi C, Buonaguro FM, Palu G. Guidelines of the Italian Society for Virology on HPV testing and vaccination for cervical cancer prevention. Infect Agent Cancer. 2008;3:14.
23. Wright TC Jr, Massad LS, Dunton CJ, Spitzer M, Wilkinson EJ, Solomon D. 2006 consensus guidelines for the management of women with abnormal cervical cancer screening tests. Am J Obstet Gynecol. 2007;197(4):346–55.
24. Meijer CJ, Berkhof J, Castle PE, et al. Guidelines for human papillomavirus DNA test requirements for primary cervical cancer screening in women 30 years and older. Int J Cancer. 2009;124(3):516–20.
25. Schiffman M, Herrero R, Hildesheim A, et al. HPV DNA testing in cervical cancer screening: results from women in a high-risk province of Costa Rica. J Am Med Assoc. 2000;283:87–93.
26. Wright TC Jr, Denny L, Kuhn L, et al. HPV DNA testing of self-collected vaginal samples compared with cytologic screening to detect cervical cancer. J Am Med Assoc. 2000;283(1):81–6.
27. Saslow D, Solomon D, Lawson HW, Killackey M, Kulasingam SL, Cain J, et al. American Cancer Society, American Society for Colposcopy and Cervical Pathology, and American Society for Clinical Pathology screening guidelines for the prevention and early detection of cervical cancer. Am J Clin Pathol. 2012;137:516–42.
28. Schiffman M, Solomon D. Findings to date from the ASCUS-LSIL triage study (ALTS). Arch Pathol Lab Med. 2003;127:946–9.
29. Paraskevaidis E, Arbyn M, Sotiriadis A, Diakomanolis E, Martin-Hirsch P, Koliopoulos G, et al. The role of HPV DNA testing in the follow-up period after treatment for CIN: a systematic review of the literature. Cancer Treat Rev. 2004;30:205–11.
30. Jones J, Saleem A, Rai N, Shylasree TS, Ashman S, Gregory K, et al. Human papillomavirus genotype testing combined with cytology as a 'test of cure' post treatment: the importance of a persistent viral infection. J Clin Virol. 2011;52:88–92.
31. Heymans J, Benoy IH, Poppe W, Depuydt CE. Type-specific HPV geno-typing improves detection of recurrent high-grade cervical neoplasia after conisation. Int J Cancer. 2011;129:903–9.
32. Verhoef VM, Bosgraaf RP, van Kemenade FJ, Rozendaal L, Heideman DA, Hesselink AT, et al. Triage by methylation-marker testing versus cytology in women who test HPV-positive on self-collected cervicovaginal specimens (PROHTECT-3): a randomised controlled non-inferiority trial. Lancet Oncol. 2014;15:315–22.
33. Coquillard G, Palao B, Patterson BK. Quantification of intracellular HPV E6/E7 mRNA expression increases the specificity and positive predictive value of cervical cancer screening compared to HPV DNA. Gynecol Oncol. 2011;120(1):89–93.
34. Cattani P, Siddu A, D'Onghia S, et al. RNA (E6 and E7) assays versus DNA (E6 and E7) assays for risk evaluation for women infected with human papillomavirus. J Clin Microbiol. 2009;47(7):2136–41.
35. Ratnam S, Coutlee F, Fontaine D, Bentley J, Escott N, Ghatage P, et al. Aptima HPV E6/E7 mRNA test is as sensitive as hybrid capture 2 assay but more specific at detecting cervical precancer and cancer. J Clin Microbiol. 2011;49(2):557–64.
36. Doorbar J. Molecular biology of human papillomavirus infection and cervical cancer. Clin Sci (Lond). 2006;110(5):525–41.
37. Munger K, Howley PM. Human papillomavirus immortalization and transformation functions. Virus Res. 2002;89:213–28.
38. Lillo FB, et al. Determination of human papillomavirus (HPV) load and type in high-grade cervical lesions surgically resected from HPV-infected women during follow-up of HPV infection. Clin Infect Dis. 2005;40:451–7.
39. Jones PA, Baylin SB. The fundamental role of epigenetic events in cancer. Nat Rev Genet. 2002;3:415428.
40. Costello JF, Fruhwald MC, Smiraglia DJ, Rush LJ, Robertson GP, Gao X, et al. Aberrant CpG island methylation has non-random and tumour-type-specific patterns. Nat Genet. 2000;24:132138.
41. Esteller M, Corn PG, Baylin SB, Herman JG. A gene hypermethylation profile of human cancer. Cancer Res. 2001;6:32253229.
42. Hanada M, Delia D, Aiello A, Stadtmauer E, Reed JC. Bcl-2 gene hypomethylation and high-level expression in B-cell chronic lymphocytic leukemia. Blood. 1993;82:18201828.
43. Esteller M, Fraga MF, Guo M, et al. DNA methylation patterns in hereditary human cancers mimic sporadic tumorigenesis. Hum Mol Genet. 2001;10:3001–7.
44. Herman JG, Graff JR, Myöhänen S, Nelkin BD, Baylin SB. Methylation-specific PCR: a novel PCR assay for methylation status of CpG islands. Proc Natl Acad Sci U S A. 1996;93(18):9821–6.
45. Eads CA1, Lord RV, Kurumboor SK, Wickramasinghe K, Skinner ML, Long TI, et al. Fields of aberrant CpG island hypermethylation in Barrett's esophagus and associated adenocarcinoma. Cancer Res. 2000;60(18):5021–6.
46. Lee TL, Leung WK, Chan MW, Ng EK, Tong JH, Lo KW, et al. Detection of gene promoter hypermethylation in the tumor and serum of patients with gastric carcinoma. Clin Cancer Res. 2002;8(6):1761–6.
47. Grady WM, Rajput A, Lutterbaugh JD, Markowitz SD. Detection of aberrantly methylated hMLH1 promoter DNA in the serum of patients with microsatellite unstable colon cancer. Cancer Res. 2001;61(3):900–2.
48. Kalantari M, Calleja-Macias IE, Tewari D, et al. Conserved methylation patterns of human papillomavirus type 16 DNA in asymptomatic infection and cervical neoplasia. J Virol. 2004;78(23):12762–72.

49. Turan T, Kalantari M, Calleja-Macias IE, et al. Methylation of the human papillomavirus-18 L1 gene: a biomarker of neoplastic progression? Virology. 2006;349(1):175–83.
50. Klaes R, Friedrich T, Spitkovsky D, Ridder R, Rudy W, Petry U, et al. Overexpression of p16(INK4A) as a specific marker for dysplastic and neoplastic epithelial cells of the cervix uteri. Int J Cancer. 2001;92:276–84.
51. Dray M, Russell P, Dalrymple C, et al. p16(INK4a) as a complementary marker of high-grade intraepithelial lesions of the uterine cervix. I: experience with squamous lesions in 189 consecutive cervical biopsies. Pathology. 2005;37(2):112–24.
52. Khleif SN, DeGregori J, Yee CL, et al. Inhibition of cyclin D-CDK4/CDK6 activity is associated with an E2F-mediated induction of cyclin kinase inhibitor activity. Proc Natl Acad Sci U S A. 1996;93(9):4350–4.
53. Yim EK, Park JS. Biomarkers in cervical cancer. Biomark Insights. 2007;l(1):215–25.
54. Kruse AJ, Baak JPA, Janssen EA, et al. Ki67 predicts progression in early CIN: validation of a multivariate progression-risk model. Cell Oncol. 2004;26:13–20.
55. Pinto AP, Schlecht NF, Woo TY, et al. Biomarker (ProExTM C, p16INK4a, and MiB-1) distinction of high-grade squamous intraepithelial lesion from its mimics. Mod Pathol. 2008;21:1067–74.
56. David O, Cabay RJ, Pasha S, et al. The role of deeper levels and ancillary studies (p16INK4a and ProExC) in reducing the discordance rate of Papanicolaou findings of high-grade squamous intraepithelial lesion and follow-up cervical biopsies. Cancer. 2009;117:157–66.
57. Shi J, Liu H, Wilkerson M, et al. Evaluation of p16INK4a, minichromosome maintenance protein 2, DNA topoisomerase IIalpha, ProEX C, and p16INK4a/ProEX C in cervical squamous intraepithelial lesions. Hum Pathol. 2007;38:1335–44.
58. Kelly D, Kincaid E, Fansler Z, et al. Detection of cervical high-grade squamous intraepithelial lesions from cytologic samples using a novel immunocytochemical assay (ProEx C). Cancer. 2006;108:494–500.
59. Hidalgo A, Schewe C, Petersen S, et al. Human papilloma virus status and chromosomal imbalances in primary cervical carcinomas and tumour cell lines. Eur J Cancer. 2000;36(4):542–8.
60. Yang YC, Shyong WY, Chang MS, et al. Frequent gain of copy number on the long arm of chromosome 3 in human cervical adenocarcinoma. Cancer Genet Cytogenet. 2001;131(1):48–53.
61. Jiang J, Wei LH, Li YL, et al. Detection of TERC amplification in cervical epithelial cells for the diagnosis of high-grade cervical lesions and invasive cancer: a multicenter study in China. J Mol Diagn. 2010;12(6):808–17.
62. Scheffner M, Werness BA, Huibregtse JM, Levine AJ, Howley PM. The E6 oncoprotein encoded by human papillomavirus types 16 and 18 promotes the degradation of p53. Cell. 1990;63:1129–36.
63. Masumoto N, Fujii T, Ishikawa M, Saito M, Iwata T, Fukuchi T, et al. P16 overexpression and human papillomavirus infection in small cell carcinoma of the uterine cervix. Hum Pathol. 2003;34:778–83.
64. Kang S, Kim J, Kim HB, Shim JW, Nam E, Kim SH, et al. Methylation of p16INK4a is a non-rare event in cervical intraepithelial neoplasia. Diagn Mol Pathol. 2006;15:74–82.
65. Kalof AN, Cooper K. p16INK4a immunoexpression: surrogate marker of high-risk HPV and high-grade cervical intraepithelial neoplasia. Adv Anat Pathol. 2006;13:190–4.
66. Shaulian E, Karin M. AP-1 in cell proliferation and survival. Oncogene. 2001;20:2390–400.
67. Bakin AV, Curran T. Role of DNA 5-methylcytosine transferase in cell transformation by fos. Science. 1999;283:387–90.
68. Hu E, Mueller E, Oliviero S, Papaioannou VE, Johnson R, Spiegelman BM. Targeted disruption of the c-fos gene demonstrates c-fos-dependent and -independent pathways for gene expression stimulated by growth factors or oncogenes. EMBO J. 1994;13:3094–103.
69. Prusty BK, Das BC. Constitutive activation of transcription factor AP-1 in cervical cancer and suppression of human papillomavirus (HPV) transcription and AP-1 activity in HeLa cells by curcumin. Int J Cancer. 2005;113:951–60.
70. Munger K, Basile JR, Duensing S, Eichten A, Gonzalez SL, et al. Biological activity and molecular targets of human papillomavirus E7 oncoprotein. Oncogene. 2001;20:788–7898.
71. Sari Aslani F, Safaei A, Pourjabali M, et al. Evaluation of Ki67, p16 and CK17 markers in differentiating cervical intraepithelial neoplasia and benign lesions. Iran J Med Sci. 2013;38:15–21.
72. McCluggage WG. Premalignant lesions of the lower female genital tract: cervix, vagina and vulva. Pathology. 2013;45:214–28.
73. Kaplanis K, Kiziridou A, Liberis V, Destouni Z, Galazios G. E-cadherin expression during progression of squamous intraepithelial lesions in the uterine cervix. Eur J Gynaecol Oncol. 2005;26(6):608–10.
74. Yaldizl M, Hakverdi AU, Bayhan G, Akku Z. Expression of E-cadherin in squamous cell carcinomas of the cervix with correlations to clinic-pathological features. Eur J Gynaecol Oncol. 2005;26(1):95–8.
75. De Boer CJ, Van Dorste E, Van Krieken H, Jansen-Van Rhijn CM, Warnaar SO, Fleuren JG, Litvinov SV. Changing roles of cadherins and catenins during progression of squamous intraepithelial lesions in the uterine cervix. Am J Pathol. 1999;155(2):505–15.
76. Birchmeier W, Behrens J. Cadherin expression in carcinomas: role in the formation of cell junctions and the prevention of invasiveness. Biochim Biophys Acta. 1994;1198(1):11–26.
77. Shukla S, Mahata S, Shishodia G, Pandey A, Tyagi A. Functional regulatory role of STAT3 in HPV16-mediated cervical carcinogenesis. PLoS One. 2013;8:e67849. https://doi.org/10.1371/journal.pone.0067849.
78. Tummers B, Van Der Burg SH. High-risk human papillomavirus targets crossroads in immune signaling.

Viruses. 2015;7:2485–506. https://doi.org/10.3390/v7052485.
79. Moody CA, Laimins LA. Human papillomavirus oncoproteins: pathways to transformation. Nat Rev Cancer. 2010;10:550–60. https://doi.org/10.1038/nrc2886.
80. Bahnassy AA, Zekri ARN, Saleh M, Lotayef M, Moneir M, Shawki O. The possible role of cell cycle regulators in multistep process of HPV-associated cervical carcinoma. BMC Clin Pathol. 2007;7:4. https://doi.org/10.1186/1472-6890-7-4.
81. Tringler B, Gup CJ, Singh M, Groshong S, Shroyer AL, Heinz DE, et al. Evaluation of p16INK4a and pRb expression in cervical squamous and glandular neoplasia. Hum Pathol. 2004;35:689–96. https://doi.org/10.1016/j.humpath.2004.02.012.
82. Cortez MA, Ivan C, Zhou P, Wu X, Ivan M, Calin GA. microRNAs in cancer: from bench to bedside. Adv Cancer Res. 2010;108:113–57.
83. Lee JW, Choi CH, Choi JJ, et al. Altered microRNA expression in cervical carcinomas. Clin Cancer Res. 2008;14(9):2535–42.
84. Lui WO, Pourmand N, Patterson BK, Fire A. Patterns of known and novel small RNAs in human cervical cancer. Cancer Res. 2007;67(13):6031–43.
85. Martinez I, Gardiner AS, Board KF, Monzon FA, Edwards RP, Khan SA. Human papillomavirus type 16 reduces the expression of microRNA-218 in cervical carcinoma cells. Oncogene. 2008;27(18):2575–82.
86. Li B, Hu Y, Ye F, Li Y, Lv W, Xie X. Reduced miR-34a expression in normal cervical tissues and cervical lesions with high-risk human papillomavirus infection. Int J Gynecol Cancer. 2010;20(4):597–604.
87. Li Y, Liu J, Yuan C, Cui B, Zou X, Qiao Y. High-risk human papillomavirus reduces the expression of microRNA-218 in women with cervical intraepithelial neoplasia. J Int Med Res. 2010;38(5):1730–6.
88. Liu C, Pan C, Shen J, Wang H, Yong L, Zhang R. Discrimination analysis of mass spectrometry proteomics for cervical cancer detection. Med Oncol. 2010;20(4):597–604.
89. Panicker G, Ye Y, Wang D, Unger ER. Characterization of the human cervical mucous proteome. Clin Proteomics. 2010;6(1–2):18–28.
90. Zegels G, Van Raemdonck GA, Coen EP, Tjalma WA, Van Ostade XW. Comprehensive proteomic analysis of human cervical–vaginal fluid using colposcopy samples. Proteome Sci. 2009;7:17.

Colposcopic Principles and Tissue Basis

11

Sumita Mehta and Ritu Khatuja

11.1 Introduction

Colposcope is an optical device used for systematic evaluation of the lower female genital tract under stereoscopic magnification (4- to 40-fold) with a powerful light source. During the procedure special emphasis is given to the superficial epithelium and blood vessels of the underlying connective tissue. Colposcopy is based on the variable absorption and reflection of its white light off these tissue interfaces [1]. Colposcopy was introduced by Hinselmann in 1925, but initially it was considered as secondary verification technique with respect to cervical cytology. But in the 1960s, it started getting the recognition when the role of transformation zone was identified in the development of carcinoma cervix. Now colposcopy is known to be an important tool that compliments cytology in the early detection, correlation with histological finding, treatment and follow-up of various lesions of the lower female genital tract. The main aim of a colposcopist is to ensure that invasive disease should not be missed [2, 3].

Thus, knowledge of the principles underlying colposcopy and its tissue basis is most important. This chapter is going to deal with basic concepts of colposcopy.

11.2 Tissue Basis of Colposcopy

In colposcopy magnified view of cervix is evaluated after application of saline, acetic acid (3–5%) and Lugol's iodine. To correctly interpret the colposcopic findings, a thorough knowledge of the histopathologic changes that occur in the epithelium and stroma of cervical tissue is required. The surface epithelium of the lower genital tract functions as a filter through which both the reflected and the incident light must pass to produce the final colposcopic picture. The epithelium does not have blood vessels which make it colourless, whereas the underlying stroma is red due to presence of blood vessels. It is the redness of the sub-epithelial stroma which is transmitted through the overlying epithelium surface and is visible through the colposcope [4].

The colposcopic image of the cervix is the result of various factors which include:

1. The architecture of the epithelium including its thickness and formation: The epithelium is colourless, while the stroma gets its colour tone from the vessels it contains. The thickness and density of the epithelium will affect

S. Mehta (✉)
Department of Obstetrics and Gynecology, Babu Jagjivan Ram Memorial Hospital, New Delhi, India

R. Khatuja
Department of Obstetrics and Gynaecology, ANIIMS, Port Blair, Andaman and Nicobar Islands, India

S. Mehta, A. Singla (eds.), *Preventive Oncology for the Gynecologist*,
https://doi.org/10.1007/978-981-13-3438-2_11

the amount of light absorbed and reflected during colposcopy. Normal ectocervical epithelium is thick and multilayered and so acts as an effective filter, appearing red to pinkish on colposcopy. The columnar epithelium is thin and translucent as it contains mucus and appears red during colposcopy. The metaplastic epithelium is thinner than the squamous epithelium and appears reddish, while rapidly regenerating epithelium may appear opaque. The squamous epithelium in postmenopausal and prepubertal girls is thinner than normal with reduced stromal blood supply and so appears pale red on colposcopy [5].

2. The composition of underlying stroma: The colposcopic appearance of the cervix is altered during inflammation because of infiltration of the stroma which is seen as a greyish white colour tone on colposcopy. Also the changes in vascular network occurring in the stroma during CIN give the characteristic image on colposcopy.
3. Surface configuration of the epithelium: This is determined by the thickness of the epithelium and surface shape which can be either smooth or papillary (Fig. 11.1). Vascular patterns of punctations and mosaic also become evident through the surface. Leukoplakia which is a white patch visible before application of acetic acid is also a determinant of surface configuration [5].

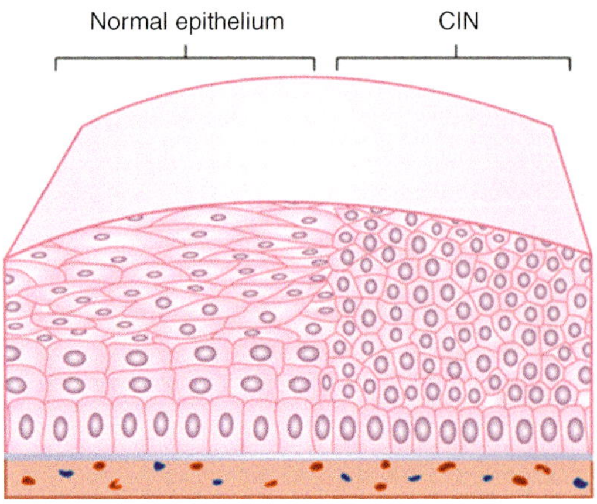

Fig. 11.1 Thickness of normal epithelium and CIN

There are three different epithelia seen during colposcopy:

- Original squamous epithelium.
- Columnar epithelium.
- Metaplastic squamous epithelium seen in transformation zone (TZ).

11.2.1 Original Squamous Epithelium

Original squamous epithelium of the ectocervix is thick, multilayered and glycogenated. The thickness of the epithelium depends on the age of the woman and ratio of estrogen and progesterone hormone. The blood vessels supplying the epithelium consist of small capillary arcade located deep within the stroma. They have branching feeder vessels which extend up to approximately one-third the thickness of epithelium. The squamous epithelium acts as filter membrane through which both the reflected and incident light pass to produce final colposcopic image. The redness of the stroma is transmitted back with modifications depending upon characteristics and thickness of epithelium.

11.2.2 Columnar Epithelium

Columnar epithelium lines the endocervix. It is thin, is single layered, contains mucus and is translucent (Fig. 11.2). The cells have moderate amount of cytoplasm and a small nucleus. The vessels supplying the columnar epithelium lie directly below the cells, and so it appears red when seen through the colposcope [6, 7].

11.2.3 Squamocolumnar Junction (SCJ)

It is important to recognize the old and new squamocolumnar junctions to delineate the transformation zone. The transformation zone is the area between the old and new squamocolumnar junctions. The columnar epithelium lines the

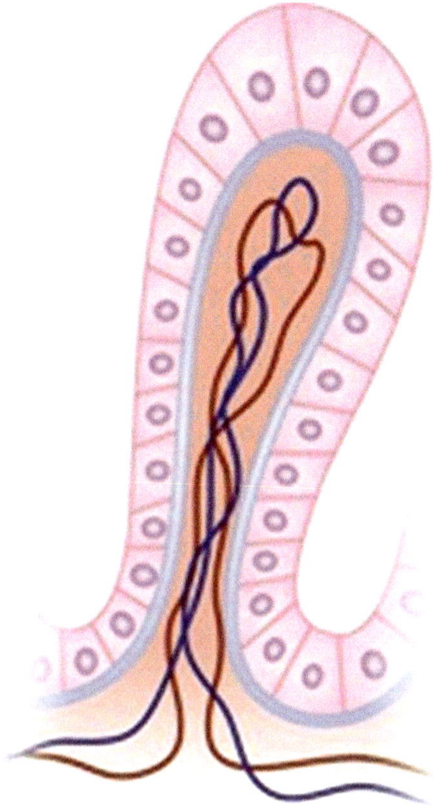

Fig. 11.2 Columnar epithelium

endocervical canal, while squamous epithelium is found on the ectocervix. The squamocolumnar junction is better defined as a dynamic point rather than static as it changes according to physiology of female during puberty, pregnancy, childbirth, hormonal stimulation, birth trauma and after menopause. In the prepubertal girls, the SCJ is located at or very close to the external os. In women in reproductive age group, the endocervical canal is everted due to the effect of endogenous estrogens. Owing to the vaginal acidity, metaplasia takes place converting the everted columnar epithelium to the squamous epithelium. The squamocolumnar junction in this age group is located away from the external os and can be recognized by the presence of crypt or gland openings [8, 9]. Thus, a new squamocolumnar junction is formed between the newly formed metaplastic squamous epithelium and the columnar epithelium. In menopausal women, new squamocolumnar epithelium moves on the ectocervix towards the external os (Fig. 11.3a–d).

11.2.4 Squamous Metaplasia Seen in Transformation Zone

Transformation zone is the area between the original and new physiological active SCJ. The outer boundary of TZ is the old SCJ which is identified by the presence of gland openings (Fig. 11.4).

The various stages of metaplasia can be seen colposcopically as (Fig. 11.5a–e):

- Stage 1: Initially the newly formed metaplastic epithelium (derived from subcolumnar reserve cells) has no stratification and is called immature metaplasia. It is seen colposcopically as progressive fusion of adjacent villi and eventual disappearance of the villous structure completely. The openings of the subepithelial glands can be seen as surface apertures.
- Stage 2: Smooth patches of immature metaplastic epithelium can be seen on colposcopy. Metaplastic epithelium can be found within the clefts of columnar epithelium.
- Stage 3: This is represented by mature squamous epithelium. At times, immature metaplastic epithelium might occlude the crypt opening leading to the development of a nabothian cyst full of mucous secretions [10].

During early stages of metaplasia, the epithelium is more vulnerable to genetic changes, and the cells at this stage may acquire a neoplastic potential and form atypical TZ. In children, the transformation zone is approximately 3 mm, whereas in adults it measures 6–8 mm.

Identifying the transformation zone is very important in colposcopy as almost all the manifestations of cervical precancer and cancer occur in this zone. The normal TZ contains mature stratified squamous epithelium, squamous metaplasia, nabothian cysts, gland openings and normal arborizing or fine reticular blood vessels.

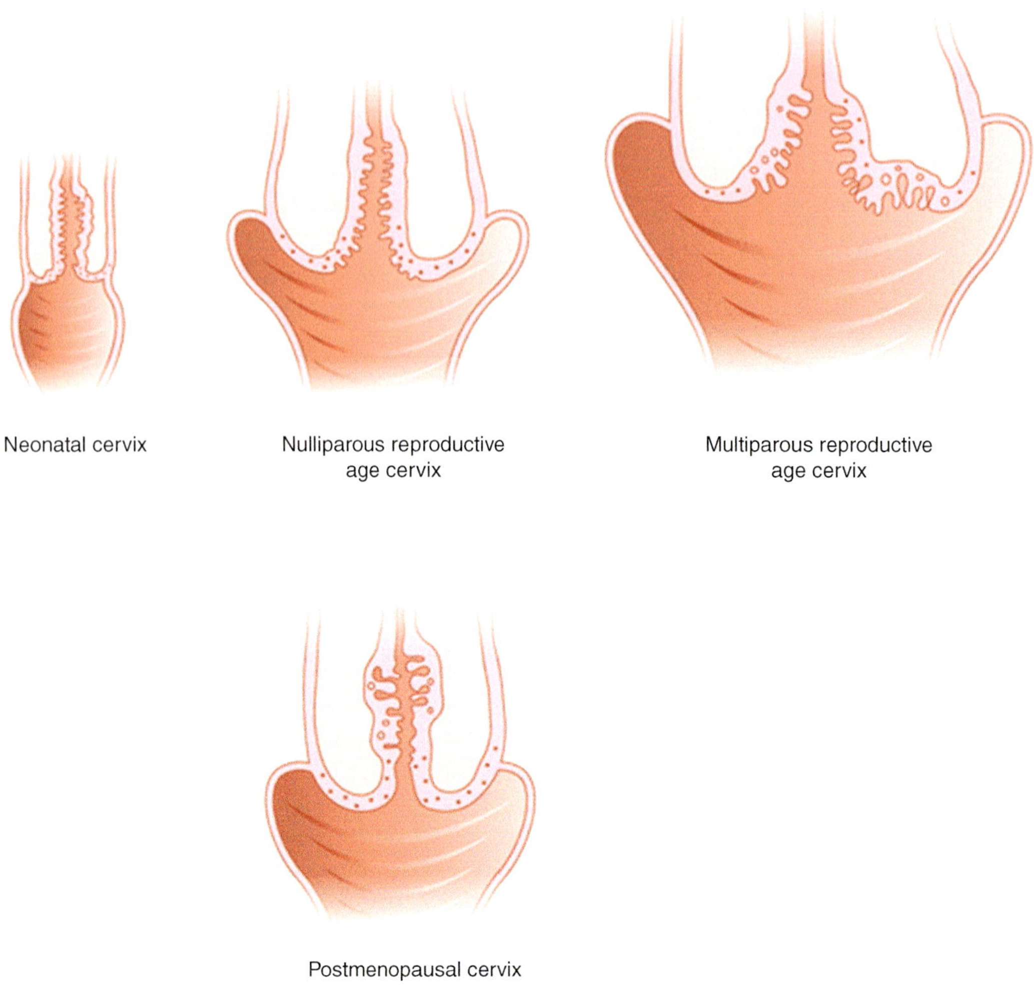

Fig. 11.3 Location of new SCJ in different age groups

The colposcopist must assess and visualize the complete transformation zone for satisfactory interpretation of colposcopic examination. Thus, according to visualization at colposcopy, TZ is divided into three types.

- Type 1 TZ—It is completely ectocervical and can be seen completely; it may be small or large.
- Type 2 TZ—It has an endocervical component also but the inner limit of the zone is fully visible and may have an ectocervical component that may be small or large.
- Type 3 TZ—It has an endocervical component that is not fully visible and may also have an ectocervical component [11, 12].

11.3 Abnormal Transformation Zone

The abnormal changes found in TZ are divided into two categories:

- *Cellular*: These changes include the colour changes seen after application of acetic acid and Lugol's iodine or the whiteness that is seen even without acetic acid application (Leukoplakia).
- *Vascular*: These include the changes seen with increased capillary growth in the form of punctations, mosaic and atypical vessels.

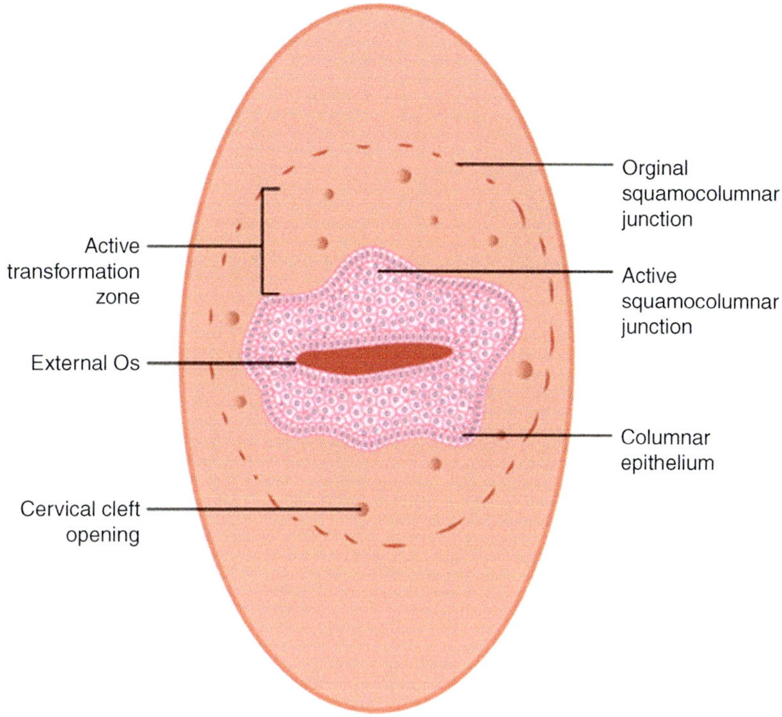

Fig. 11.4 Transformation Zone

11.3.1 Basis of Cellular Changes

The key step in colposcopic examination is to observe the cervix after application of 3–5% acetic acid. Acetic acid is mucolytic, and so it helps in clearing the mucus as well as it coagulates the nuclear protein. This coagulation is reversible and is due to precipitation of the nuclear proteins and cytokeratins [1]. The degree of coagulation depends on the amount of proteins present in the nucleus.

The squamous cells in the superficial layer of the normal epithelium have small nuclei with less nuclear proteins, and so little coagulation occurs with acetic acid. This is not opaque enough to obliterate the vascular stroma present underneath.

Areas harbouring dysplasia have higher mitotic activity and so higher amount of nuclear proteins. When acetic acid is applied to areas having CIN, this thick coagulation prevents light from passing through, and most of it is reflected back. The vessel pattern in the stroma is not seen and the epithelium appears white. The aceto-white areas are thus clearly demarcated from the surrounding pale pink healthy epithelium. Higher degrees of CIN and invasive cancer turn densely white immediately after acetic acid owing to higher amounts of nuclear proteins [13]. Also, the border between a high-grade aceto-white lesion and normal mucosa is markedly distinct. This border is most distinct in areas where the lesion ends at the new SCJ. High-grade lesions can have rolled-out margins because of dense cellularity.

In low-grade CIN, the appearance of whiteness is delayed and less in intensity due to presence of lesser amount of nuclear protein compared to areas with high-grade CIN or preclinical invasive cancer.

Aceto-whitening is not only seen in CIN and early cancer but can also be seen in other conditions associated with increased mitotic activity [14, 15]:

- Immature squamous metaplasia.
- Congenital transformation zone.
- Inflammation causing healing and regenerating changes in the epithelium.
- Leukoplakia which is associated with hyperkeratosis.
- Condylomas seen in HPV infections.

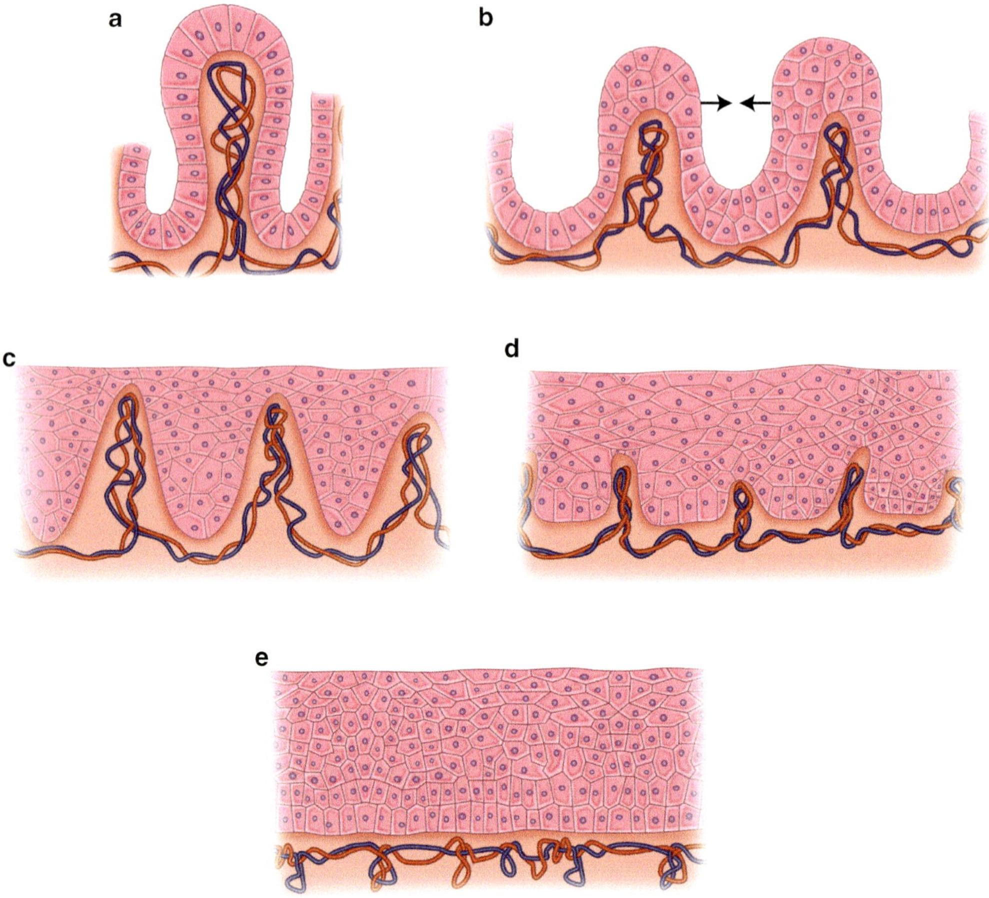

Fig. 11.5 Various stages of metaplasia

The aceto-white areas seen with the above conditions are not very dense, do not have sharp borders and are patchily distributed on the ectocervix. Also it tends to appear late and disappears quickly, usually within 30–60 s. Aceto-whitening should also be looked for in the vagina, external anogenital skin, and anal mucosa.

11.3.1.1 Leukoplakia

It is an area seen on the ectocervix which appears white on initial examination even before application of acetic acid (Fig. 11.6). It has been described on other sites such as the mouth or tongue also. The thickened surface is due to hyperkeratosis [16] (overproduction of keratin) and parakeratosis (retained nuclei in keratin which is usually acellular). This change in the epithelium is seen with HPV infection, CIN or in cases of reactive changes seen in women with prolapse. Keratin acts as a barrier for acetic acid, and it prevents from evaluation of cells underneath the leukoplakic patch. So a biopsy is advocated in such cases to document any abnormality [17].

11.3.1.2 Lugol's Iodine Application

Principle: The mature squamous epithelium of the ectocervix contains glycogen. When Lugol's iodine is applied to the ectocervix, it turns mahogany brown as iodine is taken up by glycogen. However, endocervical canal is lined by columnar epithelium which lacks glycogen. When Lugol's iodine is applied, the columnar cells do not take up iodine and remain unstained but may look slightly discoloured due to a thin film of iodine solution [18] (Fig. 11.7).

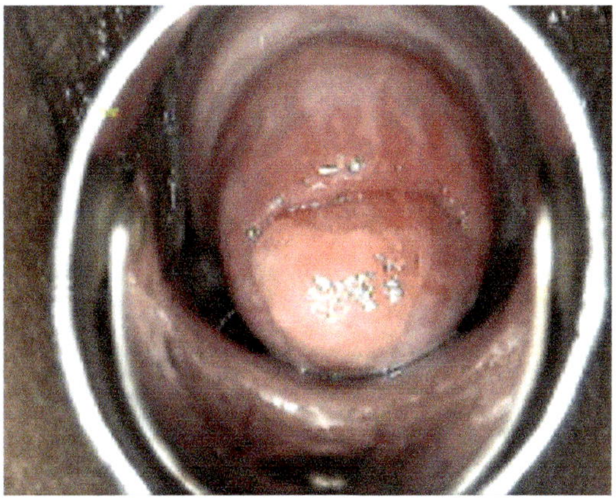

Fig. 11.6 Leukoplakia of cervix

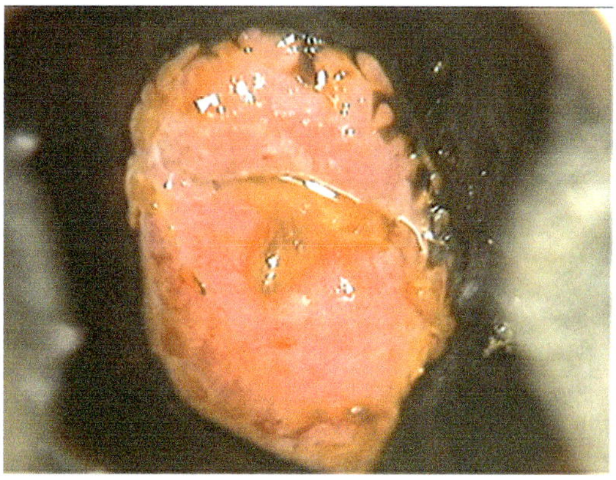

Fig. 11.7 Squamous epithelium has taken up iodine, while columnar epithelium is unstained

Immature squamous epithelium or inflammatory conditions of the cervix, leukoplakia and condylomas are associated with lack of iodine in the epithelial cells and so do not stain with Lugol's iodine or stain only patchily.

Area of dysplasias and invasive cancer also lack glycogen and do not take up iodine stain. They appear as thick mustard yellow or saffron-coloured areas on application of Lugol's iodine (Fig. 11.8).

Lugol's iodine is routinely used during the procedure of colposcopy. It helps in identifying lesions which might have been missed with acetic acid and also better delineates the anatomical extent of abnormal areas.

11.3.2 Basis of Vascular Changes in Intraepithelial Lesions

11.3.2.1 Punctation

CIN in transformation zone is associated with high rates of cell replication which in turn leads to production of angiogenic factors that help ingrowth of new feeder vessels into the surface epithelium [19, 20]. These capillary loops are seen end on by the colposcopist as punctate dots (Fig. 11.9). In cases with dysplasia, there is continued production of angiogenic factors leading to greater vascular growth and larger vessel loops and increase in size of the dots.

The distance between the capillary loops also increases with the amount of cell proliferation.

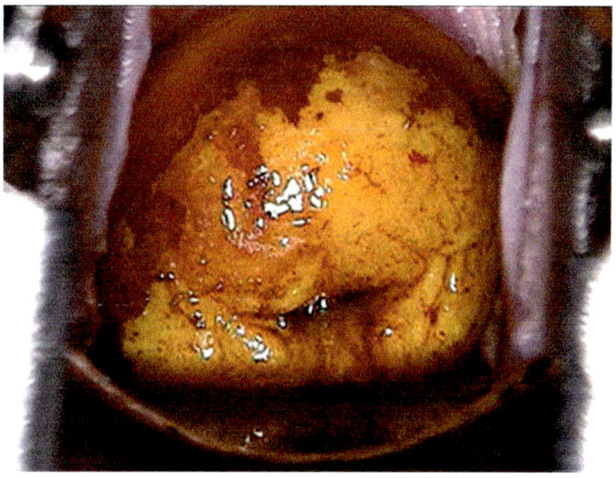

Fig. 11.8 No uptake of iodine in CIN

The cells not only increase from the basement membrane upwards but also grow laterally thereby pushing the capillary loops apart. The inter-capillary distance thereby increases with the grade of CIN; the higher the grade of CIN, the greater the inter-capillary distance [21].

The punctations are further subcategorized as:

- Fine punctations—Small uniformly sized dots with a decreased inter-capillary distance. These are mainly seen in reactive metaplasia or low-grade CIN.
- Coarse punctations—Large irregularly sized dots with an increased inter-capillary distance and the 0

11.3.2.2 Mosaicism

Punctations naturally progress to mosaicism. There is continuous production of angiogenic

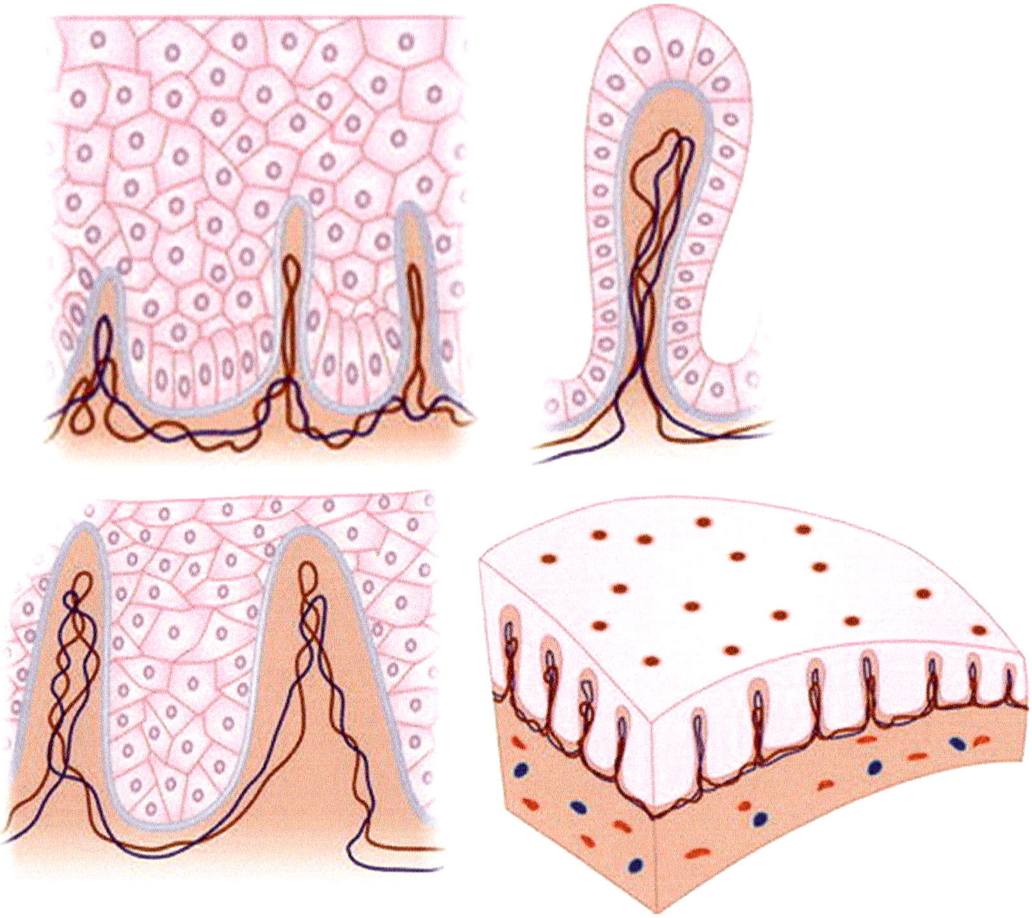

Fig. 11.9 Tissue basis of punctation

factors leading to vascular growth in intraepithelial lesions. The capillary loops arborize and coalesce, grow laterally and surround surface cells thus resembling tiles (Fig. 11.10). As atypical metaplasia proceeds further, there is compression of stromal papillae, and the network of vessels around it gives rise to a pavement-like appearance or mosaic pattern [22].

They are further categorized as:

- Fine mosaic—It consists of small tiles which are regularly shaped and have uniformly sized surrounding vessels. It is a characteristic of low-grade CIN or reactive metaplasia.
- Coarse mosaicism—It is formed by larger tiles of variable size and shape. The vessels around it are also of unequal size. It is associated with high-grade CIN [1].

11.3.2.3 Atypical Vessels (Fig. 11.11)

The cellular growth seen in invasive cancer is much more than that seen in intraepithelial lesions; the production of angiogenic factors is also abundant. Atypical vessels are abnormal with respect to:

- Haphazard arrangement—To keep up with the continued tumour expansion, the vessels lose their typical arborizing nature and arrange haphazardly.
- Atypical vessels are subcategorized on the basis of their general appearance as hairpin vessels, noodle like, glyphs or root like [23, 24].

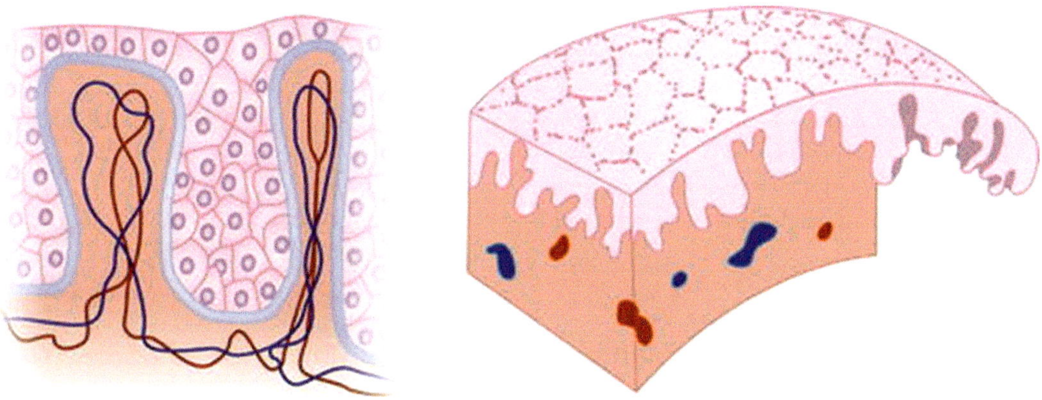

Fig. 11.10 Tissue basis of mosaic pattern

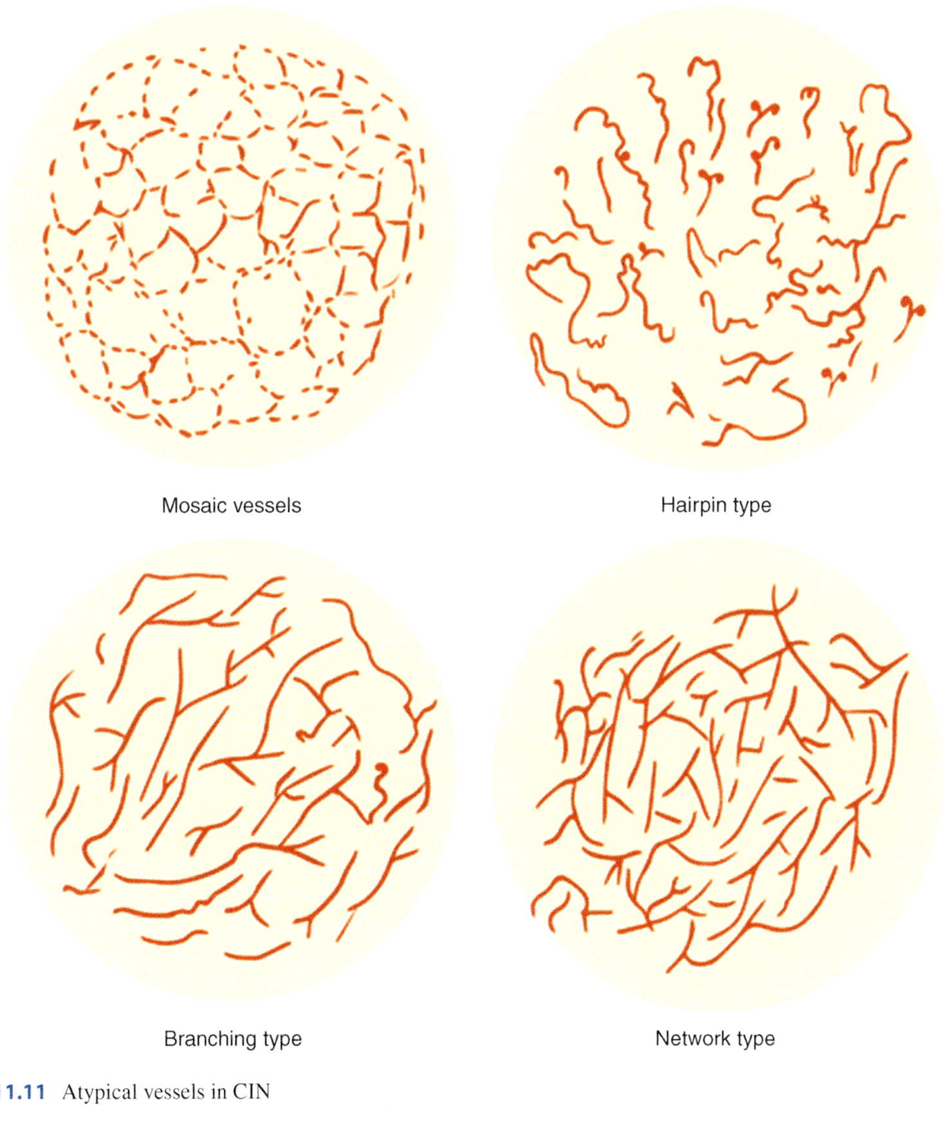

Fig. 11.11 Atypical vessels in CIN

- Abnormal branching pattern—The calibre of the vessels decreases as they branch out in normal epithelium, but in atypical vessels the size of the vessel paradoxically increases after division. The division occurs at right or obtuse angles. As they are close to surface, they bleed easily leading to postcoital bleeding [7].

11.4 Indications for Colposcopy [18, 25]

The most common reason for referral of women for colposcopy is abnormal screening test which may be abnormal cytology or positive high-risk HPV test. Some of the other indications include:

- Suspicious looking cervix.
- Persistent (for more than 12–18 months) low grade (CIN 1).
- Evaluation of squamous or glandular cell abnormality on cytology.
- Persistently unsatisfactory quality on cytology.
- Screen positive (VIA or HPV positive).
- If inflammation persists in spite of adequate treatment.
- For evaluation of postcoital bleeding, metrorrhagia and postmenopausal bleeding.
- Treatment of women with CIN.
- Follow-up of women previously treated for CIN.
- Evaluation of anogenital condylomas and subclinical human papilloma virus infection.
- In women with history of in utero exposure to diethylstilbestrol (DES).
- Evaluation of women with intraepithelial neoplasia of vulva (VIN) or vagina (VaIN).
- Forensic examination.

11.5 Contraindications for Colposcopy

- Women who cannot lie in the lithotomy position.
- Acute genital infection: vulvitis, vaginitis, cervicitis or pelvic inflammatory disease.
- Extreme difficulty in visualization of cervix on speculum.
- Severe atrophic changes in the cervix.
- Menstruating or immediate premenstrual or within 4 weeks of delivery or abortion.

11.6 Steps of Colposcopy

Proper identification of new and old SCJ is essential as the cervical intraepithelial lesions originate at the TZ. Failure to locate the squamocolumnar junction leads to unsatisfactory colposcopic examination.

- Relevant gynaecological as well as medical history should be taken. Any history of iodine reaction should be asked. A well-informed consent is mandatory. A written informed consent is also taken for the subsequent procedure such as cryotherapy, biopsy or loop electrosurgical excision procedure (LEEP) if required.
- Patient is placed in dorsal lithotomy position (extended lithotomy where cervix is pulled superior or flushed with vault) after evacuating bladder [25]. Appropriate size bivalve self-retaining vaginal speculum is inserted after inspection of the vulva and perianal area. If the vaginal walls are lax and obliterate the view, lateral wall retractors or condom (with it's tip cut off) can be used on the speculum.
- A good view of cervix and vaginal fornices should be obtained. Cervix must be adequately visualized, and cervical mucus should be removed with cotton swabs moistened with normal saline. Any gross lesions such as ectropion, polyps, ulcer, leukoplakia or growth and vascular details are noted. It is better to use green filter to evaluate the vascular details. The blood vessels appear dark black against the background of translucent epithelium.
- Using a cotton swab, apply 3–5% of acetic acid to the cervix; 3% is preferred as the 5% might cause burning sensation in some women. It is advisable not to rub or pat the swab against the cervix or vagina as this can easily abrade the abnormal epithelium resulting in bleeding. The soaked swab should be compressed against the epithelial surface for 1 min.

- The SCJ is visualized and identified, and TZ is examined till its distal end. The proximal end of TZ is identified by SCJ, whereas the distal end is identified by nabothian follicles or crypt openings. The type of transformation zone should be noted as this gives a guide for selection of the diagnostic procedure. If the TZ can be seen completely, it is labelled as adequate colposcopy (as per IFCPC terminology) [26]. This translates into 360° of visualization of columnar epithelium, squamous epithelium and newly formed SCJ and entire TZ. If the colposcopy is inadequate, an excisional procedure may be needed.
- If the inner margin of TZ has receded into the endocervical canal, it can be visualized within the cervical canal by:
  - Use of endocervical speculum of appropriate size.
  - Using dry cotton swab to retract the lips of the cervix.
  - Use of long tissue dissecting forceps with fine smooth tips.
  - Use of iris hook to retract the cervical lips.
- Examination of vagina: Vaginal fornices are also examined while withdrawing the bivalve speculum, more so when no abnormality is detected on the cervix and the woman is referred because of an abnormal Pap smear. Saline followed by 3% acetic acid is applied.
- Now cervix and vagina are swabbed with Lugol's iodine and findings are noted.
- Documentation of the colposcopic findings is done by photo or video documentation and simple hand drawing or on a preprinted diagram. There are two formats to document the results on paper, i.e., Hammond graph and Odell diagram. Most colposcopes now use a computer software to store images and patient data.
- Another important part of documentation is scoring the lesion for high grade or low grade which eventually helps in deciding the management plan. The most commonly used scoring systems are Modified Reid's Combined Colposcopic Index and Swede's Score [27].
- Endocervical curettage (ECC) should be performed in cases of inadequate colposcopy, abnormal cytology with normal ectocervix and referral cytology indicating glandular lesion.
- Colposcopy-directed biopsy can be performed if indicated. Biopsy is taken with punch biopsy forceps (Kevorkian, Tischler-Morgan) which have sharp jaws, and a sharp quick bite of the tissue should be taken including the stroma. It should be taken from the area with worst features and those abutting the SCJ. Bleeding after the procedure can be controlled with Monsel's paste or packing.

The IFCPC terminology and scoring systems are discussed in Chap. 12.

11.7 Assessment of Lesion on Colposcopy

The lesion is assessed colposcopically with respect to:

- Colour tone
- Surface contour
- Margin of aceto-white areas
- Vasculature pattern
- Iodine staining.

11.7.1 Colour Tone

Normal squamous epithelium appears smooth and translucent with pinkish appearance after application of normal saline. This is darker in comparison to metaplastic epithelium. Columnar cells appear dark red with villous appearance. Acetic acid causes reversible coagulation of nuclear and cytoplasmic proteins in the epithelium. The superficial layers of squamous epithelium are sparsely nucleated so do not undergo coagulation thereby appearing pink on colposcopy. CIN or preclinical invasive cancer appear opaque/aceto-white due to coagulation of their high nuclear content; in cases of low-grade CIN, appearance of aceto-whitening is delayed and of less intensity as compared to a high-grade lesion (Fig. 11.12).

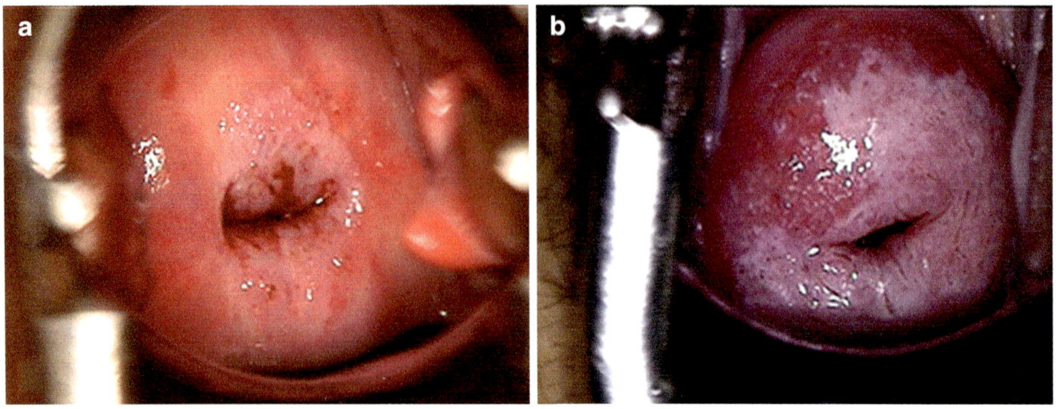

Fig. 11.12 Comparison of aceto-whitening in low- and high-grade lesion

11.7.2 Surface Contour

It may be smooth, uneven, granular or nodular. Normal squamous epithelium is smooth, while columnar epithelium has grape-like, papillomatous appearance (villi). Early invasive cancer has an uneven and elevated surface or may be nodular or polypoidal [28].

11.7.3 Margin of Aceto-White Area

The margins are sharp in high-grade lesions and normal tissue than in cases of inflammatory or mild dysplasia.

11.7.4 Iodine Staining

Normal glycogenated squamous epithelium strains mahogany brown or black on application of Lugol's iodine, whereas CIN, invasive cancers and columnar epithelium do not stain with iodine and appear as thick mustard yellow or have variegated uptake pattern.

11.7.5 Vascular Patterns

Normal vascular pattern on the ectocervix consists of tree-like branching vessels or small end-on points of hairpin capillaries seen as dots. But in dysplastic epithelium, there can be mosaic or punctations. Atypical vessels in the form of hairpin, comma shaped or noodle shaped can be seen.

11.8 Conclusion

Cervical cancer develops as a result of a series of alterations in the cervical epithelium caused by persistent infection with high-risk human papilloma virus. It develops from well-defined precancerous lesions which if not treated timely can progress to invasive cancer over a varied period of time. Detected in preinvasive stage, cervical cancer is both preventable and curable. Colposcopy with directed biopsy forms an important tool in the evaluation and management of women with preinvasive intraepithelial lesions.

Key Points

- Colposcopy and guided biopsy are considered as a diagnostic (not screening) test for evaluation of precancerous lesions of cervix.
- Identification of transformation zone (area between old and new squamocolumnar junction) is most important as maximum mitotic activity takes place in this zone, and it is the area where precancerous changes initiate.
- Systemic colposcopic examination consists of application of normal saline followed by green filter, acetic acid and Lugol's iodine in a sequential manner.
- The scoring and documentation of lesions seen colposcopically form an important aspect of diagnosis and management.
- Grade of the lesion is assessed by evaluation of the TZ in terms of aceto-whiteness, margins, vascular pattern and presence of atypical vessels.

- Vascular features such as fine punctation and fine mosaic in aceto-white area indicate low-grade lesion, while coarse punctation and mosaic are found in high-grade lesions.

References

1. Burke L, Antonioli DA, Ducatman BS. Colposcopy: text and atlas. Norwalk: Appleton and Lange; 1991.
2. Popkin RD. Colposcopy. Can Fam Physician. 1987;33:2083–8.
3. Benedet JL, Matisic JP, Bertrand MA, et al. The quality of community colposcopy practice. Obstet Gynaecol. 2004;103(1):92–100.
4. International Agency for Research on Cancer. Cervical cancer screening, Handbook of cancer prevention, vol. 10. Lyon: IARC Press; 2005.
5. Arora R, Jain S. Colposcopy: the scientific basis. In: Mehta S, Sachdeva P, editors. Colposcopy of female genital tract. 1st ed. Singapore: Springer; 2017. p. 99–109.
6. Hendrickson MR, Atkins KA, Kempson RL. Uterus and fallopian tubes. In: Mills SE, editor. Histology for pathologists. 3rd ed. Philadelphia: Lippincott, Williams and Wilkins; 2007. p. 1017–21.
7. Ferris DG, Cox JT, O'Connor DM, et al. Modern colposcopy: textbook and atlas. 2nd ed. Dubuque: Kendall/Hunt Publishing; 2004.
8. Wright TC, Ferenczy A. Anatomy and histology of the cervix. In: Kurman RJ, editor. Blaustein's pathology of the female genital tract. 4th ed. New York: Springer. p. 185–99.
9. O'Conner DM. The normal transformation zone. In: Apgar BS, Brotzman GL, Spitzer M, editors. Colposcopy principles and practice: an integrated textbook and atlas. Philadelphia: WB Saunders; 2002. p. 147–58.
10. Singh K, Badkur P. Colposcopy: the scientific basis. In: Mehta S, Sachdeva P, editors. Colposcopy of female genital tract. 1st ed. Singapore: Springer; 2017. p. 121–8.
11. Walker P, DePalo G, Campion M, Jakob C, Ray M. International terminology of colposcopy. An update report from International Federation for Cervical Pathology and Colposcopy. Obstet Gynecol. 2003;101:175–7.
12. Gilmour E, Ellerbrock TV, Koulous JP, et al. Measuring cervical ectopy: direct visual assessment versus computerized planimetry. Am J Obstet Gynecol. 1997;176:108–11.
13. Brotzman GL, Apgar BS. Abnormal transformation zone. In: Apgar BS, Brotzman GL, Spitzer M, editors. Colposcopy principles and practice: an integrated textbook and atlas. Philadelphia: WB Saunders; 2002. p. 175–82.
14. Cecchini S, Bonardi R, Iossa A, Zappa M, Tumori CS. Colposcopy as a primary screening test for cervical cancer. Tumori. 1997;83(5):810–3.
15. Frisch LE, Parmar H, Buckley LD, Chalem SA. Colposcopy of patients with Cytologic Inflammatory epithelial changes. Acta Cytol. 1990;34:1335.
16. Brown D, Kaufman R, Gardner H. Leukoplakia of the cervix. Am J Obstet Gynecol. 1973;116(2):214–21.
17. Kolstad P, Stafl A. Atlas of colposcopy. Baltimore: University Park Press; 1972.
18. Sellors JW, Sankaranarayanan R. Colposcopy and the treatment of cervical intraepithelial neoplasia: a Beginner's manual. Lyon: IARC Press; 2003. p. 30.
19. Dobbs SP, Brown LJ, Ireland D, et al. Platelet derived endothelial cell growth factor expression and angiogenesis in cervical intraepithelial neoplasia and squamous cell carcinoma of the cervix. Ann Diagn Pathol. 2000;4:286–92.
20. Dobbs SP, Hewett PW, Johnson IR, et al. Angiogenesis is associated with vascular endothelial growth factor expression in cervical intraepithelial neoplasia. Br J Cancer. 1997;76:1410–5.
21. Shahida SM, Mirza TT, Saleh AF, Islam MA. Colposcopic evaluation of pre-invasive and early cervical carcinoma with histologic correlation. Mymensingh Med J. 2012;21(2):200–6.
22. Coppelson M, Pixle E, Reid B. Colposcopy. Springfield: Charles C Thomas; 1971. p. 14–6.
23. Rokita W. Colposcopy of abnormal transformation zone. Wiad Lek. 2006;59(7):486–9.
24. O'Connor DM. A tissue basis for colposcopic findings. Obstet Gynecol Clin N Am. 2008;35:565–82.
25. Baliga BS. Step by step colposcopy, cryosurgery and LEEP. New Delhi: Jaypee Brothers Medical Publishers; 2008.
26. Bornstein J, Bentley J, Bosze P, et al. Colposcopic terminology of the international federation for cervical pathology and colposcopy. Obstet Gynecol. 2012;120:166–72.
27. Bowring J, Strander B, Young M, et al. The Swede score: evaluation of a scoring system designed to improve the predictive value of colposcopy. J Low Genit Tract Dis. 2010;14:301–5.
28. Bhaskaran S. Colposcopic evaluation of preinvasive and early cervical cancer. In: Mehta S, Sachdeva P, editors. Colposcopy of female genital tract. 1st ed. Singapore: Springer; 2017. p. 129–42.

Colposcopic Features of Cervical Intraepithelial Lesions

12

Partha Basu, Smita Joshi, and Usha Poli

Abbreviations

AIS	Adenocarcinoma-in-situ
CIN	Cervical intraepithelial neoplasia
HPV	Human papillomavirus
IFCPC	The International Federation of Cervical Pathology and Colposcopy
SCJ	Squamocolumnar junction
TZ	Transformation zone
VIA	Visual inspection with acetic acid
WHO	The World Health Organization

12.1 Introduction

The major steps in cervical carcinogenesis are persistent infection from the oncogenic types of human papillomavirus (HPV), development of cervical premalignant lesions and progression to invasion spanning over a period of 10–20 years [1]. The premalignant abnormalities of the cervical epithelium are known as cervical intraepithelial neoplasia (CIN), which if left untreated may lead to invasive cancer [2]. The precursor lesions of squamous cell carcinoma are classified into CIN 1, CIN 2 or CIN 3 depending upon the thickness of the epithelium involved with the dysplastic cells. While in CIN 1 the abnormal cells occupy the lowest third of the cervical squamous epithelium, in CIN 2 and CIN 3, the abnormal cells occupy the lower two-thirds and nearly the full thickness or full thickness of the cervical squamous epithelium, respectively. As the severity of the intraepithelial neoplasia increases from CIN 1 to CIN 3, the risk of progression to invasive cancer increases and the possibility of regression decreases. High-grade CIN usually develops from pre-existing low-grade CIN, though de novo development cannot be ruled out [3, 4]. The current accepted opinion is that CIN 3 can develop either as the consequence of progression of CIN 1 and CIN 2 or directly from a high-risk HPV infection with no detectable intermediate stages [5–7]. The precursor lesions of cervical adenocarcinoma are known as adenocarcinoma-in-situ (AIS).

Colposcopy is visualization of the cervix under magnification with appropriate illumination after application of dilute acetic acid and Lugol's iodine to observe the morphological changes of the epithelium. Almost all high-grade cervical neoplasias and cancers occur in the cervical transformation zone (TZ). Persistent

P. Basu (✉)
Screening Group, International Agency for Research on Cancer, Lyon, France
e-mail: basup@iarc.fr

S. Joshi
Department of Preventive Oncology, Prayas and HCJMRI, Pune, India

U. Poli
MNJ Institute of Oncology & Regional Cancer Center, Hyderabad, India

S. Mehta, A. Singla (eds.), *Preventive Oncology for the Gynecologist*,
https://doi.org/10.1007/978-981-13-3438-2_12

oncogenic HPV infection of the totipotent stem cells underlying the immature metaplastic epithelium over the TZ may lead to neoplastic transformation in a small proportion of the HPV-infected women [8]. The objectives of colposcopy are to examine the TZ adequately, identify any abnormal areas, rule out invasive cancer, obtain appropriate samples if required for histological assessment and guide the disease management.

12.2 Colposcopy Procedure

Colposcopy is an outpatient procedure carried out for the evaluation of women with a positive cervical cancer screening test. A colposcope is a stereoscopic, binocular telescope with variable magnification and powerful light source used for magnified visual examination of the uterine cervix. The sequencial steps of colposcopy involve cleaning of cervix and vagina with normal saline solution followed by examination with green or blue filters to look for any abnormal vasculature, application of 3–5% freshly prepared acetic acid on the cervix for a minute and painting of the cervix with Lugol's iodine. The final diagnosis is arrived at through the summation of all the findings followed by directed biopsies, if indicated.

As per the IFCPC 2011 nomenclature, all colposcopic examinations should include assessing the adequacy of colposcopy, visualization of the squamocolumnar junction (SCJ) and documenting the type of transformation zone. Every colposcopy examination should document the following:

1. Colposcopy adequate or inadequate: Colposcopic examination is inadequate when the colposcopic view is compromised by gross infection, bleeding, scarring, etc. The reason for inadequate colposcopy should be documented.
2. Visibility of SCJ: SCJ is a thin margin between the reddish, grape-like columnar epithelium of the endocervix and the smooth pinkish squamous epithelium of the ectocervix. The SCJ is not static but changes its position with the changing hormonal milieu. Depending upon the age of the woman, hormonal status, parity, birth trauma, pregnancy, etc., the location of the SCJ in relation to the external os varies. During the reproductive age, the SCJ is usually easily visible at the external os or on the ectocervix. The SCJ gets withdrawn in the endocervical canal in the post-menopausal women and may become invisible, fully or partially.
3. Transformation zone type: The transformation zone is the area of the cervix between the original SCJ and the new SCJ formed after the metaplastic process. Identifying the extent of the transformation zone is of great importance not only for a successful diagnostic evaluation of the cervix but also to make treatment decisions. Treatment of cervical intraepithelial neoplasias involves treatment of the entire TZ rather than the visible lesion alone.

The TZ is labelled as type 1 when the SCJ is seen in its entirety and is on the ectocervix. If the SCJ is seen completely but is located within the endocervix fully or partially, the TZ is considered as type 2. In type 3 TZ, the SCJ is either partially visible or is not visible at all due to its extension within the endocervix.

12.3 Features of the Atypical TZ

The colposcopic appearance of the cervical intraepithelial neoplasia (CIN) or invasive cancer is dependent on a number of factors. These include degree of neoplastic changes, thickness of the epithelium involved, alterations in the stromal blood vessels, changes in surface contour and any associated changes in the epithelium like erosion and keratinization. Such changes become more prominent after application of dilute acetic acid for 1 min.

Acetowhite Epithelium The dysplastic cervical epithelium usually appears grossly normal after cleaning with normal saline. Application of acetic acid solution (3–5%) for 1 min transforms the

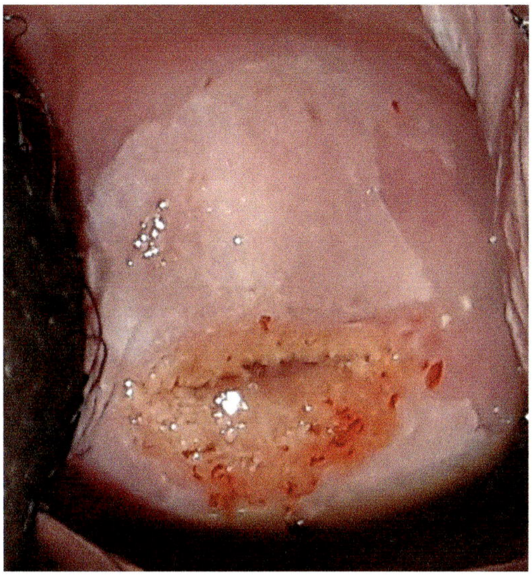

Fig. 12.1 Thin aceto-whitening at the TZ. Courtesy of Dr. Smita Joshi

epithelium white in presence of a neoplastic lesion. This transient and reversible change is called acetowhitening. Abnormal epithelial cells contain an increased amount of protein due to the increased number of cells, increased size of the nuclei and their chromatic content and intact cytoplasm. Application of dilute acetic acid results in coagulation of the cellular protein and overlapping of the enlarged nuclei. As a result light is not able to pass through the epithelium and is reflected back to the colposcope, making the abnormal epithelium appearing as opaque white areas (Fig. 12.1). Since cervical neoplasia originates at the TZ close to the squamocolumnar junction (SCJ), the acetowhitening due to the neoplastic lesions is always on the TZ. It is important to observe the real-time changes in the intensity of the whiteness. The speed of appearance of the acetowhitening and the rapidity of its disappearance are related to the number of immature, abnormal or neoplastic cells and correlate well with the grade of neoplasia. The higher the grade of CIN, the greater will be the number of such cells. As a result, in high-grade CIN, the whiteness will be more intense and the change will develop faster and last longer. The acetowhite changes are the most important of all the colposcopic features and the acetowhite epithelium should be assessed for the density, borders with surrounding tissues, surface contour, presence of vascular patterns and iodine uptake.

Density of Acetowhitening The intensity of the acetowhiteness (also known as density) may be helpful in assessing the severity of the lesion. Acetowhitening may be seen in several non-neoplastic conditions, most common of which is immature squamous metaplasia. Immature metaplastic cells also have an increased nuclear/cytoplasmic ratio and appear faintly white after acetic acid application. However, the acetowhitening of CIN is usually more dense and distinct compared to that of squamous metaplasia. Higher is the grade of neoplasia, greater is the epithelial thickness and degree of nuclear enlargement and density. The intensity of acetowhitening varies from a faint or a 'milky' white (seen in immature metaplasia and low-grade lesions) (Fig. 12.2a, b) to a dense grey white (high-grade lesions) (Fig. 12.3a, b). The faint acetowhite areas are often transparent, and the reddish colour of the cervical stroma is visible through them. Acetowhitening due to dysplastic cells appears more quickly, it is dense and appears oyster white or grey white and its border is distinct. Cervical warts are usually bright white in colour, often have multiple satellite lesions and may be located outside the TZ.

Borders The neoplastic lesions always have sharp well-demarcated smooth margins and may even be raised from the surrounding tissue in the CIN 3 lesions or invasive cancers. Squamous metaplasia has indistinct and irregular margin. The borders are often jagged, feathery or angular in low-grade lesions or in flat condylomas (lesions caused by low-risk HPV) (Fig. 12.2a, b). On the contrary CIN 2/CIN 3 has smooth, well-delineated margins (Fig. 12.3a). The acetowhite epithelium may extend into the cervical canal, and an endocervical speculum may be necessary to visualize the SCJ and identify the extent of the lesion (Fig. 12.4). A dense acetowhite area with a raised border should be carefully evaluated for invasive changes.

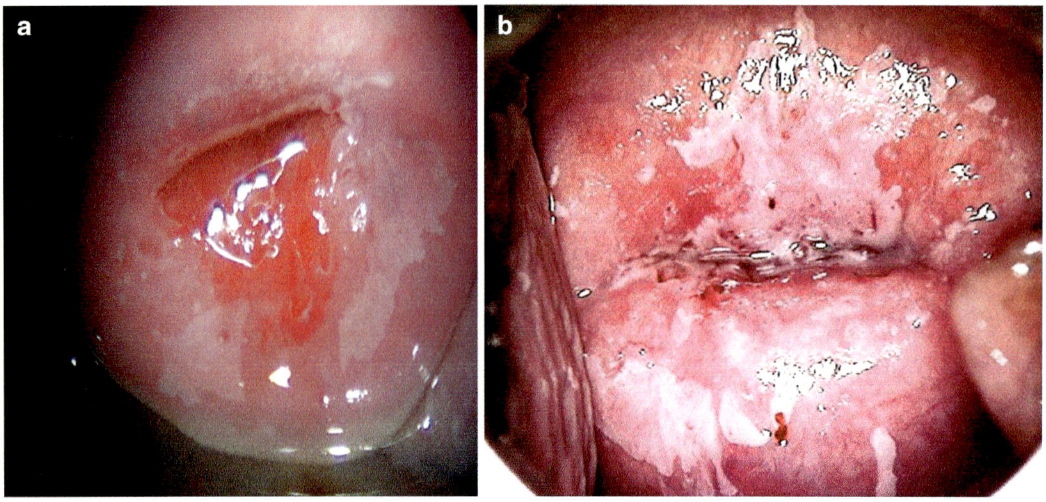

Fig. 12.2 (**a**) Faint or a "milky" white immature metaplasia and (**b**) low-grade changes. (**a**) Courtesy of Dr. Usha Poli. (**b**) Reproduced with permission from Basu P, Sankaranarayanan R (2017). Atlas of Colposcopy – Principles and Practice: IARC CancerBase No. 13 [Internet]. Lyon, France: International Agency for Research on Cancer. Available from: http://screening.iarc.fr/atlascolpo.php, accessed on 28/02/2018

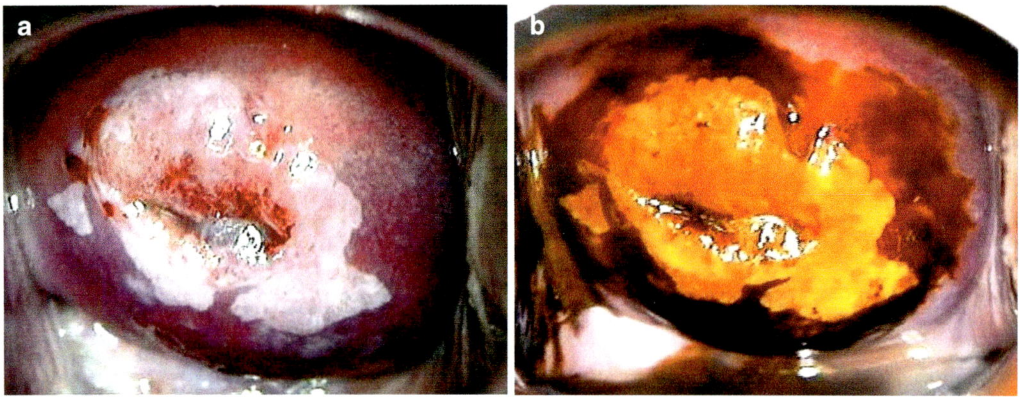

Fig. 12.3 High-grade lesion, dense aceto-whitening with sharp borders. (**a**) After application of acetic acid. (**b**) After application of Lugol's iodine. Reproduced with permission from Basu P, Sankaranarayanan R (2017). Atlas of Colposcopy – Principles and Practice: IARC CancerBase No. 13 [Internet]. Lyon, France: International Agency for Research on Cancer. Available from: http://screening.iarc.fr/atlascolpo.php, accessed on 28/02/2018

Surface Contour Normal epithelium and CIN lesions have smooth, regular surface contour. Cervical warts may have a papillary, finger-like or cauliflower-shaped surface. Uneven and raised nodular surface (mole-hill appearance) (Fig. 12.5a) that turns densely white should always raise the suspicion of invasive cancer. An exophytic growth (Fig. 12.5b) or an ulceration with everted margins is also suggestive of invasive cancer.

Vascular Patterns High-grade CIN or invasive cancer results in the formation of abnormal blood vessels in the sub-epithelial stroma that may be visible through the transparent epithelium during colposcopy prior to application of acetic acid. The formation of abnormal vessels is due to the expression of the vascular endothelial growth factor (VEGF) and other angiogenic factors, and the process is called neovascularization. The fine network of normal vessels may be visible in immature

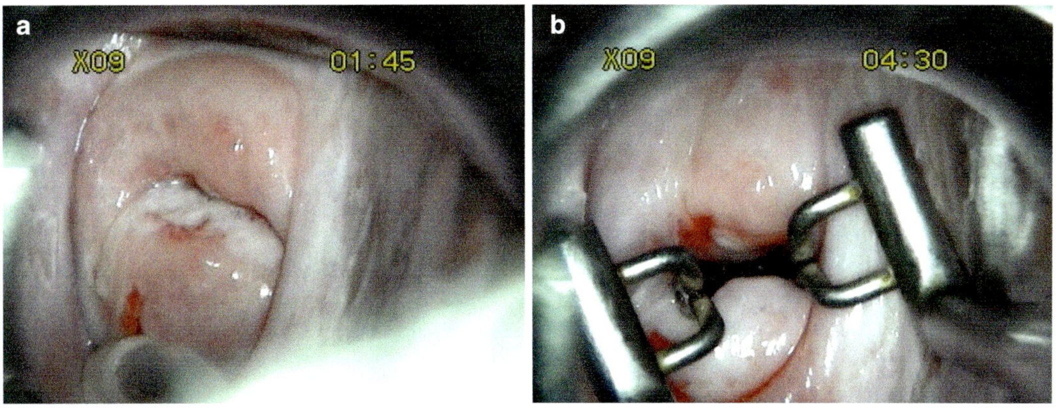

Fig. 12.4 (**a**, **b**) Endocervical lesion, endocervical speculum is being used to visualize the SCJ and to identify the extent of the lesion. Reproduced with permission from Basu P, Sankaranarayanan R (2017). Atlas of Colposcopy – Principles and Practice: IARC CancerBase No. 13 [Internet]. Lyon, France: International Agency for Research on Cancer. Available from: http://screening.iarc.fr/atlascolpo.php, accessed on 28/02/2018

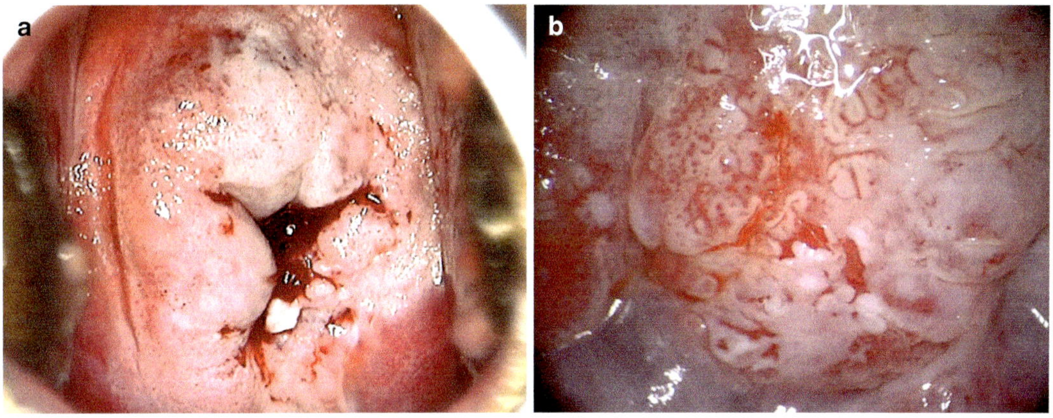

Fig. 12.5 (**a**) Invasive cancer, grossly uneven with raised nodular areas. Reproduced with permission from Basu P, Sankaranarayanan R (2017). Atlas of Colposcopy – Principles and Practice: IARC CancerBase No. 13 [Internet]. Lyon, France: International Agency for Research on Cancer. Available from: http://screening.iarc.fr/atlascolpo.php, accessed on 28/02/2018. (**b**) Invasive cancer with ulceration. Reprinted with permission from Prendiville W, Sankaranarayanan R. Colposcopy and treatment of cervical precancer. IARC technical publications, 45. Lyon: IARC, 2017

metaplasia due to the lower thickness of the epithelium. This regular network of normal vessels is called 'fine mosaic'. The stromal vessels also form loops towards the epithelial surface, and they appear colposcopically as fine red dots. This pattern is called punctation, which is fine and regular in the normal epithelium or in immature metaplasia. The abnormal blood vessels formed in the high-grade neoplastic tissues are usually prominent and irregularly spaced and may bulge out from the surface. The capillary loops are visible on colposcopy as irregularly placed red dots of various sizes and are known as coarse punctations (Fig. 12.6). As with punctation, mosaicism can be also be graded as coarse (Fig. 12.7) if the diameter of the vessels is uneven and they are irregularly distributed. Coarse punctation or mosaics are hallmarks of higher-grade lesions or invasive cancers. Fine punctation and mosaic are more commonly seen in immature metaplasia or low-grade lesions. A normal stromal

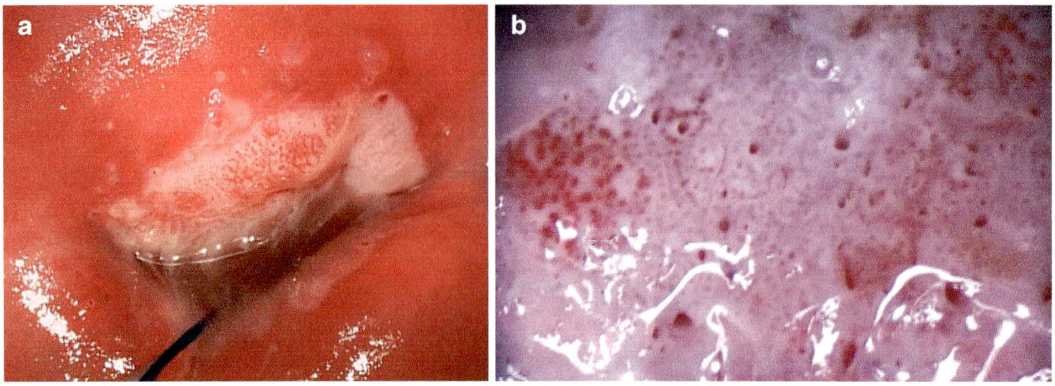

Fig. 12.6 (a, b) High-grade lesion with coarse punctations. Reprinted with permission from Prendiville W, Sankaranarayanan R. Colposcopy and treatment of cervical precancer. IARC technical publications, 45. Lyon: IARC, 2017

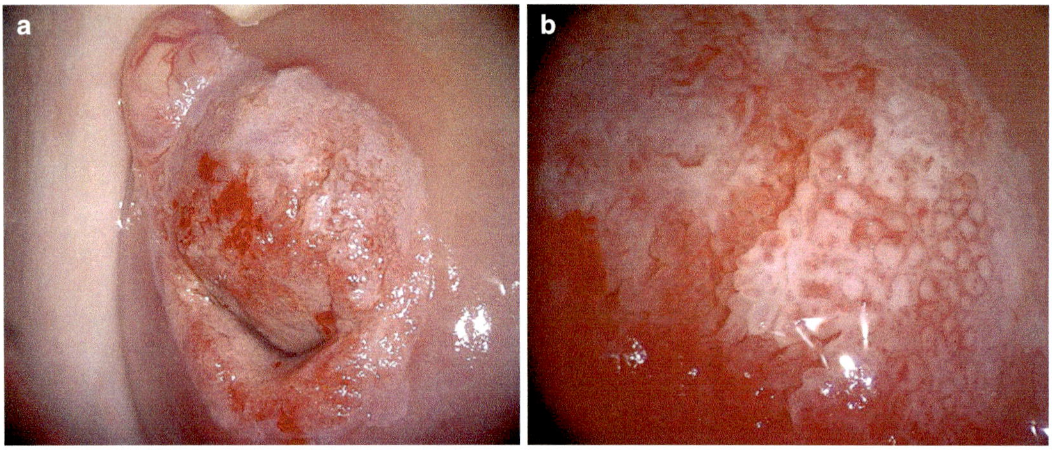

Fig. 12.7 (a) Coarse mosaic (under low power). (b) Coarse mosaic (under high power). Reprinted with permission from Prendiville W, Sankaranarayanan R. Colposcopy and treatment of cervical precancer. IARC technical publications, 45. Lyon: IARC, 2017

blood vessel has a typical branching pattern with a central stem that branches off to thinner blood vessels before finally disappearing. In presence of microinvasive or invasive cancer, the vascular pattern is often 'atypical' (Fig. 12.8). The atypical vessels do not follow the typical branching patterns of the normal vessels and often have bizarre shapes and uneven calibres. Atypical vessels are often friable and bleed to touch.

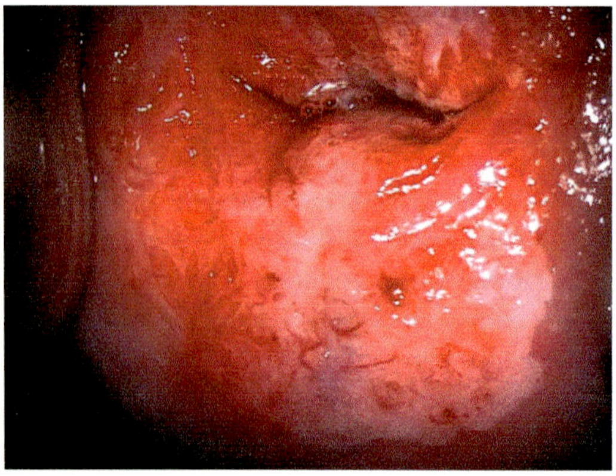

Fig. 12.8 Invasive cancer with atypical vessels. Reprinted with permission from Prendiville W, Sankaranarayanan R. Colposcopy and treatment of cervical precancer. IARC technical publications, 45. Lyon: IARC, 2017

Lugol's Iodine Uptake Lugol's iodine is a solution of 10 g potassium iodide dissolved in 100 mL distilled water with 5 g iodine crystals. The iodine stains the glycogen in normal squamous epithelium to make it appear dark brown. The poorly differentiated epithelium of the CIN lesions is devoid of glycogen, and hence they do not turn brown with Lugol's solution. The Lugol's negative areas appear yellow in colour (Fig. 12.3b). The cervical epithelium may not be stained with Lugol's iodine or may have patchy uptake of the stain in presence of inflammation, metaplasia or atrophy.

12.4 Colposcopic Features of Low-Grade Lesions (CIN 1 and Condylomas)

The low-grade lesions or the flat condylomas are usually due to transient HPV infections and may be seen adjacent to the squamocolumnar junction (SCJ) or even away from the transformation zone (TZ). The CIN 1 lesions are often confused with the flat condylomas or the immature metaplastic epithelium. The CIN 1 lesions usually appear thin but opaque acetowhite. They usually have irregular borders, which may be geographic, feathered, flocculated or indistinct (Fig. 12.9). The acetowhite changes on CIN1 lesions take longer time to appear and disappear early compared to that seen in CIN 2 or CIN 3. Low-grade lesions may have fine punctations and mosaics. CIN lesions appear iodine negative and are light mustard yellow in colour (Fig. 12.3b).

Condylomas may present on the cervix as flat or slightly raised lesions that turn acetowhite or as exophytic condylomata acuminate (Fig. 12.10). These may be found inside or beyond the TZ.

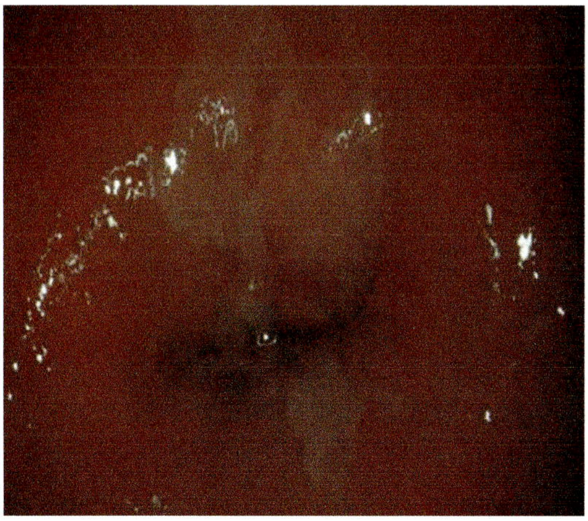

Fig. 12.9 CIN 1 lesion with thin, opaque acetowhitening. Reprinted with permission from Prendiville W, Sankaranarayanan R. Colposcopy and treatment of cervical precancer. IARC technical publications, 45. Lyon: IARC, 2017

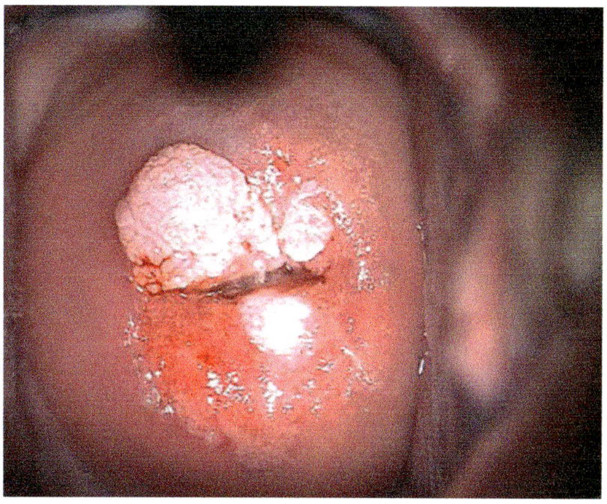

Fig. 12.10 Colposcopic view of cervical condyloma at low-power magnification. Reprinted with permission from Prendiville W, Sankaranarayanan R. Colposcopy and treatment of cervical precancer. IARC technical publications, 45. Lyon: IARC, 2017

12.5 Colposcopic Features of High-Grade Lesions (CIN 2 and CIN 3)

High-grade lesions usually originate from the SCJ and, depending on the type of TZ, may or may not extend to the endocervical canal. Acetowhite areas are dense and dull white and may have raised margins. The abnormal epithelium could be peeled away from the underlying stroma forming an area of erosion (Fig. 12.11). Such lesions may occupy three or four quadrants of the cervix. In type 2 or type 3 TZ, the lesion will extend to the endocervical canal, and the upper limit may not be visible on colposcopy. The margins of high-grade lesions are generally smooth with a distinct demarcation between the normal epithelium and neoplastic epithelium. The CIN 3 lesions are particularly opaque and have a 'dull oyster-grey' appearance. Moreover, the acetowhite effect persists longer in CIN 2/CIN 3 lesions than in CIN 1 lesions. Extensive lesions with higher-grade lesion located centrally and lesser grade located peripherally ('lesion within a lesion') can be also seen. The sharp demarcation between the thin and dense acetowhite

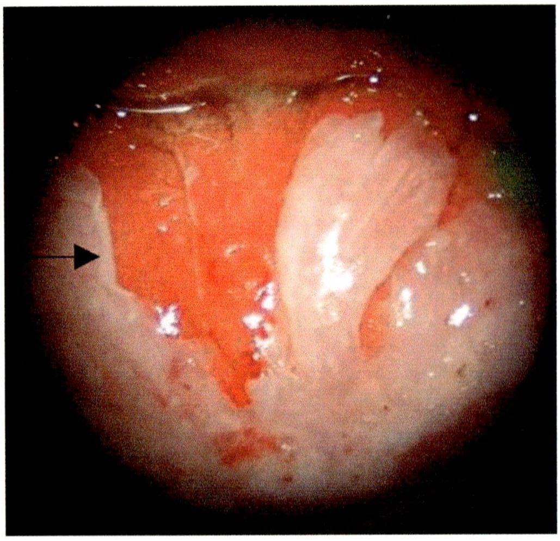

Fig. 12.11 High-grade lesion with peeling/Rag sign. Arrow indicates peeling of the epithelium. Courtesy of Dr. Usha Poli

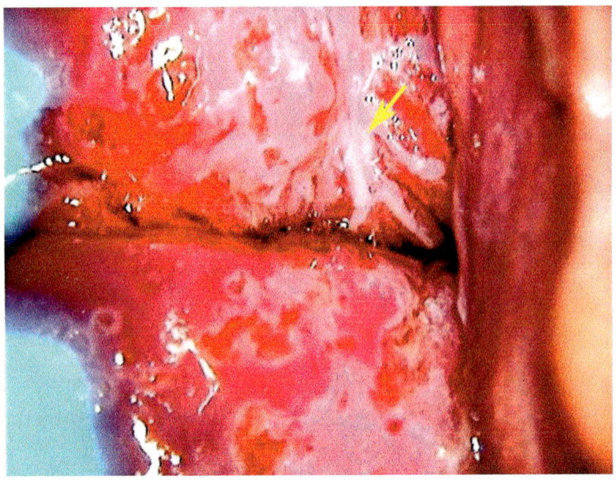

Fig. 12.12 High-grade lesion with ridge sign (opaque protuberance within a white lesion within the TZ). Reproduced with permission from Basu P, Sankaranarayanan R (2017). Atlas of Colposcopy – Principles and Practice: IARC CancerBase No. 13 [Internet]. Lyon, France: International Agency for Research on Cancer. Available from: http://screening.iarc.fr/atlascolpo.php, accessed on 28/02/2018

areas that exists within the same lesion is known as the 'inner border sign'.

CIN 3 may be characterized by a 'ridge sign', (Fig. 12.12) which is an opaque lesion, directly adjacent to the squamocolumnar junction, resembling a ridge or a table top. CIN 3 lesions may

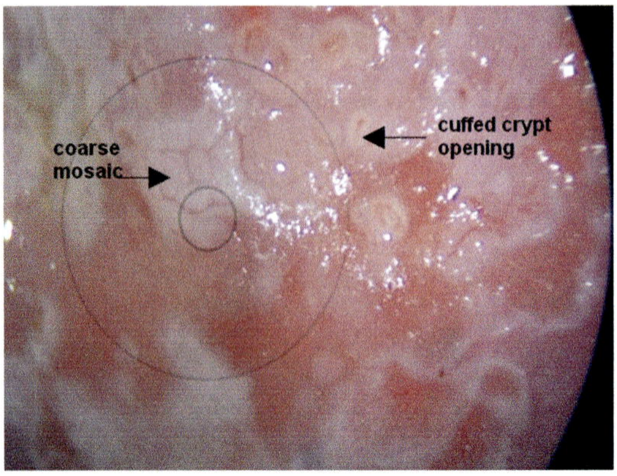

Fig. 12.13 High-grade lesion with cuffed crypt openings. Courtesy of Dr. Usha Poli

also have peeling edges, also known as 'rag sign' (Fig. 12.11). The thickened epithelium of CIN 3 can be peeled from the underlying stroma because of the poor cohesiveness among the dysplastic cells. The neoplastic epithelium may get abraded during the introduction of the speculum, collection of the smear for cytology or HPV testing or applying acetic acid or Lugol's solution. The raw naked stroma without any epithelial covering and revealing the fine capillaries is known as 'erosion'.

A raised acetowhite band around crypt opening is known as 'cuffed' crypt opening or 'doughnut appearance' and indicates extension of the high-grade lesion into the epithelial crypts (Fig. 12.13).

The coagulation caused by the acetic acid may mask the blood vessel pattern in a high-grade lesion, and they may not be apparent when observed immediately after application of acetic acid. The vessels will become apparent once the acetic acid effect begins to wear out after a few seconds.

There is little or no glycogen in the epithelium of high-grade lesions. Hence, a yellow iodine-negative area appears over the acetowhite lesion following the application of Lugol's solution (Fig. 12.3b). The colour is uniformly bright yellow ('canary yellow') in a CIN 3 on an invasive cancer.

12.6 Colposcopic Features of Preclinical Invasive Cancer

One of the major responsibilities of a colposcopist is to correctly identify the microinvasive and the early invasive cancers, though it may be challenging at times. Quite often such lesions are hidden in large CIN 3 lesions. Large lesion, with dull dense acetowhitening, extending to the canal, with irregular surface, erosions, coarse mosaics and punctations and atypical blood vessels, is always suspicious for microinvasive or early invasive cancer (Fig. 12.14). Diagnostic excision (cold knife conization) of the whole transformation zone is required, if colposcopy-guided punch biopsies do not confirm cancer.

A nodular, papillary, papular, or exophytic contour with necrosis and other features of high-grade lesion suggest the presence of frankly invasive cancer (Fig. 12.15). Atypical vessels (Fig. 12.8) are the hallmark of invasive cancer and may obtain the shape of corkscrew, spaghetti, comma, tendril and waste thread.

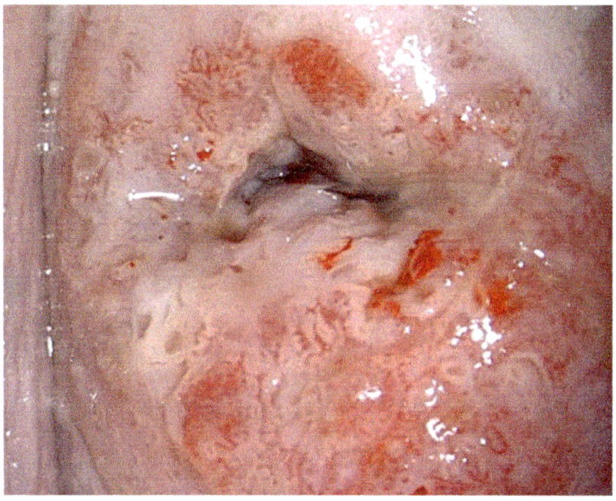

Fig. 12.14 Microinvasive cancer. Reprinted with permission from Prendiville W, Sankaranarayanan R. Colposcopy and treatment of cervical precancer. IARC technical publications, 45. Lyon: IARC, 2017

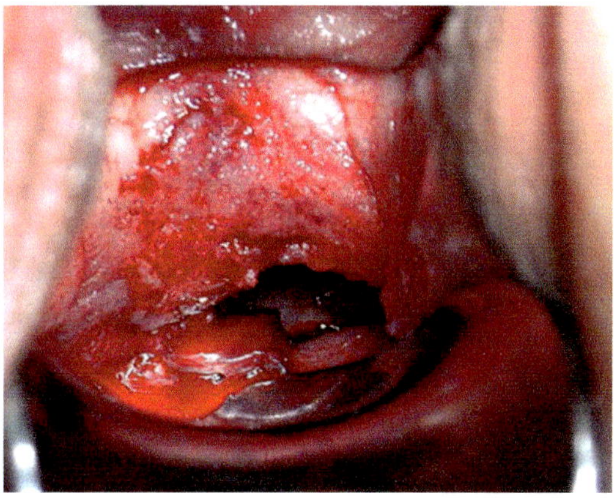

Fig. 12.15 Frank invasive cancer. Reprinted with permission from Prendiville W, Sankaranarayanan R. Colposcopy and treatment of cervical precancer. IARC technical publications, 45. Lyon: IARC, 2017

12.7 Documentation of Colposcopic Findings

It is important to document the colposcopic findings not only for appropriate diagnosis and management but also for future follow-up. Saving of the images in digital formats allows comparison of the findings at follow-up. A simple diagrammatic representation of the transformation zone and the abnormalities detected can also be very useful for future comparison. A uniform terminology and uniform scoring system reduce the variability and improve the objectivity of reporting and also help in the comparison between published reports on test performance. To improve the diagnostic accuracy of colposcopy and make it more objective, the International Federation of Cervical Pathology and Colposcopy (IFCPC) introduced a new system of nomenclature in 2011. The Reid score has been replaced by Swede score to grade the severity of abnormalities.

IFCPC 2011 Classification of Colposcopic Terminology The 2011 IFCPC nomenclature aims to standardize the colposcopic examination findings. At the outset the colposcopist must comment on the adequacy of the examination. The examination should be considered inadequate if the cervix cannot be exposed properly due to adhesions, atrophy or lax vaginal wall. Sometimes the features on the transformation zone may not be satisfactorily visible due to surface bleeding and/or extensive inflammation, and

Table 12.1 IFCPC 2011 classification

Abnormal colposcopic findings	**General principles**	*Location of lesion*: inside or outside the T-zone, location by clock position *Size of lesion*: number of cervical quadrants the lesion covers, size of lesion in percentage of cervix	
	Grade 1 (minor)	Thin acetowhite epithelium	Fine mosaic
		Irregular, geographic border	Fine punctation
	Grade 2 (major)	Dense acetowhite epithelium	Coarse mosaic
		Rapid appearance of acetowhitening	Coarse punctation, sharp border, inner
		Cuffed crypt (gland) openings	Border, ridge sign
	Non-specific	Leukoplakia (keratosis, hyperkeratosis), erosion, Lugol's staining (Schiller's test): stained/unstained	

Table 12.2 Swede scoring system

Swede score	0	1	2
Aceto uptake	Zero or transparent	Shady, milky Neither transparent nor opaque	Distinct Opaque White
Margins/ surface	Diffuse	Sharp but irregular, jagged, geographic satellites	Sharp, even, difference in surface level, includes cuffing
Vessels	Fine, regular	Absent	Coarse or atypical
Lesion size	<5 mm	5–15 mm or Two quadrants	>15 mm or Three to four quadrants or undefined endocervically
Iodine staining	Brown	Faintly or patchy yellow	Distinct yellow
Total score			

the examination is considered inadequate. It is mandatory to document the location of the SCJ and its visibility. Depending on the location and the visibility of the SCJ, the TZ should be classified as TZ type 1 (SCJ fully visible on the ectocervix or at the external os), TZ type 2 (SCJ fully visible but is situated in the endocervical cancer either fully or partially) or type 3 (the SCJ is partially or completely invisible due to its location inside the canal). The colposcopist should comment on the normal squamous epithelium (whether any features of metaplasia, atrophy or pregnancy are present) and the normal columnar epithelium (presence of ectropion), even if the colposcopy is completely normal.

The abnormal colposcopic findings are classified as minor (grade 1) or major (grade 2), depending on their severity, the minor and the major findings being predictive of low-grade and high-grade lesions, respectively (Table 12.1). It is important to describe the location of the lesion in relation to the TZ and also the size of the lesion, as described in the table.

Swede Scoring System The Swede scoring system takes into account the five main characteristics of the lesion described in Table 12.2. These are the density of acetowhitening, margin and surface of the abnormality, presence or absence of blood vessels, lesion size and the changes after iodine staining; each feature is ascribed a score of 0, 1 or 2. A total score of less than 5 reasonably excludes the presence of high-grade lesions. A score of either 5 or 6 indicates high-grade lesion; invasive cancer is very unlikely. A high-grade lesion or even an invasive cancer should be suspected if the score exceeds 6.

12.8 Accuracy of Colposcopy

Colposcopy is a highly subjective procedure, and the interobserver agreement in the assessment of components of colposcopic grading using static/digital cervical images remains poor between providers [9–11]. In order to reduce the interobserver variability, it is important to adapt a uniform reporting and grading system suggested by the IFCPC. When the 2011 IFCPC classification is used, colposcopic accuracy by examiners with differing amounts of experience has no significant difference [12–14]. The diagnostic accuracy of colposcopic examination, like that of any subjective test, varies according to the training and expertise of the colposcopist, the prevalence of the disease and the knowledge of the referral screening test report [15]. Even when performed by experienced colposcopists, when colposcopy is used as a triaging tool, its specificity is very low and is around 50% [16]. A systematic, pooled analysis of the accuracy of colposcopy observed that 46.4% screen-positive women undergoing colposcopy would be falsely diagnosed to have CIN 2/CIN 3 and would be unnecessarily treated (in a 'colposcopy-and-treat' scenario) [17]. Finally, colposcopy performs better at the extremes of abnormality: excluding the normal cervix and identifying the CIN 3 and invasive cancer [15].

12.9 Limitations of Colposcopy

The purpose of colposcopy is to define which women need further diagnostic evaluation by a biopsy and treatment and which women do not need the same.

The technique of performing colposcopy requires a thorough knowledge of the pathophysiology of HPV infection, cervical abnormalities, good training and mentoring, continued learning, improvement in skills and frequent colposcopic-histopathological correlation to improve one's performance. The accuracy of colposcopy also depends upon the adequacy of colposcopy, visualization of SCJ and TZ type. The adequacy of colposcopy may be affected when there is inflammation, bleeding, atrophy, previous treatment, etc.

Studies of loop excision after colposcopy have identified women with high-grade disease missed colposcopically [18]. Blind biopsies from the apparent normal TZ on colposcopy may detect unsuspected CIN2+ [19]. Therefore a colposcopist should be liberal in obtaining biopsies specially from the equivocal changes [20].

Colposcopy is also expensive and time-consuming and requires a dedicated setup and a well-trained team. Such infrastructure may not always be available in many low- and middle-income countries. The retrospective analysis of a large study conducted in South India showed that the risk of cervical cancer among women who tested positive by visual inspection with acetic acid (VIA) and underwent colposcopy and who did not undergo colposcopy was the same [21]. This suggests that colposcopy triage has limited value in VIA screening, especially in limited resourced settings. Moreover, colposcopy requires an additional visit to the health facilities that reduces the compliance of the women. The world Health Organization (WHO) has recommended a 'screen and treat' strategy using VIA or HPV testing (when affordable) in settings where organizing colposcopy and histopathology services is difficult. The main disadvantage of exclusion of colposcopy in the 'see and treat' strategy is that a large number of women may be overtreated.

12.10 Summary

Colposcopy is a triage tool between a positive cervical cancer screening test (or a suspicious looking cervix) and the histopathological diagnosis. The essential characteristics noted during colposcopy are acetowhiteness, vessel types, margin status, lesion size and iodine staining. Adapting a uniform reporting system, the

Swede scoring system helps in improving the yield and reduces the variability of reporting. A high-grade lesion on colposcopy appears distinct, opaque white; it has a sharp and even border, has coarse punctation and mosaic pattern, involves three or four quadrants, may be >15 mm in longest diameter and may have endocervical extension which cannot be defined; and it appears distinct yellow after application of Lugol's iodine. Inner border sign and ridge sign are two more pathognomonic criteria that are highly associated with the presence of high-grade CIN.

Key Points

- IFCPC nomenclature and Swede scoring system should be adapted for uniform reporting of colposcopy findings.
- Although acetowhitening itself cannot distinguish between dysplastic cells and non-dysplastic cells, acetowhitening due to dysplastic cells appears more quickly, it is dense, it appears oyster white or grey white and its border is distinct and lasts longer.
- The characteristics of the vessels are punctations, mosaicism and atypical vessels. These are seen when there is abnormal epithelium or dysplastic epithelium.
- Abnormal cells/cancerous cells do not contain glycogen and hence do not stain mahogany brown or black and remain mustard or saffron yellow in colour.
- Generally sharp margin status is associated with a high-grade lesion. As the sharpness of the margin increases, the possibility of a high-grade lesion increases. Low-grade lesions are associated with geographic, jagged margins.
- A small geographic lesion with fine punctation and/or fine mosaic is likely to be a low-grade lesion, whereas a large lesion involving more than two quadrants with coarse punctations and coarse mosaic is likely to be a high-grade lesion.
- The colposcopic abnormalities within the transformation zone and large lesions are more closely related to high-grade lesion/carcinoma.
- Grade 1 (minor) abnormalities have fine mosaic, fine punctation, thin acetowhite epithelium and irregular, geographic border.
- Grade 2 (major) abnormalities have sharp border, inner border sign, ridge sign, dense acetowhite epithelium, coarse mosaic, coarse punctations, rapid appearance of acetowhitening and cuffed crypt (gland) openings.
- Screening, either evaluation of screen positives or immediate treatment of screen positives, and recall of screen negatives at regular interval are essential to ultimately reduce cervical cancer incidence and mortality.

References

1. Schiffman M, Kjaer SK. Chapter 2: Natural history of anogenital human papillomavirus infection and neoplasia. J Natl Cancer Inst Monogr. 2003;31:14–9.
2. Wheeler CM. Natural history of human papillomavirus infections, cytologic and histologic abnormalities, and cancer. Obstet Gynecol Clin N Am. 2008;35(4):519–36.
3. Koutsky LA, Holmes KK, Critchlow CW, Stevens CE, Paavonen J, Beckmann AM, et al. A cohort study of the risk of cervical intraepithelial neoplasia grade 2 or 3 in relation to papillomavirus infection. N Engl J Med. 1992;327(18):1272–8.
4. Kiviat NB, Koutsky LA. Specific human papillomavirus types as the causal agents of most cervical intraepithelial neoplasia: implications for current views and treatment. J Natl Cancer Inst. 1993;85(12):934–5.
5. Kiviat NB, Critchlow CW, Kurman RJ. Reassessment of the morphological continuum of cervical intraepithelial lesions: does it reflect different stages in the progression to cervical carcinoma? IARC Sci Publ. 1992;119:59–66.
6. Park J, Sun D, Genest DR, Trivijitsilp P, Suh I, Crum CP. Coexistence of low and high grade squamous intraepithelial lesions of the cervix: morphologic progression or multiple papillomaviruses? Gynecol Oncol. 1998;70(3):386–91.
7. Winer RL, Kiviat NB, Hughes JP, Adam DE, Lee SK, Kuypers JM, et al. Development and duration of human papillomavirus lesions, after initial infection. J Infect Dis. 2005;191(5):731–8.
8. Crum CP. Contemporary theories of cervical carcinogenesis: the virus, the host, and the stem cell. Mod Pathol. 2000;13(3):243–51.
9. Jeronimo J, Massad LS, Castle PE, Wacholder S, Schiffman M. Interobserver agreement in the evaluation of digitized cervical images. Obstet Gynecol. 2007;110(4):833–40.
10. Ferris DG, Litaker M. Interobserver agreement for colposcopy quality control using digitized colposcopic images during the ALTS trial. J Low Genit Tract Dis. 2005;9(1):29–35.

11. Massad LS, Jeronimo J, Schiffman M. Interobserver agreement in the assessment of components of colposcopic grading. Obstet Gynecol. 2008;111(6):1279–84.
12. Hammes LS, Naud P, Passos EP, Matos J, Brouwers K, Rivoire W, et al. Value of the International Federation for Cervical Pathology and Colposcopy (IFCPC) Terminology in predicting cervical disease. J Low Genit Tract Dis. 2007;11(3):158–65.
13. Li Y, Duan X, Sui L, Xu F, Xu S, Zhang H, et al. Closer to a uniform language in colposcopy: study on the potential application of 2011 International Federation for Cervical Pathology and Colposcopy Terminology in clinical practice. Biomed Res Int. 2017;2017:8984516.
14. Cristiani P, Costa S, Schincaglia P, Garutti P, de Bianchi PS, Naldoni C, et al. An online quality assurance program for colposcopy in a population-based cervical screening setting in Italy: results on colposcopic impression. J Low Genit Tract Dis. 2014;18(4):309–13.
15. Prendiville W, Sankaranarayanan R. Colposcopy and treatment of cervical precancer, IARC technical publications, 45. Lyon: IARC; 2017.
16. Mitchell MF. Accuracy of colposcopy. Consult Obstet Gynecol. 1994;6:70–3.
17. Mustafa RA, Santesso N, Khatib R, Mustafa AA, Wiercioch W, Kehar R, et al. Systematic reviews and meta-analyses of the accuracy of HPV tests, visual inspection with acetic acid, cytology, and colposcopy. Int J Gynecol Obstet. 2016;132:259–65.
18. Massad LS, Halperin CJ, Bitterman P. Correlation between colposcopically directed biopsy and cervical loop excision. Gynecol Oncol. 1996;60:400–3.
19. Pretorius RG, Zhang WH, Belinson JL, Huang MN, Wu LY, Zhang X, et al. Colposcopically directed biopsy, random cervical biopsy, and endocervical curettage in the diagnosis of cervical intraepithelial neoplasia II or worse. Am J Obstet Gynecol. 2004;191:430–4.
20. Massad LS, Jeronimo J, Katki HA, Schiffman M, National Institutes of Health/American Society for Colposcopy and Cervical Pathology Research Group. The accuracy of colposcopic grading for detection of high-grade cervical intraepithelial neoplasia. J Low Genit Tract Dis. 2009;13(3):137–44.
21. Shastri SS, Mittra I, Mishra GA, Gupta S, Dikshit R, Singh S, et al. Effect of VIA screening by primary health workers: randomized controlled study in Mumbai, India. J Natl Cancer Inst. 2014;106(3):dju009.

Further Reading

Basu P, Sankaranarayanan R. Atlas of colposcopy: Principles and practice. Lyon: IARC; 2017. http://screening.iarc.fr/atlascolpo.php.

Sellors JW, Sankaranarayanan R. Colposcopy and treatment of cervical intraepithelial neoplasia: a beginners' manual. Lyon: IARC; 2003.

Cervical Cancer Screening in Pregnancy

13

Dipanwita Banerjee, Ranajit Mandal, and Alpana Chhetri

13.1 Introduction

Cervical cancer is the most common genital malignancy diagnosed during pregnancy. Around 3% of newly diagnosed invasive cervical cancer occurs in pregnant women [1]. The prevalence of abnormal Papanicolaou (Pap) test result in pregnancy does not differ from the age-matched non-pregnant population. In some populations up to 20% of pregnant women have an abnormal Pap test result during pregnancy [2]. The objective of this chapter is to review the existing guidelines on cervical cancer screening in pregnancy and also diagnosis and management of cervical intraepithelial neoplasias (CIN) in pregnancy.

D. Banerjee (✉) · R. Mandal
Department of Gynaecological Oncology, Chittaranjan National Cancer Institute, Kolkata, West Bengal, India

A. Chhetri
Department of Obstetrics and Gynaecology, Chittaranjan Seva Sadan College of Obstetrics, Gynaecology and Child Health, Kolkata, West Bengal, India

13.2 Current Scenario of Screening Programs in Developed and Low- and Middle-Income Countries

Annual incidence of 122,000 new cervical cancer cases and 67,000 cervical cancer-related deaths clearly show the burden of this totally preventable cancer in India [3]. The screening program available in India is very sporadic, opportunistic, and non-population based. According to the India HPV report, in 2012, only 2.6% of the rural women and 4.9% of the urban women have been screened in the country [4]. Tamil Nadu is the only state in the country that has initiated systematic screening of the women after conducting a pilot project in three districts [4]. In high-income countries, a Pap test linked with definitive treatment has prevented millions of women from cervical cancer but failed to achieve optimum utilization in most developing countries. In the last two decades, various research works have convincingly established the utility of visual inspection on acetic acid (VIA) and human papillomavirus test (HPV) in low- and middle-income countries (LMICS) including India [5–7]. The evidence was evaluated by the World Health Organization (WHO) in recently published recommendations for comprehensive cervical cancer control strategies for the low- and middle-income countries [8]. The existing guidelines are almost the same for the specified age

S. Mehta, A. Singla (eds.), *Preventive Oncology for the Gynecologist*,
https://doi.org/10.1007/978-981-13-3438-2_13

group of 21–65 years irrespective of the pregnancy status with few modifications according to the gestational age of the women and severity of abnormality on screening test.

Prenatal care provides an opportunity for screening because many women seek health care only when they are pregnant. This is especially true for low- and middle-income countries where catching up the reproductive age group women may be the only opportunity to screen all pregnant women who are older than 21 years when they present for their first prenatal visit.

13.3 Physiological Changes of the Cervix in Pregnancy

Due to increased estrogen and progesterone, the cervix becomes soft and swollen with resultant hypertrophy and hyperplasia of the elastic and connective tissues. Estradiol stimulates growth of columnar epithelium resulting in exposure of the columnar line of endocervical canal into the vaginal secretions. This condition is also known as ectropion. Due to increased mucus production, clinical examination of the cervix becomes difficult (Fig. 13.1). Decidualization of the cervical stroma often causes increased friability, polyps, and plaque-like changes that can be seen grossly and also on colposcopy examination (Fig. 13.2).

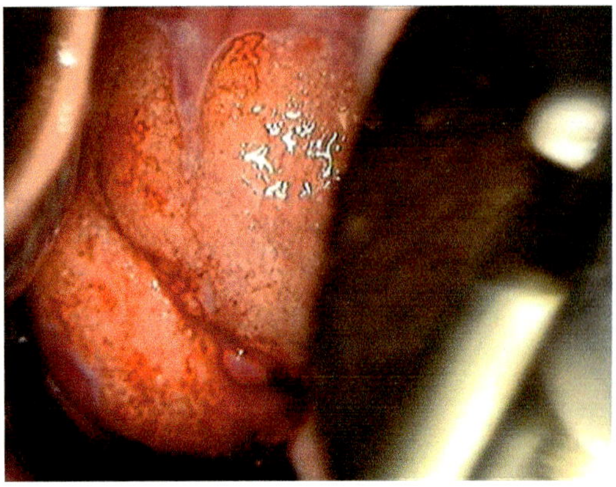

Fig. 13.1 Difficult colposcopy examination due to large ectropion in pregnancy

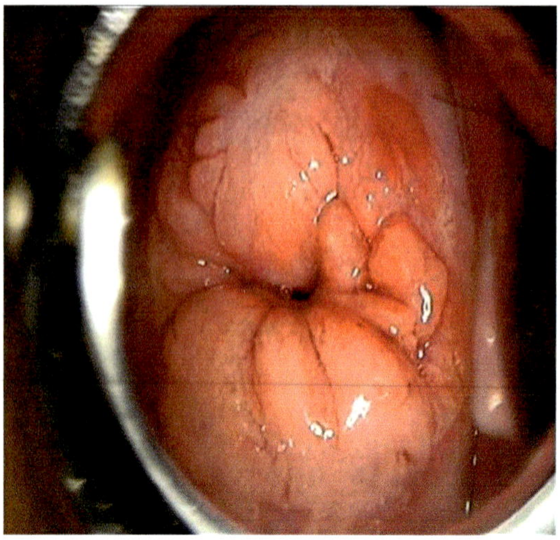

Fig. 13.2 Hypertrophy of columnar epithelium in pregnancy

13.4 Guiding Principles of Cervical Cancer Screening in Pregnancy

The cervical cancer screening algorithm has undergone significant changes after the introduction of HPV DNA and VIA tests as an option. Both anatomical and physiological changes in the cervix during pregnancy make the screening procedure a different scenario altogether as the management principles are directly related to obstetric outcome of the women.

13.4.1 Screening Methods

13.4.1.1 Cytological Tests

In the developed countries with an established cytology-based screening program, the need of opportunistic screening by Pap smear as a routine prenatal examination to increase rate of detection of cervical abnormalities is rarely necessary. Due to availability of routine screening covered up by health insurance, the incidence of cervical cancer has dramatically gone down and rarely addressed in high-resource countries. But for low-resource countries, visit to the antenatal clinic may be the only time, when women will attend the healthcare facility and will remain compliant to her clinician's advice. Thus opportunistic screening at the time of their routine prenatal visit is required, and this plays a key role in diagnosis and management of cervical pre-cancers. However, interpretation of conventional or liquid-based Pap testing is difficult due to high mucus production and large number of navicular, reactive glandular, and even trophoblastic cells in the smear. To rule out misdiagnosis and resultant over treatment, interpretation of Pap test results should be done carefully especially during pregnancy and postpartum period.

13.4.1.2 Noncytological Tests

Under the hormonal influence, significant change in anatomy and physiology of the cervix during pregnancy can make the result of any visual screening tests like VIA with 5% freshly prepared acetic acid or visual inspection with Lugol's iodine (VILI) harder to interpret and could be inaccurate. Moreover, the younger the age, the probability of false-positive VIA test is also high. The role of molecular tests like HPV mRNA test and hybrid capture 2 (HC2) test, which detects 13 high-risk types of oncogenic HPV DNA (HPV types 16, 18, 31, 33, 35, 39, 45, 51, 52, 56, 58, 59, 68) by nuclear hybridization technique, is more reliable. The interpretation of results with these tests is not observer-dependant, and results are highly sensitive and specific [9].

Various researchers in different studies have shown that the pooled estimates of sensitivity and specificity of VIA, Pap smear cytology, and human papillomavirus DNA to be 67.65% and 84.32%, 62.11% and 93.51%, and 77.81% and 91.54%, respectively [9, 10].

13.4.2 Time to Perform Screening Tests During Pregnancy

During pregnancy, the time of performing cervical cancer screening tests also depends on which trimester the lady is reporting to the clinic. The National Health Service (NHS) trust cervical screening program recommends that routine cervical screening tests can usually be delayed in pregnant women till 6 weeks postpartum provided they are up to date with their routine Pap test prior to the conception [11]. Apart from suspicion of invasive cancer definitive diagnostic tests and further management can be postponed till delivery. This is because of the fact that even left untreated, only 2–5% of CIN3 cases will progress to invasive cancer in the future [12, 13].

13.4.3 Screening Interval

The current recommendation of screening interval for pregnant women remains same as the non-pregnant individuals.

13.4.4 ASCCP Guidelines on Cervical Cancer Screening in Pregnancy

In 2012, the American Cancer Society (ACS), the American Society for Colposcopy and Cervical Pathology (ASCCP), American Society for Clinical Pathology (ASCP), United States Preventive Services Task Force, and ACOG released updated recommendations for cervical cancer screening in pregnancy [14, 15]. As there is an already established cytology-based screening practice available, the recommendations are strongly based on abnormal Pap smear results. The following are the special recommendations for management of abnormal cytological findings in pregnancy (Table 13.1):

1. Management of screen test positive result depends on the severity of abnormality on cytology.
2. In case of any suspicion of invasive cancer, further referral for colposcopy and biopsy is mandatory.
3. Treatment of any grade of CIN is contraindicated during pregnancy as there is no immediate harm to the mother or fetus, while unnecessary treatment may be associated with adverse fetal and maternal outcome.
4. In case of CIN2 and CIN3 lesions, repeat colposcopy and cytology can be done at a minimum of 6 weeks interval.

Table 13.1 Summary of abnormal Pap smear management in pregnancy

Pap test result	Management
Atypical squamous cells of undetermined significance (ASC-US)	• Defer colposcopy 6 weeks postpartum • No ECC
Low-grade squamous intraepithelial lesion (LSIL)	• Colposcopy 6 weeks postpartum acceptable • No ECC • If no evidence of high-grade lesion follow-up as per non-pregnant guidelines
High-grade squamous intraepithelial lesion (HSIL)	• Colposcopy • No ECC • Diagnostic excision only if suspected invasive disease • Treatment only in case of invasive cancer
Atypical glandular cells (AGC)	• Colposcopy • No ECC • If no evidence of high-grade lesion, repeat cytology and HPV postpartum

5. Treatment by excision methods is only recommended to rule out suspected invasive cancer.
6. Glandular abnormality in Pap smear should be referred for further evaluation by colposcopy; however, endocervical curettage (ECC) is not recommended during pregnancy.
7. Plan for pregnancy and/or mode of delivery should not be altered unless invasive disease is present.
8. The 2012 recommendations include the utility of molecular testing as an adjunct test to cytology screening for certain women and provide guidance to the treating physicians based on different risk-benefit considerations for different ages [16].

The increase in cost with very few benefits of picking up true high-risk cases which require further evaluation makes co-testing with HPV DNA and Pap smear a questionable method in a resource-constrained setup. The World Health Organization (WHO) has strongly recommended HPV DNA test as a primary screening test if feasible [17, 18]. However, the main objective of preventing cervical cancer should be addressed by using any screening method according to public health resources and country-specific need.

13.4.5 Age of Screening

According to the ASCCP guidelines, cervical carcinoma screening by cytology should begin at 21 years of age, regardless of age of coitus or vaccination status, until age 30. For women more than 30 years of age, co-testing with cytology and HPV testing every 5 years is the preferred method of screening [14, 15], although cytology screening every 3 years is acceptable. When HPV testing is used as a primary screening test, the screening should start at 30 years of age. Majority of studies utilizing VIA as a screening method has reported the starting age of VIA at more than 25 years [19, 20]. This is to avoid unnecessary false-positive results due to immature squamous metaplasia and inflammation at younger age.

Studies report that 10–70% of cervical intraepithelial neoplasias, CIN1 and CIN2, diagnosed during pregnancy regress and sometimes even disappear postpartum, while persistence in the severity of cervical neoplasia is reported in 25–47% of cases and progression in 3–30% of cases [21, 22]. In absence of strong recommendations, data obtained are mainly based on personal experiences and retrospective studies of pregnant women.

13.5 Colposcopy Examination in Screen-Positive Cases

Indications for colposcopy in pregnant and non-pregnant women are same. The only exception in the ASCCP guidelines is that colposcopy examination may be deferred until the postpartum period in low-grade squamous intraepithelial lesions (LSIL) or atypical squamous cells of undetermined significance (ASC-US) with HPV-positive status (Fig. 13.3). As more than 80% of HPV infection gets cleared within a year, the co-testing for HPV DNA is recommended after 6 weeks in the postpartum period if early trimester co-testing with cytology and HPV DNA were positive [23]. Due to hormonal changes interpretation of colposcopy, findings are difficult during pregnancy. The pregnant cervix may be easily seen or may be difficult to visualize than the non-pregnant state. It is usually easier to see the entire

TZ due to eversion of cervical epithelium colposcopically described as large ectropion which reverts postpartum. On colposcopy, the cervix becomes more hyperemic with prominent ectropion, and the vaginal rugosities also are more prominent and hyperemic. As pregnancy progresses, vaginal walls may become highly patulous especially in multiparous women making visualization of cervix more difficult. The use of lateral vaginal speculum or condom may help to hold back the vaginal walls. Vulvovaginal varices may also become prominent in pregnancy due to high blood supply.

As the pregnancy progresses, decidualization of stroma often becomes prominent, appearing as hyperemic-raised plaque-like lesions, which becomes acetowhite after application of 5% acetic acid. Even in the first trimester, edema and increased vascularity make colposcopy examination difficult. Active immature metaplasia often produces thin patchy acetowhite areas with fine mosaics and fine punctations, making it difficult to distinguish between low-grade dysplasia and squamous metaplasia. Due to vasodilation, intraepithelial blood vessels become larger, which makes the low-grade lesions look more severe (Fig. 13.3). Subtle signs of invasive cancer can be easily missed within a high-grade intraepithelial lesion. Regarding the positioning of the patient, no changes in position is required in early pregnancy, whereas in late trimester, lying down in left lateral position is preferable to avoid supine hypotension during colposcopic examination.

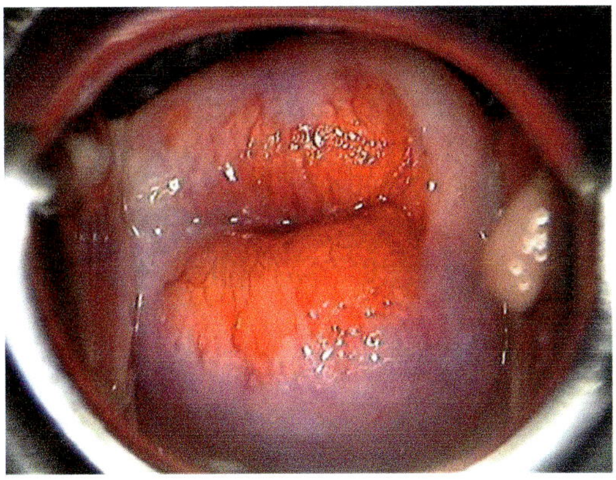

Fig. 13.3 Vasodilatation of intraepithelial blood vessels due to hormonal changes in pregnancy

13.6 Hispathological Examination

A sharp cut with a punch biopsy from the worst affected area under colposcopy guidance is recommended. Biopsy should only be done in high-grade lesions on colposcopic examination to rule out invasive cancer. As cytology test results, interpretation of histopathological findings is also challenging with prominent decidual changes and Arias-Stella reaction in the pregnant cervix. Due to high vascularity of the cervix, securing hemostasis becomes difficult but should be obtained with pressure gauze or Monsel's solution.

13.7 Management of CIN Lesions in Pregnancy

Repeated colposcopy examination with no evidence of high-grade lesions on colposcopy and biopsy is unnecessary and is categorized as unacceptable in ASCCP guideline. The majority of CIN lesions regresses in the postpartum period. The reasons for the regression may be the following [21, 22]:

- Due to natural history of the disease itself.
- The typical hormonal pattern during pregnancy may induce a viral activation that spontaneously leads to higher clearance rates postpartum.
- Misinterpretation of histopathological findings in antenatal period.
- The process of childbirth possibly leads to loss of abnormal cervical epithelium in intrapartum period.

Only high-grade lesions need further evaluation by colposcopy and guided biopsy to rule out invasive cancer. In case of absence of any invasive component in histology, treatment of even high-grade pre-cancers CIN2 and CIN3 can be deferred until 6 weeks postpartum with reevaluation by colposcopy and/or biopsy. Treatment methods available are as same as in non-pregnant women. Ablative methods by cryotherapy, thermocoagulation, laser ablation or excisional method by loop electrosurgical excision procedure (LEEP), cold knife conization (CKC), and laser conization are the standard modes of treatment available for management of cervical pre-cancerous lesions.

13.7.1 Ablative Treatment

In case of high probability of loss to follow-up or if additional opportunities to treatment are unlikely, treatment during pregnancy by ablative method can be considered [24, 25]. The limited evidence does not suggest that either cryotherapy or thermocoagulation treatment during pregnancy is related to any adverse pregnancy outcomes; however, an increased risk of pregnancy loss cannot be ruled out, and further evidence is required. There also are possible negative perceptions if ablative treatment is accidentally associated with pregnancy loss by women.

13.7.2 Excision Method

Both LEEP and CKC in pregnancy should be performed if required to rule out invasive cancers. LEEP in the first trimester is a safe procedure with unclear evidences regarding comparison of obstetric outcome between cryotherapy and LEEP [25–27]. Meta-analysis on early pregnancy outcomes for CIN states increased risk of miscarriages when LEEP is performed in the second trimester possibly as a result of cervical incompetence after proportionally large excision during the LEEP procedure [27–29]. However, cold knife conization is associated with increased second-trimester miscarriages and more chances of cesarean delivery [30]. This may be due to larger depth of cone than the LEEP specimen with increased risk of cervical incompetence.

Unnecessary treatment of cervical pre-cancers can lead to cervical stenosis, preterm delivery, and preterm premature rupture of membranes [31]. The treatment of cervical pre-cancers in young women should be minimized with individual case assessment of risk-benefit ratio and chances of future fertility and adverse obstetric outcome.

13.8 Treatment of Invasive Cancer

Biopsy-proven invasive cancer cervix (ICC) in pregnancy should be referred to an oncology center. ICC requires a multidisciplinary approach according to the stage of the disease and gestational age of the current pregnancy.

13.9 Mode of Delivery

An abnormal screening test is not an indication for cesarean delivery. Even histologically proven high-grade pre-cancer is not a contraindication for vaginal delivery. In case of invasive cancers only, delivery by cesarean section is advised due to high probability of micrometastasis in locoregional area and/or obstruction of birth canal due to large growth [32].

13.10 Screening for HPV-Vaccinated Pregnant Women

After the introduction of HPV vaccination in 2007, there is a cohort of women who are vaccinated against high-risk oncogenic types 16 and 18 of HPV. Irrespective of their pregnancy status, current recommendation is as same as the routine screening protocol of non-vaccinated women [33, 34]. More studies are required to establish an evidence-based cervical cancer screening strategies for the HPV-vaccinated girls.

13.11 Conclusion

Cervical cancer screening guidelines are not different in pregnant population from non-pregnant population. In low-grade abnormalities, colposcopy and/or biopsy may be deferred until 6 weeks postpartum. In case of high-grade lesions, biopsy should be performed to rule out invasive cancers. Treatment options are also same as non-pregnant women but shall be reserved for highly selected cases and in suspicion of invasive cancers. In invasive cancer cases, appropriate referral to oncology center with multidisciplinary team approach can influence the obstetric outcome as well as the prognosis of the disease.

Key Points

- The current indication for cervical cancer screening is same in both pregnant and non-pregnant women.
- Colposcopy may be deferred at least 6 weeks postpartum for atypical squamous cells of undetermined significance and low-grade squamous intraepithelial lesions but should be used to triage high-grade abnormalities.
- Cervical biopsy in pregnancy is indicated only in suspicion of invasive cancer.
- Cervical pre-cancers should be monitored during pregnancy and reevaluated after delivery, which may be done vaginally.
- The treatment of cervical pre-cancers in young women should be minimized with individual case assessment of risk-benefit ratio and chances of future fertility and adverse obstetric outcome.
- More studies are required to establish evidence-based cervical cancer screening strategies for the HPV-vaccinated girls.

References

1. McIntyre-Seltman K, Lesnock JL. Cervical cancer screening in pregnancy. Obstet Gynecol Clin N Am. 2008;35(4):645–58.
2. Economos D, Perez VN, Delke I, Collado ML, Tancer ML. Abnormal cervical cytology in pregnancy: a 17-year experience. Obstet Gynecol. 1993;81:915–8.
3. WHO/ICO Information Centre on HPV and Cervical Cancer (HPV Information Centre). Summary report on HPV and cervical cancer statistics in India 2012.
4. http://www.hpvcentre.net/statistics/reports/IND.pdf. Accessed 12 Aug 2017.
5. Shastri SS, Mittra I, Mishra GA, Gupta S, Dikshit R, Singh S, et al. Effect of VIA screening by primary health workers: randomized controlled study in Mumbai, India. J Natl Cancer Inst. 2014;106(3):dju009. https://doi.org/10.1093/jnci/dju009. Epub 2014 Feb 22
6. Mittal S, Ghosh I, Banerjee D, Singh P, Biswas J, Nijhawan R, et al. Reproducibility of cervical intraepithelial neoplasia diagnosis on histological review of cervical punch biopsies from a visual inspection with acetic acid and HPV detection-based screening program. Int J Gynaecol Obstet. 2014;126(3):227–31. https://doi.org/10.1016/j.ijgo.2014.03.037. Epub 2014 May 29
7. Basu P, Mittal S, Banerjee D, Singh P, Panda C, Dutta S, et al. Diagnostic accuracy of VIA and HPV detection as primary and sequential screening tests in a Cervical Cancer Screening Demonstration Project in India. Int J Cancer. 2015; https://doi.org/10.1002/ijc.29458.
8. IARC handbook of cancer prevention. Vol. 10. https://www.iarc.fr/en/publications/pdfs-online. Accessed 12 Aug 2017.
9. Bobdey S, Sathwara J, Jain A, Balasubramaniam G. Burden of cervical cancer and role of screening in India. Indian J Med Paediatr Oncol. 2016;37(4):278–85. https://doi.org/10.4103/0971-5851.195751.
10. Gravitt PE, Paul P, Katki HA, Vendantham H, Ramakrishna G, Sudula M, et al. Effectiveness of VIA, Pap, and HPV DNA testing in a cervical cancer screening program in a peri-urban community in Andhra Pradesh, India. CATCH Study Team. PLoS One. 2010;5(10):e13711.
11. Cervical screening - NHS.UK. https://www.nhs.uk/conditions/cervical-screening.
12. Vink MA, Bogaards JA, van Kemenade FJ, de Melker HE, Meijer CJ, Berkhof J. Clinical progression of high-grade cervical intraepithelial neoplasia: estimating the time to preclinical cervical cancer from doubly censored national registry data. Am J Epidemiol. 2013;178(7):1161–9.
13. Committee on Practice Bulletins—Gynecology. ACOG Practice Bulletin Number 131: screening for cervical cancer. Obstet Gynecol. 2012;120(5):1222–38.
14. Saslow D, Solomon D, Lawson HW, Killackey M, Kulasingam SL, Cain J, et al. American Cancer Society, American Society for Colposcopy and Cervical Pathology, and American Society for Clinical Pathology screening guidelines for the prevention and early detection of cervical cancer. CA Cancer J Clin. 2012;62:147–72. https://doi.org/10.3322/caac.21139.
15. Moyer VA. U.S. Preventive Services Task Force Screening for cervical cancer: U.S. Preventive Services Task Force recommendation statement. Ann Intern Med. 2012;156:880–91. https://doi.org/10.7326/0003-4819-156-12-201206190-00424.
16. https://www.nhp.gov.in/national-programme-for-prevention-and-control-of-c_pg. Accessed 19 Nov 2017.
17. Arbyn M, Sasieni P, Meijer CJ, Clavel C, Koliopoulos G, Dillner J. Chapter 9: Clinical applications of HPV testing: a summary of meta-analyses. Vaccine. 2006;24(Suppl 3):S78–89.
18. Sankaranarayanan R, Swaminathan R, Brenner H, Chen K, Chia KS, Chen JG, et al. Cancer survival in Africa, Asia, and Central America: a population-based study. Lancet Oncol. 2010;11:165–73.
19. Sankaranarayanan R, Chatterji R, Shastri SS, Wesley RS, Basu P, Mahe C, et al. Accuracy of human papillomavirus testing in primary screening of cervical neoplasia: results from a multicenter study in India. Int J Cancer. 2004;112:341–7.

20. Manikkam B. Screening for cervical cancer during pregnancy. Int J Commun Med Public Health. 2016;3(9) https://doi.org/10.18203/2394-6040.ijcmph20163059.
21. Dinc A. Pap smear screening results for Turkish pregnant women. Asian Pac J Cancer Prev. 2012;13(11):5835–8.
22. Lorincz A, Castanon A, Lim AWW, Sasieni P. New strategies for HPV-based cervical screening. Women's Health (Lond Engl). 2013;9(5) https://doi.org/10.2217/whe.13.48.
23. WHO guidelines: use of cryotherapy for cervical intraepithelial neoplasia. Recommendations. Geneva: World Health Organization; 2011. https://www.ncbi.nlm.nih.gov/books/NBK138474.
24. WHO guidelines. WHO guidelines for screening and treatment of pre-cancerous lesions for cervical cancer prevention. http://apps.who.int/iris/bitstream/10665/94830/1/9789241548694_eng.pdf. Accessed 31 Dec 2017.
25. Kyrgiou M, Mitra A, Arbyn M, Stasinou SM, Martin-Hirsch P, Bennett P, et al. Fertility and early pregnancy outcomes after treatment for cervical intraepithelial neoplasia: systematic review and meta-analysis. BMJ. 2014;349:g6192. https://doi.org/10.1136/bmj.g6192.
26. Khalid S, Dimitriou E, Conroy R, Paraskevaidis E, Kyrgiou M, Harrity C, et al. The thickness and volume of LLETZ specimens can predict the relative risk of pregnancy-related morbidity. Br J Obstetr Gynaecol. 2012;119:685–91.
27. Arbyn M, Kyrgiou M, Gondry J, Petry KU, Paraskevaidis E. Long term outcomes for women treated for cervical pre-cancer. BMJ. 2014;348:f7700.
28. Kyrgiou M, Valasoulis G, Stasinou SM, Founta C, Athanasiou A, Bennett P, et al. Proportion of cervical excision for cervical intraepithelial neoplasia as a predictor of pregnancy outcomes. Int J Gynaecol Obstet. 2015;128(2):141–7. https://doi.org/10.1016/j.ijgo.2014.07.038. Epub 2014 Oct 2
29. Jakobsson M, Gissler M, Sainio S, Paavonen J, Tapper AM. Preterm delivery after surgical treatment for cervical intraepithelial neoplasia. Obstet Gynecol. 2007;109(2 Pt 1):309–13.
30. Schlichte MJ, Guidry J. Current cervical carcinoma screening guidelines. J Clin Med. 2015;4(5):918–32. https://doi.org/10.3390/jcm4050918.
31. Mailath-Pokorny M, Schwameis R, Grimm C, Reinthaller A, Polterauer S. Natural history of cervical intraepithelial neoplasia in pregnancy: postpartum histo-pathologic outcome and review of the literature. BMC Pregnancy Childbirth. 2016;16:74. Published online 2016 Apr 7. https://doi.org/10.1186/s12884-016-0861-8.
32. Zhang X, Gao Y, Yang Y. Treatment and prognosis of cervical cancer associated with pregnancy: analysis of 20 cases from a Chinese tumor institution. J Zhejiang Univ Sci B. 2015;16(5):388–94. https://doi.org/10.1631/jzus.B1400251.
33. Rossi PG, Carozzi F, Federici A, Ronco G, Zappa M, Franceschi S. Cervical cancer screening in women vaccinated against human papillomavirus infection: recommendations from a consensus conference. Prev Med. 2017;98:21–30.
34. Herweijer E, Feldman AL, Ploner A, Arnheim-Dahlström L, Uhnoo I, Netterlid E, et al. The participation of HPV-vaccinated women in a national cervical screening program: population-based cohort study. PLoS One. 2015;10(7):e0134185. https://doi.org/10.1371/journal.pone.0134185.

14 Cervical Cancer Screening in Low-Resource Settings

Ashrafun Nessa, Begum Rokeya Anwar, and Shirin Akter Begum

14.1 Introduction

The incidence of cervical cancer (CC) varies greatly between developing and developed countries, where CC cases have been considerably reduced due to effective implementation of screening programs. CC is one of the most common cancers in women across the globe, with an estimated prevalence of 1,547,161 cases worldwide in 2012 [1]. A large fraction of the world's population lives in low- and middle-income countries (LMICs) and contributes to a significant burden of CC. This increase is mostly related to growing aging population, inadequate treatment facilities, and poor involvement of the community in cancer control [2]. Almost 80% of cervical cancer occurs in developing countries such as Southeast Asia, Western Pacific regions, India, and Africa, the regions of very high mortality rate [3]. LMICs have high burden of cervical cancer due to lack of screening; high prevalence of risk factors like early marriage, early initiation of sexual activity, multiparity, and sexually transmitted diseases (STDs) and low socioeconomic status. Treatment of CC is expensive and requires radical operative procedures and/or radiotherapy and prolonged hospital stay. In many low-resource countries, facilities for radical surgery and radiotherapy are inadequate and expensive.

Presently, several developing countries are trying to adopt a CC screening program to ensure wide coverage of the target population with on-site, low-cost screening with minimum infrastructure requirement. Management of screen-positive cases and adequate follow-up with proper linkage to immediate treatment are essential to make all these efforts successful.

Two main approaches have been adopted for cancer screening programs: organized and opportunistic [4]. An organized cancer screening program should be population-based, be managed through the public health delivery system, follow a uniform guideline, achieve a reasonable coverage of the target population, and have efficient linkage between screening and treatment of the positive cases. On the other hand, in opportunistic screening, a doctor or health professional offers the test when a woman visits health facilities for other reasons. In opportunistic screening, cases may not be checked or monitored. In LMICs, organized population-based screening needs to be introduced at national level with good population coverage to make the program successful.

A. Nessa · S. A. Begum
Department of Obstetrics and Gynaecology, Bangabandhu Sheikh Mujib Medical University (BSMMU), Dhaka, Bangladesh

B. R. Anwar (✉)
Department of Gynaecological Oncology, National Institute of Cancer Research and Hospital, Dhaka, Bangladesh

S. Mehta, A. Singla (eds.), *Preventive Oncology for the Gynecologist*,
https://doi.org/10.1007/978-981-13-3438-2_14

In LMICs, CC screening started sporadically in one or two tertiary health-care centers in the mid-1980s by conventional cervical cytology. However, the United Kingdom and some other developed countries developed a systemic call and recall system in the late 1980s and reduced the death rate of CC by conventional cytological test [5]. Tertiary centers of low-resource countries became familiar with cytological test and started opportunistic screening in the mid-1990s, but several difficulties were encountered in implementing the cytology-based screening program in a low-resource setting. As a result, the CC burden remained unchanged.

In the mid-1990s, developed countries initiated research on HPV DNA test, and by 2005 many developed countries started using HPV DNA test as the primary screening test [6]. In the meantime, liquid-based cytology (LBC) replaced conventional cytology in some developed countries due to its higher sensitivity and specificity [7]. Several studies in LMICs have suggested the feasibility of primary screening by HPV test in terms of decreased program costs and increased screening interval [8]. However, the test is too expensive for introduction in the screening program of many LMICs due to resource shortage at the present moment. LMICs need to adopt an affordable, accessible way of cervical cancer screening. The best available evidence supports visual inspection with acetic acid (VIA) testing as a primary screening modality for cervical precancer screening in low-resource countries, as it requires minimum infrastructure support, and the result of the procedure is available immediately.

In most LMICs, population-based cervical cancer screening is still nonexistent. In these countries, CC screening remains opportunistic due to competing health-care priorities, insufficient financial resources, and a limited number of trained providers. Hence, a significant number of cases are detected at advanced stages, leading to increased mortality. To implement successful CC screening program in LMICs, support and funding from the Ministry of Health are essential. The Middle East and North Africa have taken steps to implement national screening programs based on VIA [9].

India is carrying the largest burden of disease in the world. India developed guidelines for a population-based screening program for cervical cancer detection based on visual inspection tests more than 10 years ago. Despite introduction of the national guidelines, important demonstration projects, and a number of well-conducted research studies showing feasibility and cost-effectiveness, very little scale-up of CC screening services has been developed in the country [10]. The government of Bangladesh (GOB) evaluated the feasibility of screening with VIA in 2005 and initiated to scale up the program in 2006 to the district level and is now expanding the program to the sub-district level [11, 12]. In Bangladesh, screening is practiced currently by 411 centers at primary, secondary and tertiary health-care facilities [13].

14.2 Screening in LMICs

14.2.1 Choice of Screening Test in LMICs

Despite the attractiveness of the vaccination program, CC screening is still recognized as the most successful approach for CC control. The available methods of CC screening are cervical cytology (Pap smear), HPV test, VIA, visual inspection of the cervix with Lugol's iodine (VILI), and colposcopy. An ideal screening test should be simple, painless, less time-consuming, cost-effective, and accurate. Pap smear has been used most frequently in cervical cancer screening programs of different high-resource countries. However, cytology-based screening has several drawbacks that limit its usefulness. The technical and monetary constrains of implementing cytology-based screening programs in LMICs initiated the development of simple screening tests. VIA and HPV testing have been suggested as suitable tests for primary screening methods in low-resource countries.

14.2.1.1 Cytology-Based Screening

Cytology-based CC screening is the oldest and most widespread cancer screening technique.

It began in the United Kingdom in the 1960s as opportunistic screening. In 1988, a systemic call and recall program was developed that significantly reduced cervical cancer and subsequently has led to effective reduction in the incidence and mortality from CC in many developed countries [14, 15]. In the United Kingdom, from 1990 to 2008, women aged 35–64 years participating in a CC screening program had a reduced risk of CC of 60–80% and a reduced risk of developing an advanced CC of 90% over the next 5-year period [16].

Introduction of conventional cytology services in Cameroon, a low-resource country, reduced cervical cancer rates by 60–90% within 3 years of implementation [17]. However, the widespread opportunistic screening and the large-scale national or regional cytology screening programs in Brazil, Cuba, Costa Rica, Chile, and Mexico, among others, in Latin America and the Caribbean have been largely ineffective in reducing the CC burden compared with high-income developed countries [18].

A combination of suboptimal cytology testing, lack of quality assurance, poor coverage of women, and inadequate follow-up of screen-positive women were the main reasons for lack of success of cytology programs in low-resource countries which are mainly due to the inadequate health-care infrastructure, human resource, and program logistics.

Drawbacks and limitations of cytology-based screening are as follows:

- Sensitivity is inadequate to detect cervical intraepithelial neoplasia (CIN) 2+ disease (approximately 50%).
- Needs expensive laboratory infrastructure and highly skilled manpower that may not be easily available.
- The strict quality control required for optimum performance of the test cannot be ensured.
- Does not provide the result immediately, and the positive women need to be recalled after the results are available.
- A repeat visit is inconvenient for the women and increases the dropout rates.

Table 14.1 Sensitivity and specificity of cytology-based screening in different LMICs

Author, year, country	Sensitivity (%)	Specificity (%)
Nessa et al., 2013, Bangladesh [19]	33.3	95.8
Sankaranarayanan et al., 2003, India [20]	81.9	87.8
Karimi et al., 2013, Iran [21]	51	66.6

Even if high-quality cytology programs were implemented in low-resource countries, the cytology-based programs would only be moderately effective. The cytology test misses approximately 50% of high-grade precursor lesion and cancers with a single screening [6]. In low-resource settings, women would probably only be screened once or twice in their lifetime making cytology screening less effective. Sensitivity and specificity of cytology-based screening in different low-resource settings are shown in Table 14.1.

14.2.1.2 Human Papillomavirus (HPV) Test

Infection by the high-risk (hr) HPV is needed for the development of CC. So detection of hrHPV DNA should be a good approach to identifying women with CIN. HPV causes cellular changes very slowly. The time from HPV infection to development of CC is about 10–20 years [22]. Therefore, a woman who is HPV negative is extremely unlikely to develop cervical cancer over the next 5–10 years, and infrequent screening would be safe. Thus, there are two potential uses for HPV testing: to identify those likely to have the disease presently and those who may develop the disease after few years. The HPV test has been proved more effective than cytology for CC screening, providing increased reassurance and allowing longer screening intervals [23]. Though many types of HPV tests are available, only several commercial HPV tests have documented clinical performance compared with the standard HPV test. According to guidelines, an ideal test should have at least 90% clinical sensitivity for CIN 2+ and clinical specificity of at least 98% [24, 25]. However, too many options of HPV tests make selection of a suitable one difficult. Due to high sensitivity, HPV tests have replaced cervical cytology for primary screening in many countries.

Several studies have confirmed that HPV testing is feasible in low-resource settings and appears to be the best strategy for CC screening [26, 27]. A large-cluster randomized trial from rural India has shown approximately 50% reduction of CC after a single round of HPV screening (Hybrid Capture II) [28]. HPV testing is time-consuming, and expensive laboratory infrastructure is required, but development of new rapid molecular methods for detecting HPV DNA initiated a new horizon in CC screening in low-resource settings. As a result of introduction of rapid molecular methods with high sensitivity, HPV test became the most efficient and cost-effective strategy for use in low-resource settings [29]. Moreover, the use of "screen-and-treat" and "see-and-treat" approaches requiring minimum visits made HPV test more cost-effective. Even then, affordability and sustainability using HPV test for primary CC screening in some low-resource settings are difficult to implement.

14.2.1.3 Visual Inspection of the Cervix with Acetic Acid (VIA)

VIA, also known as "the acetic acid test," involves naked eye inspection of the cervix under bright light at least 1 min after the application of 3% to 5% dilute acetic acid using a cotton swab or a spray. It involves non-magnified visualization of the uterine cervix and search for the appearance of acetowhite areas in the transformation zone (TZ), close to the squamocolumnar junction (SCJ) or the external os. The identification of acetowhite lesions helps in early diagnosis of preinvasive disease and early preclinical, asymptomatic invasive cancer.

The test can be categorized as VIA positive or VIA negative. A positive test is the detection of well-defined, densely opaque dull acetowhite lesions in the TZ of the cervix. The faint, ill-defined, translucent acetowhite areas, faint acetowhitening of endocervical polyps, nabothian cysts, dot-like acetowhite appearance, and prominent SCJ are categorized as negative. However, immature squamous metaplasia and inflamed and regenerating cervical epithelium may appear as faint acetowhite areas, and therefore these are not specific to cervical neoplasia.

A major benefit of VIA is that the result of screening test is available without delay, and therefore additional investigations/management can be planned and carried out during the same visit. All these advantages lead to VIA being considered as the primary cervical screening tool.

The advantages of VIA in programmatic context are as follows:

- Sensitivity better than cytology (80% to detect CIN 2+ disease).
- Can be performed at primary and secondary health centers.
- Paramedical staff (nurses, female health workers) and nonspecialist doctors can be trained to do the test.
- The procedure is simple, and the test providers can be trained through a 1 to 2 weeks course.
- The equipment is inexpensive and the consumables can be made available very easily.
- The test result is available immediately.

Studies indicate that VIA is at least as sensitive as conventional cytology in detecting high-grade lesions, but its specificity is lower. VIA appears to be the most promising low-technology alternative to cytology [29, 30]. Table 14.2 compares the sensitivity and specificity of VIA in detecting CIN 2 and CIN 3 and invasive cancer in different low-resource countries.

For countries in resource-constrained settings, where screening with an HPV test is not feasible, the World Health Organization (WHO) recommends screening with VIA and treatment with cryotherapy. However, if the lesion is not eligible for treatment by cryotherapy, she should be referred to a higher center [39, 40].

Several countries in Asia, Africa, and Central America initiated scale-up of the program after gaining some experience from the pilot program.

Table 14.2 Accuracy of VIA in detecting CIN 2–3 and invasive cancer [38]

Author, year, country	Number of participants	Sensitivity (%)	Specificity (%)
Denny et al., 2000, South Africa [8]	2885	67	84
Nessa et al., 2010, Bangladesh [12]	104,098	93.6	58.3
University of Zimbabwe, 1999, Zimbabwe [31]	2148	77	64
Denny et al., 2002, South Africa [32]	2754	70	79
Sankaranarayanan et al., 2004, India [33]	54,981	79	86
Braganca et al., 2005, Brazil [34]	809	54	88
Ngoma et al., 2010, Tanzania [35]	10,378	60.6	98.2
Muwonge et al., 2010, Angola [36]	8851	70.7	94.5
Sauvag et al., 2011 [37]		80	92
Sankaranarayanan et al., 2011 [18]		80 (14–95)	92 (14–98)

The government of Zambia has initiated a large-scale screening program using VIA [41, 42]. Characteristics of the screening programs of the mentioned countries including the management algorithm for screen-positive women are given in Table 14.3 [42]. Bangladesh evaluated the feasibility of screening with VIA within the existing government health infrastructure in 16 districts in 2005 [11] and scaled up the program to all the districts and is now expanding the program to the sub-district level. In Bangladesh, screening is practiced currently by 411 centers at primary-, secondary-, and tertiary-level health-care facilities [13]. Bangladesh has adopted CC screening for the women of 30 years and above with VIA, and positive cases are being referred to the higher facilities, where colposcopy and management are carried out. In Bangladesh, colposcopy became an important part of this prevention program both for diagnosis and guiding the treatment [12, 43, 44]. However this is predominantly an opportunistic screening program [42, 43]. In India also the government has advocated VIA as the screening modality for women more than 30 years of age.

Procedure of VIA

VIA has become the screening test of choice for the CC screening program in several low-resource countries due to its simplicity and affordability. If a woman wishes to undergo VIA test, she needs counseling along with taking a brief reproductive, contraceptive, and menstrual history including date of last menstrual period. The criteria to categorize the observations into negative, positive, or suspected cancer after VIA are given in Table 14.4.

The steps of VIA are as follows:

- Select a bivalve speculum of appropriate size to see the vagina and cervix adequately (Fig. 14.1).
- Use a good focusing light preferably with halogen or LED or 100 W tungsten bulb.
- The woman should be informed before inserting the speculum in the vagina.
- When inserting the speculum, ask the woman to breathe in deeply and then breathe out slowly through her mouth. This helps her to relax and not contract her vaginal muscles.
- Insert the blades fully or until resistance is felt.
- If difficulty is faced in exposing the cervix because of lax vaginal walls, a non-lubricated condom over the speculum blades can be used with cutting the tip of the condom.
- Examine the vagina. Note for inflammation, ulcers, or sores.
- Examine the cervix and locate the cervical opening (external os) (Fig. 14.2).
  - Note the color of the cervix. The surface should be smooth and pink. The area of the cervix where the color changes from pink to red is the squamocolumnar junction, which is usually close to the external cervical os (Fig. 14.3).
  - Note if there is bleeding or discharge from the cervix. Normal cervical secretions should be clear and odorless.
  - To perform VIA, apply 5% freshly prepared dilute acetic acid solution liberally on the cervix using a cotton swab (Fig. 14.4).

Table 14.3 Characteristics of country screening programs [42]

Country	Year pilot project initiated	Year program scale-up began	Screening policy and protocol	Screening test used	Target age	Management algorithm for screen-positive women	Health information system capabilities	Institution responsible for program coordination
Bangladesh	2004	2006	Cervical and Breast Cancer Screening Program: Standard & Guidelines (2005)	VIA	≥30 years	VIA+ women referred for colposcopy and treated immediately	Electronic template recently introduced; generates key system indicators; does not yet enable tracking of women	Ministry of Health and Family Welfare, Bangabandhu Sheikh Mujib Medical University and UNFPA
Guatemala	2015	2016	National Guidelines for Screening and Treatment of Precancerous Lesions for the Prevention of Cervical Cancer (2014)	HPV DNA	30–65 years	Varies by health facility • HPV screen-and-treat, using VIA to determine treatment eligibility only • HPV+ VIA+ women treated; HPV+ VIA– women rescreened in 1 year • HPV+ Pap ASCUS+ women referred for colposcopy and treatment; HPV+ normal Pap rescreened in 1 year	Electronic; generates key system indicators; limited functionality for tracking of women	Ministry of Public Health and Social Assistance
Honduras	2015	2016	Protocol for Screening and Treatment of Precancerous Lesions for Cervical Cancer Prevention (2015)	HPV DNA	30–64 years	HPV+ VIA+ women treated; HPV+ VIA– women rescreened in 1 year	Electronic template recently introduced; generates key system indicators; limited functionality for tracking of women	Secretary of Health

Nicaragua	2015	2016	Norm and Protocol for Cervical Cancer Prevention and Control (not yet published)	HPV DNA	30–59 years	Varies by health facility • HPV+ VIA+ women treated; HPV+ VIA− women rescreened in 1 year • HPV+ Pap ASCUS+ women referred for colposcopy and treatment; HPV+ normal Pap rescreened in 1 year	Electronic; generates key system indicators; enables tracking of women	Ministry of Health
Zambia	2006	2012	Visual Inspection with Acetic Acid (VIA) and Cryotherapy: A Reference Manual for Trainers and Health Care Providers (2015)	VIA aided by digital cervicography	25–59 years	VIA+ women treated immediately	Electronic; generates key system indicators; enables tracking of women	Ministry of Health

Table 14.4 Criteria for categorizing VIA test results

VIA category	Description of the findings
Negative	No acetowhite area
	Transparent or faint patchy acetowhite areas without definite margins
	Nabothian cysts becoming acetowhite
	Faint line like acetowhitening at the junction of the columnar and squamous epithelium
	Acetowhite lesions far away from the transformation zone
Positive	Distinct, opaque acetowhite area
	Margin should be well-defined, may or may not be raised
	Abnormality close to the squamocolumnar junction in the transformation zone and not far away from the os
Suspected cancer	Obvious growth or ulcer on the cervix
	Acetowhite area may not be visible because of bleeding

- After at least 1 min, inspect the cervix to reconfirm the position of the SCJ and also to look for features of the transformation zone (TZ) (Fig. 14.5).
- Carefully look for any abnormality, especially an acetowhite area on the TZ (Figs. 14.6, 14.7, and 14.8).
- After completion of the test, wipe out the excess acetic acid, and gently remove the speculum, keeping the blades partially closed.
- Inform the woman of the test results and appropriately counsel her.
- Fill out appropriate forms and registers. Document the findings clearly.

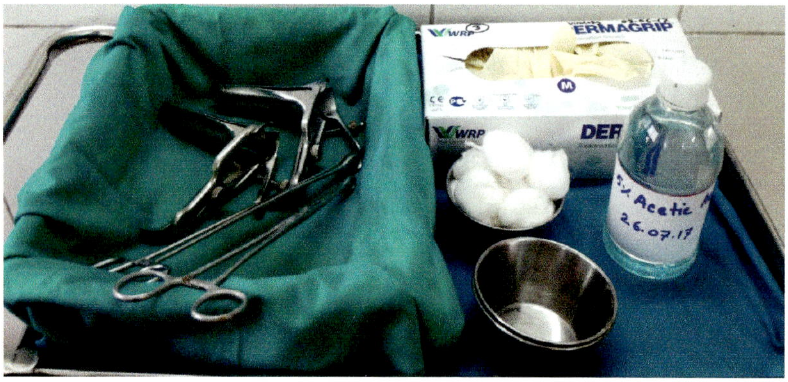

Fig. 14.1 Instrument tray for VIA

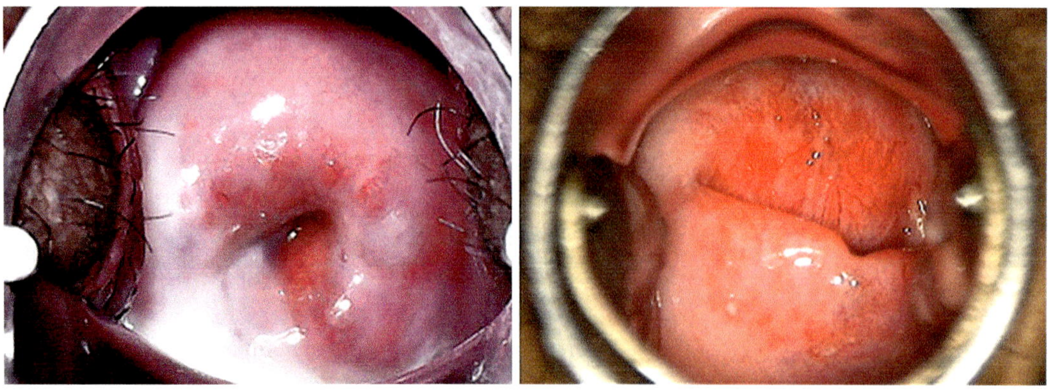

Fig. 14.2 Exposing the cervix and noting the type of vaginal discharge if any

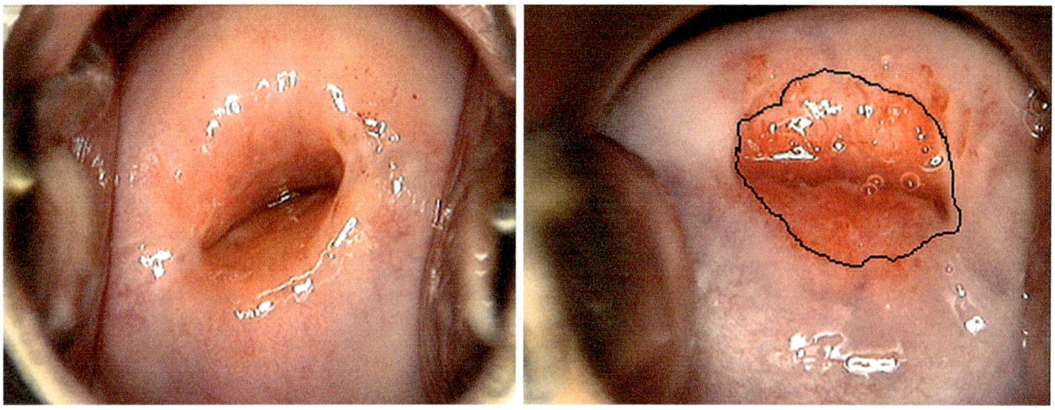

Fig. 14.3 Identifying the squamocolumnar junction

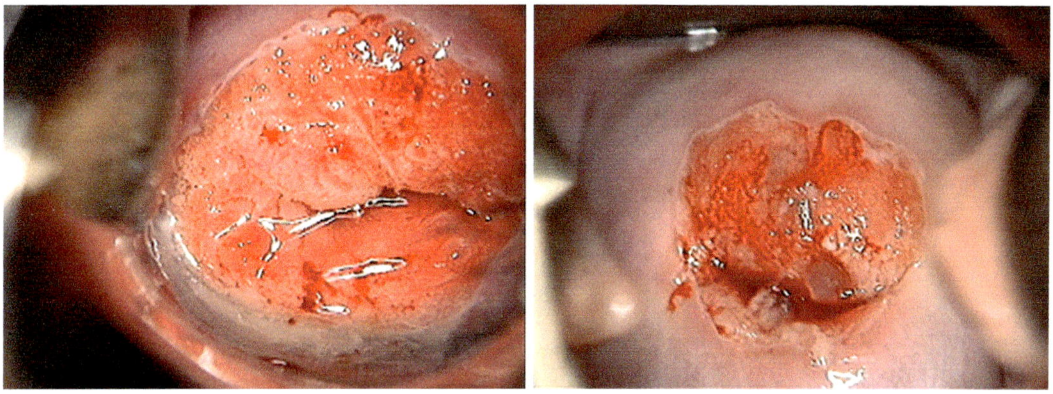

Fig. 14.4 The cervix after application of acetic acid

Fig. 14.5 Identifying the TZ

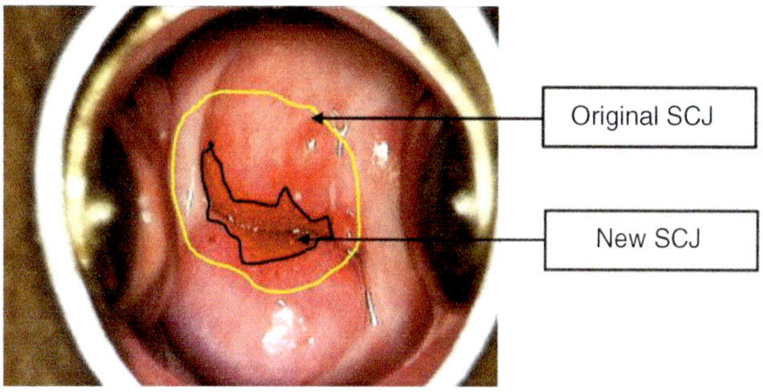

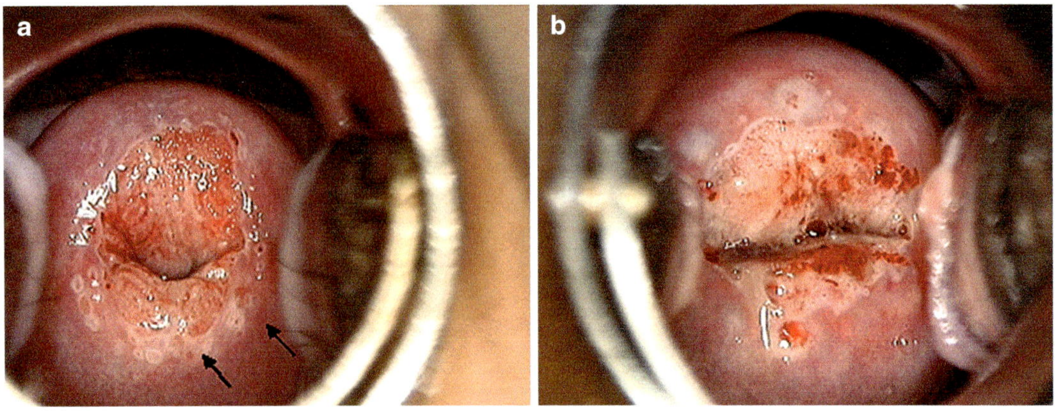

Fig. 14.6 VIA category—negative. (**a**) Blanching of the columnar epithelium noted. Crypt openings are seen prominently. (**b**) The columnar epithelium temporarily becomes patchy acetowhite

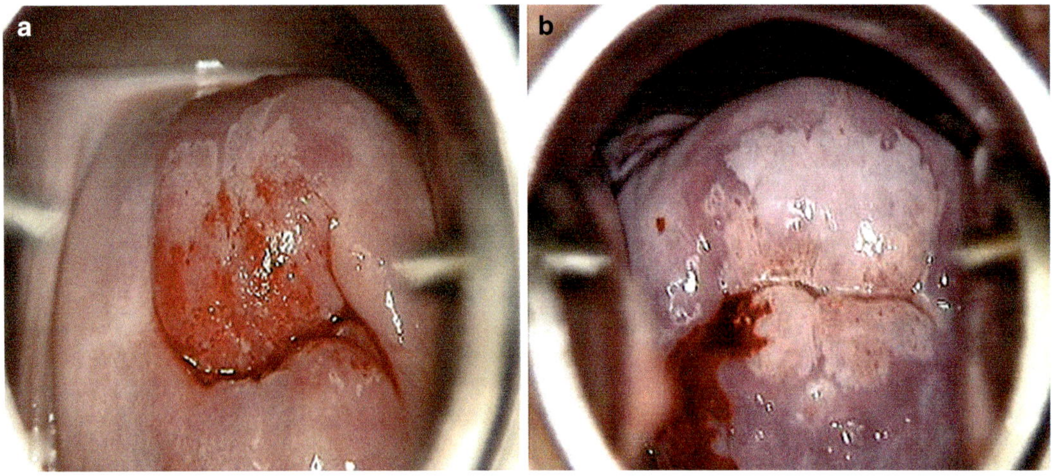

Fig. 14.7 VIA category—positive. (**a**) Thin acetowhite area seen on the anterior lip in the transformation zone attached to the SCJ. (**b**) Dense acetowhite area seen on both the anterior and posterior lip in the transformation zone

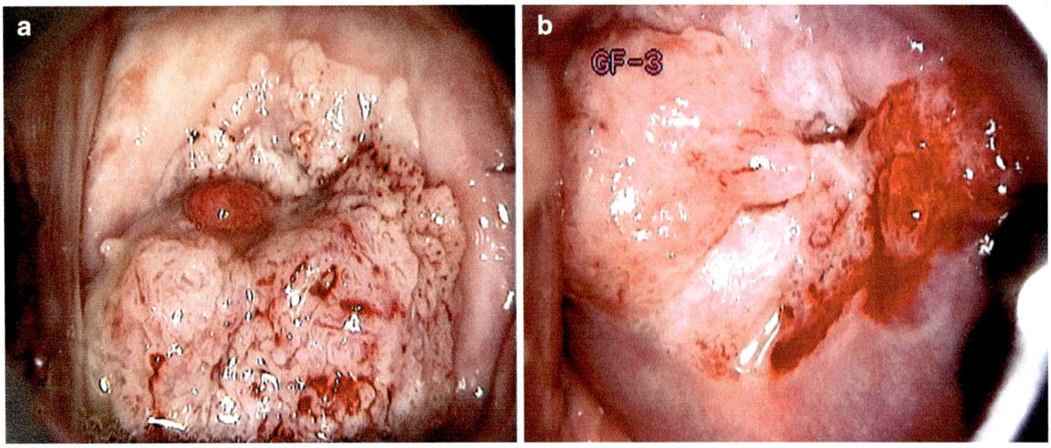

Fig. 14.8 VIA category—suspected cancer. (**a**) Dense acetowhite area with surface irregularity and bleeding points seen mostly on the posterior lip. (**b**) Raised nodular growth with dense acetowhite area and contact bleeding

14.2.2 Components of Screening Program

14.2.2.1 Defining the Target Population, Frequency of Screening, and Population Coverage

The target age group for CC screening and the frequency of screening should be based on the reasonable estimation of the capabilities and resources available for the program. In LMICs, utilization of the limited resources should be planned to provide benefit to the maximum number of women who are at risk of the disease. CC screening should be started at the age of 30 years in programs with limited resources as this disease is rare before the age of 30 years and screening women at a younger age detects many low-grade lesions that never progress to cancer.

WHO recommends screening from 30 years of age, with population screening coverage of women aged 30–49 years of age [39, 40]. Best utilization of the resources is possible if screening is limited to the age group with maximum possibility of detecting the high-grade precancer lesions (CIN 2 and 3), which is between 30 and 49 years of age. Individual countries may adopt variations depending on the government's attitude and political will, stakeholder's view, economic situation, budgetary allocation, etc.

The screening should be performed every 5 years. All efforts should be made to achieve high coverage of the target population. For test-negative women on VIA or cytology, the screening interval for repeat screening should be every 3–5 years. However, in case of HPV test, women with negative result should have rescreening after a minimum interval of 5 years. In women who are HIV-positive or with unknown HIV status in areas with endemic HIV infection, the screening interval should be more frequent [40].

Too frequent screening of women such as every year or every 2 years causes a heavy burden on the limited manpower and financial resources of low-resource settings. Frequent screening does not add extra benefit over 3-yearly or 5-yearly screening. It has been estimated that screening women with VIA even twice in their lifetime is highly cost-effective. In countries of low-resource settings, achieving a good coverage (more than 70%) of the target women determines the success of the screening program rather than too frequent screening.

14.2.2.2 Screening Test Facilities

The CC screening program of low-resource settings should be integrated into the existing government health-care delivery system. This is convenient and cost-effective. For convenience and to ensure better compliance, the screening tests should be done close to the residence of the women. Primary and secondary health-care facilities are best suited for this purpose. However, if the health facilities are too far from a particular locality or are in hard-to-reach areas, mobile clinics (screening camps) can be set up on a temporary basis at a suitable place in the village.

14.2.2.3 Capacity Building of Test Providers

The nurses, female health workers, and other paramedical staff or the physicians at the primary and secondary health-care level can do the screening test. They require training and certification before they start the procedure. One essential component is the development of a strong screening implementation infrastructure.

Adequate number of trained manpower for service delivery should be developed at all levels of the health-care system to achieve optimum screening coverage. Competency-based training for service providers at designated training centers should be ensured with proper resource persons and training materials. Good-quality training with appropriate post-training follow-up should be ensured. Only certified providers should perform the tests. After training, the service providers need to be supervised until they achieve a satisfactory level of competency. All test providers should receive a short refresher training, initially every year and later every alternate year.

14.2.2.4 Ensuring Management of the Screen-Positive Women

All screen-positive women should have adequate counseling, further evaluation, and treatment at appropriate facilities. In low-resource settings, equipment for evaluation and treatment (colposcope, electrosurgical equipment, cryotherapy equipment, thermocoagulator) and trained expertise (colposcopists, gynecologists) are less available. Therefore "screen-and-treat" and "see-and-treat" strategy is being introduced as alternative approach of management. Women should have easy access to treatment services to ensure high compliance. In low-resource settings, an approach requiring fewer visits should be adopted to achieve better compliance for the screen-positive cases. They can be managed during the first visit with or without evaluation by colposcopy/histopathology report. However, selected cases need referral to the colposcopy clinics/higher-level health-care facilities (secondary/tertiary level) where further evaluation and management can be carried out.

14.2.2.5 Screen-and-Treat Protocol

The purpose of a "screen-and-treat protocol" is to link screening test to appropriate treatment of precancer with less adverse effects. However, women who are not eligible to receive treatment at the respective facility need referral to higher centers. WHO mentions cryotherapy as the preferred method of treatment in the "screen-and-treat" protocol. WHO algorithm for screen-and-treat strategy at the program level is shown in Fig. 14.9. Using this chart, program managers and decision-makers can determine the best option for screen and treat, in context to their country. Cryotherapy has fewer side effects and nurse/paramedics can perform the procedure at

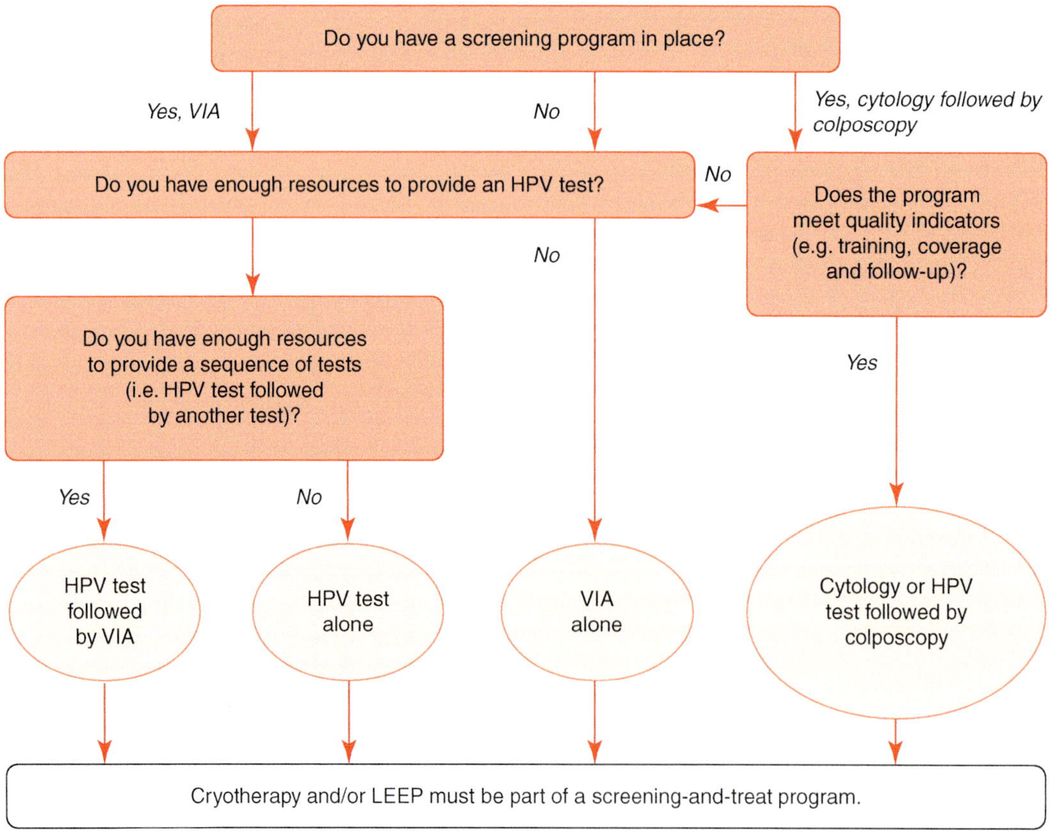

Fig. 14.9 Decision-making flowchart for program managers [39]

the lower level of the health-care system [39]. However, when women are not eligible for cryotherapy, loop electrosurgical excision procedure (LEEP) is the preferred method of treatment.

All HPV-positive women should be treated, and VIA should be used to determine eligibility for treatment with cryotherapy or LEEP [39]. A demonstration project on "prevention of cervical cancer through screening using VIA and treatment with cryotherapy" involving seven sites in six African countries (Madagascar, Malawi, Nigeria, Uganda, United Republic of Tanzania, and Zambia), from 2005 to 2009, revealed that the "screen-and-treat" approach can be introduced in the existing reproductive health services in low-resource countries. Screening for precancerous lesions using VIA and treatment with cryotherapy were well accepted by women and have been incorporated into the cervical cancer-prevention services in existing reproductive health services in these countries [45]. However, though cryotherapy is the primary treatment option for many countries, procuring the gas required for freezing is a significant obstacle. Low quality of carbon dioxide gas also damages equipment. To overcome the barriers, different low-resource countries are trying to adopt use of thermocoagulator to treat CIN. The Guatemalan government has taken steps to introduce thermocoagulation, which needs only electricity [42]. Thermocoagulation is safe, simple, and an effective technique to treat selected CIN lesions of any grade, and it can be used in the single-visit "screen-and-treat" approach and "see-and-treat" approach in the management of CIN in the cervical cancer control program [46].

Sequential testing with VIA and VILI is the most feasible screening approach for cervical cancer screening for HIV-infected women in low-resource countries. When HPV testing becomes feasible and affordable, HPV testing followed by VIA/VILI may be considered [47].

14.2.2.6 See-and-Treat Protocol

In LMICs, where facilities are available, the screen-positive women can be further evaluated following "see-and-treat protocol," and diseased cases can be treated during the same visit for better compliance of treatment. Women with VIA-, HPV-, or Pap-positive report can have further evaluation using colposcopy through addition of a second visit at a higher referral system where colposcopy facilities are available. The women suspected to have high-grade CIN on colposcopy may be treated at the same visit without any histopathological confirmation of the disease. This strategy is called "see-and-treat" or also "colposcopy-and-treat" approach. The "see-and-treat" approach is convenient for the woman; it reduces her anxiety, it improves compliance to treatment, and it is cost-effective for the program. LEEP has been used as the treatment modality for such protocols. A population-based large randomized screening trial in Osmanabad district in Maharashtra, India, was conducted during 2000–2004. The study confirmed that a "see-and-treat" approach using cryotherapy by nurses is acceptable to women, is safe, and ensures satisfactory participation of screen-positive women for diagnosis and treatment [48–50]. Another randomized trial in India has shown a significant reduction in cervical cancer mortality following a single round of screening with HPV testing or VIA screening [51].

In Bangladesh, the government has adopted "see-and-treat" approach combining VIA with colposcopy and LEEP since the year 2010 to improve compliance to treatment [52]. The program is also using thermocoagulation in "see-and-treat" protocols in selected centers. Pooled data from five sites in Asia and South America for women treated for CIN with thermocoagulation from 2010 to 2015, and followed up within 6–12 months of treatment, showed cure after thermocoagulation treatment was 88% (475/543) for CIN 1, 83% (113/137) for CIN 2, and 83% (79/95) for CIN 3 lesions. No serious adverse effect or complications were observed throughout the follow-up period. Thermocoagulation was effective, safe, and accepted in treatment of women diagnosed with CIN and can be used in the single-visit "screen-and-treat" approach or "see-and-treat" approach in management of CIN in the cervical cancer control program [46]. The major benefits are shorter treatment time, easy portability of the equipment to field, use of easily available electricity than gas refills, is noiseless and produces less smoke, and there is no need for general anesthesia.

14.2.2.7 Posttreatment Follow-up

The treated women should receive posttreatment follow-up screening at 1 year to ensure effectiveness of treatment [39]. Follow-up of treated patients can be continued at all levels of facilities by available methods. VIA, colposcopy, or HPV DNA test can be used during follow-up on an annual basis for 3 years. Women tested negative on three consecutive rounds should be returned to the routine screening protocol applicable to the normal population.

14.2.2.8 Record-Keeping and Data Management

Maintenance of records, storage of data related to various components of screening, and periodic reports are essential for an organized screening program. For population-based organized screening, countries need to develop an electronic database for all women of target age. This database should include women's basic information, screening, colposcopy, treatment, and follow-up records. The computerized database should be maintained at each screening center and all colposcopy centers. A mechanism to check the compliance of screen-positive women to colposcopy and/or treatment should be established by the government.

14.2.2.9 Monitoring, Evaluation, and Quality Assurance

Reduction of CC incidence and death from the disease can be assessed by impact indicators. It can be obtained through a population-based cancer registry or organized health information system. Outcome indicators should be monitored on a regular basis to identify gaps and to identify ways of improvement.

14.2.3 Overcoming Challenges for Cancer Screening Services in LMICs

The main challenges to improve CC screening services include:

- Lack of initiation of a demonstration /pilot program and scale-up of program
- Low level of community awareness on the importance of screening for this cancer
- Poor health system in low-resource settings with insufficient number of skilled manpower and inadequate treatment facilities when there is precancer or cancer diagnosis
- Lack of an effective health information system to facilitate referral and tracking of noncompliant women
- Lack of well-coordinated monitoring and evaluation plan, especially for data collection and management

14.2.3.1 Initiation of a Pilot Program and Scaling Up CC Screening Strategies in LMICs

A pilot program should be initiated by the government and can be supported by nonprofit or international organizations. An advocacy meeting to initiate a pilot program should be organized by the government in countries where piloting has not been performed. The advocacy document should include focused country-specific messages and data on CC incidence and deaths. It should also clearly identify strategies and service delivery guidelines based on the country's needs and priorities. Advocacy meetings should focus on the elimination of policy barriers, allotment of adequate monetary, and human resources for the CC control program. Working with other government sectors and nongovernmental agencies, developing materials to increase public awareness on CC and its prevention, mobilizing eligible women to utilize CC control services, and encouraging communities to assist women with cervical cancer are important.

Although pilot or demonstration programs have taken place in several LMICs, only a few countries have experienced scale-up of evidence-based screening strategies. These countries selected screening modalities recommended by the WHO to avoid budgetary constraints and other health system bottlenecks [42]. The gathered experience may help other countries plan for large-scale implementation. In Bangladesh scale-up efforts began in 2006. About 411 VIA centers are operational throughout the country, and 1,386,887 VIA tests were performed from 2005 to 2016 at different service centers. Among them 65,247 (4.7%) women were found VIA-positive. The coverage of the screening tests is increasing every year. VIA+ve cases are referred to the colposcopy clinic of Bangabandhu Sheikh Mujib Medical University (BSMMU) and different medical college hospitals. In Bangladesh, LEEP acquired acceptability as a commonly used outpatient treatment procedure for CIN under local anesthesia and thermocoagulation without local anesthesia.

In Central America, governments are implementing HPV testing using a low-cost assay. HPV testing enables women to collect their own vaginal samples in a variety of settings. Several common challenges remain for continued scale-up in these countries such as training and maintaining a manpower to carry out screening and treatment activities and monitoring and improving the quality of screening and treatment services to bring an impact on CC mortality rates. Governments must begin to move beyond pilot testing and opportunistic efforts to implementing large-scale, population-based approaches where possible.

14.2.3.2 Development of Organized CC Screening Program

In LMICs, a mass screening policy should be taken along with developing a population-based screening program. Low-resource countries should have an organized screening program, in which all eligible women would be systematically invited to have the screening test through extensive community mobilization.

The essential components of an organized screening program:

- A protocol and guideline that will clearly spell out the target population, frequency of screening, screening test, and management of screen-positive population.
- A definite plan for broad-based community mobilization to ensure high participation rate of the target population.
- Ensuring access to screening as well as detection services at the grassroot level so that a high coverage (at least 70% of the target population) can be achieved.
- Linkage between screening and treatment to ensure that the positive cases detected through the program are treated appropriately.
- All categories of service providers should be trained and certified.
- A plan for supportive supervision and quality assurance should be inbuilt in the program.

14.2.3.3 Health Education and Awareness Creation

In low-resource countries, awareness programs conducted by NGOs and government are inadequate to increase awareness among women about CC and its risk factors. Awareness programs remain out of reach of target groups, because they live in villages and rural and urban slums. Programs conducted on special dates, like World Cancer Day, World Health Day, CC Awareness Day, etc., may create more awareness.

Health education and awareness are important elements of a cervical cancer control program, particularly in LMICs where education and health service-seeking attitude is low. Awareness should be created to develop service-seeking behavior among the community. Health education should be delivered both at the community and health facilities. In many LMICs, the existing health infrastructure has manpower and volunteers to increase public awareness, and health education messages in such situations can be imparted through direct face-to-face meetings. Health workers at community or primary health facilities are the first point of contact with the community, and this is particularly true for LMICs where a large number of women do not have access to the electronic media, and the government has less allocation on these expensive media.

At health facilities, health education and counseling can be given by trained service providers. Service providers can develop special skills on counseling techniques and should be well conversed with methods to ask and answer questions about CC screening in a well-informed, honest, and culturally sensitive way. Health educators need to realize that most precancerous lesions of the cervix and early cervical cancer do not have clinical symptoms. Thus, most women being tested need to be informed that the disease may be silent for a long time without causing any problem, and the tests are for preventing CC and better treatment of the disease.

Flip charts should be developed for use by the health-care providers for counseling both at the screening center and in the community using their own language with consideration of cultural factors.

Posters in the local language aided by pictures, diagrams, and charts should be used to propagate the messages. A broad-based media campaign utilizing print and electronic media will be used to improve the visibility of the program and enhance participation rates.

Some basic principles and suggestions are listed below:

- Inform the community about the risk factors and common signs and symptoms of CC.
- Promote screening for women aged 30 to 60 years.
- Reduce ignorance, fear, embarrassment, and stigma related to cancer.
- Inform the community of available services and where to get them.
- Involvement of community leaders is critical to gain support for the outreach efforts and for adequate allocation of local resources.
- Male partners and other community members must support women's decisions to seek screening and to go for treatment when required.
- Multi-sectorial involvement of governmental and nongovernmental agencies is imperative for the success of this strategy.

14.2.3.4 Strengthening the Health Infrastructure

Patients are reluctant to attend the primary health-care centers in due time for many reasons. The main reasons are lack of awareness, poor knowledge, bad communication and transport facility, financial constrain, etc. In many centers health-care professionals poorly follow the referral system, mostly due to weak coordination with tertiary health-care center. Most of the South Asian countries and some countries of sub-Saharan Africa have insufficient number of pathologists, laboratories, colposcopists, and other health-care providers, which limits the services. Poor resource allocation and suboptimal infrastructure also hinder screening programs.

Strengthening various services within the existing health infrastructure, ensuring supply and maintenance of equipment, and uninterrupted supply of consumables are important factors for success of the screening program in LMICs. Appropriate referral system for screening and management within the existing health system should be organized. Development of a strong screening implementation infrastructure is an essential component for success in LMICs. The number of trained manpower for CC screening, including community health workers and administrators, should be increased. Improvement of coverage is important for the success of the program. Policies should be reviewed from time to time to reduce obstacles to improving coverage. Outreach clinics and health camps should be arranged to improve coverage, particularly at hard-to-reach and/or low-performing areas.

14.2.3.5 Strengthening Record-Keeping and Data Management

For population-based organized screening, countries need to develop an electronic database for all women of target age. The computerized database should be maintained at each screening center and all colposcopy centers. A mechanism to check the compliance of screen-positive women to colposcopy and/or treatment should be established by the government.

14.2.3.6 Strengthening Monitoring, Evaluation, and Quality Assurance

Reduction of CC incidence and death from the disease can be assessed by impact indicators. It can be obtained through a population-based cancer registry or organized health information system. Outcome indicators should be monitored on a regular basis to identify gaps and to identify ways of improvement. Head of the respective health facilities, gynecology consultants, and program managers should be responsible for implementation of services, coordination between various levels of service delivery, and quality assurance.

The indicators to be used for monitoring and quality assurance of the program, and how they will be monitored periodically, should be clearly defined. The performance indicatos are coverage of the target population, screening test positivity, compliance to treatment, and detection rate of CIN 2 or worse.

14.3 Conclusion

In order to improve screening programs for cervical cancer in low-resource countries, it is imperative to increase access to accurate and timely information on CC, mobilize the community through a specific action plan, generate more trained human resources on priority basis, strengthen partnerships between stakeholders, mobilize resources for long-term continuity of the program, and establish a monitoring and evaluation framework.

Key Points

- CC can be prevented through implementing population-based organized CC screening program along with development of electronic data tracking for all women of target age group.
- HPV DNA test has proved more effective than other screening methods as it has a high negative predictive value.
- VIA is accepted as a method of screening in many countries with low-resource settings as it needs minimum infrastructure support and the results are available immediately.
- LMICs need to organize a stakeholders meeting to choose a method of screening suitable for the country's socioeconomic status wherever necessary, followed by a demonstration program and gradual nationwide scale-up.
- All low-resource countries need to develop national CC control strategies focusing age of initiation of screening, mechanism of awareness creation, method of screening, and mechanism of population coverage.
- All screen-positive cases should be treated following "screen-and-treat" strategy or "see-and-treat" strategy.
- Strengthening health infrastructure, ensuring supply and maintenance of equipment, and uninterrupted supply of consumables are important factors for CC screening program in LMICs.
- Strengthening monitoring, evaluation, and quality assurance and monitoring outcome indicators on a regular basis to identify gaps are important factors to reduce CC death.
- Multi-sectorial involvement of governmental and nongovernmental agencies is imperative for the success of this strategy.

Acknowledgments We are very much grateful to the International Agency for Research on Cancer (IARC), Lyon, France, including Dr. R. Sankaranarayanan and Dr. Partha Basu, and the World Health Organization for permitting us to use photographs, cancer statistics, and figures in the manuscript.

References

1. Ferlay J, Soerjomataram I, Ervik M, Dikshit R, Eser S, Mathers C, et al. GLOBOCAN 2012 v1.0, cancer incidence and mortality worldwide: IARC cancer base no. 11. Lyon: International Agency for Research on Cancer; 2013.
2. Farmer P, Frenk J, Knaul FM, Shulman LN, Alleyne G, Armstrong L, et al. Expansion of cancer care and control in countries of low and middle income: a call to action. Lancet. 2010;376(9747):1186–93.
3. IARC: GLOBOCAN 2012 Cervical cancer: estimated incidence, mortality and prevalence worldwide in 2012.
4. Sullivan T, Sullivan R, Ginsburg OM. Screening for cancer: considerations for low- and middle-income countries. In: Gelband H, Jha P, Sankaranarayanan R, Horton S, editors. Cancer: disease control priorities, vol. 3. 3rd ed. Washington: The International Bank for Reconstruction and Development/The World Bank; 2015.
5. Albow R, Kitchener H, Gupta N, Desai M. Cervical screening in England: the past, present, and future. Cancer Cytopathol. 2012;120:87–96.
6. Cuzick J, Clavel C, Petry KU, Meijer CJ, Hoyer H, Ratnam S, et al. Overview of the European and North American studies on HPV testing in primary cervical cancer screening. Int J Cancer. 2006;119:1095–101.
7. Haghighi F, Ghanbarzadeh N, Ataee M, Sharifzadeh G, Mojarrad JS, Najafi-Semnani F. A comparison of

liquid-based cytology with conventional Papanicolaou smears in cervical dysplasia diagnosis. Adv Biomed Res. 2016;5:162. e Collection 2016.
8. Denny L, Kuhn L, Pollack A, Wainwright H, Wright TC. Evaluation of alternative methods of cervical cancer screening for resource-poor settings. Cancer. 2000;89:826–33.
9. Sancho-Garnier H, Khazraji YC, Cherif MH, Mahnane A, Hsairi M, El Shalakamy A, et al. Overview of cervical cancer screening practices in the extended Middle East and North Africa countries. Vaccine. 2013;31(Suppl 6):G51–7.
10. Aswathy S, Quereshi MA, Kurian B, Leelamoni K. Cervical cancer screening: current knowledge & practice among women in a rural population of Kerala, India. Indian J Med Res. 2012;136:205–10.
11. Ahmed T, Ashrafunnessa RJ. Development of a visual inspection programme for cervical cancer prevention in Bangladesh. Reprod Health Matters. 2008;16(32):78–85.
12. Nessa A, Hussain MA, Rahman JN, Rashid MH, Muwonge R, Sankaranarayanan R. Screening for cervical neoplasia in Bangladesh using visual inspection with acetic acid. Int J Gynaecol Obstet. 2010;111:115–8.
13. Heath Bulletin, MIS, Directorate General of Health Services, Dhaka, Bangladesh, 2017; Preliminary Pre-Print Version.
14. Arbyn M, Rebolj M, De Kok IM, Fender M, Becker N, O'Reilly M, et al. The challenges of organising cervical screening programmes in the 15 old member states of the European Union. Eur J Cancer. 2009;45:2671–8.
15. Adegoke O, Kulasingam S, Viring B. Cervical cancer trends in the United States: a 35-year population-based analysis. J Women Health (Larchamt). 2012:21:1031–7.
16. Sasieni P, Castanon A, Cuzick J. Effectiveness of cervical screening with age: population-based case-control study of prospectively recorded data. BMJ. 2009;339:b2968.
17. Robyr R, Nazeer S, Vasoilakos P, Matute JC, Sando Z, Halle G, et al. Feasibility of cytology-based cervical cancer screening in rural Cameroon. Acta Cytol. 2002;46:1110–6.
18. Sankaranarayanan R, Nessa A, Esmy PO, Dangou JM. Visual inspection methods for cervical cancer prevention. Best Pract Res Clin Obstet Gynaecol. 2012;26(2):221–32.
19. Nessa A, Nahar KN, Begum SA, Anwary SA, Hossain F, Nahar K. Comparison between visual inspection of cervix and cytology-based screening procedures in Bangladesh. Asian J. 2013;14(12):7607–11.
20. Sankaranarayanan R, Wesley R, Thara S, Dhakad N, Chandralekha B, Sebastian P, et al. Test characteristics of visual inspection with 4% acetic acid (VIA) and Lugol's iodine (VILI) in cervical cancer screening in Kerala, India. Int J Cancer. 2003;106:404–8.
21. Karimi-Zarchi M, Peighmbari F, Karmi N, Rohi M, Chiti Z. A comparison of 3 ways of conventional pap smear, liquid-based cytology and colposcopy vs cervical biopsy for early diagnosis of premalignant lesions or cervical cancer in women with abnormal conventional pap test. Int J Biomed Sci. 2013;9(4):205–10.
22. Holowaty P, Miller AB, Rohan T, To T. Natural history of dysplasia of the uterine cervix. J Natl Cancer Inst. 1999;91(3):252–8.
23. Ronco G, Dillner J, Elfström KM, Tunesi S, Snijders PJ, Arbyn M, et al. Efficacy of HPV-based screening for prevention of invasive cervical cancer: follow-up of four European randomised controlled trials. Lancet. 2014;383:524–32.
24. Meijer CJ, Berkhof J, Castle PE, Hesselink AT, Franco EL, Ronco G, et al. Guidelines for human papillomavirus DNA test requirements for primary cervical cancer screening in women 30 years and older. Int J Cancer. 2009;124:516–20.
25. Cuzick J, Arbyn M, Sankaranarayanan R, Tsu V, Ronco G, Mayrand MH, et al. Overview of human papillomavirus-based and other novel options for cervical cancer screening in developed and developing countries. Vaccine. 2008;26(Suppl 10):K29–41.
26. Sankaranarayanan R, Basu P, Wesley RS, Mahe C, Keita N, Mbalawa CC, et al. Accuracy of visual screening for cervical neoplasia: results from an IARC multicenter study in India and Africa. Int J Cancer. 2004;110:907–13.
27. Sankaranarayanan R, Gaffikin L, Jacob M, Sellors J, Robles S. A critical assessment of screening methods for cervical neoplasia. Int J Gynaecol Obstet. 2005;89(Suppl 2):S4–12.
28. Sankaranarayanan R, Nene BM, Shastri SS, Jayant K, Muwonge R, Budukh AM, et al. HPV screening for cervical cancer in rural India. N Engl J Med. 2009;360:1385–94.
29. Jeronimo J, Bansil P, Lim J, Peck R, Paul P, Amador JJ, et al. A multicountry evaluation of care HPV testing, visual inspection with acetic acid, and papanicolaou testing for the detection of cervical cancer. Int J Gynecol Cancer. 2014:24(3):576–85.
30. Shastri SS, Mittra I, Mishra GA, Gupta S, Dikshit R, Singh S, et al. Effect of VIA screening by primary health workers: randomized controlled study in Mumbai, India. J Natl Cancer Inst. 2014;106(3). https://doi.org/10.1093/jnci/dju009.
31. University of Zimbabwe, JHPIEGO Cervical Cancer Project Visual inspection with acetic acid for cervical cancer screening: test qualities in a primary-care setting. Lancet. 1999;353:869–73.
32. Denny L, Kuhn L, Pollack A, Wright TC Jr. Direct visual inspection for cervical cancer screening: an analysis of factors influencing test performance. Cancer. 2002;94:1699–707.
33. Sankaranarayanan R, Thara S, Anjali S, Roy C, Shastri S, Mahé C, et al. Accuracy of conventional cytology: results from a multicenter screening study in India. J Med Screen. 2004;11:77–84.
34. Braganca JF, Derchain SFM, Sarian LO, Messias da Silva SM, Labatte S, Zeferino LC. Aided visual inspection with acetic acid (VIA) and HPV detec-

tion as optional screening tools for cervical cancer and its precursor lesions. Clin Exp Obstet Gynecol. 2005;32:225–9.

35. Ngoma T, Muwonge R, Mwaiselage J, Kawegere J, Bukori P, Sankaranarayanan R. Evaluation of cervical visual inspection screening in Dar es Salaam, Tanzania. Int J Gynecol Obstet. 2010;109:100–4.
36. Muwonge R, Manuel MG, Filipe AP, Dumas JB, Frank MR, Sankaranarayanan R. Visual screening for early detection of cervical neoplasia in Angola. Int J Gynecol Obstet. 2010;111:68–72.
37. Sauvaget C, Fayette JM, Muwonge R, Wesley R, Sankaranarayanan R. Accuracy of visual inspection with acetic acid for cervical cancer screening. Int J Gynaecol Obstet. 2011;113:14–24.
38. Bradford L, Goodman A. Cervical cancer screening and prevention in low-resource setting. Clin Obstet Gynecol. 2013;56:76–87.
39. World Health Organization. WHO guidelines for screening and treatment of precancerous lesions for cervical cancer prevention. Geneva: World Health Organization; 2013.
40. World Health Organization. Comprehensive cervical cancer control: a guide to essential practice. 2nd ed. Geneva: World Health Organization; 2014.
41. Parham GP, Mwanahamuntu MH, Kapambwe S, Muwonge R, Bateman AC, Blevins M, et al. Population-level scale-up of cervical cancer prevention services in a low-resource setting: development, implementation, and evaluation of the cervical cancer prevention program in Zambia. PLoS One. 2015;10:e0122169.
42. Holme F, Kapambwe S, Nessa A, Partha B, Murillo R, Jeronimo J. Scaling up proven innovative cervical cancer screening strategies: challenges and opportunities in implementation at the population level in low and lower-middle income countries. Int J Gynecol Obstet. 2017;138(Suppl 1):63–8.
43. Basu P, Nessa A, Majid M, Rahman JN, Ahmed T. Evaluation of the National Cervical Cancer Screening Programme of Bangladesh and the formulation of quality assurance guidelines. J Fam Plann Reprod Health Care. 2010;36:131–4.
44. Nessa A, Wistrand C, Begum SA, Thuresson M, Shemer I, Thorsell M, et al. Evaluation of stationary colposcope and the Gynocular, by the Swede score systematic colposcopic system in VIA positive women: a crossover randomized trial. Int J Gynecol Cancer. 2014;24(2):339–45.
45. Prevention of cervical cancer through screening using visual inspection using acetic acid (VIA) and treatment with cryotherapy: a demonstration project in six African countries: Malawi, Madagascar, Nigeria, Uganda, the United Republic of Tanzania and Zambia. World Health Organization (WHO), International Agency for Research on Cancer (IARC), African Population and Health Research Center (APHRC). Geneva: World Health Organization; 2012.
46. Nessa A, Naud P, Esmy PO, Joshi S, Rema P, Wesley R, et al. Efficacy, safety, and acceptability of thermal coagulation to treat cervical intraepithelial neoplasia: pooled data from Bangladesh, Brazil and India. Clin Gynecol Obstet. 2017;6(3–4):58–64.
47. Josi S, Kulkarni V, Somanathan T, Divate U. Screening of cervical neoplasia in HIV-infected women in India. AIDS. 2013;27(4):607–15.
48. Sankaranarayanan R, Keshkar V, Kothari A, Kane S, Fayette JM, Shastri S. Effectiveness and safety of loop electrosurgical excision procedure for cervical neoplasia in rural India. Int J Gynaecol Obstet. 2009;104:95–9.
49. Nene BM, Hiremath PS, Kane S, Fayette JM, Shastri SS, Sankaranarayanan R. Effectiveness, safety, and acceptability of cryotherapy by midwives for cervical intraepithelial neoplasia in Maharashtra, India. Int J Gynaecol Obstet. 2008;103:232–6.
50. Sankaranarayanan R, Rajkumar R, Esmy PO, Fayette JM, Shanthakumary S, Frappart L, et al. Effectiveness, safety and acceptability of 'see and treat' with cryotherapy by nurses in a cervical screening study in India. Br J Cancer. 2007;96:738–43.
51. Sankaranarayanan R, Esmy PO, Rajkumar R, Muwonge R, Swaminathan R, Shanthakumari S, et al. Effect of visual screening on cervical cancer incidence and mortality in Tamil Nadu, India: a cluster-randomised trial. Lancet. 2007;370:398–406.
52. Nessa A, Rashid MH, Ferdous NE, Chowdhury A. Screening for and management of high-grade cervical intraepithelial neoplasia in Bangladesh: a cross-sectional study comparing two protocols. J Obstet Gynaecol Res. 2013;39:564–71.

15 Ablative Methods for Treatment of Intraepithelial Lesions

Shruti Bhatia

15.1 Introduction

Intraepithelial neoplasia is the development of dysplasia in an epithelium. It is distinct from cancer but has the potential to evolve into the latter. Because these are premalignant lesions, treatment is usually indicated. Lower genital tract (cervix, vulva, vagina) neoplasias (intraepithelial and invasive) are associated with human papilloma virus (HPV) infection. Among these three genital areas, cervical intraepithelial neoplasia (CIN) is the most common but fortunately least difficult to cure. Vulvar intraepithelial neoplasia (VIN), on the other hand, is often multifocal and much more difficult to treat. Vaginal intraepithelial neoplasia (VAIN) is least common among the three sites and usually coexists with CIN. Treatment modalities for intraepithelial neoplasias can be excisional or ablative (destructive). In this chapter, various ablative procedures that are used for treatment of intraepithelial lesions of the cervix, vulva, and vagina are discussed.

S. Bhatia (✉)
Department of Gynaecological Oncology, Action Cancer Hospital, New Delhi, India

15.1.1 Cervical Intraepithelial Neoplasia

Incidence of invasive cervical cancer and mortality from it has decreased over the past decades due to widespread use of cytology-based screening programs and HPV testing. Women with abnormal screening results are referred for colposcopy and directed biopsies for confirmation of histological diagnosis. Based on the degree of cellular and epithelial abnormalities, lesions are graded as CIN 1, 2, or 3. CIN 1 lesions are generally manifestation of HPV infection and are spontaneously cleared by the innate immune system within 1–2 years. Hence, surveillance rather than active treatment of CIN 1 lesions is appropriate. CIN 3 lesions have high chances of progression to invasive cancer as neoplastic changes are present throughout the full thickness of the epithelium. CIN 2 lesions have an intermediate biological behavior between CIN 1 and 3, with up to 40% regressing spontaneously over long follow-up. Thus, the cornerstone of cervical cancer prevention is detection and treatment of CIN 2 and CIN 3 lesions.

CIN should be considered as a morphological manifestation of persisting HPV infection in the epithelial cells. Invasive cancer is related to accumulation of increasing mutational burden, longer duration of infection, and multiple other permissive cofactors. CIN can extend into the cervical

S. Mehta, A. Singla (eds.), *Preventive Oncology for the Gynecologist*,
https://doi.org/10.1007/978-981-13-3438-2_15

stromal glands, and so their treatment requires to extend below the epithelial surface. Morphometric studies guide the clinicians in the appropriate method of treatment.

Anderson et al. examined 343 women who had undergone conization for CIN and found that the mean depth of glands containing CIN was 1.24 mm from the surface, with the deepest gland involvement extending up to 5.22 mm [1]. Abdul-Karim et al. found that there is a direct relationship between lesion grade and the vertical and horizontal extent of the lesion. In 319 conization specimens, they reported the mean depth of CIN 1, CIN 2, and CIN 3 was 0.42 mm, 0.93 mm, and 1.35 mm, respectively, and the mean linear extent was 4.10 mm, 5.84 mm, and 7.60 mm, respectively. So the authors recommended a treatment depth of 4.8 mm to eradicate 99.7% of high-grade lesions [2] (Fig. 15.1).

The conclusion from these studies has the following important clinical applications for the practitioners:

- Given that CIN 3 lesions are located within 4.8 mm of the surface of the cervix and the deepest gland containing CIN 3 is 5.2 mm from surface, a treatment depth of 6–7 mm below the epithelium will be successful in majority of patients with satisfactory colposcopy [1, 2].
- The aim of ablative therapy should be to destroy full thickness of the abnormal epithelium including glandular crypts up to a depth of 5–7 mm, as CIN has a tendency to extend into glandular crypts.

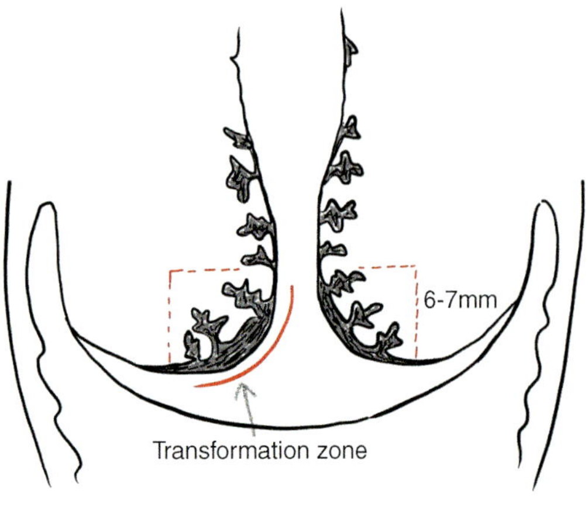

Fig. 15.1 Schematic presentation of cervical glands

The prerequisites for ablative therapy include:

- The entire transformation zone can be visualized.
- Lesion is fully visualized.
- There is no suggestion of microinvasive or invasive disease.
- There is no suspicion of glandular disease.
- Cytology and histology are concordant.

Ablative methods are not recommended in the following situations:

- In cases of recurrence of CIN.
- Endocervical sampling shows CIN/lesion extending into endocervical canal.
- Cytology or colposcopy suggests cancer.
- Histology is CIN 2 or CIN 3 and colposcopy is inadequate.

When the patient is not a candidate for ablative treatments, excisional therapies like LEEP (loop electrosurgical excision procedure) or conization may be used. In addition, if there is recurrence of CIN after ablation, excision may be preferred over repeated ablation procedures. Randomized trials comparing LEEP, conization, and cryotherapy have shown similar efficacy, ranging from 90% to 95% [3–5]. Whatever the treatment chosen, the entire transformation zone must be treated.

Several techniques for ablation are available, like cryotherapy, laser ablation, and thermocoagulation. Each of these techniques has its own advantages and disadvantages. Selection of appropriate treatment depends on various factors like operator's experience, available equipment, and location and size of lesion. The ideal time to do any ablative procedure is post-menstrual phase of the menstrual cycle.

Disadvantages and adverse effects of ablative procedures include non-availability of tissue specimen for histology, bleeding, infection, scarring, and cervical stenosis.

15.2 Types of Ablative Procedures

15.2.1 Cryotherapy

Cryotherapy is an old technique and was introduced in the late 1960s to treat CIN. Thousands of patients have been treated by this method worldwide, and it still remains popular as it is easy to perform in outpatient setting and causes minimal discomfort. It is an appropriate technique for use in low-resource settings as it does not require electricity, instruments are not expensive, and procedure is technically simple. A recent WHO report called cervical precancer screening using visual inspection with acetic acid (VIA) and cryotherapy a "best buy" for the control of noncommunicable diseases [6].

During cryotherapy, the lesion is cooled to extremely low temperature using a cryoprobe. Cellular destruction is by intracellular crystallization of water and through rapid freeze-thaw cycles. Cryotherapy typically generates an ice ball that is 5–7 mm deep, which is sufficient for treatment, given the morphometric data enumerated above [7].

The size of the cryoprobe and lateral spread of the freeze zone determines the area of destruction of the transformation zone. For example, if the freeze zone extends 5 mm beyond the probe, then it ensures 5 mm depth of freeze [8]. Two methods are used to cool the cryoprobe:

- When a compressed gas is expanded by passing through a nozzle, it causes cooling by the Joule-Thomson effect.
- Use of cryogenic liquids such as liquid nitrogen.

The cryogenic liquid-based procedure is associated with several problems like damage to surrounding tissue and problem of delivery, storage, and handling of liquid nitrogen. Hence, compressed gas-based cryosurgical equipment is recommended for treatment of CIN. The gas passes through the cryoprobe and causes ice formation on the probe tip and the tissue surface in contact. A temperature of less than −20 °C to −30 °C should be reached for tissue destruction.

The most widely used compressed gasses for the procedure are carbon dioxide (CO_2) and nitrous oxide (N_2O), and temperatures of −60 °C and −90 °C, respectively, can be reached. Most equipment manufacturers offer the option of using either of the two gasses. The choice of gas does not alter the success rate of treatment, although few studies like Mariategui et al. [9] and Cremer et al. [10] have shown that CO_2 causes 1 mm shallower depth of necrosis as compared to N_2O. However, CO_2 is more widely available and lower in cost and hence most widely used.

The cervix heals by reepithelialization, which occurs in most patients by 6 weeks and in all patients by 3 months. There may also be activation of local mucosal immunity after cryotherapy, with an increase in IgA, contributing to clearance of HPV infection [11].

Cryotherapy is an appropriate treatment for CIN if the following conditions are met:

- Entire squamocolumnar junction is visualized.
- Entire lesion is visible.
- Lesion is confined to the ectocervix.
- Lesion involves <75% area of the cervix.
- Lesion does not extend >2 mm beyond the tip of cryotherapy probe.
- There is no suspicion of invasive lesion.

15.2.1.1 Procedure

The equipment consists of a hand held unit with a shaft to which detachable probe tips can be attached. A hose assembly connects the hand unit to a connector/pressure gauge assembly and a high-pressure gas cylinder. The tips of the cryoprobes are round in shape and approximately 20 mm in diameter. They are detachable and can be sterilized/autoclaved. The surface of the cryoprobe tip that contacts the tissue is either flat or with a nipple-shaped cone extrusion. This extrusion of probe tip should not be more than 5 mm, as longer tips can lead to higher incidence of cervical stenosis (Figs. 15.2 and 15.3).

There is no requirement of anesthesia, and an analgesic may be used as needed. After placing the patient in lithotomy position, the lesion is identified after applying acetic acid and Lugol's

Fig. 15.2 Cryotherapy apparatus including the cryoprobe attached to pressure gauge assembly and gas cylinder

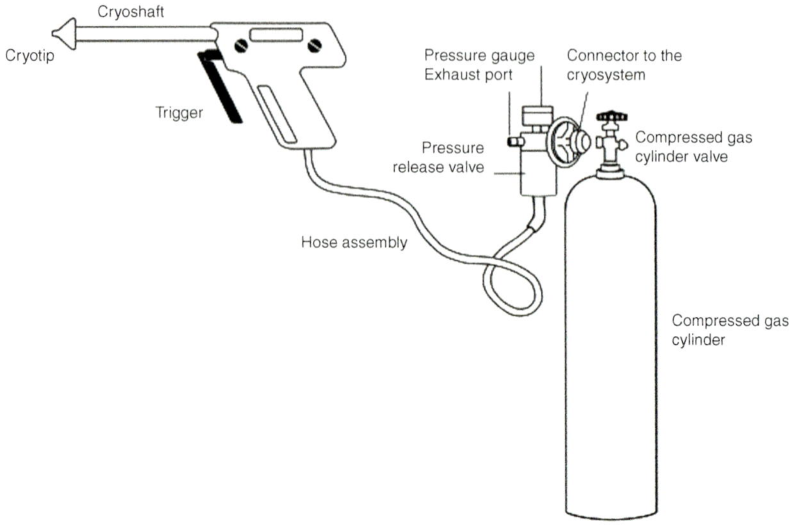

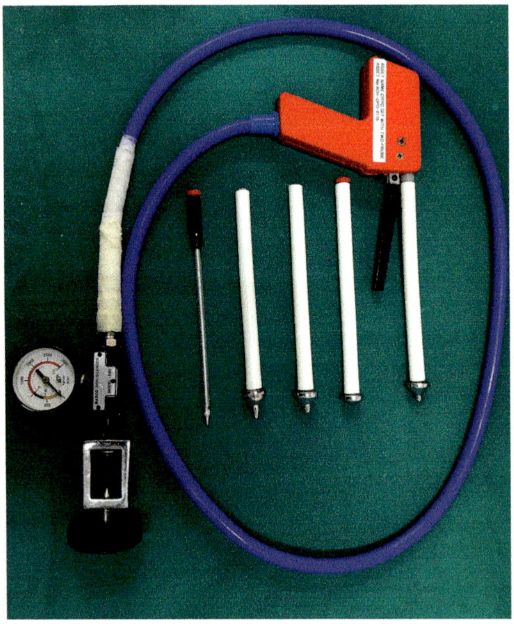

Fig. 15.3 Cryotherapy gun and different size probes

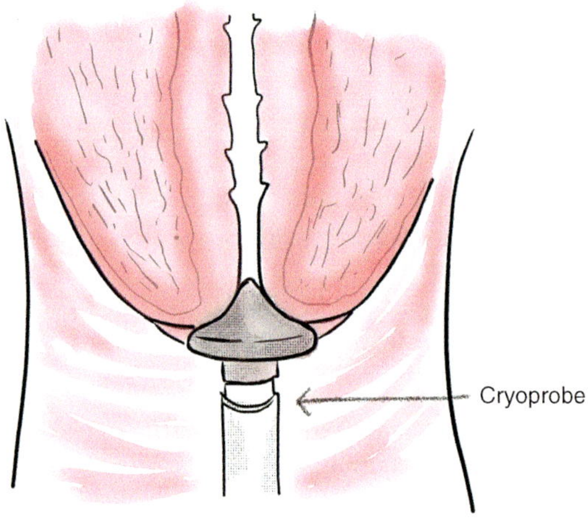

Fig. 15.4 Diagram depicting the correct way of cryoprobe application on cervical os

iodine. Appropriate size probe is selected, and a thin film of lubricant jelly is applied. This removes any "air gaps" and improves thermal contact of the probe with the surface of the cervix. The probe tip is applied in the center of os, taking care to ensure that the probe adequately covers the lesion and the vaginal walls are not in contact so as to avoid injury to the vagina (Fig. 15.4). The gas trigger of the gun is released to cool the probe. Pressure gauge attached to the cylinder is a visual indicator of the pressure in tank and should be in green zone at the time of procedure for adequate ice formation. The appropriate pressure should be above 40 kg/cm^2 to achieve satisfactory results. The time taken for ice ball formation is approximately 1.5–2 min. If 4–5 mm ice ball is not formed within this time, equipment is probably malfunctioning. When the frozen area extends 4–5 mm beyond the edge of the cryoprobe, freezing is adequate (Fig. 15.5).

Cryotherapy can be done using single-freeze technique or double-freeze technique. Various studies have shown that double-freeze technique gives better results than single-freeze technique [12, 13]. In the former technique, a 3 min freezing cycle is followed by 5 min thawing, followed by further 3 min of freezing. Once the second freezing cycle is complete, time is allowed for thawing before removing the probe. The frozen area appears white (Fig. 15.6a, b).

Patients usually experience some lower abdominal cramps or minor bleeding during the procedure which subsides afterwards. During the 2 weeks post-procedure, many will have profuse watery discharge that may even require wearing a pad. Some will have light spotting, especially 12–15 days after the procedure. Although infections following cryotherapy are rare, especially if there was no evidence of infection prior to the procedure, the patient is informed of possible complications like high-grade fever, severe abdominal pain, foul-smelling discharge, or heavy vaginal bleeding. Instructions are also given regarding self-hygiene and abstinence for 4 weeks.

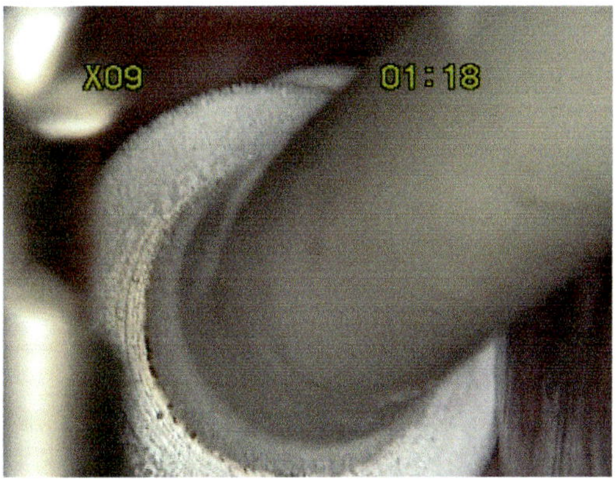

Fig. 15.5 Ice ball formation during cryotherapy

Follow-up visit is done at 4–6 weeks after procedure to check for healing. Long-term complications of cryotherapy are minimal, most common being cervical stenosis seen in 1–4% of patients.

15.2.1.2 Results

CIN lesions have been divided as small lesion (<25% area covered, 1 quadrant), moderate lesion (25–75% area covered, 2 quadrants), and large lesion (>75% area covered, >2 quadrants). At 1 year post cryotherapy, recurrence rate has been found to be maximum in women with large lesions. Recurrence rate of all grades of CIN in women with a small lesion is 6% (from 5 to 7%), with a moderate size lesion is 7% (from 6 to 8%), and with large lesion is 18% (from 13 to 23%) [8]. According to a meta-analysis done by Sauvaget, including 77 studies, cryotherapy achieved cure rates of approximately 94%, 92%, and 85% for CIN 1, CIN 2, and CIN 3, respectively [14]. The complications were very few and minor, which included local infection (<5% of patients), cervical stenosis (<1%), severe pain abdomen (<1%), and rarely obstetric complications. The main adverse effect was watery vaginal

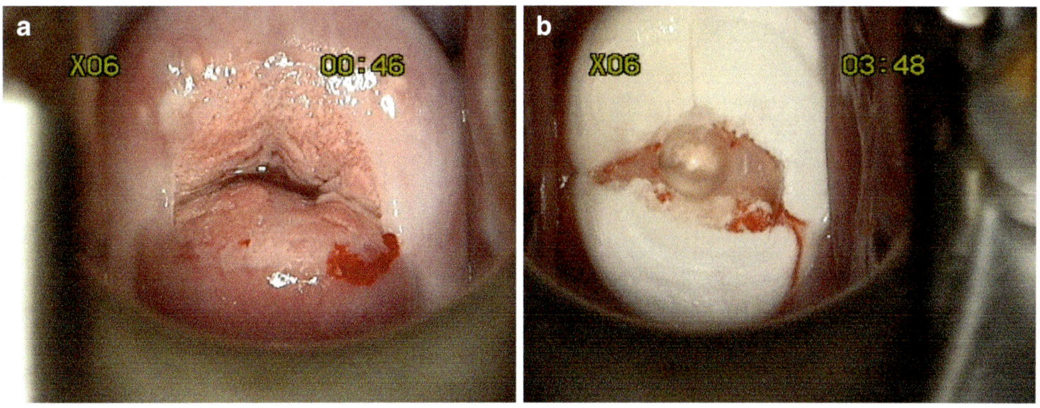

Fig. 15.6 (**a**) Colposcopic image of cervical lesion, before cryotherapy. (**b**) Colposcopic image of cervical lesion, after cryotherapy

discharge. The effectiveness of all treatment modalities like cryotherapy, cold knife or laser conization and LEEP were comparable. They concluded that cryotherapy is an effective, acceptable, and safe outpatient treatment for CIN and the cure rates are further increased by use of double-freeze method and absence of endocervical disease.

The advantages and disadvantages of the various treatment modalities for CIN including cryotherapy, LEEP, and cold knife conization were compared by Santesso et al. They suggested that recurrence of CIN 2 and CIN 3 is probably reduced with LEEP, although there are lesser complications with cryotherapy [15]. Due to its safety profile and ease of use, cryotherapy has been used successfully for "see-and-treat policy" for cervical cancer prevention worldwide [16–18].

WHO cancer prevention guidelines recommend use of cryotherapy over no treatment for women who have histologically confirmed CIN 2+ disease [19]. According to a 2010 Cochrane review, cryotherapy was as effective and acceptable as other ablative and excisional techniques for treatment of CIN [3].

New cryotherapy devices are being developed which are easy to transport and do not rely on large tanks of gas. A new device called CryoPen, which uses battery for cooling, does not require gas or liquids, is more portable, and can be used in peripheral areas, is being evaluated (ClinicalTrials.gov identifier: NCT03084081). Another device called CryoPop is also under evaluation (ClinicalTrials.gov identifier: NCT02367625). Although it uses gas for cooling, it is not tethered to gas cylinder during the procedure. It is also more durable and less costly [20].

15.2.2 Thermal Coagulation

Thermal coagulation or cold coagulation, as it was called earlier, was developed by Kurt Semm in 1966. Though it has been used in the UK for several decades, it is not very popular worldwide. Because of this infrequent use, it was also not included in the recent updated WHO guidelines for screening and treatment of precancerous lesions. However, it is a useful tool in the management of ectocervical CIN and can be integrated into the cervical cancer prevention program, especially in low- and middle-income countries.

It utilizes electricity to heat a thermoprobe to temperatures of 100–120 °C. The treatment is based on contact thermal heating to destroy cells by heat-induced coagulation; no current flows through the patient.

The eligibility criteria for thermal coagulation are same as cryotherapy: lesion should be fully visible and involve ≤ three quadrants of the transformation zone with no evidence of invasive cancer. It should be of the size so that it can be completely covered by the probe.

The main advantages of this procedure are:

- Procedure is rapid and easy to learn.
- Instrument is small, portable, and with minimum infrastructure requirement.
- Self-sterilizing by heating.
- Adequate treatment depth (4–7 mm).
- No tissue scarring and low bleeding
- Low rates of watery discharge.
- Low pain scores and quick healing.

15.2.2.1 Procedure

The apparatus consists of a control unit and autoclavable instrument cable and therapy probes of various sizes. These probes are made of stainless steel and are coated with Teflon to provide an anti-stick surface (Figs. 15.7 and 15.8). There is a thermocouple inside the probe to regulate the probe temperature. The patient is placed in lithotomy position, and the lesion is identified using colposcope or visual inspection with acetic acid. The cervix may be infiltrated with local anesthesia if required. The probe is heated to temperature of 100 °C and applied on the lesion for a minimum of 20 s. There can be minimum of two and maximum of four applications in order to cover the transformation zone adequately.

After the procedure hemostasis is confirmed and any thermal burns to the vagina are ruled out, the probe is decontaminated with alcohol and heated to 100 °C for sterilization before reuse.

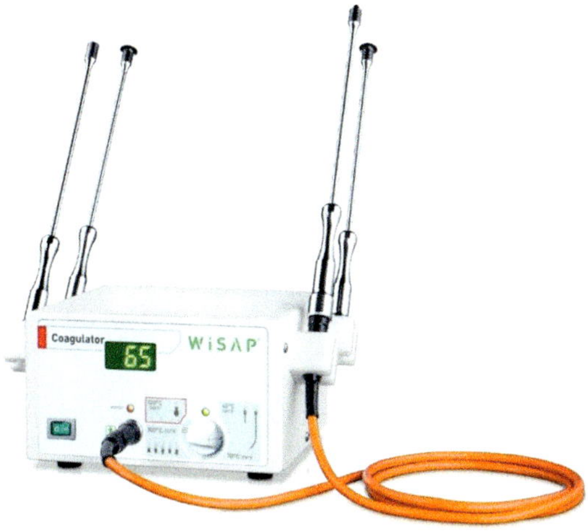

Fig. 15.7 Thermal coagulation machine. Courtesy of WISAP Medical Technology

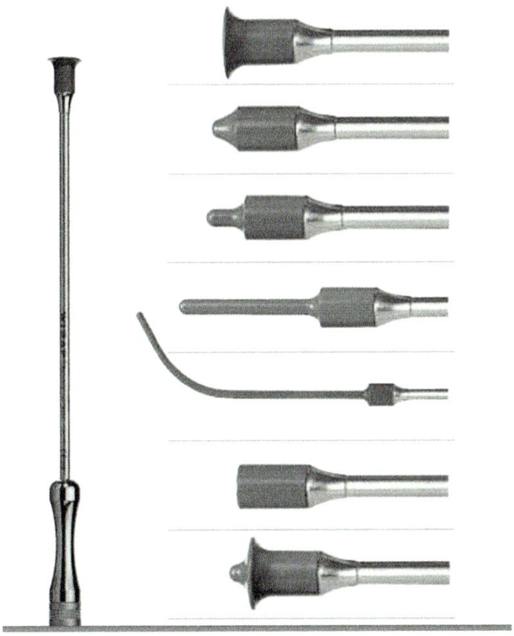

Fig. 15.8 Thermoprobes of various sizes. Courtesy of WISAP Medical Technology

Patients are advised regarding self-hygiene and to avoid douching and use of tampons for 1 month. They are advised to report in case of severe pain or cramps, heavy vaginal bleeding, foul-smelling discharge, and/or fever for more than 2 days. Follow-up is done at 4 weeks and then at 6 months.

15.2.2.2 Results

Dolman et al. published their meta-analysis of 13 studies (4569 patients with CIN 1 to CIN 3) on efficacy of cold coagulation in treatment of CIN [21]. They reported cure rates of 96% and 95% for CIN 1 and CIN 2 and 3, respectively. There were no major complications including any obstetric complications. A recent retrospective analysis compared the effectiveness of thermal coagulation and large loop excision of transformation zone (LLETZ) in the treatment of CIN 2 and CIN 3. They found similar efficacy in both the groups at 12-month follow-up [22]. Naud et al. reported that in a group of 52 women, 84% with CIN 2 and 3 lesions were cured using thermal coagulation, without any serious adverse effects or complications [23].

At present, newer versions of the device which are portable, battery powered, and handheld are being developed and evaluated. These will be able to treat approximately 20–30 women per battery life (Liger Thermal coagulator; ClinicalTrials.gov identifier: NCT02956239).

15.2.3 Laser Vaporization

Laser vaporization or ablation is a very effective tool for CIN lesions that extend onto the vagina as it can be tailored to the lesion and has excellent depth control. Of the various lasers available, CO_2 laser has limited depth of penetration (0.1–0.5 mm) and lateral thermal damage (0.5 mm) and is very safe for use. It can be used for both vaporization and excision by changing the power density.

The major advantages of CO_2 laser treatment of CIN are:

- Clinical efficacy is high.
- High precision with minimal damage to normal tissue.
- Good healing and less scar formation.
- Minimal complications.
- Outpatient procedure.
- Ablative procedure of choice if lesion extends onto the vagina.

15.2.3.1 Procedure

The procedure is performed on outpatient basis and does not require general or regional anesthesia. Local anesthesia in form of 1% lidocaine can be used as intracervical injection. The patient is placed in dorsal lithotomy position, and an adequate size bivalve speculum is inserted. A suction line with laser filter is attached to the speculum. This is required to maintain clear view of the operative field. A laser-mounted colposcope is used. The lesion is defined using acetic acid. Power setting of 30–40 W and spot size of 1.5–2 mm are generally used. Tissue destruction occurs mainly by vaporization, with the degree of tissue destruction dependent on power, spot size, and duration of the laser beam. The margins of the transformation zone are circumferentially outlined with a 3–5 mm margin around the lesion. The craters are connected and the cervix is divided into four quadrants. Beginning in the lower quadrants and using a circular pattern, vaporization is carried to depth of 7 mm (Fig. 15.9). The depth can be measured with a calibrated measuring device. The endocervical button is spared to ensure patency of the endocervical canal. The treatment causes minor discomfort in form of uterine cramps. Bleeding is not usually encountered and if occurs can be managed by using wet cotton swab as tamponade.

Postoperative follow-up is done at 2 and 4 weeks. Coitus is avoided for at least 4 weeks. Patient is asked to report in case of high fever or heavy bleeding during menstrual cycle.

15.2.3.2 Results

Baggish and Dorsey [24] reported a series of more than 4000 cases of CIN treated with laser with overall success rate between 96% and 97%. Persad and colleagues reported 1126 patients with CIN treated over 13 years by laser with no evidence of recurrence or persistence in 92% cases [25].

There are few complications of laser ablation procedure. Cervical stenosis has been seen in 1.3% of cases and major bleeding in less than 1% of cases [26].

The disadvantages of laser ablation include increased procedure time; expense of the laser unit, including its maintenance; increased time to acquire operative skills; and increased patient discomfort and bleeding complications.

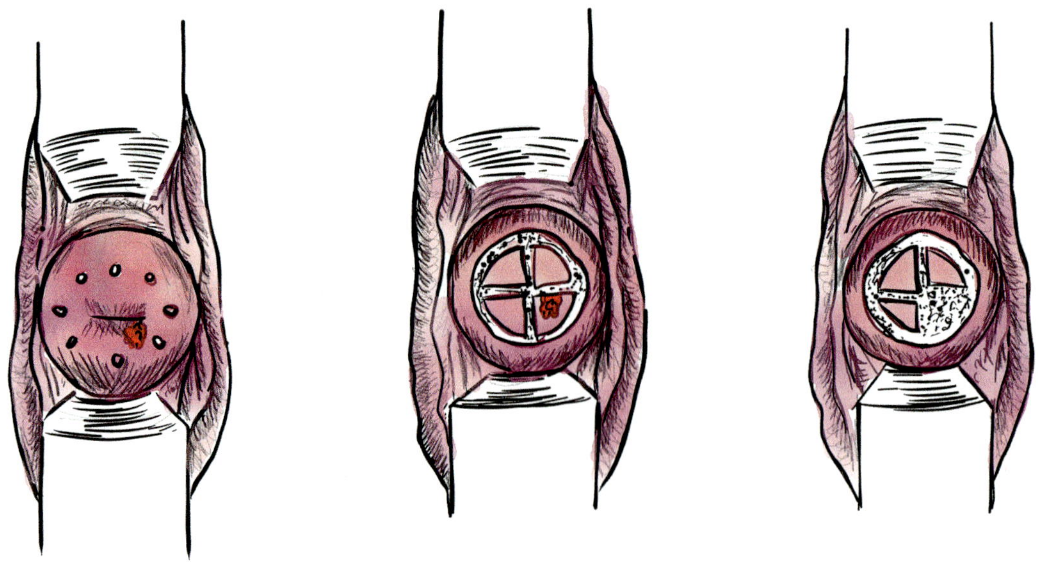

Fig. 15.9 Use of laser on cervical lesion. The margins of the transformation zone are marked. The craters are connected and the cervix is divided into four quadrants. Ablation is started from the lower quadrant and then extended to all

15.2.4 Electrocoagulation

Electrocautery has been used for many years to eradicate CIN. Historically it was used to destroy the "abnormal" epithelium found on the cervix after delivery. This technique uses a straight electrodiathermy needle to destroy the tissue.

15.2.4.1 Procedure

The patient is placed in lithotomy position, and an abnormal area of cervix is visualized using colposcope or visual inspection with acetic acid. Since this is a painful procedure, to achieve an adequate ablation depth of 5 mm and cover the entire transformation zone, anesthesia (general/regional) is required.

There are no major side effects. Postoperative pain is managed with analgesics. Dilatation and curettage may be done in the same sitting to prevent cervical stenosis.

15.2.4.2 Results

Chanen and Rome [27] reported their 15 years of experience with the use of electrocautery for treatment of CIN. They recommend doing the procedure in the operating room under anesthesia, so that adequate depth of cervical tissue can be burned. They reported a success rate of 97.3% with single diathermy treatment.

15.2.5 Photodynamic Therapy

Photodynamic therapy (PDT) is a conservative treatment modality using a photosensitizer and irradiation with laser or light energy at a low intensity which enables selective destruction of cancerous or dysplastic cells while preserving the uterus. PDT does not cause any cervical stenosis or scarring, which is a major advantage for management of CIN in young patients, where fertility needs to be preserved.

15.2.5.1 Procedure

Prior to PDT procedure, a definitive colposcopic and histopathologic diagnosis must be made. PDT can be used for type I and type II lesions based on colposcopy. PDT of type III lesions is contraindicated since laser irradiation of the lesion will be without visual control. Blood biochemistries including hepatic function should be tested, since the photosensitizer drugs are excreted via the biliary tract. The first-generation photosensitizers were administered systemically (e.g., Photofrin) and had significant side effects [28]. 5-Aminolevulinic acid (5-ALA), a substrate from heme cycle, was used as a local application, but it led to accumulation of photoactive porphyrins in the cervical epithelium [29]. Other salts like hexyl aminolevulinate (HAL) and methyl aminolevulinate (MAL), which are derivatives of 5-ALA, have also been used as local photosensitizers [30].

The freshly prepared drug solution is applied to the cervix using a cervical cap, 12 hours before the PDT. The procedure is done under general or regional anesthesia, under colposcopic guidance. The patient is placed in lithotomy position. After visualization of the lesion, laser emission at an energy density of 100 J/cm^2 per spot is performed. For the endocervix, a specialized laser probe, called the cervical probe, is used.

Post procedure, patient may have plenty of mucoid discharge. If an intravenous photosensitizer is used, it leads to cutaneous photosensitivity, and patients must avoid direct sunlight and bright indoor light for at least 6 weeks. Patients need to be followed up monthly for any side effects and photosensitivity. Healing usually takes place in 6 months.

15.2.5.2 Results

Various studies have shown response rates between 33% and 90% [31, 32]. These authors used PDT as an alternative to LEEP/conization for CIN. However, photosensitivity was a major side effect, and obstetric outcomes were not followed. Moreover, colposcopy-directed punch biopsy without LEEP/cone in high-grade CIN has a possibility to miss microinvasive cancer.

Currently, the possible use of PDT in management of CIN is in margin positive cases or recurrence after LEEP/cone. In these situations, repeating LEEP/cone or hysterectomy will compromise their fertility. Hence, PDT offers a potential alternative for effective conservative treatment of CIN [33].

15.3 Special Situations

HIV-positive females: Progression to cancer and recurrent disease is more common in women who are HIV positive. Though recurrence of disease is high despite treatment, it should still be undertaken as it can effectively interrupt progression to invasive cancer [34]. When two screening tests (co-test) are normal, the woman can return to annual screening.

Pregnant females: A pregnant woman with CIN 1 does not require any treatment and can be kept on follow-up. Most of these lesions will regress in the postpartum period. Cytology and colposcopy should be repeated after 6 weeks in the postpartum period. If the histology during pregnancy is high grade with exclusion of invasive disease, cytology and colposcopy are to be done every 12 weeks. There is no role of any ablative therapy during pregnancy. Reevaluation at 6 weeks postpartum is to be done in all cases. Treatment of CIN should not be commenced during pregnancy unless there is suspicion of invasive disease as various modalities of management can lead to preterm delivery and even fetal loss [35].

15.4 Posttreatment Monitoring

Long-term surveillance is required for women who have been treated for dysplasia. Most cases of recurrent or persistent CIN are found within the first 2 years of treatment, though data has shown cancer developing even 20 years after treatment [36].

Co-testing at 1 and 2 years is recommended for women who have been treated for CIN2/CIN3. If both co-tests are negative, then retesting is recommended after 3 years. If any test is abnormal, then colposcopy and endocervical sampling is to be done. Routine screening in these women has to continue for at least the next 20 years [37].

15.5 Which Ablative Method Is Better?

Cryotherapy is reliable, easy to use, and cost-effective. Its major disadvantage is that there is no tissue for histopathology. Though in laser vaporization, also there is lack of tissue specimen but with laser the treatment can be tailored to the size of the lesion. The disadvantages of laser are that it is expensive, moderate training is required to operate it, and it can cause burns or eye injuries [38]. There is no statistical significant difference in cure rates between cryotherapy and laser treatment [39].

Meta-analysis of four trials assessing 73, 289, and 205 women with CIN 1, CIN 2, and CIN 3, respectively, showed no statistically significant differences between cure rates and risk of residual disease in laser ablation and cryotherapy. The side effects of both the treatment modalities with respect to pain, vaginal bleeding, or cervical stenosis were also comparable. However, there were significantly fewer vasomotor symptoms and vaginal discharge or inadequate colposcopy with laser ablation [38].

15.6 Vulvar Intraepithelial Neoplasia

Vulvar intraepithelial neoplasia (VIN) is considered a precursor to invasive vulvar cancer. It is often multifocal, with a high risk of recurrence. Colposcopy of the vulva and directed biopsy are particularly helpful in confirming the diagnosis. VIN is now classified into two types, "usual VIN," associated with HPV infection, and "differentiated VIN," usually seen in older women with lichen sclerosus or squamous cell hyperplasia. The International Society for the Study of Vulvovaginal Diseases (ISSVD) recommends the terms low-grade squamous intraepithelial lesion of the vulva (vulvar LSIL) and high-grade squamous intraepithelial lesion of the vulva (vulvar HSIL) for histopathologic diagnoses of productive HPV infections. The "usual-type VIN" is now classified as vulvar HSIL, and "differentiated VIN" remains the same. Also, lesions classified as VIN 1 earlier are now classified as LSIL according to the current 2015 ISSVD classification system.

Treatment of VIN needs to be individualized depending on patient's age, symptoms, distribution and size of lesions, malignant potential, psychological issues, and recurrence rates. Treatment is recommended for all women with vulvar HSIL (usual VIN). As there is risk of occult invasion, wide local excision is preferred. However, if occult invasion is not a concern, laser ablation or topical imiquimod can be used.

Treatment options for low-grade VIN are:

1. Close observation: VIN 1 lesions are associated with HPV infection and may regress spontaneously, especially in women <40 years of age. They can be observed closely, and therapy may be done in persistent lesions.
2. Cryocautery: This is used for vulval warts and low-grade vulval lesions. These lesions are destroyed by cytolysis using liquid nitrogen applied directly to the lesion using a cotton-tipped applicator. Metal probes or cryotweezers can also be used. This procedure does not require anesthesia and can be done easily on an outpatient basis. Healing takes place in 2–4 weeks, and there are few side effects.
3. Electrocautery: Monopolar electrocautery can be used to ablate vulvar lesion. As it is painful, local/regional or even general anesthesia may be required. It is difficult to use in cases with extensive and/or multiple lesions. It causes scarring, sometimes extensive, because of damage to surrounding tissues. Electrocautery used to be the mainstay of treatment previously but is not commonly used now.
4. Tri- or bi-chloroacetic acid (TCA or BCA) topical application: This chemical is used commonly for treatment of vulvar warts. Before application, the surrounding normal epithelium is coated with a protective substance like 5% lidocaine gel. The TCA/BCA solution is then applied to the warts with a cotton-tipped applicator. It is tolerated well except local burning for few minutes. The procedure may be repeated weekly until all warts are gone.
5. 5-Fluorouracil (5-FU): This has been used for local application in VIN. However, it causes severe pain and has high recurrence rate.
6. Laser vaporization: Laser uses high-intensity beam to burn the lesion. As it is an expensive method, it is rarely used as the first-line therapy for vulval warts.

Treatment options for high-grade VIN are:

1. Topical imiquimod cream: Application of 5% imiquimod topically has found to be effective in vulvar HSIL. It is an immune response modulator and acts locally to cause cytolysis. It should be applied three times a week to the affected area for 12–20 weeks. It can be applied by the patient herself. It causes erythema and local pain. If severe, then treatment needs to be discontinued [40]. Repeated colposcopy examinations are done to assess the response. Residual lesions will require excision. This drug has not been approved yet by US Food and Drug Administration for this indication.
2. Laser vaporization: CO_2 laser ablation can be used for the treatment of vulvar HSIL (VIN usual type), when cancer is not suspected. It can be used for single, multifocal, or confluent lesions, although the risk of recurrence may be higher compared to excision for multifocal disease. Procedure is done under colposcopy guidance after adequate biopsy. Local or general anesthesia is required, depending on lesion extent. A micromanipulator or a handpiece with a depth gauge should be used. Appropriate power density of 600–1000 W/cm^2 is required to avoid coagulation injury; too deep wound can result in long-term ulcers. The lesion is outlined with the laser and the area inside is then ablated. A small margin (0.5–1 cm) of normal-appearing skin adjacent to the lesion should also be treated. For optimal treatment, full thickness destruction of the epithelium is required. Care must be taken to ablate hair follicles in hair-bearing areas as the disease can extend into the subcutaneous fat for 3 mm or more. In the non-hair-bearing areas, ablation should extend through the dermis up to 2 mm.

Reid [41] had defined surgical planes in the vulva to guide laser therapy. The first plane is the surface epithelium only, including the basement membrane. The second plane involves the dermal papillae, where both the epidermis and papillary dermis are treated. The third plane involves the upper and mid-reticular area

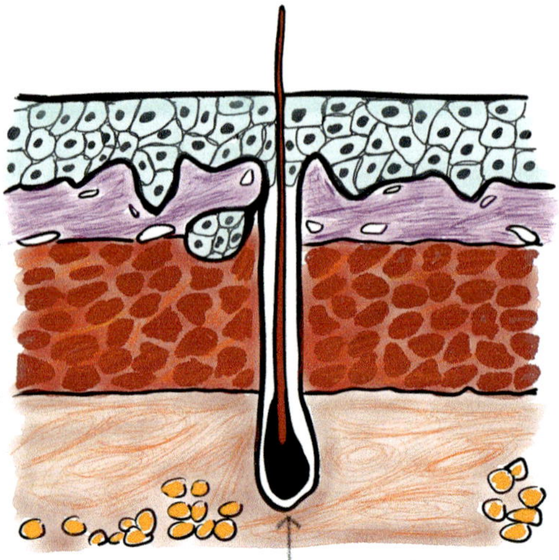

Fig. 15.10 Planes for therapy for vulvar intraepithelial neoplasia using a laser

where the pilosebaceous glands are located. The fourth surgical plane involves complete removal of the skin up to the underlying subdermal fat (Fig. 15.10). Destruction up to depth of plane one to two is needed for non-hair-bearing areas, and destruction to third plane is adequate for hair-bearing areas. If the fourth plane is reached, healing is slow and skin grafting may be required.

Postoperatively, patient is advised regarding local hygiene and sitz baths. Antibacterial ointment/cream is applied locally and oral analgesics are given. If a large area is ablated, Foley's catheter may be required for few days. Most common side effects are pain, bleeding, and infection. Rapid healing usually occurs because of relatively little residual thermal damage. One of the greatest benefits of vulval laser surgery, in comparison with skinning vulvectomy, is that vulvar anatomy, particularly the labia minora and clitoris, are maintained.

As compared to excision, recurrence is more common with laser ablation. Leufflen et al. achieved disease-free rates of 65% with laser and 91% with excision, at 1 year. At 5 years, the rate was the same for excision group but dropped to 51% for the laser group [42].

3. CUSA (cavitational ultrasonic surgical aspirator): CUSA has been used for the treatment of VIN, especially in multifocal lesions, in non-hair bearing vulvar skin. The depth of destruction can be more easily controlled than with laser. Ultrasonic sound waves cause the slender tip of the CUSA probe to vibrate at approximately 23 kHz. The probe shatters any section of the lesion that it touches, and the fragments are flushed out. The procedure is done under anesthesia. Healing takes place in 4–6 weeks and cosmesis is good. Postoperative care is similar to that described for laser ablation above. Miller treated 37 patients of VIN with CUSA and followed them for an average of 33 months. Thirty-five percent of patients developed recurrence in 16 months. Recurrences were significantly more if VIN involved hair-bearing areas [43].
4. Photodynamic therapy: PDT has advantage of preserving the normal anatomy and sexual function with equivalent therapeutic efficacy [44].
5. Wide local excision or skinning/simple vulvectomy: These procedures can cause disfigurement and are not recommended routinely. They are to be used when risk of invasion is very high or when there is recurrence of VIN which cannot be treated by other procedures.

Lifetime follow-up is required for these patients due to high risk of recurrence. Recurrences are more common after ablative procedure and less in surgically treated patients.

Higher recurrence rates are also seen in multiple lesions. Women, with a complete response and no new lesion at 6 and 12 months after treatment, can be followed annually. Follow-up is done by visual inspection and colposcopy of the vulva whenever required.

15.7 Vaginal Intraepithelial Neoplasia

Intraepithelial lesions of the vagina (VAIN) are less common than that of the cervix and vulva. They are usually associated with concomitant cervical lesions. The lesions can be identified on colposcopy and confirmed by biopsy. Almost all lesions are asymptomatic, although they may present with excessive vaginal discharge or abnormal bleeding per vaginum. In most cases, the upper third of vagina is involved. However, disease-free skip areas may be present with additional lesion in the lower vagina. Patients with VAIN tend to have either an antecedent or coexistent neoplasia in the lower genital tract. In contrast to CIN, VAIN presents with certain specific challenges:

- The vagina has a large surface area, with many rugae and folds, which are difficult to visualize with colposcope.
- Lesions tend to be multifocal, even if a lesion is identified, and the entire vagina needs to be examined for skip lesions.
- Colposcopic appearance of VAIN varies greatly and often goes unrecognized.

In the updated WHO 2014 classification, VAIN lesions are graded as vaginal low-grade squamous intraepithelial lesions (LSIL), which include VAIN 1, and vaginal high-grade intraepithelial lesions (HSIL), which include VAIN 2 and VAIN 3. VAIN 1 can also be considered as a productive HPV infection with a spontaneous regression rate of 50% and can therefore be managed expectantly. VAIN 2 and 3 are considered precancerous lesions and require treatment.

Treatment options of low-grade VAIN are:

1. Cryotherapy: Use of cryoprobe in the vagina is not recommended because of the risk of vaginal perforation and fistula formation.
2. Tri- or bichloroacetic acid (TCA/BCA): These can be used for small lesions. TCA and BCA are applied under colposcopic guidance with a wooden end of cotton tip applicator.
3. 5-Fluorouracil (5-FU): Applied directly on the lesion under coloscopic guidance.
4. Imiquimod: Applied directly to the lesions under coloscopic guidance [45].

Treatment options for high-grade VAIN are:

1. Laser: It involves focused laser destruction of the identified lesions. Destruction of 1–1.5 mm depth is sufficient to destroy the epithelium without damaging the underlying structures. Laser is very effective in achieving the required depth and width of destruction. The procedure is used only for those lesions that are visible and accessible and where malignancy has been ruled out by colposcopy-directed biopsy. The abnormal areas in the folds can be missed often due to rugae in the vagina. This problem can be solved by manipulating the speculum to smooth out the rugae. The procedure is usually done under general anesthesia. Prior to the procedure, the lesion is injected with saline that acts as a protective buffer that prevents penetration of laser to deeper tissues. A spot size of 2 mm and power settings of 15 to 30 W are used. If the lesion is large, it is subdivided so that ablation is more accurate. A wet sponge or cotton is used intermittently to wipe away eschar and coagulated epithelium. Most common side effects are pain and bleeding. Treated areas generally heal well and therapy is well tolerated. Patients are advised regarding sitz baths and use of antiseptic vaginal creams, postoperatively. Many patients may require more than one session. Laser is a good option for multifocal disease and especially in young women. Tainio et al. observed 100% regression of VAIN in patients treated with laser [46].

2. CUSA: It allows selective removal of diseased tissue with minimal damage to surrounding healthy tissues and does not cause any scarring or stenosis [47].
3. Local excision using loop or knife or cautery: Useful option when malignancy is suspected.

Contemporary treatment of choice for VAIN is laser vaporization, which is effective especially in case of multiple lesions. Recurrent VAIN lesions are common and require repeat treatments. This may cause vaginal scarring or mutilation. Risk factors for relapse have been shown to be persistent high-risk HPV infection and severity of VAIN.

15.8 Conclusion

Cervical cancer is a preventable disease. This can be achieved through screening, detection of preinvasive lesions, and their treatment. The choice of treatment depends on local resources, especially in low- and middle-income countries, along with trained persons and extent of lesion. Treatment options for high-grade CIN have changed over the last few decades. It is now generally accepted that only a small percentage of women with CIN need excisional procedures. Majority can be treated with ablative procedures, which are increasingly being used for "screen-and-treat" approach. Cryotherapy and thermal coagulation are easily learnt procedures which can be used at resource-limited health facilities. Laser ablation, though expensive and requiring more extensive training, can be used for all types of cervical, vaginal, and vulvar intraepithelial lesions. Therefore, the choice of treatment must be individualized based on cost considerations, available equipment, morbidity, and efficacy of the particular method in treating the intraepithelial lesion.

Key Points

- Cryotherapy is easy to use, inexpensive, and associated with low morbidity. It is a good treatment modality for ectocervix confined, small-volume disease, particularly in low-resource settings. For all screen-and-treat recommendations, cryotherapy is the first-choice treatment for women who have screened positive and are eligible for cryotherapy.
- Laser ablation is an expensive method which requires training to use. However, it is very useful when a large area of the cervix or vaginal fornices is involved. It is also very useful for vaginal and vulvar intraepithelial neoplasia.
- Thermal coagulation is an attractive option as it requires minimal supplies, is easy to use, and can be used in low-resource settings.
- Topical applications of TCA/BCA, 5-FU, and imiquimod are good options for managing low-grade VAIN and VIN.

References

1. Anderson MC, Hartley RB. Cervical crypt involvement by intraepithelial neoplasia. Obstet Gynecol. 1980;55(5):546–50.
2. Abdul-Karim FW, Fu YS, Reagan JW, Wentz WB. Morphometric study of intraepithelial neoplasia of the uterine cervix. Obstet Gynecol. 1982;60(2):210–4.
3. Martin-Hirsch PP, Paraskevaidis E, Bryant A, Dickinson HO. Surgery for cervical intraepithelial neoplasia. Cochrane Database Syst Rev. 2013;12:CD001318.
4. Kyrgiou M, Koliopoulos G, Martin-Hirsch P, Arbyn M, Prendiville W, Paraskevaidis E. Obstetric outcomes after conservative treatment for intraepithelial or early invasive cervical lesions: systematic review and meta-analysis. Lancet. 2006;367(9509):489–98.
5. Kalliala I, Nieminen P, Dyba T, Pukkala E, Anttila A. Cancer free survival after CIN treatment: comparisons of treatment methods and histology. Gynecol Oncol. 2007;105(1):228–33.
6. Miranda D. Screening still the "best buy" for tackling cervical cancer. Bull World Health Organ. 2011;89(9):628–9.
7. Khan MJ, Smith-McCune KK. Treatment of cervical precancers: back to basics. Obstet Gynecol. 2014;123(6):1339–43.
8. Santesso N, Schünemann H, Blumenthal P, De Vuyst H, Gage J, Garcia F, et al. World health Organization Steering Committee for Recommendations on Use of Cryotherapy for Cervical Cancer Prevention. World Health Organization Guidelines: use of cryotherapy for cervical intraepithelial neoplasia. Int J Gynaecol Obstet. 2012;118(2):97–102.

9. Mariategui J, Santos C, Taxa L, Jeronimo J, Castle PE. Comparison of depth of necrosis achieved by CO2- and N2O-cryotherapy. Int J Gynaecol Obstet. 2008;100(1):24–6.
10. Cremer M, Ditzian L, Winkler JL, Jerónimo J, Singleton J, Franco HV, et al. Comparison of depth of necrosis using cryotherapy by gas and number of freeze cycles. J Low Genit Tract Dis. 2015;19(1):1–6.
11. Luciani S, Gonzales M, Munoz S, Jeronimo J, Robles S. Effectiveness of cryotherapy treatment for cervical intraepithelial neoplasia. Int J Gynaecol Obstet. 2008;101(2):172–7.
12. Creasman WT, Hinshaw WM, Clarke-Pearson DL. Cryosurgery in the management of cervical intraepithelial neoplasia. Obstet Gynecol. 1984;63(2):145–9.
13. Schantz A, Thormann L. Cryosurgery for dysplasia of the uterine ectocervix. A randomized study of the efficacy of the single- and double-freeze techniques. Acta Obstet Gynecol Scand. 1984;63(5):417–20.
14. Sauvaget C, Muwonge R, Sankaranarayanan R. Meta-analysis of the effectiveness of cryotherapy in the treatment of cervical intraepithelial neoplasia. Int J Gynaecol Obstet. 2013;120(3):218–23.
15. Santesso N, Mustafa RA, Wiercioch W, Kehar R, Gandhi S, Chen Y, et al. Systematic reviews and meta-analyses of benefits and harms of cryotherapy, LEEP, and cold knife conization to treat cervical intraepithelial neoplasia. Int J Gynaecol Obstet. 2016;132(3):266–71.
16. Chumworathayi B, Srisupundit S, Lumbiganon P, Limpaphayom KK. One-year follow-up of single-visit approach to cervical cancer prevention based on visual inspection with acetic acid wash and immediate cryotherapy in rural Thailand. Int J Gynecol Cancer. 2008;18(4):736–42.
17. Sankaranarayanan R, Rajkumar R, Esmy PO, Fayette JM, Shanthakumary S, Frappart L, et al. Effectiveness, safety and acceptability of 'see and treat' with cryotherapy by nurses in a cervical screening study in India. Br J Cancer. 2007;96(5):738–43.
18. Blumenthal PD, Gaffikin L, Deganus S, Lewis R, Emerson M, Adadevoh S, Ghana Cervicare Group. Cervical cancer prevention: safety, acceptability, and feasibility of a single-visit approach in Accra, Ghana. Am J Obstet Gynecol. 2007;196(4):407.e1–8.
19. World Health Organization. Treatment of cervical intraepithelial neoplasia 2-3 and adenocarcinoma in situ: cryotherapy, large loop excision of the transformation zone, and cold knife conisation. http://www.who.int/reproductivehealth/publications/cancers/treatment_CIN_2-3/en/. Published 2014.
20. Castle PE, Murokora D, Perez C, Alvarez M, Quek SC, Campbell C. Treatment of cervical intraepithelial lesions. Int J Gynaecol Obstet. 2017;138(Suppl 1):20–5.
21. Dolman L, Sauvaget C, Muwonge R, Sankaranarayanan R. Meta-analysis of the efficacy of cold coagulation as a treatment method for cervical intraepithelial neoplasia: a systematic review. BJOG. 2014;121(8):929–42.
22. Papoutsis D, Underwood M, Parry-Smith W, Panikkar J. Comparison of cure rates in women treated with cold-coagulation versus LLETZ cervical treatment for CIN2-3 on pretreatment cervical punch biopsies: a retrospective cohort study. Arch Gynecol Obstet. 2017;295(4):979–86.
23. Naud PS, Muwonge R, Passos EP, Magno V, Matos J, Sankaranarayanan R. Efficacy, safety, and acceptability of thermocoagulation for treatment of cervical intraepithelial neoplasia in a hospital setting in Brazil. Int J Gynaecol Obstet. 2016;133(3):351–4.
24. Baggish MS, Dorsey JH, Adelson M. A ten-year experience treating cervical intraepithelial neoplasia with the CO2 laser. Am J Obstet Gynecol. 1989;161(1):60–8.
25. Persad VL, Pierotic MA, Guijon FB. Management of cervical neoplasia: a 13-year experience with cryotherapy and laser. J Low Genit Tract Dis. 2001;5(4):199–203.
26. Indman PD, Arndt BC. Laser treatment of cervical intraepithelial neoplasia in an office setting. Am J Obstet Gynecol. 1985;152(6 Pt 1):674–6.
27. Chanen W, Rome RM. Electrocoagulation diathermy for cervical dysplasia and carcinoma in situ: a 15-year survey. Obstet Gynecol. 1983;61(6):673–9.
28. Yamaguchi S, Tsuda H, Takemori M, Nakata S, Nishimura S, Kawamura N, et al. Photodynamic therapy for cervical intraepithelial neoplasia. Oncology. 2005;69(2):110–6.
29. Hillemanns P, Korell M, Schmitt-Sody M, Baumgartner R, Beyer W, Kimmig R, et al. Photodynamic therapy in women with cervical intraepithelial neoplasia using topically applied 5-aminolevulinic acid. Int J Cancer. 1999;81(1):34–8.
30. Soergel P, Loehr-Schulz R, Hillemanns M, Landwehr S, Makowski L, Hillemanns P. Effects of photodynamic therapy using topical applied hexylaminolevulinate and methylaminolevulinate upon the integrity of cervical epithelium. Lasers Surg Med. 2010;42(9):624–30.
31. Barnett AA, Haller JC, Cairnduff F, Lane G, Brown SB, Roberts DJ. A randomised, double-blind, placebo-controlled trial of photodynamic therapy using 5-aminolaevulinic acid for the treatment of cervical intraepithelial neoplasia. Int J Cancer. 2003;103(6):829–32.
32. Istomin YP, Lapzevich TP, Chalau VN, Shliakhtsin SV, Trukhachova TV. Photodynamic therapy of cervical intraepithelial neoplasia grades II and III with Photolon. Photodiagnosis Photodyn Ther. 2010;7(3):144–51.
33. Choi MC, Jung SG, Park H, Lee SY, Lee C, Hwang YY, Kim SJ. Photodynamic therapy for management of cervical intraepithelial neoplasia II and III in young patients and obstetric outcomes. Lasers Surg Med. 2013;45(9):564–72.
34. Fruchter RG, Maiman M, Sedlis A, Bartley L, Camilien L, Arrastia CD. Multiple recurrences of

cervical intraepithelial neoplasia in women with the human immunodeficiency virus. Obstet Gynecol. 1996;87(3):338–44.
35. Boardman LA, Goldman DL, Cooper AS, Heber WW, Weitzen S. CIN in pregnancy: antepartum and postpartum cytology and histology. J Reprod Med. 2005;50(1):13–8.
36. Jakobsson M, Gissler M, Paavonen J, Tapper AM. Long-term mortality in women treated for cervical intraepithelial neoplasia. BJOG. 2009;116(6):838–44.
37. American College of Obstetricians and Gynecologists. Practice Bulletin No. 140: management of abnormal cervical cancer screening test results and cervical cancer precursors. Obstet Gynecol. 2013;122(6):1338–67.
38. Mitchell MF, Tortolero-Luna G, Cook E, Whittaker L, Rhodes-Morris H, Silva E. A randomized clinical trial of cryotherapy, laser vaporization, and loop electrosurgical excision for treatment of squamous intraepithelial lesions of the cervix. Obstet Gynecol. 1998;92(5):737–44.
39. Mitchell MF. Preinvasive diseases of the female genital tract. In: Gershenson DM, De Cherney AH, Curry SL, editors. Operative gynecology. Philadelphia: WB Saunders Co.; 1993. p. 231–56.
40. American College of Obstetricians and Gynecologists' Committee on Gynecologic Practice; American Society for Colposcopy and Cervical Pathology (ASCCP). Committee opinion no. 675: management of vulvar intraepithelial neoplasia. Obstet Gynecol. 2016;128(4):e178–82.
41. Reid R. Laser surgery of the vulva. Obstet Gynecol Clin North Am. 1991;18(3):491–510.
42. Leufflen L, Baermann P Jr, Rauch P, Routiot T, Bezdetnava L, Guillemin F, et al. Treatment of vulvar intraepithelial neoplasia with CO_2 laser vaporization and excision surgery. J Low Genit Tract Dis. 2013;17(4):446–51.
43. Miller BE. Vulvar intraepithelial neoplasia treated with cavitational ultrasonic surgical aspiration. Gynecol Oncol. 2002;85(1):114–8.
44. Choi MC, Kim MS, Lee GH, Jung SG, Park H, Joo WD, et al. Photodynamic therapy for premalignant lesions of the vulva and vagina: a long-term follow-up study. Lasers Surg Med. 2015;47(7):566–70.
45. Gurumurthy M, Cruickshank ME. Management of vaginal intraepithelial neoplasia. J Low Genit Tract Dis. 2012;16(3):306–12.
46. Tainio K, Jakobsson M, Louvanto K, Kalliala I, Paavonen J, Nieminen P, et al. Randomised trial on treatment of vaginal intraepithelial neoplasia-imiquimod, laser vaporisation and expectant management. Int J Cancer. 2016;139(10):2353–8.
47. Matsuo K, Chi DS, Walker LD, Rosenshein NB, Im DD. Ultrasonic surgical aspiration for vaginal intraepithelial neoplasia. Int J Gynaecol Obstet. 2009;105(1):71–3.

Management of High-Grade Lesions

16

Neha Gami and Kanika Gupta

16.1 Introduction

According to the Bethesda system [1], high-grade lesions refers to high-grade squamous intraepithelial lesion (HSIL) on cytology (which includes what is used to be known as moderate to severe dysplasia) and CIN 2/CIN 3 on histology.

Among the precursors to cervical cancer, the high-grade lesions are considered most significant as they have a high chance of either harboring malignant disease or progressing to cervical cancer if left untreated. The risk of developing cervical cancer in the next 5 years in women 30 years or older has been reported to be 8% [2] (Table 16.1). However, this risk may be modified, depending on the HPV status of the woman.

The management of high-grade lesions begins from the finding of a HSIL result on cytology. According to various studies, HSIL is seen in 0.5% of all the Pap smears done for screening [3].

Table 16.1 Effect of HPV infection on disease progression

	5 year risk of CIN 3+ (%)	5 year risk of cancer (%)
HSIL, HR HPV negative	29	7
HSIL, HR HPV positive	50	7

16.2 Management of High-Grade Lesions

The aim of management of high-grade lesions is to prevent the progression of these lesions to malignancy without excessive harm to the woman. It is imperative to carefully select cases to avoid overtreatment of such women.

16.2.1 Management of HSIL on Cytology

At colposcopy, CIN 2+ is found in approximately 60% of the cases with HSIL on cytology [3], and invasive cervical cancer is found in approximately 2% of these women [4]. That is the reason why HSIL should be referred for further assessment of the cervix and the requisite treatment.

The assessment of the cervix includes visual inspection of the cervix and vagina followed by colposcopy. Both immediate referral for colposcopy and immediate loop electrosurgical excision of the

N. Gami (✉)
Department of Obstetrics and Gynecology, Healthplus Clinic and Danat al Emarat Hospital, Abu Dhabi, UAE

K. Gupta
Department of Obstetrics and Gynecology, Medcare Multispeciality Hospital, Sharjah, UAE

S. Mehta, A. Singla (eds.), *Preventive Oncology for the Gynecologist*,
https://doi.org/10.1007/978-981-13-3438-2_16

lesion are acceptable alternatives as per ASCCP guidelines [5]. Monitoring by repeat Pap smear and reflex HPV testing are not acceptable options to manage a woman with HSIL on cytology [5].

Earlier punch biopsy was the method to obtain a tissue sample from the cervix of women presenting with HSIL and abnormal colposcopy. However, this may result in the loss to follow-up of approximately one in four women [1]. Considering that six out of ten of these women may be having concurrent CIN 2 or worse on histology [4], it is now recommended to offer excisional biopsy using large loop excision of the transformation zone (LLETZ) as a one-step approach.

The advantages of this method are a reduced loss to follow-up and one-step diagnosis and possible treatment. This is only recommended in women with HSIL on cytology with lesions suggestive of high-grade CIN on colposcopy but no evidence of invasive cancer [1].

16.2.1.1 Colposcopy

Salient points while doing colposcopy for HSIL:

1. Have a pre-colposcopy consultation with the woman, explain the procedure to her, and discuss the possible treatment options depending on what you may find.
2. Examine the external genitalia for evidence of vulval disease or warts.
3. While inserting the speculum, assess the vaginal wall as well.
4. Ensure the colposcopy is satisfactory and that the entire lesion can be seen.

Findings on Colposcopy Suggestive of CIN 2 and 3

Four features are looked at while deciding on the grade of lesion during colposcopy. These are the intensity or whiteness of the acetowhitening, margins and surface contour of the acetowhite lesion, vascular patterns of the lesion, and the color changes that accompany application of iodine [6].

CIN 2 or 3 is likely when the lesions appear thick, dull grayish white areas with well-demarcated, sharp, and regular margins. The margins may sometimes be raised and rolled out. They may be complex with different shades of whitening within them (lesion within a lesion). The surface is more irregular and nodular and less smooth [6] as shown in Figs. 16.1, 16.2, and 16.3.

Vascular patterns of coarse mosaic and punctations in the acetowhite areas also usually signify high-grade lesion (Fig. 16.4). On application of Lugol's iodine, these lesions do not take up the iodine and remain a mustard or saffron yellow [6].

Findings on Colposcopy Suggestive of Invasive Cancer

Lesions, which could be harboring invasive carcinoma, are large, densely acetowhite in color, sometimes obliterating the os, with atypical vessels and rolled out margins (Fig. 16.5). Lesions which bleed on touch should also raise suspicion. Atypical vessels may be seen in the form of hairpins, corkscrew, waste thread, commas, tadpole, and strange irregular patterns with irregular caliber of the vessels [6].

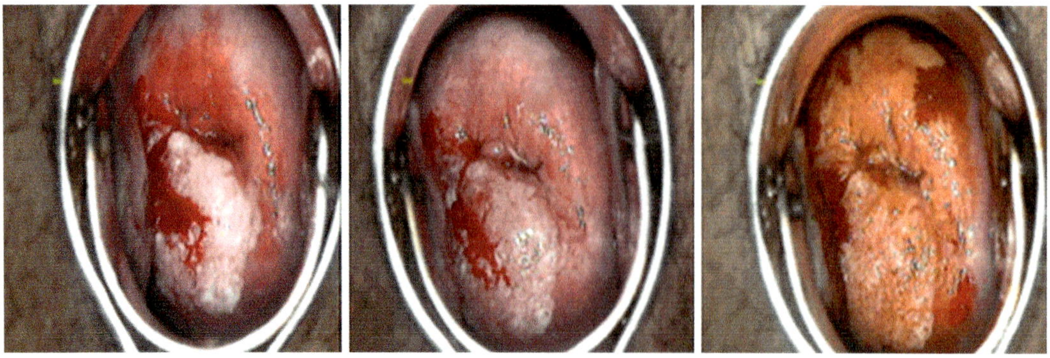

Fig. 16.1 Colposcopy of high-grade lesion; biopsy confirmed CIN 2

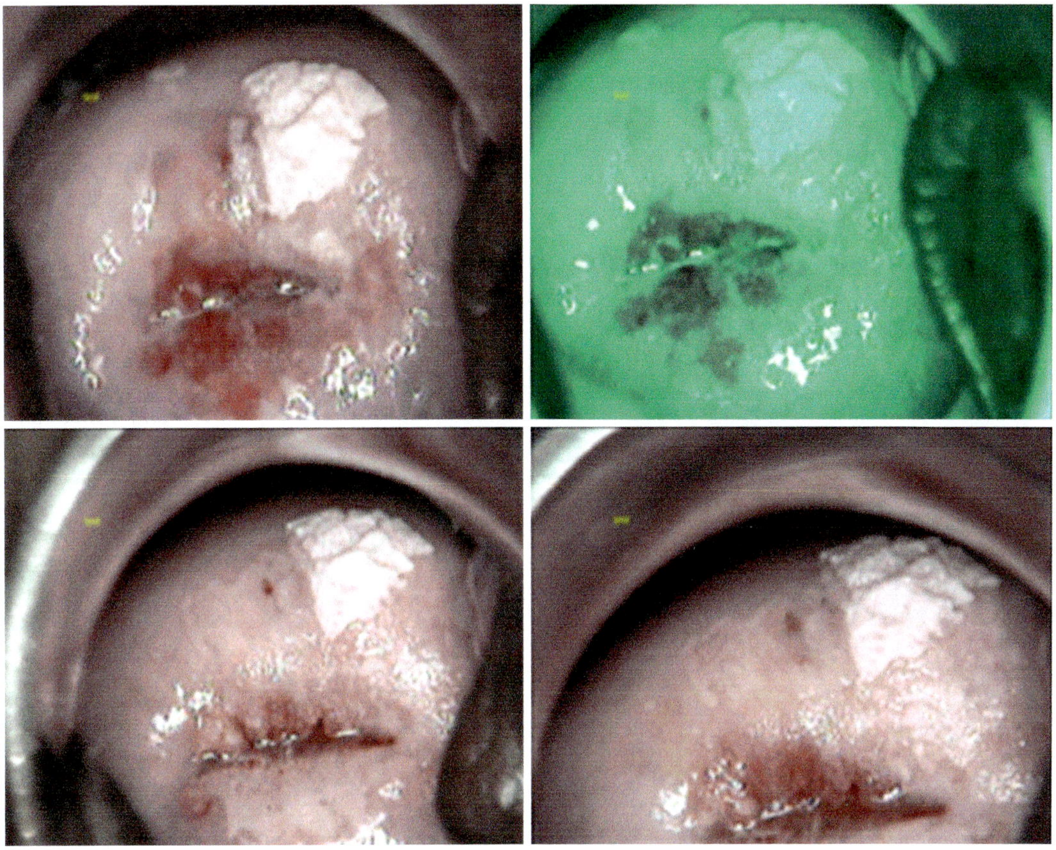

Fig. 16.2 Colposcopy of high-grade lesion; biopsy confirmed CIN 3

When such features are seen on colposcopy, punch biopsy from the most sinister areas should be taken, and further treatment should only be planned after ruling out invasive carcinoma.

If the colposcopy is inadequate, a diagnostic excisional procedure is acceptable [4] except if the woman is pregnant. Ablation is not acceptable if colposcopy has not been done and when the biopsy does not show CIN 2,3 but the endocervical curettings show CIN 2,3. Algorithm 16.1 shows management of HSIL as per ASCCP guidelines.

16.2.2 Management of HSIL in Young Women (21–24 Years)

When HSIL is reported in young women, referral for colposcopy is recommended, but immediate LLETZ at the same sitting is not recommended. If high-grade disease is identified on the biopsy, it should be managed by either observation or treatment; both are acceptable. If the biopsy does not show CIN 2 or 3, the woman can be monitored every 6 months with cytology and colposcopy, only if the colposcopic examination is adequate with negative endocervical cytology [4].

16.2.3 Management of CIN 2 and CIN 3 on Histology

Once CIN 2 or 3 has been confirmed by biopsy, the choice of management depends upon many factors. The age; parity; risk factors for progression; prior treatment for cervical disease; size, location, and appearance of the lesion; and the likelihood of follow-up all determine what modality is finally chosen.

As per the ASCCP guidelines, the modalities that currently exist for treating CIN 2, 3 are excisional methods, ablative methods, and hysterectomy. If the woman has a satisfactory colposcopy, CIN 2 or CIN 3 on biopsy, and no evidence of invasive cancer on colposcopy, excisional and ablative treatment are both acceptable choices [4]. If however the colposcopy is inadequate or the endocervical sampling shows CIN 2 or 3, then excisional method is recommended. A diagnostic excisional procedure is the method of choice for recurrent CIN 2 or 3 [4] (Algorithm 16.2).

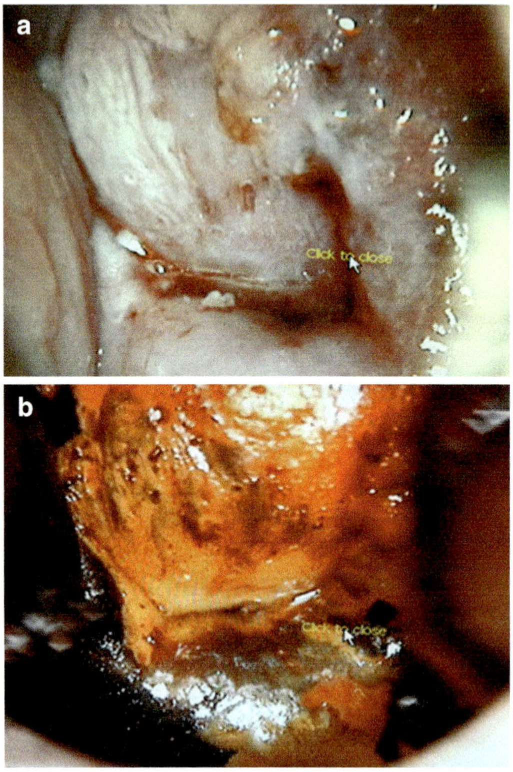

Fig. 16.3 (**a**, **b**) High-grade lesion on anterior lip and has not taken up Lugol's iodine

16.2.4 Excisional Methods

The commonly used excisional methods include:

- LLETZ/LEEP
- Cold knife cone
- Laser cone biopsy

The advantages of excisional methods include:

- Tissue for histopathologic examination—Excisional methods provide a good specimen for histopathology so as to accurately stage the disease.
- "See-and-treat" protocol—They also offer the possibility of a one-step diagnosis and treatment.
- Technically easy—LLETZ and laser cone biopsy can be done under local anesthesia as well, thus reducing cost of the treatment.
- Minimal effect on future pregnancy rates—LLETZ and laser have minimal effect on the cervical function, hence suitable even for young patients, keen on maintaining their fertility.

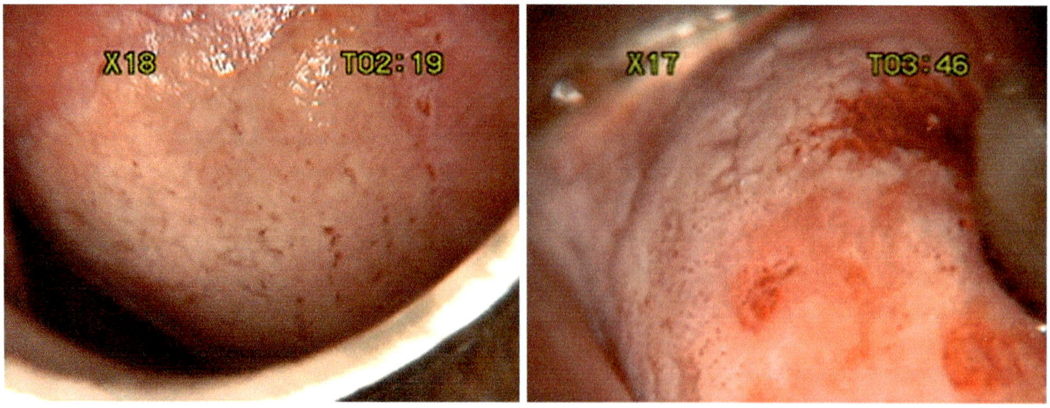

Fig. 16.4 Coarse punctations

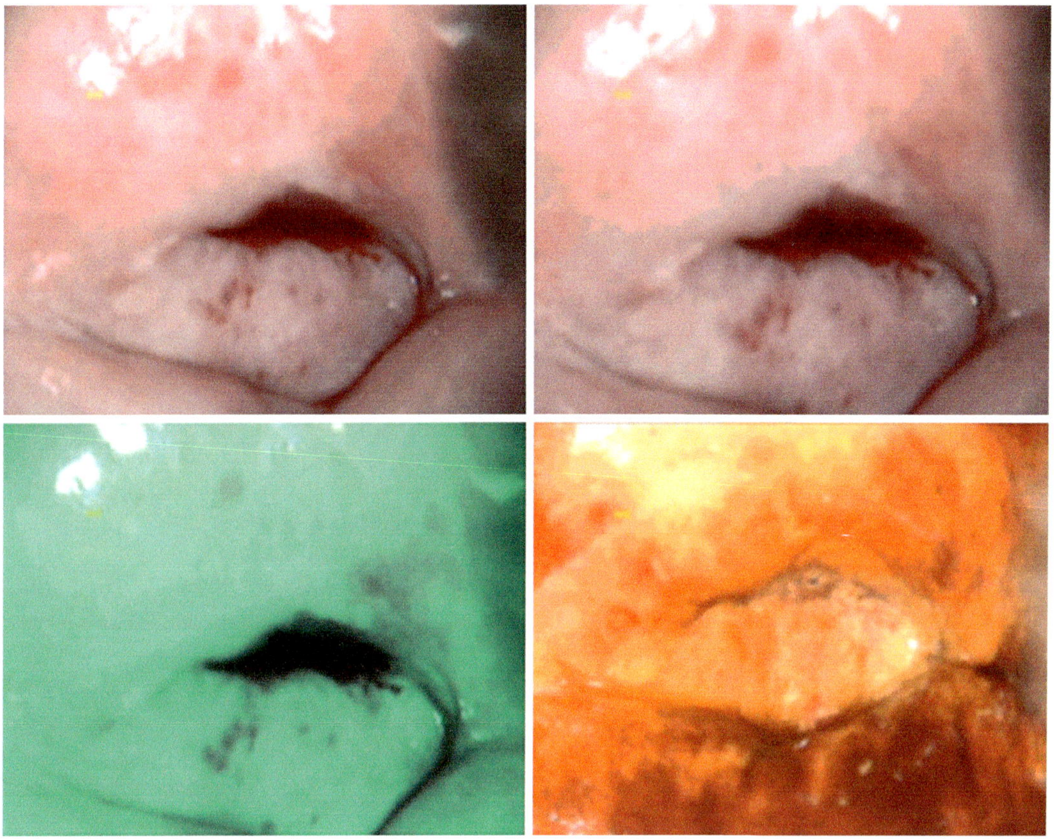

Fig. 16.5 Colposcopy, cervical biopsy, and ECC showing keratinizing squamous cell carcinoma

The actual choice of the method used depends on factors like type of transformation zone, size of lesion, skill and comfort of operator, equipment available, and age and choice of the patient.

Types of transformation zone: There are three types of transformation zone as per the International Federation for Colposcopy and Cervical Pathology [7].

Type 1—where the entire transformation zone (TZ) is ectocervical and can be seen on colposcopy

Type 2—where the TZ extends into the cervical canal but the upper limit of the TZ can be seen during colposcopy

Type 3—where part of TZ is endocervical and the upper limit of the TZ cannot be seen on colposcopy

For type 1 and type 2 TZ, LLETZ and laser are acceptable methods of choice. The aim is to remove a tissue of 8 mm depth in center and 5 mm at the periphery. For type 2 TZ, LLETZ and laser are again good methods, but a second central excision of about 7–10 mm depth should be done with a smaller loop so as to obtain the tissue that is extending into the cervical canal. For type 3 TZ, excision of the ectocervix should be followed by an excision of the endocervical canal to a greater depth to get an inverted hat-shaped specimen [7].

16.2.5 Large Loop Excision of the Transformation Zone (LLETZ)

LLETZ and loop electrosurgical excision procedure (LEEP) both refer to excision of the transformation zone with electrocautery. They have now become the standard of care for high-grade cervical premalignant lesions.

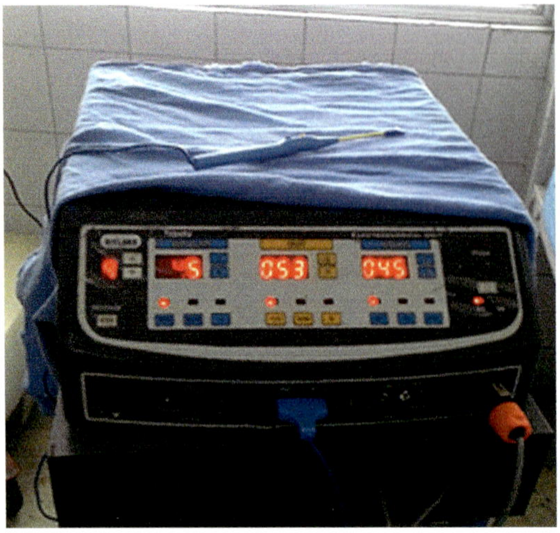

Fig. 16.6 Bipolar electrocautery system

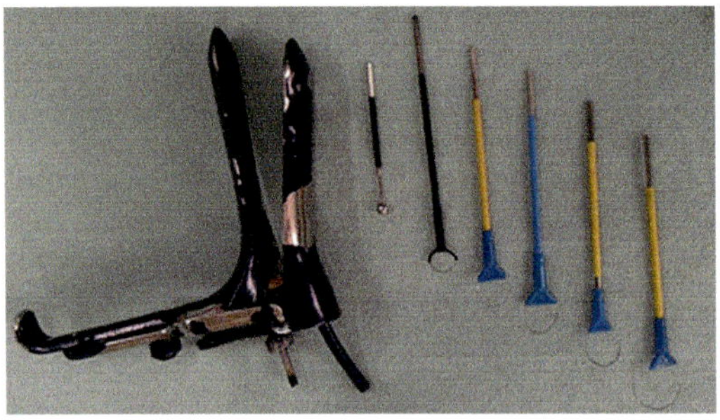

Fig. 16.7 Insulated speculum and wire loops of various sizes

Equipment needed for LLETZ: A bipolar, electrocautery system with cutting and coagulation functions (Fig. 16.6)

1. Cusco's speculum with attachment for suction tubing
2. Insulated handpiece, with handheld cautery control
3. Thin, wire loops of various sizes (Fig. 16.7)
4. Ball cautery electrodes
5. Earth plate

16.2.5.1 Procedure of LLETZ

LLETZ can be performed under local anesthesia. General anesthesia may be used in certain situations, like when patient is uncomfortable undergoing the procedure.

The patient is positioned in lithotomy position after she has emptied her bladder. An insulated self-retaining, double-blade, vaginal speculum is then inserted to visualize the cervix. Ideally it should have an attachment for the smoke evacuator where the suction tubing can be attached.

If the LLETZ is taking place in the second sitting, then a colposcopy should preferably be done just before the LLETZ. Otherwise application of Lugol's iodine can help to delineate the lesion. For local anesthesia, 1% lidocaine solution is injected in a circular manner all around the circumference of the cervix, using a thin needle and a dental syringe. Injecting 2–4 mL of 1:20 diluted ornipressin into the cervical tissue will help reduce the bleeding.

LEETZ is performed, by placing the loop of appropriate size, 1–2 mm beyond the edge of the lesion. Using either blend or coagulation current, the loop is gently passed through the cervical tissue in such a way that a cone-shaped tissue is excised. The loop is then brought out beyond the other edge of the lesion, again leaving a 1–2 mm margin. It is important to let the current cut the tissue and not by mechanical pull on the loop. Pulling the loop before the tissue is cut will lead to unnecessary bleeding. The tissue so obtained is labeled and sent for histopathology. The crater is then examined for any bleeding, and the bleeding points are cauterized using ball cautery electrodes (Figs. 16.8, 16.9, 16.10, and 16.11). If the lesion is large, then it might have to be excised in multiple passes (Fig. 16.12).

If LEETZ is being performed in patients where the upper limit of the lesion cannot be seen on colposcopy, a deeper resection of the central area should be done.

In women who have extension of the lesion up to the vaginal fornix, the cervical lesion should be excised as usual, and the vaginal extension can be cauterized with ball cautery. These women will require a close follow-up.

16.2.5.2 Postoperative Care

Immediately after the procedure, a tampon or vaginal swab can be inserted for few hours to prevent bleeding. This should be removed in 4 h. Patient can be

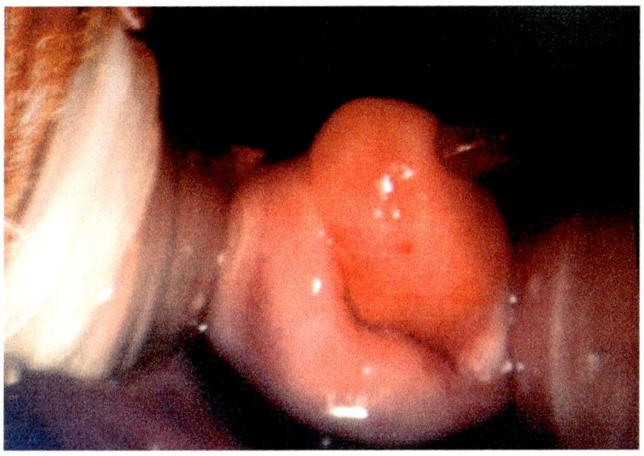

Fig. 16.8 Large ectropion on the anterior lip

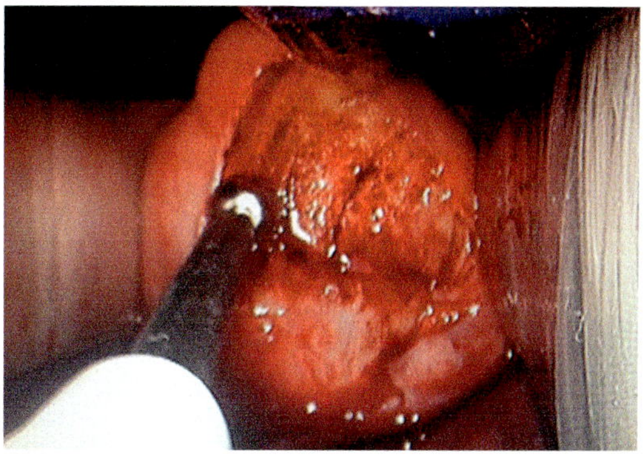

Fig. 16.10 Ball cautery being used to control bleeding

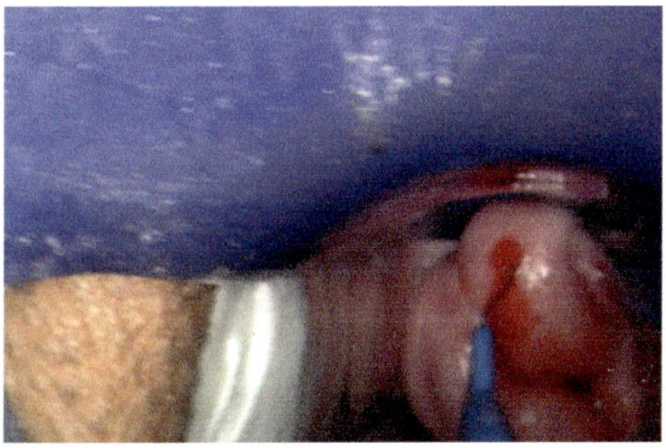

Fig. 16.9 Cautery loop in position

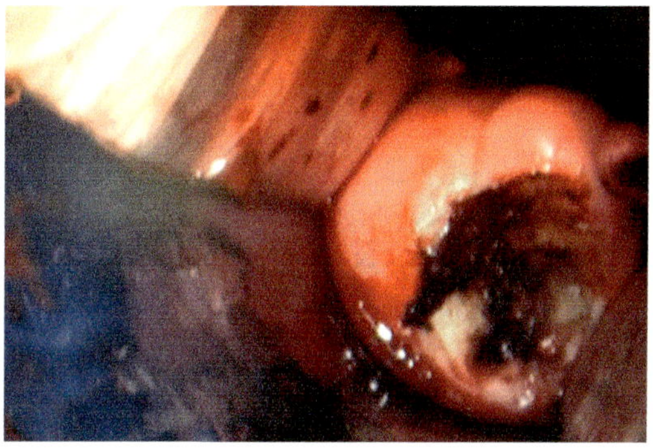

Fig. 16.11 Final crater

Fig. 16.12 Excision of an ectocervical lesion with multiple passes

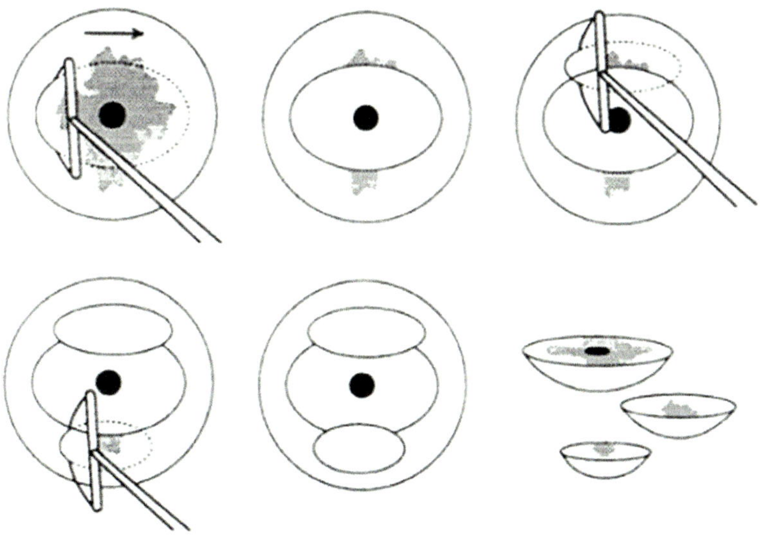

discharged or sent home soon after with a follow-up planned after 4 weeks to review the crater. She should be advised to avoid intercourse for 4 weeks.

16.2.5.3 Post-op Complications

Some minor and major complications associated with LLETZ are:

a. Minor complications—They may occur in about 0.6% of the cases [8]. These are abdominal pain, vaginal bleeding or discharge, and bladder spasm.
b. Major complications are seen in 9.1% of the cases [8]. These could be excessive vaginal bleeding requiring further procedure, bowel, or bladder injury.
c. Post-op cervical stenosis—This may occur if a larger volume of cervical tissue has been removed. It was seen in 6% of the women in a study by Suh-Burgmann et al. [9].
d. Some studies have reported an increased risk of late miscarriages [10, 11], preterm labor [12, 13], preterm prelabor rupture of membranes [12, 13], and a statistically insignificant increased risk of low birth weight babies in women who had undergone LLETZ previously. There was no increased risk of cesarean section, precipitate labor, or need for induction of labor.

16.2.5.4 Disadvantages of LLETZ

Cauterization artifact: As the tissue is removed using both coagulation and cutting current, a little bit of thermal artifact is unavoidable. This may lead to uncertainty while reporting the histopathology, especially the status of the margins. In a study by Montz et al., although 92% of the 50 cases reported were considered sufficient for interpretation, full assessment of the ectocervical margin was not possible in 20% cases and that of the endocervical margin in 44% cases.

16.2.5.5 Follow-Up After LLETZ

Women are to be followed up after treatment of high-grade lesions to ensure completeness of therapy. After LLETZ for high-grade CIN, the follow-up cytology and colposcopy are recommended at 3–12 months depending on the margin status. This may be increased to 6–12 months for the next 5–10 years, depending on the risk factors.

If the histopathology shows involved margins at LLETZ, then the woman should be followed up with colposcopy and cytology at 3, 9, and 15 months.

If the margins are free, co-testing with Pap smear and HPV is recommended at 12 and 24 months [4]. If both are negative, then the woman can return to routine screening for the next 20 years, even if that goes beyond the 65 years age limit [4].

Factors that increase the chances of recurrence are:

- Positive margins at the primary excision.
- High-grade lesion: CIN 3 lesions have a higher chance of recurrence than lower-grade lesions [1].
- Advanced age of the patient: Highest chance of recurrence was found in women older than 50 years with positive endocervical margins [1].
- High-risk HPV-positive status.
- HIV-positive status: Patients who were HR HPV negative at their first follow-up had a significantly lower risk of persistent or recurrent disease [1].

16.2.6 Cold Knife Cone Biopsy (CKC)

Although CKC has mostly given way to LLETZ or laser cone, it may still be used in certain situations. It is preferred in postmenopausal women with high-grade cytology and narrow vagina, which makes LLETZ difficult. It may also be a better choice in women with cytology showing adenocarcinoma in situ (AIS) or malignant cells without any identifiable lesion on the ectocervix. In women with an endocervical extension of the lesion of more than 1.5 cm, CKC is a better option than LLETZ cone. The main indications for conization are:

- Colposcopy is inadequate, and the squamocolumnar junction cannot be seen entirely.
- CIN 2/3 is seen on endocervical curettage.
- There is discordance between the results of cytology, biopsy, and colposcopy.
- Microinvasion is suspected or colposcopy cannot rule out invasive cancer.

Equipment:

1. Vaginal speculum
2. Allis forceps
3. Knife and blade (No. 11)
4. Artery forceps
5. Cervical dilators

16.2.6.1 Procedure

Patient is placed in lithotomy position after regional or general anesthesia. After cleaning and draping the parts, a speculum is inserted to retract the posterior vaginal wall. The uterus is sounded and cervical length is estimated using a sound. Lugol's iodine may now be applied to the cervix to delineate the lesion. To reduce the bleeding, stitches can be taken at 3 and 9 o'clock position on the cervix. The cervical canal is first dilated. The conization is now done by incising with the blade pointing toward the apex of the planned cone. It is better to start at 3 or 9 o'clock position to avoid loss of vision due to bleeding. The incision should include the lesion and 2–3 mm of the normal tissue around it (Fig). The apex of the cone should ideally be 1 cm below the level of the internal os. One should try to remove the specimen in one piece as far as possible [7] (Figs. 16.13 and 16.14).

After removing the cone, the endocervical canal above it should be curetted to exclude presence of disease in the canal. A suture is put at 12 o'clock position of the excised cone specimen to help the pathologist in specimen orientation (Fig. 16.15). To reduce postoperative bleeding, ball cautery or Monsel's solution may be used.

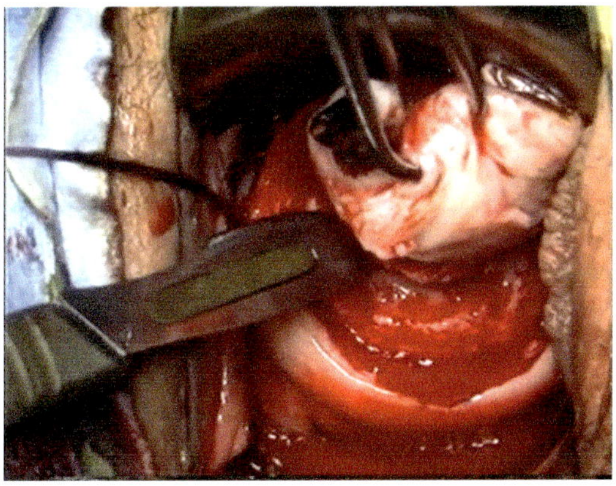

Fig. 16.13 Technique of cone biopsy

16.2.6.2 Postoperative Care

Complete healing of the cervix may take up to 6 weeks. Patient is advised to abstain from intercourse and not to use vaginal tampons as it may lead to significant bleeding and infection.

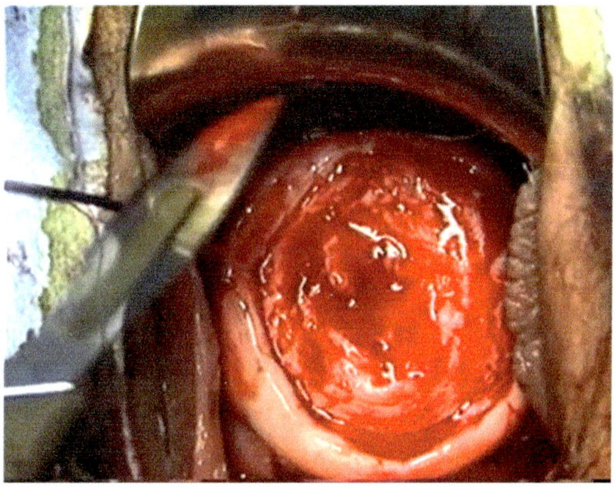

Fig. 16.14 Crater after cone biopsy

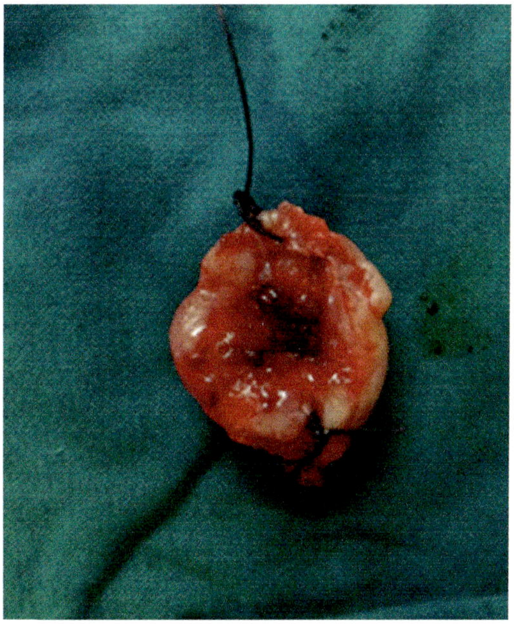

Fig. 16.15 Cone specimen with knot indicating 12 "o'clock" position

16.2.6.3 Follow-Up

Patients should be called back for the first follow-up after 2 weeks. A final postoperative examination is recommended at 6 weeks. To rule out residual or recurrent CIN, cytology is done every 3 months during the first postoperative year and every 6 months thereafter.

16.2.6.4 Complications

Immediate:

- Anesthetic risk
- Hemorrhage
- Uterine perforation

Delayed:

- Secondary hemorrhage
- Cervical stenosis
- Incompetence of the cervix
- Risk of preterm delivery or premature rupture of membranes in future pregnancy

16.2.7 LEEP Versus CKC

There is hardly any differences in the occurrence of complications after LEEP or cryotherapy, but they are seen more frequently after CKC [17].

	LEEP (%)	CKC (%)	Cryotherapy (%)
Recurrence of CIN 2/3	5.3	1.43	5.3
Major bleeding	0.22	0.85	0.03
Major infections	0.12	0.08	0.01
Premature delivery	1.85	3.41	2.25
HPV clearance	64.7	72.2	–

16.2.8 Straight Wire Excision of TZ (SWETZ)

Straight wire excision of transformation zone (TZ) or SWETZ is an electrosurgical excision of the endocervical TZ or type 3 TZ and glandular disease with 1 cm straight wire electrode. The specimen obtained is a cone, but it involves using the activated wire instead of a cold knife. Needle excision of transformation zone (TZ) or NETZ is a synonym for SWETZ.

16.2.8.1 Indications for SWETZ

- Some type 2 or type 3 TZ
- Glandular disease
- Suspicion of microinvasion

16.2.8.2 Procedure

It uses a 1 cm straight wire electrode and a blend cutting, and coagulation setting is used at 40 W (Fig. 16.16).

16.2.8.3 Advantages

Lower morbidity

Less chances of incomplete removal and segmentation of specimen

Less chances of excessive removal

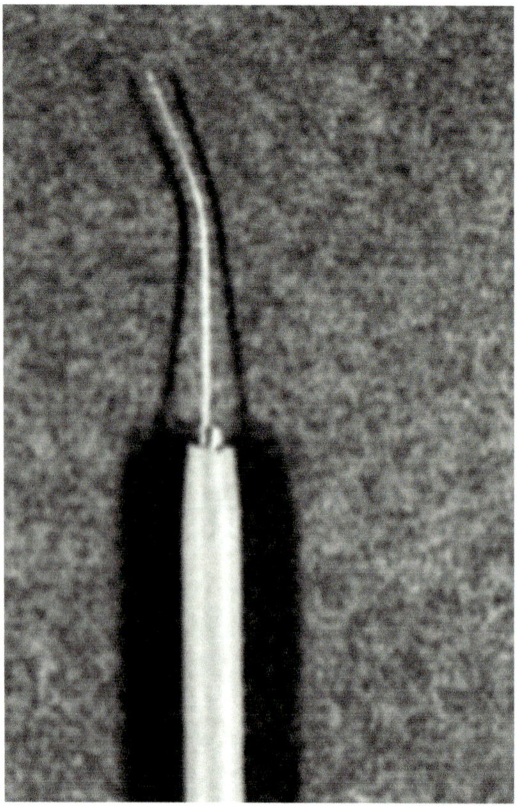

Fig. 16.16 Straight wire electrode

According to Pansokaltsis et al., the performance of NETZ was better in regard to specimen fragmentation, free margins, and risk of residual disease [14]. Camargo and colleagues in their randomized controlled trial observed no statistical difference between SWETZ and LLETZ cone in achieving clear histological margins. But SWETZ resulted in a higher blood loss and an increased operating time [15]. Fabio Russomano concluded that LLETZ had a higher compromised endocervical margins in the specimen than SWETZ [16].

16.2.9 Laser Cone Biopsy

Laser cone is comparable to LLETZ for its ability to effectively treat CIN 2 and 3. However, it needs intensive training and special equipment [7].

Equipment required for laser conization is shown in Table 16.2.

The operative and post-procedure complications of all three methods of obtaining a cone have been compared in Table 16.3.

Table 16.2 Equipment required for laser conization

Instruments	CO_2 laser, colposcope
Power output	25–30 W
Spot size	0.5 mm
Operating mode	Continuous
Lateral margins	5 mm around the lesion
Endocervical margin	Excised surgically
Hemostasis	By sutures
Anesthesia	Either general or local

Table 16.3 Comparison of LEEP, CKC, and laser [18, 19]

Parameters	LEEP	CKC	Laser conization
Blood loss	5.4 cm^3	16.2 cm^3	21.5 cm^3
Operating time (min)	5.4	14	15.6
Volume of cone	Small	Good	Small
Thermal artifact	53%	–	57%
Postoperative bleeding	Similar	Similar	Similar
Post-procedural TZ visibility (%)	19	50	20
Cervical stenosis (%)	1	4	0
PROM/PTL	1%	–	–
Recurrence (%)	2	1	2

16.3 Ablative Methods

16.3.1 Cryotherapy

Ablation of the transformation zone is considered an effective method to treat CIN [1]. The main advantage of cryotherapy as a treatment modality is that it does not have any known adverse effect on fertility and during future pregnancy. But the no specimen is available for histopathology.

Cryotherapy uses a cryoprobe with a tip made of highly conductive metal. When a compressed refrigerant gas (nitrous oxide or carbon dioxide) is allowed to pass through a small aperture in the cryoprobe, it results in a substantial drop in temperature of the tip. This causes cryonecrosis of the cells in contact with the probe. This is the principle behind its use to destroy cells with CIN changes.

16.3.1.1 Indications for Cryotherapy

- CIN is confirmed by cervical biopsy/colposcopy, and invasive cancer has been ruled out.
- The entire lesion is ectocervical, and there is no extension to the vagina and/or endocervix.
- The size of the lesion is such that it can be covered entirely by the cryoprobe.
- The woman is not pregnant or at least 3 months postpartum.
- There is no active genital infection.

Details regarding equipment and procedure are discussed in Chap. 15.

16.3.1.2 Procedure

The procedure is discussed in short here.

After obtaining informed consent, the woman is asked to lie down in a modified lithotomy position after emptying her bladder. The largest size speculum that can be comfortably inserted is used to visualize the cervix. Any secretions are then removed with Q-tips. Lugol's iodine may be applied to delineate the lesion.

The cryoprobe surface should be cleaned with saline before applying it firmly in contact with the ectocervix. Ensure that the center of the tip is placed at the os.

The trigger is then pressed to release the gas and timer is started. We must ensure that we can see the icicles forming around the probe tip and that it is not touching the vagina.

As the gas passes though the tip, it causes immediate cooling to sub-zero temperatures. The temperatures achieved at the center of the ice ball are −89 °C and −60 °C with the nitrous oxide-based cryotherapy and the carbon dioxide-based system, respectively. The temperatures reached at the edges of the frozen tissue may be around −20 °C.

Adequate destruction of the transformation zone is achieved by two sequential cycles of freeze-thaw with each freeze lasting for 3 min followed by 5 min for the cervix to thaw. Freezing is said to be adequate when the margin of the ice ball extends around 4–5 mm beyond the CryoTip.

After the freeze is finished, we should wait for the tip to get separated from the cervix on its own, as pulling it forcefully may cause bleeding.

At the time of discharge from the clinic, women should be told that they may have excessive vaginal secretions or blood-stained watery vaginal discharge for up to 4–6 weeks. They should be advised to avoid tampon use and intercourse for about 4 weeks after the procedure and to return in case they develop high-grade fever, purulent discharge, or severe lower abdominal pain.

16.3.1.3 Post-op Complications

1. Patient may have some lower abdominal pain or cramps during and after cryotherapy.
2. Bleeding is extremely rare after cryotherapy; however, she may have blood-tinged watery discharge for 4–6 weeks after the procedure.
3. Cervical stenosis is seen in less than 1% of women; 5–10% of women may have decreased mucus production [10].

16.3.1.4 Follow-Up

As for other treatment modalities, the adequacy of treatment may be assessed by cytology and HPV testing 4–6 months after treatment. If there is persistence of a high-grade abnormality, colposcopy and biopsy should be repeated. If they are normal even at 9–12 months, the patient may return to routine screening.

16.4 Hysterectomy

Hysterectomy is not the first choice for treatment of high-grade cervical lesions as more conservative methods like LLETZ and laser are now widely available. Some special indications where hysterectomy may still be used are:

- HSIL in a woman who has completed her family and in whom follow-up may be difficult
- If the margins are involved at LLETZ or CKC and the woman has completed her family
- HSIL or a high-grade CIN in a postmenopausal woman
- HSIL on cytology or high-grade CIN on biopsy, in a woman who needs definitive treatment for other benign pathology like fibroids

16.4.1 Managing High-Grade Lesions in Young Women

More than 20% of women aged 21–24 years may be infected by high-risk HPV infection, but incidence of cervical cancer is very low in them. Most low-grade lesions including CIN 2 lesions will regress in them without any intervention. Therefore, such women are managed more conservatively. As HPV infection is common in this age group, testing for high-risk HPV is not advocated, and if tested the results should not modify management. Even high-grade lesions (HSIL or CIN 2/3) can be managed conservatively with only observation, provided colposcopy is satisfactory [20].

16.4.2 WHO Guidelines for Treatment of CIN 2/3 and AIS (2014) [21]

16.4.2.1 Strong Recommendation

LEEP to be used over no treatment.

Cryotherapy to be used rather than no treatment.

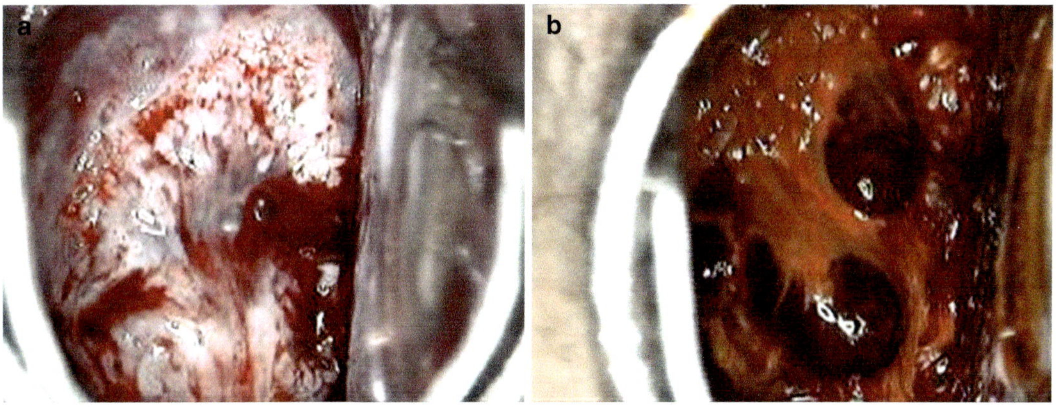

Fig. 16.17 (**a**, **b**) Thick tenacious mucus over the cervix

Cold knife conization to be used over no treatment.

If both cryotherapy and CKC can be used in a patient, cryotherapy to be used.

If both LEEP and CKC are appropriate to use in a patient, LEEP is to be preferred.

16.4.2.2 Conditional Recommendation

CKC to be used in women with histologically proven diagnosis of adenocarcinoma in situ instead of LEEP.

16.4.3 Managing High-Grade Lesions in Pregnancy

The main purpose of cervical cancer screening and management of cervical dysplasia during pregnancy is to be able to pick up early invasive cancer [14]. Up to 5% pregnant women may have cervical dysplasia; however, the progression to cancer within the duration of the pregnancy is very rare.

Colposcopy can be safely performed in pregnancy, but significant expertise is required for interpreting colposcopic findings in pregnancy. This is due to the following reasons:

Technically difficult – The cervix is hypertrophied, hyperemic, and friable and so can bleed easily during manipulation. Also, the lax vaginal walls and thick tenacious mucus (Fig. 16.17) may cause difficulty in visualization.

Difficulty in interpretation—The vascular changes and features of metaplasia appear exaggerated which one can confuse with high-grade lesions. Deciduosis in pregnancy also mimics a high-grade lesion thereby adding to the difficulty in interpreting the results.

If colposcopy is done in pregnancy for a cytology showing a high-grade lesion, biopsy should be taken with a Tischler forceps. Only one biopsy is sufficient due to the risk of bleeding. The purpose of the biopsy is only to rule out invasive cancer. Endocervical curettage is contraindicated in pregnancy. Decision regarding whether biopsy is needed should be taken by an experienced clinician with relevant expertise. If CIN 2 or 3 is confirmed in the biopsy, the woman may be followed by a colposcopy in each trimester, and repeat biopsy should be done only if colposcopy drastically worsens. The treatment should be planned only after delivery, and reevaluation at 6 weeks postpartum is also acceptable. At postpartum follow-up, a repeat cytology and colposcopy are done to confirm the disease or regression of the lesion (Algorithm 16.3).

16.5 Conclusion

For all women with HSIL on cytology, colposcopy referral is a must. Women with a high-grade lesion on colposcopy should have a diagnostic excisional procedure to confirm the grade of lesion and offer treatment as well. Diagnostic excisional methods are preferred to ablative methods in CIN 2/3 although both are acceptable if the colposcopy is adequate. Less aggressive treatment is recommended for young women and pregnant women. Follow-up after treatment is essential to ensure freedom from disease and no recurrence.

Key Points

- According to the Bethesda system, high-grade lesions refer to high-grade squamous intraepithelial lesion (HSIL) on cytology (which includes what is used to be known as moderate to severe dysplasia) and CIN 2 or CIN 3 on histology.
- At colposcopy, CIN 2+ is found in approximately 60% of the cases with HSIL on cytology, and invasive cervical cancer is found in approximately 2% of women undergoing colposcopy for HSIL. That is the reason why HSIL should be referred for further assessment of the cervix and the requisite treatment.
- The aim of management of high-grade lesions is to prevent the progression of these lesions to malignancy without excessive harm to the woman.
- Offer excisional biopsy using large loop excision of the transformation zone (LLETZ) as a one-step approach to women with HSIL on cytology.
- Excisional methods available to treat CIN 2/3 on biopsy are LLETZ, cold knife cone, and laser cone biopsy.
- Ablative methods available are cryotherapy and laser.
- When HSIL is reported in young women, referral for colposcopy is recommended, but immediate LLETZ at the same sitting is not recommended.
- The main purpose of cervical cancer screening and management of cervical dysplasia during pregnancy is to be able to pick up early invasive cancer.
- Follow-up with cytology and HPV DNA testing can help predict or rule out chances of recurrence.

Algorithm 16.1 Management of Women with High-grade Squamous Intraepithelial Lesions (HSIL)*

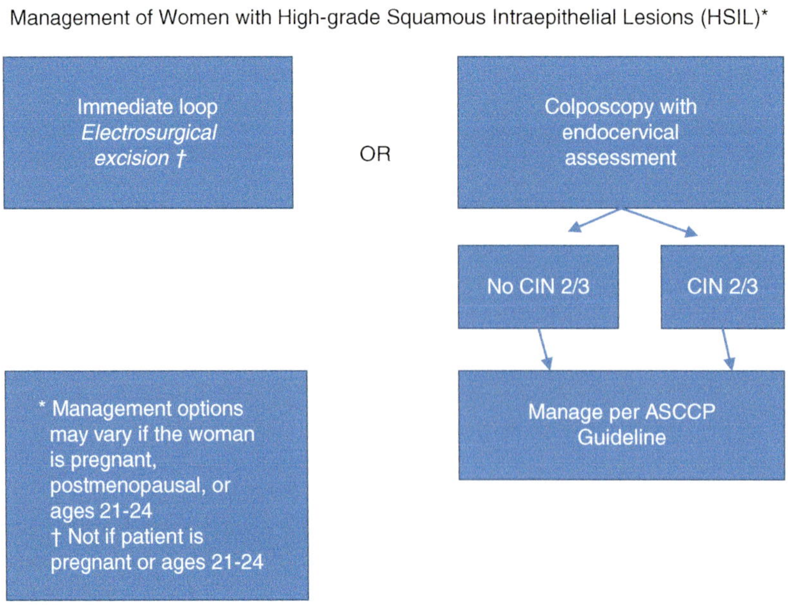

Algorithm 16.2 Management of Women with Biopsy-Confirmed CIN 2 and CIN 3*

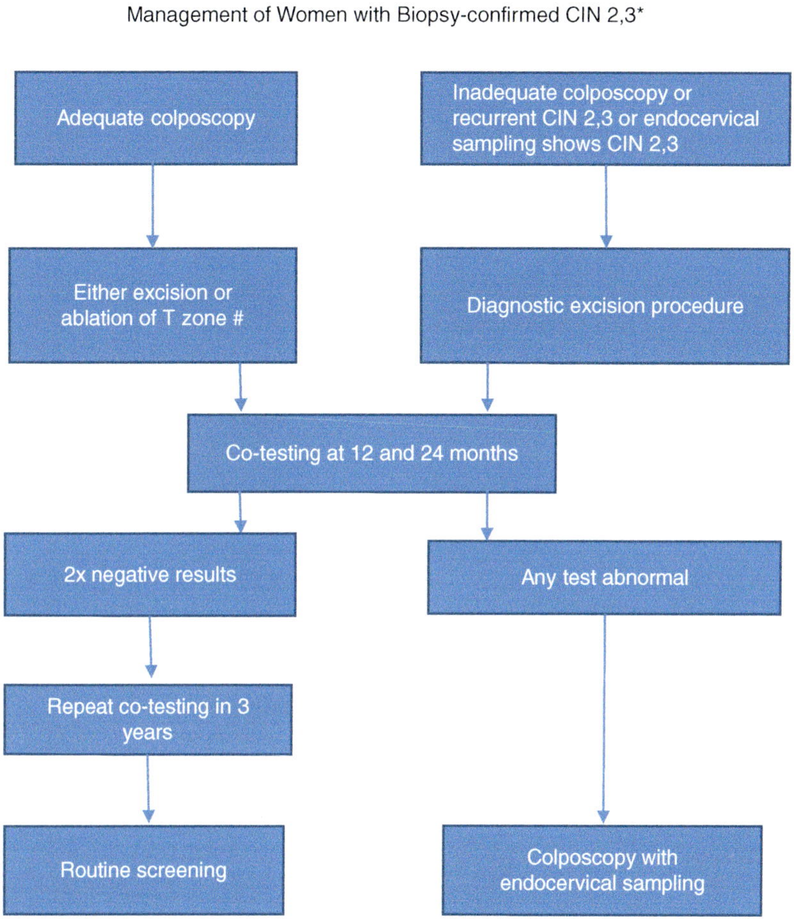

Algorithm 16.3 Management of ASC-H and HISL During Pregnancy

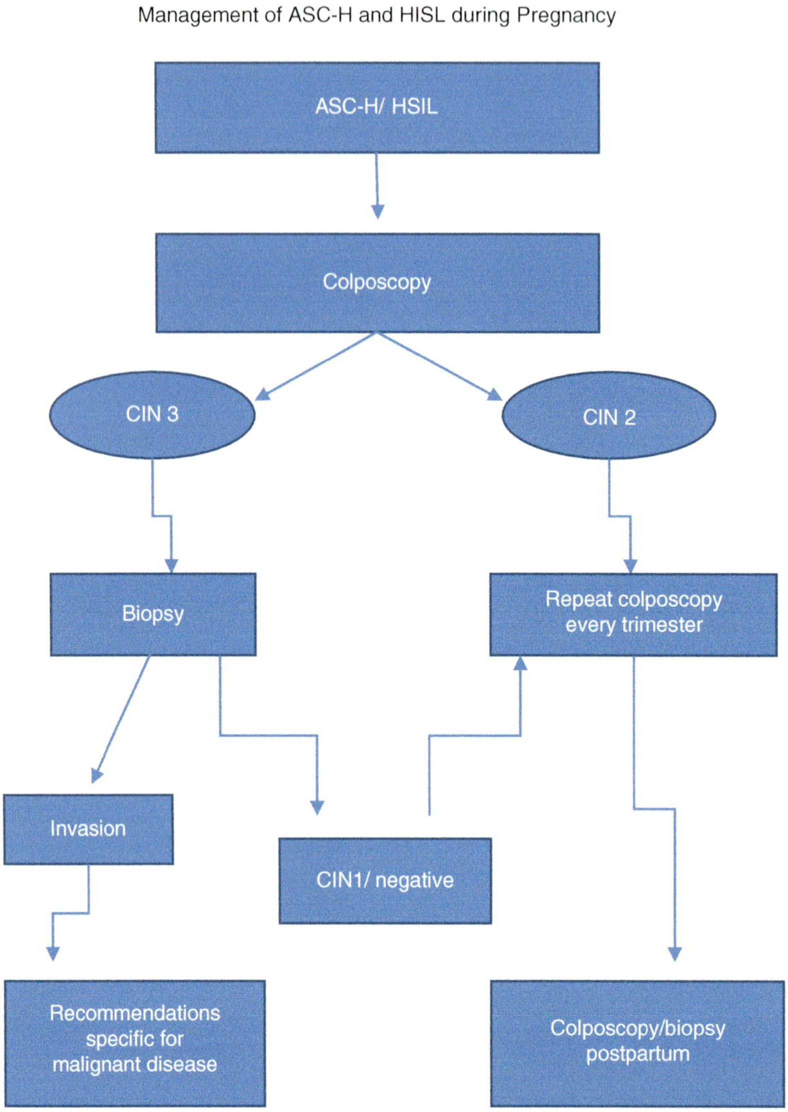

References

1. Lindeque B. Management of cervical premalignant lesions. Best Pract Res Clin Obstet Gynaecol. 2005;19(4):545–61.
2. Katki H, Schiffman M, Castle P, Fetterman B, Poitras N, Lorey T, et al. Five-year risks of CIN 3+ and cervical cancer among women with HPV-positive and HPV-negative high-grade pap results. J Low Genit Tract Dis. 2013;17:S50–5.
3. Medicine U. Abnormal Pap Smear. UW Medicine [Internet]. Uwmedicine.org. 2018. http://www.uwmedicine.org/health-library/pages/abnormal-pap-smear.aspx. Cited 17 Feb 2018.
4. Massad L, Einstein M, Huh W, Katki H, Kinney W, Schiffman M, et al. 2012 updated consensus guidelines for the management of abnormal cervical cancer screening tests and cancer precursors. Obstet Gynecol. 2013;121(4):829–46.
5. Massad L, Collins Y, Meyer P. Biopsy correlates of abnormal cervical cytology classified using the Bethesda system. Gynecol Oncol. 2001;82(3):516–22.
6. Sellors J, Sankaranarayanan R. Colposcopia e tratamento da neoplasia intra-epitelial cervical. Lyon: Centro Internacional de Pesquisas sobre o Câncer; 2004.

7. Petry K. Management options for cervical intraepithelial neoplasia. Best Pract Res Clin Obstet Gynaecol. 2011;25(5):641–51.
8. Dunn T, Killoran K, Wolf D. Complications of outpatient LLETZ procedures. Obstet Gynecol Surv. 2004;59(6):431–2.
9. Suh-Burgmann E. Risk factors for cervical stenosis after loop electrocautery excision procedure. Obstet Gynecol. 2000;96(5):657–60.
10. Santesso N, Mustafa R, Wiercioch W, Kehar R, Gandhi S, Chen Y, et al. Systematic reviews and meta-analyses of benefits and harms of cryotherapy, LEEP, and cold knife conization to treat cervical intraepithelial neoplasia. Int J Gynecol Obstet. 2015;132(3):266–71.
11. Arbyn M, Kyrgiou M, Simoens C, Raifu A, Koliopoulos G, Martin-Hirsch P, et al. Perinatal mortality and other severe adverse pregnancy outcomes associated with treatment of cervical intraepithelial neoplasia: meta-analysis. BMJ. 2008;337:a1284.
12. CRANE J. Pregnancy outcome after loop electrosurgical excision procedure: a systematic review. Obstet Gynecol. 2003;102(5):1058–62.
13. Sadler L. Treatment for cervical intraepithelial neoplasia and risk of preterm delivery. JAMA. 2004;291(17):2100.
14. Panoskaltsis T, Ind TE, Perryman K, Dina R, Abrahams Y, Soutter WP. Needleversus loop diathermy excision of the transformation zone for the treatment of cervical intraepithelial neoplasia: a randomised controlled trial. BJOG. 2004;111(7):748–53.
15. Camargo MJ, Russomano FB, Tristão MA, Huf G, Prendiville W. Large loop versus straight-wire excision of the transformation zone for treatment of cervical intraepithelial neoplasia: a randomised controlled trial of electrosurgical techniques. BJOG. 2015;122(4):552–7.
16. Russomano F, Tristao MA, Côrtes R, de Camargo MJ. A comparison between type 3 excision of the transformation zone by straight wire excision of the transformation zone (SWETZ) and large loop excision of the transformation zone (LLETZ): a randomized study. BMC Womens Health. 2015;15:12.
17. Santesso N, Mustafa RA, Wiercioch W, Kehar R, Gandhi S, Chen Y, et al. Systematic reviews and meta-analyses of benefits and harms of cryotherapy, LEEP, and cold knife conization to treat cervical intraepithelial neoplasia. Int J Gynaecol Obstet. 2016;132(3):266–71.
18. Mathevet P, Dargent D, Roy M, Beau G. A randomized prospective study comparing three techniques of conization: cold knife, laser, and LEEP. Gynecol Oncol. 1994;54(2):175–9.
19. Mathevet P, Chemali E, Roy M, Dargent D. Long-term outcome of a randomized study comparing three techniques of conization: cold knife, laser, and LEEP. Eur J Obstet Gynecol Reprod Biol. 2003;106(2):214–8.
20. di Saia P, Morrow C, Townsend D. Synopsis of gynecologic oncology. New York: Wiley; 1975.
21. World Health Organization. WHO guidelines. Guidelines for screening and treatment of precancerous lesions for cervical cancer prevention. 2013. http://apps.who.int/iris/bitstream/handle/10665/94830/9789241548694_eng.pdf;jsessionid=8E43D2FBAEAE4BDE3C2D1CD1B1E4641C?sequence=1. Accessed 24 Mar 2018.

Part III

Ovary

Epidemiology and Risk Factors for Ovarian Cancer

17

Anshuja Singla

17.1 Introduction

The International Agency for Research on Cancer reported that in 2012 gynecological cancers accounted for 20% of the 14.1 million new cancer cases and 8.2 million cancer deaths in females. Of this, 239,000 new cases were diagnosed as OC and caused 1,52,000 deaths [1].

By 2020, an estimated 182,602 cases of gynecological cancer will be diagnosed in Indian women which would be 30% of the total cancers among females [2].

In the United States, an estimated 22,440 new cases of OC were diagnosed in 2017 accounting for 5% of the total cancer-related deaths. Over the past two decades, OC rates have declined by about 1.1% per year in whites and 0.4% per year in black women with a similar decrease in mortality (2% per year versus 1% per year) [3].

The median age at diagnosis is 63 years, and the lifetime risk of having OC is 1 in 75 (1.3%) with the mortality rate of approximately 25% for all stages of OC. The 5-year survival rate for OC is low (46.5%) as 60% of women are diagnosed in later stages where the survival incidence is on an average 29%. Early-stage cancer is diagnosed only in 15% women though the survival rate is as good as 92% [4].

17.2 Geographic Distribution

A wide geographic variation is observed for OC with the highest rates (>8 per lakh) being observed from developed nations like North and Central America and Eastern Europe. South Asia and Africa account for the lowest incidence of less than 3 per lakh with South America being between the two (5.8 per lakh) [5] which are in congruence with the variations observed across the globe [4]. Figure 17.1 exhibits the wide geographic distribution of ovarian cancer all over the globe [1].

Maximum decline in OC-related mortality has been seen in major developed countries like the European Union, America, and Australia (10%, 16%, 12%, respectively). The fall was larger for the young and the middle-aged women. Latin American countries had lower rates with a modest decline of only 2.1% noted in Japan [6].

A. Singla (✉)
Department of Obstetrics and Gynecology, University College of Medical Sciences and Guru Teg Bahadur Hospital, New Delhi, India

S. Mehta, A. Singla (eds.), *Preventive Oncology for the Gynecologist*,
https://doi.org/10.1007/978-981-13-3438-2_17

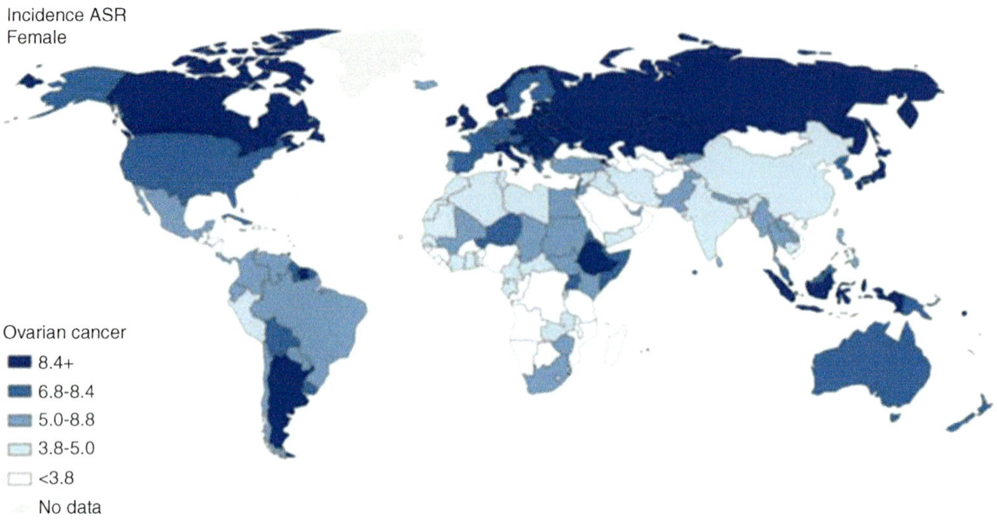

Fig. 17.1 Geographic distribution of ovarian cancer. Adapted with permission from Ferlay J., Soerjomataram I., Ervik M., Dikshit R., Eser S., Mathers C., Rebelo M., Parkin D.M., Forman D., Bray, F. GLOBOCAN 2012 v1.0, Cancer Incidence and Mortality Worldwide: IARC CancerBase No. 11 [Internet]. Lyon, France: International Agency for Research on Cancer; 2013. Available from: http://gco.iarc.fr/today/home

17.3 Risk Factors

The two predominant hypotheses for OC that have emerged after decades of research are the incessant ovulation and the gonadotropin hypothesis. According to the former theory, with the increasing number of ovulatory cycles, there is an increase in the rate of cellular division associated with the repair of ovarian epithelium in turn increasing the chances of spontaneous mutations [7]. Entrapment of the ovarian surface epithelium within the ovarian stroma and its subsequent differentiation, proliferation, and malignant transformation may occur due to estrogen stimulation. These occur more likely especially with high gonadotropin levels (luteinizing hormone [LH] and follicle-stimulating hormone [FSH]) and form the basis of gonadotropin hypothesis [8, 9].

17.3.1 Age

Early age at menarche and late age of menopause increase the number of ovulatory cycles, thereby increasing the risk of development of OC, though many studies do not support the same [10]. Gong et al. analyzed 22 case-control and five cohort studies in their meta-analysis and reported a statistically significant inverse association between menarcheal age and OC risk (RR = 0.85; 95% CI, 0.75–0.97), but the association was restricted to invasive and borderline serous ovarian cancer [11].

Similar inconsistent results have been reported with regard to age at menopause. In the EPIC cohort of 327,396 women, menopausal age more than 52 had an increased risk compared to <45 years (>52 vs ≤45: HR, 1.46; 95% CI, 1.06–1.99; P-trend 0.02) [12]. A collaborative report from NHS and NHS-II found an increased association of increasing age at menopause with endometrioid tumors and not serous invasive or mucinous tumor [13]. To conclude, with all the available evidence, the effect of age at the ends of the reproductive spectrum is small.

17.3.2 Pregnancy and Parity

Pregnancy exerts a strong protective effect on ovarian cancer by causation of anovulation and decreased pituitary gonadotropins. Gaitskell et al. in their prospective Million Women Study (MWS) showed that nulliparous females had a 29% increase of ovarian cancer risk compared to women even with a single child with significant variation for histological subtype. There was no significant increase in serous to a modest increase for mucinous but a substantial increase for clear cell and endometrioid tumors [14].

A large case-control study from Denmark found a significant decrease in the risk of serous borderline OCs with increasing parity ($p < 0.01$), whereas infertility was associated with an increased risk (OR = 3.31; 95% CI, 2.44–4.49) [15]. Similar results were reported by Koushik et al. [16].

17.3.3 Breastfeeding

Prolactin release after delivery helps in the establishment of lactation and switches off LH and FSH secretion in turn causing anovulation. So breastfeeding (BF) has a protective effect in the development of ovarian cancer [9]. Tsilidis and colleagues showed that there was no significant association of risk of OC with breastfeeding [12]. In a recent meta-analysis by Li et al. including 17,137 women with ovarian malignancy, a 30% risk reduction was seen with up to 6 months of BF as compared to no BF with a significant decrease in epithelial variety. When duration of BF was considered, the relative risks for <6 months, 6–12 months, and >12 months were 0.85, 0.73, and 0.64, respectively, thus showing that there is a linear trend toward ovarian cancer risk and duration of BF [17]. Sung et al. observed that first birth and first 6 months of BF had a greater protective effect than subsequent births and additional months of BF [18].

17.3.4 Oral Contraception

Consistent reports of the protective effect of oral contraception on development of ovarian cancer exist in the literature with the protective effect increasing with the duration of use [16, 19, 20].

Koushik et al. reported that ever use was not associated with risk overall but >10 years of use versus no use reduced the risk especially for invasive OC [16], whereas another study showed that if use was 5 years or more, the risk was halved [9].

The EPIC trial showed that oral contraceptive use for ≥10 years decreased the risk of ovarian cancer by 45% compared to ≤1 year of use, though ever users had significant lower risk of OC [12].

No particular oral contraception formulation or ovarian cancer histiotype is associated with risk reduction [21]. A lower risk of ovarian cancer with progestin only contraception has also been seen [22].

Across the globe, the choice of contraceptive method usage varies. Huang et al. in the prospective Shanghai Women's Health Study showed that with intrauterine device use of longer than 20 years, there was a reduction of 38% for OC compared to never users [23]. With levonorgestrel intrauterine system (LNG-IUS), a lower incidence of OC has been seen [24]. To conclude, still further research is needed to establish the effect of different formulations and modes of contraception on ovarian cancer risk.

17.3.5 Hormone Replacement Therapy (HRT)

Despite the well-known ill effects of HRT on women's health, Ness et al. reported that 12% postmenopausal women with a mean age of 66 years still take HRT [21]. The evidence suggest that HRT is the risk factor for ovarian cancer. Initial studies mainly focused on unopposed estrogen therapy (ET) and OC risk. Studies both support [25–27] and refute [28, 29] the association of OC risk with unopposed ET therapy. But a recent reanalysis of 52 epidemiological studies reported that 55% women who used HRT develop OC and the risk was increased even with <5 years of use. The risk mostly increased for serous and endometrioid type, and the risk remained despite stoppage of HRT even up to the next 10 years [30].

Combined estrogen and progestin therapy (EPT), though initially deemed to have no association or was weakly protective [31, 32], has been shown to have increased risks as well.

Greiser and colleagues observed that risk of ovarian cancer was increased 1.28-fold with ET compared to 1.1-fold increase with EPT, though no differential impact of the formulation was noted on histological subtypes [26].

Thus, HRT use in women is associated with a small but significant risk of OC.

17.4 Lifestyle Factors

17.4.1 Smoking

Cigarette smoke contains carcinogenic chemicals like benzo[a]pyrenes, which is a potent mutagen and carcinogen found in cigarettes. Women exposed to cigarette smoke have benzo[a]pyrene DNA adducts in their ovarian follicular cells which may increase the risk of DNA damage [33].

Some studies [34–36] reported that smoking was not a risk factor for ovarian cancer. A study published in *The Lancet* journal analyzed the effect of smoking on ovarian cancer for 28,000 women from a total of 51 studies. They reported that current smoking rather than past history was associated with an excess of mucinous tumors mainly of the borderline histology (49% mucinous invasive and 125% borderline). A reported decrease in endometrioid and clear cell tumors was noted which is in congruence with the fact that smoking decreases the risk of endometrial cancer. Thus, the overall increase in incidence is small though nonsignificant [37].

Mettler and colleagues in their pooled analysis showed that cigarette smoking had differing strengths of association with different histological subtypes of ovarian cancer. Maximum association was with invasive and borderline mucinous tumors to the tune of 31% and 83%, respectively, in current smokers. The association between smoking and risk of low- and high-grade serous OC was insignificant though a significant increase was noted for serous borderline tumors among former and not current smokers [38].

There has been a global increase in female smoking. Serous ovarian cancers are the most lethal of them, but most studies have found that this histological type does not have an increased association with smoking [37, 39–41].

Various studies have shown a protective effect of smoking on endometrioid OC, but quite a good number found no association between the same [39, 41–44].

A decreased risk for clear cell ovarian cancer was seen in some studies [37, 39, 44], though others found an increased but nonsignificant association between the same [42, 43].

17.4.2 Diet and Vitamin Intake

A null association was observed with intake of vitamins A, C, and E and folate and ovarian cancer though some association was observed with greater vitamin intake especially carotenoids with endometrioid histology [45]. Schulz et al. noted that higher intake of vegetables, whole grain foods, and low-fat milk have some evidence for decrease in OC risk [46]. The meta-analysis of EPIC cohort and the Netherlands cohort including 430,476 women with 1522 OC cases found that high intake of saturated fats elevates the OC risk (HR = 1.21, 95% CI, 1.04–1.41) [47]. Yin et al. found no strong evidence of vitamin D decreasing the risks [48]. A very recent Mendelian randomization study found single nucleotide polymorphisms (SNPs) that were associated with circulating levels of vitamin D and increased risk of OC [49].

17.4.3 Asbestos and Talc

IARC has notified that evidence suggested that exposure to asbestos in humans causes OC [50]. A 75% excess risk of OC with asbestos exposure occurs though the effect is negated upon histopathological confirmation of the reported OC cases [51].

Talc like asbestos is a silicate mineral. Though mechanistic, pathological, and animal studies are not supportive of the carcinogenic properties of talc on ovarian epithelium [52], studies both supporting [53, 54] and refuting the same have been reported in literature [55]. Thus IARC classified genital talc use as possibly carcinogenic in humans [56].

17.4.4 Obesity

Adipose tissue converts androgens to estrogens, and increase in body mass index (BMI) has been associated with OC risk mainly in premenopausal women [57, 58], but some studies also found an association with postmenopausal women [59, 60]. Increase in different histological types of OC has been also seen [59, 61, 62].

17.4.5 Physical Activity

Olsen and colleagues suggested a modest inverse relationship between the level of physical activity and the risk of ovarian cancer, though the benefit did not vary for different histological subtypes. Thus, regular physical activity should be the norm considering its beneficial outcome on weight control and hence a better bone and heart health [63].

17.4.6 Drugs

The inflammatory etiology of ovarian cancer [64] wherein inflammatory mediators released during ovulation initiate cell transformation and a similar inflammatory process in endometriosis support the protective anti-inflammatory role of aspirin and NSAIDs. Aspirin is an irreversible COX-1 inhibitor, and this inhibition is more important for decrease in risk for ovarian malignancy as OC tissue overexpress COX-1.

In the analysis of more than 7500 patients, aspirin use was associated with decreased risk of OC, more so for regular users of low dose [65]. Aspirin use for cardiovascular disease prevention has reported a 12% reduction in cancer incidence with ≥3 years of daily aspirin use, especially for female genital cancers [66]. In contrast regular use of NSAIDs was seen as protective in comparison to aspirin [67].

Interestingly, evidence is emerging for the role of metformin in OC prevention and treatment. In a very recent retrospective study by Wang et al., patients with OC who regularly use metformin had a longer progression-free survival and overall survival than who did not take or discontinued metformin and in nondiabetic OC controls [68].

Thus, further research is warranted, keeping in mind potential drug adverse effects on long-term use.

17.5 Gynecological Conditions and Risk of Ovarian Cancer

Benign conditions like endometriosis, pelvic inflammatory diseases (PID), and PCOS have all been evaluated as potential risk factors for development of OC.

Endometriosis has been long linked to the development of OC. A systematic review reported increased risk of OC especially of endometrioid, clear cell, and low-grade serous tumors [69, 70].

PCOD is known to be associated with endometrial cancer due to unopposed estrogens and androgens. Literature is scarce on the association of PCOD with OC [71, 72].

Studies are inconclusive about the association between PID and ovarian cancer [73–77]. PID was found to be a risk factor especially in women <35 years [75] though an increased association was seen with borderline tumors [76], especially of the serous variety and not mucinous [77].

17.6 Gynecological Surgery and Ovarian Cancer

Various mechanisms by which tubal ligation acts as a protective barrier are an early screening effect, alteration of ovarian function, mechanical barrier against ascending carcinogenic agents, and prevention of endometrial and proximal fallopian tube ascent [78]. Tubal ligation has been shown to decrease the risk of ovarian cancer. Cibula and colleagues showed a decreased risk for epithelial OC by 34% though a risk reduction was also noted for endometrioid and serous variety and not mucinous OC [79].

The role of prophylactic oophorectomy in decreasing OC has been well established especially among high-risk women [80, 81]. This is discussed in detail in Chap. 20.

Hysterectomy has also been identified to reduce OC risk of endometrioid and clear cell type as is with tubal ligation [82, 83].

17.7 Conclusion

Ovarian cancer is one of the common cancers in women and the leading cause of mortality. Lifestyle modification with avoidance of occupational hazards and appropriate and timely prophylaxis in high-risk women can go a long way in decreasing the risk and mortality associated with ovarian cancer. Promotion of breastfeeding for a minimum of 6 months, regular and consistent use of contraception, prescription of HRT to women who are in actual need of it, and, most importantly, monitoring of one's own health will help prevent many more cases.

Key Points

- Ovarian cancer is one of the most commonly diagnosed cancers and the cancer-related cause of mortality among women.
- The highest rates have been recorded from the most developed nations probably because of the increased screening protocols.
- Early and increased use of oral contraceptives has contributed to declining rates observed in developed countries.
- In developing countries reduced parity, decreased physical activity, and a higher dietary saturated fat intake may be playing a crucial role in the increasing trends observed.
- Lifestyle modifications will play a definitive role in further decreasing the associated morbidity and mortality.

References

1. Ferlay J, Soerjomataram I, Ervik M, Dikshit R, Eser S, Mathers C, et al. GLOBOCAN 2012 v1.0, Cancer incidence and mortality worldwide: IARC cancer base no. 11. Lyon: International Agency for Research on Cancer; 2013.
2. Takiar R, Nadayil D, Nandakumar A. Projections of number of cancer cases in India (2010-2020) by cancer groups. Asian Pac J Cancer Prev. 2010;11(4):1045–9.
3. American Cancer Society. Cancer facts & figures 2017. Atlanta: American Cancer Society; 2017.
4. Howlader N, Noone AM, Krapcho M, Neyman N, Aminou R, Waldron W, et al. SEER Cancer Statistics Review, 1975–2008. Bethesda: National Cancer Institute; 2010.
5. Ferlay JSH, Bray F, Forman D, Mathers C, Parkin DM. GLOBOCAN 2008 v 1.2: Cancer incidence, mortality, and prevalence worldwide: IARC cancer base no. 10. International Agency for Research on Cancer: Lyon; 2008. http://globocan.iarc.fr
6. Malvezzi M, Carioli G, Rodriguez T, Negri E, La Vecchia C. Global trends and predictions in ovarian cancer mortality. Ann Oncol. 2016;27(11):2017–25.
7. Fathalla MF. Incessant ovulation—a factor in ovarian neoplasia? Lancet. 1971;2(7716):163.
8. Cramer DW, Hutchison GB, Welch WR, Scully RE, Ryan KJ. Determinants of ovarian cancer risk. I. Reproductive experiences and family history. J Natl Cancer Inst. 1983;71(4):711–6.
9. Riman T, Nilsson S, Persson IR. Review of epidemiological evidence for reproductive and hormonal factors in relation to the risk of epithelial ovarian malignancies. Acta Obstet Gynecol Scand. 2004;83:783–95.
10. Whittemore AS, Harris R, Itnyre J. Characteristics relating to ovarian cancer risk: collaborative analysis of 12 US case-control studies. II. Invasive epithelial ovarian cancers in white women. Collaborative Ovarian Cancer Group. Am J Epidemiol. 1992;136:1184–203.
11. Gong TT, Wu QJ, Vogtmann E, Lin B, Wang YL. Age at menarche and risk of ovarian cancer: a meta-analysis of epidemiological studies. Int J Cancer. 2013;132(12):2894–900.
12. Tsilidis KK, Allen NE, Key TJ, Dossus L, Lukanova A, Bakken K, et al. Oral contraceptive use and reproductive factors and risk of ovarian cancer in the European Prospective Investigation into Cancer and Nutrition. Br J Cancer. 2011;105:1436–42.
13. Gates MA, Rosner BA, Hecht JL, Tworoger SS. Risk factors for epithelial ovarian cancer by histologic subtype. Am J Epidemiol. 2010;171:45–53.
14. Gaitskell K, Green J, Pirie K, Barnes I, Hermon C, Reeves GK, Beral V, Million Women Study Collaborators. Histological subtypes of ovarian cancer associated with parity and breastfeeding in the prospective Million Women Study. Int J Cancer. 2018;142(2):281–9.

15. Rasmussen EL, Hannibal CG, Dehlendorff C, Baandrup L, Junge J, Vang R, et al. Parity, infertility, oral contraceptives, and hormone replacement therapy and the risk of ovarian serous borderline tumors: a nationwide case-control study. Gynecol Oncol. 2017;144(3):571–6.
16. Koushik A, Grundy A, Abrahamowicz M, Arseneau J, Gilbert L, Gotlieb WH, et al. Hormonal and reproductive factors and the risk of ovarian cancer. Cancer Causes Control. 2017;28(5):393–403.
17. Li DP, Du C, Zhang ZM, Li GX, Yu ZF, Wang X, et al. Breastfeeding and ovarian cancer risk: a systematic review and meta-analysis of 40 epidemiological studies. Asian Pac J Cancer Prev. 2014;15(12):4829–37.
18. Sung HK, Ma SH, Choi JY, Hwang Y, Ahn C, Kim BG, et al. The effect of breastfeeding duration and parity on the risk of epithelial ovarian cancer: a systematic review and meta-analysis. J Prev Med Public Health. 2016;49(6):349–66.
19. Risch HA, Marrett LD, Howe GR. Parity, contraception, infertility, and the risk of epithelial ovarian cancer. Am J Epidemiol. 1994;140:585–97.
20. Franceschi S, Parazzini F, Negri E, Booth M, La Vecchia C, Beral V, et al. Pooled analysis of 3 European case-control studies of epithelial ovarian cancer: III. Oral contraceptive use. Int J Cancer. 1991;49:61–5.
21. Ness RB, Grisso JA, Klapper J, Schlesselman JJ, Silberzweig S, Vergona R, et al. Risk of ovarian cancer in relation to estrogen and progestin dose and use characteristics of oral contraceptives. Am J Epidemiol. 2000;152:233–41.
22. Rosenberg L, Palmer JR, Zauber AG, Warshauer ME, Lewis JL Jr, Strom BL, et al. A case-control study of oral contraceptive use and invasive epithelial ovarian cancer. Am J Epidemiol. 1994;139:654–61.
23. Huang ZZ, Gao YT, Wen WQ, Li HL, Zheng W, Shu XO, et al. Contraceptive methods and ovarian cancer risk among Chinese women: a report from the Shanghai Women's Health Study. Int J Cancer. 2015;137:607–14.
24. Soini T, Hurskainen R, Grénman S, Mäenpä J, Paavonen J, Pukkala E. Cancer risk in women using the levonorgestrel-releasing intrauterine system in Finland. Obstet Gynecol. 2014;124:292–9.
25. Kaufman DW, Kelly JP, Welch WR, Rosenberg L, Stolley PD, Warshauer ME, et al. Noncontraceptive estrogen use and epithelial ovarian cancer. Am J Epidemiol. 1989;130:1142–51.
26. Greiser CM, Greiser EM, Dören M. Menopausal hormone therapy and risk of ovarian cancer: systematic review and meta-analysis. Hum Reprod Update. 2007;13:453–63.
27. Zhou B, Sun QM, Cong RH, Gu HJ, Tang NP, Yang L, et al. Hormone replacement therapy and ovarian cancer risk: a meta-analysis. Gynecol Oncol. 2008;108:641–51.
28. Coughlin SS, Giustozzi A, Smith SJ, Lee NC. A meta-analysis of estrogen replacement therapy and risk of epithelial ovarian cancer. J Clin Epidemiol. 2000;53:367–75.
29. Garg PP, Kerlikowske K, Subak L, Grady D. Hormone replacement therapy and the risk of epithelial ovarian carcinoma: a meta-analysis. Obstet Gynecol. 1998;92:472–9.
30. Collaborative Group on Epidemiological Studies of Ovarian Cancer. Menopausal hormone use and ovarian cancer risk: individual participant meta-analysis of 52 epidemiological studies. Lancet. 2015;385:1835–42.
31. Lacey JV Jr, Mink PJ, Lubin JH, Sherman ME, Troisi R, Hartge P, et al. Menopausal hormone replacement therapy and risk of ovarian cancer. JAMA. 2002;288:334–41.
32. Hildebrand JS, Gapstur SM, Feigelson HS, Teras LR, Thun MJ, Patel AV. Postmenopausal hormone use and incident ovarian cancer: associations differ by regimen. Int J Cancer. 2010;127:2928–35.
33. Zenzes MT, Puy LA, Bielecki R. Immunodetection of benzo[a]pyrene adducts in ovarian cells of women exposed to cigarette smoke. Mol Hum Reprod. 1998;4(2):159–65.
34. Whittemore AS, Wu ML, Paffenbarger RS Jr, Sarles DL, Kampert JB, Grosser S, et al. Personal and environmental characteristics related to epithelial ovarian cancer. II. Exposures to talcum powder, tobacco, alcohol, and coffee. Am J Epidemiol. 1988;128:1228–40.
35. Franks AL, Lee NC, Kendrick JS, Rubin GL, Layde PM. Cigarette smoking and the risk of epithelial ovarian cancer. Am J Epidemiol. 1987;126:112–7.
36. Smith EM, Sowers MF, Burns TL. Effects of smoking on the development of female reproductive cancers. J Natl Cancer Inst. 1984;73:371–6.
37. Collaborative Group on Epidemiological Studies of Ovarian Cancer, Beral V, Gaitskell K, Hermon C, Moser K, Reeves G, Peto R. Ovarian cancer and smoking: individual participant meta-analysis including 28,114 women with ovarian cancer from 51 epidemiological studies. Lancet Oncol. 2012;13(9):946–56.
38. Faber MT, Kjær SK, Dehlendorff C, Chang-Claude J, Andersen KK, Høgdall E, et al. Cigarette smoking and risk of ovarian cancer: a pooled analysis of 21 case-control studies. Cancer Causes Control. 2013;24(5):989–1004.
39. Jordan SJ, Whiteman DC, Purdie DM. Does smoking increase risk of ovarian cancer? A systematic review. Gynecol Oncol. 2006;103(3):1122–9.
40. Gram IT, Lukanova A, Brill I. Cigarette smoking and risk of histological subtypes of epithelial ovarian cancer in the EPIC cohort study. Int J Cancer. 2012;130(9):2204–10.
41. Soegaard M, Jensen A, Hogdall E. Different risk factor profiles for mucinous and nonmucinous ovarian cancer: results from the Danish MALOVA study. Cancer Epidemiol Biomark Prev. 2007;16(6):1160–6.
42. Baker JA, Odunuga OO, Rodabaugh KJ. Active and passive smoking and risk of ovarian cancer. Int J Gynecol Cancer. 2006;16(Suppl 1):211–8.
43. Riman T, Dickman PW, Nilsson S. Some life-style factors and the risk of invasive epithelial ovar-

ian cancer in Swedish women. Eur J Epidemiol. 2004;19(11):1011–9.
44. Nagle CM, Olsen CM, Webb PM. Endometrioid and clear cell ovarian cancers: a comparative analysis of risk factors. Eur J Cancer. 2008;44(16):2477–84.
45. Koushik A, Wang M, Anderson KE, van den Brandt P, Clendenen TV, Eliassen AH, et al. Intake of vitamins A, C, and E and folate and the risk of ovarian cancer in a pooled analysis of 10 cohort studies. Cancer Causes Control. 2015;26(9):1315–27.
46. Schulz M, Lahmann PH, Riboli E, Boeing H. Dietary determinants of epithelial ovarian cancer: a review of the epidemiologic literature. Nutr Cancer. 2004;50:120–40.
47. Merritt MA, Tzoulaki I, van den Brandt PA, Schouten LJ, Tsilidis KK, Weiderpass E, et al. Nutrient-wide association study of 57 foods/nutrients and epithelial ovarian cancer in the European Prospective Investigation into Cancer and Nutrition study and the Netherlands Cohort Study. Am J ClinNutr. 2016;103(1):161–7.
48. Yin L, Grandi N, Raum E, Haug U, Arndt V, Brenner H. Meta-analysis: circulating vitamin D and ovarian cancer risk. Gynecolc Oncol. 2011;121:369–75.
49. Ong JS, Cuellar-Partida G, Lu Y, Australian Ovarian Cancer Study, Fasching PA, Hein A, et al. Association of vitamin D levels and risk of ovarian cancer: a Mendelian randomization study. Int J Epidemiol. 2016;45:1619–30.
50. International Agency for Research on Cancer. IARC monographs on the evaluation of carcinogenic risks to humans. Overall evaluations of carcinogenicity: an updating of IARC monographs supplement 7. International Agency for Research on Cancer 1987. Lyon: International Agency for Research on Cancer; 1987.
51. Reid A, de Klerk N, Musk AW. Does exposure to asbestos cause ovarian cancer? A systematic literature review and meta-analysis. Cancer Epidemiol Biomark Prev. 2011;20:1287–95.
52. Cibula D, Widschwendter M, Zikan M, Dusek L. Underlying mechanisms of ovarian cancer risk reduction after tubal ligation. Acta Obstet Gynecol Scand. 2011;90(6):559–63.
53. Langseth H, Hankinson SE, Siemiatycki J, Weiderpass E. Perineal use of talc and risk of ovarian cancer. J Epidemiol Commun Health. 2008;62:358–60.
54. Cramer DW, Vitonis AF, Terry KL, Welch WR, Titus LJ. The association between talc use and ovarian cancer: a retrospective case-control study in two US States. Epidemiology. 2016;27:334–46.
55. Houghton SC, Reeves KW, Hankinson SE, Crawford L, Lane D, Wactawski-Wende J, et al. Perineal powder use and risk of ovarian cancer. J Natl Cancer Inst. 2014;106(9):dju208.
56. Baan R, Straif K, Grosse Y, Secretan B, El Ghissassi F, Cogliano V. Carcinogenicity of carbon black, titanium dioxide, and talc. Lancet Oncol. 2006;7:295–6.
57. Schouten LJ, Rivera C, Hunter DJ, Spiegelman D, Adami HO, Arslan A, et al. Height, body mass index, and ovarian cancer: a pooled analysis of 12 cohort studies. Cancer Epidemiol Biomark Prev. 2008;17:902–12.
58. Olsen CM, Nagle CM, Whiteman DC, Ness R, Pearce CL, Pike MC, et al. Obesity and risk of ovarian cancer subtypes: evidence from the Ovarian Cancer Association Consortium. Endocr Relat Cancer. 2013;20:251–62.
59. Lahmann PH, Cust AE, Friedenreich CM, Schulz M, Lukanova A, Kaaks R, et al. Anthropometric measures and epithelial ovarian cancer risk in the European Prospective Investigation into Cancer and Nutrition. Int J Cancer. 2010;126:2404–15.
60. Kotsopoulos J, Baer HJ, Tworoger SS. Anthropometric measures and risk of epithelial ovarian cancer: results from the nurses' health study. Obesity. 2009;18:1625–31.
61. Collaborative Group on Epidemiological Studies of Ovarian Cancer. Ovarian cancer and body size: individual participant meta-analysis including 25, 157 women with ovarian cancer from 47 epidemiological studies. PLoS Med. 2012;9:e1001200.
62. Dixon SC, Nagle CM, Thrift AP, Pharoah PDP, Pearce CL, Zheng W, et al. Adult body mass index and risk of ovarian cancer by subtype: a Mendelian randomization study. Int J Epidemiol. 2016;45:884–95.
63. Olsen CM, Bain CJ, Jordan SJ, Nagle CM, Green AC, Whiteman DC, et al. Recreational physical activity and epithelial ovarian cancer: a case-control study, systematic review, and meta-analysis. Cancer Epidemiol Biomark Prev. 2007;16:2321–30.
64. Ness RB, Cottreau C. Possible role of ovarian epithelial inflammation in ovarian cancer. J Natl Cancer Inst. 1999;91(17):1459–67.
65. Trabert B, Ness RB, Lo-Ciganic WH, Murphy MA, Goode EL, Poole EM, Ovarian Cancer Association Consortium, et al. Aspirin, nonaspirin nonsteroidal anti-inflammatory drug, and acetaminophen use and risk of invasive epithelial ovarian cancer: a pooled analysis in the Ovarian Cancer Association Consortium. J Natl Cancer Inst. 2014;106(2):djt431.
66. Rothwell PM, Price JF, Fowkes FG, Zanchetti A, Roncaglioni MC, Tognoni G, et al. Short-term effects of daily aspirin on cancer incidence, mortality, and non-vascular death: analysis of the time course of risks and benefits in 51 randomised controlled trials. Lancet. 2012;379(9826):1602–12.
67. Pinheiro SP, Tworoger SS, Cramer DW, Rosner BA, Hankinson SE. Use of nonsteroidal antiinflammatory agents and incidence of ovarian cancer in 2 large prospective cohorts. Am J Epidemiol. 2009;169:1378–87.
68. Wang SB, Lei KJ, Liu JP, Jia YM. Continuous use of metformin can improve survival in type 2 diabetic patients with ovarian cancer: a retrospective study. Medicine (Baltimore). 2017;96(29):e7605.
69. Sayasneh A, Tsivos D, Crawford R. Endometriosis and ovarian cancer: a systematic review. ISRN Obstet Gynecol. 2011;2011:140310.
70. Pearce CL, Templeman C, Rossing MA, Lee A, Near AM, Webb PM, et al. Association between endometri-

osis and risk of histological subtypes of ovarian cancer: a pooled analysis of case-control studies. Lancet Oncol. 2012;13:385–94.
71. Schildkraut JM, Schwingl PJ, Bastos E, Evanoff A, Hughes C. Epithelial ovarian cancer risk among women with polycystic ovary syndrome. Obstet Gynecol. 1996;88:554–9.
72. Fauser BCJM, Tarlatzis BC, Rebar RW, Legro RS, Balen AH, Lobo R, et al. Consensus on women's health aspects of polycystic ovary syndrome (PCOS): the Amsterdam ESHRE/ASRM-sponsored 3rd PCOS Consensus Workshop Group. Fertil Steril. 2012;97:28–38.
73. Parazzini F, La Vecchia C, Negri E, Moroni S, dal Pino D, Fedele L. Pelvic inflammatory disease and risk of ovarian cancer. Cancer Epidemiol Biomark Prev. 1996;5:667–9.
74. Merritt MA, Green AC, Nagle CM, Webb PM. Talcum powder, chronic pelvic inflammation and NSAIDs in relation to risk of epithelial ovarian cancer. Int J Cancer. 2008;122:170–6.
75. Lin HW, Tu YY, Lin SY, Su WJ, Lin WL, Lin WZ, et al. Risk of ovarian cancer in women with pelvic inflammatory disease: a population-based study. Lancet Oncol. 2011;12:900–4.
76. Rasmussen CB, Faber MT, Jensen A, Høgdall E, Høgdall C, Blaakær J, et al. Pelvic inflammatory disease and risk of invasive ovarian cancer and ovarian borderline tumors. Cancer Causes Control. 2013;24:1459–64.
77. Rasmussen CB, Jensen A, Albieri V, Andersen KK, Kjaer SK. Increased risk of borderline ovarian tumors in women with a history of pelvic inflammatory disease: a nationwide population-based cohort study. Gynecol Oncol. 2016;143:346–51.
78. Muscat JE, Huncharek MS. Perineal talc use and ovarian cancer: a critical review. Eur J Cancer Prev. 2008;17(2):139–46.
79. Cibula D, Widschwendter M, Májek O, Dusek L. Tubal ligation and the risk of ovarian cancer: review and meta-analysis. Hum Reprod Update. 2011;17:55–67.
80. Temkin SM, Bergstrom J, Samimi G, Minasian L. Ovarian cancer prevention in high-risk women. Clin Obstet Gynecol. 2017;60(4):738–57.
81. Berek JS, Chalas E, Edelson M, Moore DH, Burke WM, Cliby WA, Society of Gynecologic Oncologists Clinical Practice Committee, et al. Prophylactic and risk-reducing bilateral salpingo-oophorectomy: recommendations based on risk of ovarian cancer. Obstet Gynecol. 2010;116(3):733–43.
82. Rosenblatt KA, Thomas DB. Reduced risk of ovarian cancer in women with a tubal ligation or hysterectomy. The World Health Organization Collaborative Study of Neoplasia and Steroid Contraceptives. Cancer Epidemiol Biomark Prev. 1996;5:933–5.
83. Rice MS, Murphy MA, Vitonis AF, Cramer DW, Titus LJ, Tworoger SS, et al. Tubal ligation, hysterectomy and epithelial ovarian cancer in the New England Case-Control Study. Int J Cancer. 2013;133:2415–21.

Role of Tumor Markers

18

Sarah Lynam and Shashikant Lele

18.1 Introduction

Tumor markers are substances or molecules produced by the body and found in blood, urine, or peripheral tissue that may be elevated in the presence of malignancy. Detectable levels of tumor markers can suggest presence of underlying pathology requiring further evaluation, provide insight into nature of disease, or monitor treatment response in patients with cancer. Markers are in the form of enzymes, conjugated proteins, hormones, receptors, growth factors, or carbohydrates. Serum assays of these factors have been used in the management of ovarian, primary peritoneal, fallopian tube, uterine, cervical, and trophoblastic neoplasms.

Cancer is the second leading cause of death globally and was responsible for 8.8 million deaths in 2015, and approximately 70% of deaths from cancer occur in low- and middle-income countries. This is so because of lack of cancer awareness and inadequate screening facilities in developing countries leading to more women reporting at advanced stages of the disease [1]. The poor prognosis facing these women reinforces the need to identify patients at earlier stages of disease. World Health Organization guidelines for effective screening strategies include the ability to recognize diseases in a manner acceptable for the population at large to prevent or mitigate early-stage conditions when medical intervention may be more successful [2]. An ideal screening test would be sensitive in correctly identifying patients with disease and specific in ruling out unaffected individuals with a high positive predictive value (Table 18.1). The reliability of current serum marker-based strategies is limited by a lack of specificity to discrete pathology and can be affected by benign or malignant processes in multiple sites.

This chapter will discuss markers pertinent to assessment and management of benign and malignant gynecologic diseases. With thorough medical assessment, a high index of suspicion, and judicious use of tumor markers, providers can potentially diagnose early-stage disease in patients with gynecologic pathology.

Table 18.1 Characteristics of effective screening test

	Disease status	
Test result	Present	Absent
Positive	a (true positive)	b (false positive)
Negative	c (false negative)	d (true negative)

Sensitivity = a/a + c *or* true positive/all patients with disease—reflects ability to reliably diagnose disease if present. *Specificity* = d/b + d *or* true negative/all patients without disease—ability to reliably exclude disease when it is not present in population

S. Lynam · S. Lele (✉)
Department of Gynecologic Oncology, Roswell Park Cancer Institute, Buffalo, NY, USA
e-mail: shashi.lele@roswellpark.org

S. Mehta, A. Singla (eds.), *Preventive Oncology for the Gynecologist*,
https://doi.org/10.1007/978-981-13-3438-2_18

18.2 Tumor Markers in Ovarian Malignancy

18.2.1 CA125

Cancer antigen 125 (CA125) is a 200 kD glycoprotein encoded by the *MUC16* gene (19p13.2) produced by coelomic epithelium during embryologic development. This membrane-associated mucin contains extracellular highly glycosylated N-terminal, tandem repeat, and C-terminal domains with a cytoplasmic tail [3]. This marker was initially described in 1981 by Bast and colleagues whereby a murine monoclonal antibody, OC125, was found to bind multiple cell lines of epithelial ovarian carcinoma (EOC) [4]. Modern commercially available assays detect both OC125 and M11 epitopes of CA125. To date, it serves as the single most commonly used biomarker in the diagnosis, management, and surveillance of ovarian cancer. Serum CA125 elevations have also been reported in advanced-stage uterine and cervical cancers.

CA125 is expressed by mesothelial cells in the pleura, pericardium, peritoneum, and ocular epithelia as well as tubal, endometrial, and endocervical tissues. Of note, pathologic analysis of normal adult ovarian surface epithelium has not demonstrated expression of CA125 with the exception of inclusion cysts, areas of metaplastic change, and papillary excrescences [5]. Levels of CA125 may also be affected by benign gynecologic conditions including endometriosis, pelvic inflammatory disease, and adenomyosis as well as cirrhosis, pulmonary disease, congestive heart failure, systemic lupus erythematosus, inflammatory bowel diseases, and nongynecologic malignancy (Table 18.2). Physiologic increase in CA125 is seen during first trimester of pregnancy with reported levels as high as 550 U/mL, generally regressing to within normal limits over second and third trimesters with slight increases in puerperium [10]. Marked elevations in CA125 >1000 U/mL are generally in association with ovarian cancers, and roughly 80% of patients with ovarian cancer will present with elevated levels of CA125.

Table 18.2 CA125 in various disease sites (based on FIGO stage)

		% with CA125 >35 U/mL
Benign gynecologic disorders	Menstruation [6]	5.2
	Ovarian cysts [7]	14
	Endometriosis [7]	67
	Pelvic inflammatory disease [7]	37
	Leiomyomas [7]	26
Benign ovarian tumors	Serous epithelial tumors [7]	20
	Mucinous epithelial tumors [7]	18
	Germ cell tumors (mature teratoma) [7]	21
	Sex cord stromal tumors (thecoma, fibrothecoma) [7]	52
	Cystadenoma, cystadenofibroma, adenofibroma [7]	20
	Serous epithelial tumors [7]	20
	Mucinous epithelial tumors [7]	18
Ovarian cancer	Stage I [8]	50
	Stage II [8]	90
	Stage III [8]	92.1
	Stage IV [8]	93.9
	All stages [8]	85.1
Systemic diseases	Congestive heart failure [9]	14.7
	Lung disease [9]	18
	Cirrhosis [8]	67.1
	Acute pancreatitis [8]	32.2
	Renal failure [8]	14.6

Serum marker testing with CA125 primarily aids in evaluation of adnexal masses to distinguish patients at increased risk of malignancy. Given the widespread distribution of CA125 in various organ sites, a lack of both sensitivity for early-stage EOC and specificity in premenopausal patients has deleteriously impacted its use as an independent screening test. A study of 888 healthy donors with a median age of 34 years demonstrated 1% of individuals had CA125 levels greater than 35 U/mL, establishing the universally accepted cutoff for normal values of this marker [11]. Lower reference values have been suggested in postmenopausal patients (26 U/mL) with improved specificity in this population [12]. The sensitivity and specificity for prediction of ovarian cancer using CA125 are 50–74% and 26–92%, respectively, in premenopausal women versus 69–87% and 81–100% in postmenopausal women [13]. Given the low prevalence of epithelial ovarian cancers and risk of false-positive testing leading to invasive diagnostic procedures, the United States Preventive Services Task Force advises against screening asymptomatic average-risk women using serum tumor markers or ultrasonography [14].

18.2.1.1 Benign Gynecological Conditions

The use of CA125 in nonmalignant gynecologic disease has historically been in the evaluation of endometriosis. Inflammation of peritoneal surfaces secondary to ectopic endometrial glandular tissue causing dysmenorrhea, dyspareunia, and subfertility is frequently associated with elevations in CA125. Pathologic confirmation of endometriosis remains the gold standard of diagnosis for this disease. Serum elevations of CA125 greater than 30 U/mL are suggestive of endometriosis in symptomatic patients thereby expediting time to diagnosis and treatment [15]. A meta-analysis of 3626 patients found a sensitivity of 52.4% with specificity of 92.7% for advanced endometriosis using this cutoff [15]. While marked elevations in CA125 are suggestive of the presence of endometriomas and deep infiltrative endometriosis, CA125 levels have not been shown to be an independent predictor of malignant transformation to carcinoma of the ovary [16, 17]. Fluctuations of this marker with menses and ovulation may limit interpretation of CA125 in premenopausal women, but its role as a noninvasive tool in initial evaluation of patients with pelvic pain should be considered.

Association between CA125 and uterine pathology is mixed, particularly with respect to evaluation of leiomyoma. While some series have identified elevated CA125 in up to 26% of patients with uterine leiomyoma, these findings have been inconsistent between study populations [7, 18, 19]. Presence of lesions larger than 5 cm or concomitant adenomyosis has been associated with significantly higher levels of CA125 in patients with uterine fibroids [19]. While CA125 levels can be considered in initial evaluation of women with suspected adenomyosis, diagnostic accuracy may be limited. Investigation has been performed in the role of CA125 in differentiation of leiomyoma from uterine sarcoma; however there has been no consistent data to suggest a clear role of CA125 in differentiating these lesions [20, 21].

18.2.1.2 Ovarian Cancer Screening

Identification of effective screening for evaluation of early-stage ovarian cancer in postmenopausal women has been attempted through prospective analysis in several major trials, using a combination of transvaginal ultrasonography and CA125 in concurrent or sequential fashion. The Prostate, Lung, Colorectal and Ovarian Cancer Screening Trial (PLCO) randomized 78,216 postmenopausal women to annual transvaginal sonography screening with CA125 versus usual care over a median 12.4-year follow-up period [22]. Ovarian cancer was diagnosed in 212 women in the intervention group compared to 176 in the usual care group, with no reduction in ovarian cancer mortality and a 15% surgical complication rate for women with a false-positive screening test [22]. In the larger UK Collaborative Trial of Ovarian Cancer Screening (UKCTOCS), 202,638 women were randomized to control, annual screening with sonography or multimodal screening with CA125 to stratify low-, intermediate-, and high-risk patients [23]. Women in multimodal screening received annual CA125 with subsequent transvaginal sonography and reevaluation of CA125. Multimodal screening was more likely to detect ovarian cancer at an early stage with higher specificity compared to controls with a statistically nonsignificant reduction in ovarian cancer mortality apparently only after 7–14 years of trial participation [23]. Further interim analysis is planned. At present, it remains unclear if the harms of screening using sonography with CA125 and subsequent false-positive results leading to invasive surgical procedures outweigh the benefits of universal screening.

18.2.1.3 Ovarian Cancer

The role of CA125 in identification and risk stratification for women with adnexal masses concerning for gynecologic malignancy cannot be understated. The risk of malignancy index (RMI), combining CA125 with ultrasound characterization of adnexal masses as initially described by Jacobs et al., demonstrates a sensitivity of 85% and specificity of 97% in the detection of malignancy for postmenopausal women [24]. Variations of this index remain central to preoperative evaluation of adnexal masses with RMI as one of the most validated models for prediction of gynecologic malignancy. Several prognostic models using a combination of serum tumor markers including CA125 and radiographic findings have been developed for clinical use and are beyond the scope of this discussion. In addition to disease identification, CA125 is used for treatment monitoring, surveillance, and detection of recurrent disease in patients with EOC.

The prognostic role of CA125 in patients with EOC has been well characterized in women with ovary-confined (stage I) disease. Preoperative CA125 >65 U/mL confers a 6.37-fold higher risk of death for women with stage I disease [25]. For women with advanced-stage EOC, CA125 levels greater than 500 U/mL were historically associated with unsuccessful cytoreduction. Critique of modern surgical techniques and implementation of neoadjuvant chemotherapy for patients with advanced-stage disease have demonstrated limited role for preoperative CA125 in the prediction of surgical outcomes [26, 27]. The prognostic role of CA125 in patients with advanced-stage disease is largely reflected in perioperative changes in this tumor marker. Failure of CA125 levels to regress greater than 80% after primary surgery, including patients with optimal resection, is strongly associated with increased risk of relapse and reduced disease-specific survival [28, 29].

Routine assessment of serum CA125 is crucial to assess disease response in patients receiving active treatment as well as monitoring for disease recurrence in approximately 90% of patients who demonstrate elevations in this marker at time of diagnosis. Increase in serum CA125 levels precedes clinical evidence of disease recurrence by physical examination or imaging in an estimated 80% of patients with ovarian cancer but should not be used as a sole indicator for recurrence [30]. Of note, treatment of recurrent disease at the time of increased CA125 prior to clinical or symptomatic relapse has not been shown to confer a survival benefit [31]. Patients should be thoroughly counseled regarding use and limitations of CA125 in surveillance of ovarian and associated Müllerian malignancies.

18.2.1.4 Endometrial Cancer

Although the role of tumor markers in clinically evident uterine carcinomas is largely limited, CA125 has proven a useful tool in disease prognosis. Elevations in this tumor marker have been well described in advanced and recurrent disease and found in 10–31% of patients [32–34]. For women with newly diagnosed endometrial cancer, preoperative CA125 levels greater than 65 U/mL are associated with a 6.5-fold higher risk of extrauterine disease [32]. Correlation between CA125 and survival has also been demonstrated, as patients with a preoperative serum CA125 less than or equal to 28.5 U/mL have a significantly higher 5-year disease-free survival of 85.6% vs 60% for women with levels above this threshold [35]. While CA125 may serve as a prognostic tool for endometrial cancers, its utility is largely supplemental to existing imaging techniques and surgical staging practices.

18.2.2 HE4

Overexpression of the human epididymis protein 4 (HE4) has recently been identified in epithelial ovarian cancers and may represent a promising opportunity for earlier detection of gynecologic malignancy and disease recurrence. HE4 is among the four-disulfide core family of proteins, composed of two whey acidic protein domains encoded by the *WFDC2* gene (20q12–13.1) and typically confined to urogenital and respiratory epithelia [36]. Similar to CA125, this protein has not been identified on immunohistochemical analysis of normal ovarian surface epithelium but noted to have frequent overexpression within cortical inclusion cysts [36]. HE4 overexpression has been identified in 100% of endometrioid, 93% of serous, and 50% of clear cell ovarian carcinomas but is not characteristically elevated in mucinous tumors [36]. Elevated circulating levels of HE4 have been identified in women with ovarian carcinoma compared to controls as well as patients with endometrial, pulmonary, and breast carcinomas [37, 38].

HE4 interpretation is largely affected by patient menopausal status. An analysis of 1101 healthy women and 67 pregnant women by Moore and colleagues established an HE4 threshold of 89 pmol/L for premenopausal women and 128 pmol/L for postmenopausal women using the 95th percentile as upper limit of normal [39]. Renal failure and advancing age after controlling for menopausal status are associated with an elevated serum HE4 concentration while pregnancy significantly lowers levels [39]. Comparative analyses between HE4 and CA125 of patients with benign gynecologic processes have demonstrated lower HE4 levels in pathologies usually associated with elevated CA125 [7, 40]. Endometriosis is associated with an elevated CA125 in 67% of pathologically confirmed cases compared to 3% for HE4, suggesting improved specificity of this marker in premenopausal women [7]. A meta-analysis demonstrates a pooled sensitivity using HE4 for detection of borderline or invasive ovarian tumors of 75% (95% CI, 0.72–0.76) and pooled specificity of 87% (95% CI, 0.85–0.89) [41]. Approximately 58% of patients with stage I–II EOC will have elevated serum levels of HE4 >140 pmol/L compared to 75.2% of all patients with ovarian malignancy [40].

Given the limitations of CA125 in evaluation of adnexal masses, combined serum testing using CA125 and HE4 to improve accurate detection of early-stage disease has been investigated. Among 233 patients undergoing surgical management for adnexal masses with preoperative CA125, HE4, inhibin, epidermal growth factor, and additional investigational markers, combined CA125 and HE4 demonstrated highest sensitivity of 76.4% (specificity 95%) for ovarian cancer detection [42]. These findings were not supported in a larger analysis conducted by Partheen and colleagues; however further evidence has reinforced improved sensitivity and specificity of HE4 particularly when combined with CA125 [43–46].

Several clinical algorithms using HE4 in combination with other tumor markers have been investigated to stratify patients at increased risk of malignancy with pelvic masses. The risk of ovarian malignancy algorithm (ROMA) incorporates CA125 and HE4 with menopausal status to triage low-risk versus high-risk adnexal masses with a predicted probability of ovarian cancer ranging from 0 to 100% [47]. Among a cohort of 531 women, ROMA preoperatively classified 93.8% of cases of epithelial ovarian cancer as high risk with a sensitivity of 92.3% (95% CI, 85.9–96.4) and specificity of 75% (95% CI, 66.9–81.4) in postmenopausal patients [47]. Subsequent prospective analysis of ROMA did not demonstrate increased detection of ovarian malignancy when compared to CA125 or HE4 alone [48]. The clinical impact of these testing strategies on improved detection of early-stage EOC remains to be elucidated, but evaluation of HE4 may be considered for the differential diagnosis of pelvic masses for postmenopausal women.

HE4 has additionally served a prognostic role in patients with ovarian cancer and may be used to detect disease recurrence. Marked elevations in serum HE4 levels in patients with newly diagnosed ovarian cancer have been associated with higher volume of residual disease after cytoreductive surgery as well as shorter progression-free and overall survival, serving as independent risk factor for poor prognosis [49, 50]. For patients that achieve disease remission, monitoring with regular clinical examination and serum assessment with CA125 levels is standard of care. Evaluations into the incorporation of HE4 into disease surveillance have demonstrated a lead time of 4.5–8 months prior to disease recurrence in patients with ovarian cancer using HE4, generally in advance of rising serum concentrations of CA125 [51, 52].

Further investigational roles for HE4 include evaluation of patients with endometrial cancer as well as differentiation of gastrointestinal carcinomas. While a majority of patients with endometrial cancer will present with abnormal uterine bleeding, upregulation in HE4 has been identified in women with early-stage endometrial cancer compared to benign uterine disease with correlation to depth of myometrial invasion and tumor size [53, 54]. HE4 may additionally aid in differentiation between advanced-stage EOC and ovarian metastases of gastrointestinal carcinomas. Cytologic assessment of patients presenting with malignant ascites secondary to adenocarcinoma of Müllerian or gastrointestinal origin has demonstrated HE4 positivity in 100% of patients with high-grade serous ovarian carcinoma versus 25 and 21% for gastric and colorectal cancers, respectively [55].

18.2.3 Alpha-Fetoprotein

Alpha-fetoprotein (AFP) is an oncofetal protein produced by the fetal yolk sac, liver, and gastrointestinal tract with structural similarity to albumin. AFP reaches peak serum concentration in the fetus at 12 weeks gestation and nadir during infancy. Serum levels are elevated in pregnancy as well as in patients with liver disease and gastric, pancreatic, or colon cancers. Elevations in AFP attributed to gynecologic malignancy are characteristically associated with malignant germ cell tumors of the ovary, particularly endodermal sinus or yolk sac tumors where 90–100% of patients express this marker (Table 18.3) [56, 57]. High levels of AFP have also been identified in approximately 20% of immature teratomas and 10% of embryonal carcinomas. Pretreatment elevation in serum levels of AFP and hCG has been shown to be a significant predictor of overall survival in patients with malignant germ cell tumors of the ovary, and posttreatment surveillance suggests AFP may be used as a reliable indicator of disease recurrence [58, 59].

Table 18.3 Tumor marker expression in ovarian germ cell tumors[a]

	CA125	AFP	hCG	LDH
Dysgerminoma	–	–	±	++
Endodermal sinus tumor (yolk sac tumor)	–	++	±	+
Choriocarcinoma	–	–	++	±
Embryonal carcinoma	–	±	+	–
Immature teratoma	+	+	–	±

AFP alpha-fetoprotein, *hCG* human chorionic gonadotrophin, *LDH* lactate dehydrogenase
[a]Adapted from [56]

18.2.4 Human Chorionic Gonadotropin

Produced by the syncytiotrophoblast in pregnancy, human chorionic gonadotropin (hCG) is a heterodimeric glycoprotein with alpha- and beta-subunits. While the alpha-subunit shares homology with luteinizing hormone, follicle-stimulating hormone, and thyroid-stimulating hormone, the beta-subunit is unique to hCG and degrades into a beta-core fragment detectable in urine assays. Elevations in hCG are alpha characteristically seen in pregnancy, as well as hypothalamic hypogonadism and gynecologic malignancy. hCG primarily serves as a tumor marker for patients with gestational trophoblastic disease, where aberrant expression of hyperglycosylated hCG arising from abnormal proliferation of placental trophoblasts promotes growth and invasion of malignant cells [60]. Current staging criteria for patients with gestational trophoblastic disease incorporate serum hCG levels in risk assessment to guide treatment planning [61]. Continued monitoring of serum quantitative hCG at regular intervals after completion of therapy is crucial to detection of persistent or recurrent disease.

Elevated serum hCG can be detected in patients with malignant germ cell tumors including non-gestational choriocarcinoma, embryonal carcinomas, and occasionally endodermal sinus tumors, with roughly half of patients with stage IC to IV disease expressing this marker [56, 58]. Serum beta-hCG or urinary beta-core fragment has been detected in 68% of ovarian, 51% of endometrial, and 46% of cervical malignancies where it is thought to act as a growth factor or in autocrine fashion to promote angiogenesis and is associated with poorer disease prognosis [62].

18.2.5 Lactate Dehydrogenase

Lactate dehydrogenase (LDH) is a glycolytic enzyme used in conversion of pyruvate to lactate that is often elevated in patients with dysgerminoma of the ovary as well as other disease sites. Multiple isoforms of this enzyme have been identified although greater elevations in LDH1 and LDH2 have been noted in patients with dysgerminomas [63]. Investigations into changes in LDH concentration at time of treatment and disease recurrence suggest that this marker can be effective in surveillance of patients after primary treatment of dysgerminoma, particularly given the paucity of AFP and hCG expression in this tumor type [64, 65].

18.2.6 Inhibin

Inhibin is a heterodimeric peptide hormone produced by granulosa cells of the ovary, acting as an inhibitory signal to prevent secretion of follicle-stimulating hormone from the anterior pituitary gland as well as a paracrine factor regulating folliculogenesis. Expressed with a common alpha-subunit with one of two beta-subunits giving rise to inhibin A and inhibin B isoforms, serum concentration of inhibins A and B varies throughout the menstrual cycle in reproductive-aged women [66]. Granulosa cell tumors of the ovary, even when steroidogenically inactive and lacking estradiol production, are associated with an elevated serum concentration of inhibin [67]. Inhibin levels may be elevated in postmenopausal women with mucinous epithelial cancers, while high preoperative serum concentrations serve as an independent risk factor for survival in women with EOC [68, 69].

Prolonged surveillance of patients with ovarian granulosa cell tumor is essential given an extended median time to disease recurrence of approximately 4.4 years with roughly half of recurrences occurring greater than 5 years from initial diagnosis [70]. Inhibin B has been established as the superior isoform with respect to reflection of disease burden as well as detection of recurrence, which may be identified 11.5 months prior to clinical evidence of disease recurrence [71, 72]. Measurement of anti-Müllerian hormone (AMH), an inhibitory protein also produced by granulosa cells of the ovary in conjunction with inhibin B levels in diagnosis and surveillance of patients with granulosa cell tumors, has been proposed with promising results [73].

18.2.7 Carcinoembryonic Antigen

Carcinoembryonic antigen (CEA) is an oncofetal protein produced by the gastrointestinal system during organogenesis and isolated in small amounts on the luminal side of normal epithelial intestinal cells in the adult colon. This glycoprotein family is involved in cell adhesion, innate immunity, and signal transduction pathways of the gastrointestinal tract [74]. CEA was originally described in 1965 by Gold and Freedman as a serum marker produced in large quantities by carcinoma of the pancreas and colon and is the most commonly elevated marker in colorectal cancers [75]. Current management practices for colorectal cancers include baseline determination of serum CEA with surveillance levels every 3–6 months after completion of therapy [76]. Borderline elevations in this marker can be seen in patients with inflammatory bowel disease, cirrhosis, pancreatitis, and chronic obstructive pulmonary disease as well as heavy tobacco use.

CEA also has clinical utility in evaluation of adnexal masses. Elevations in CEA have been demonstrated in 25–50% of women with EOC, particularly in mucinous carcinomas with as many as 88% demonstrating serum CEA levels greater than 5 ng/mL [77–79]. Patients with mucinous histology and abnormal elevations in CEA may achieve better disease surveillance and detection of recurrence with serial detection of CEA in lieu of CA125. Mucinous borderline ovarian tumors and Brenner tumors of the ovary are also associated with abnormal elevations in CEA. Preoperative elevations in this marker can be identified in 11–33% of women with mucinous borderline ovarian tumors and have been described in up to 80% of patients with Brenner tumors [80–82].

Risk of ovarian metastasis from primary gastrointestinal tumors must also be considered, as 6–9% of ovarian malignancies represent metastasis from primary breast or gastrointestinal disease sites [83]. Women undergoing primary surgical treatment for colorectal cancer will have ovarian metastasis demonstrated in 3.6–7.4% of patients [84]. Findings that are more suggestive of nongynecologic metastasis include younger, premenopausal patients with bilateral adnexal masses with a CA125:CEA ratio less than 25. While serum CEA levels may aid in the differentiation between primary ovarian carcinoma and ovarian metastases of gastrointestinal origin, patterns of CEA expression in benign and malignant gynecologic processes must be considered.

In addition to evaluation of adnexal masses, the use of CEA as a tumor marker in adenocarcinoma of the cervix has been reported but with limited clinical application. An estimated 48% of patients will have increase in serum CEA concentrations in comparison to 71% of patients with elevated CA125 suggesting the latter could be considered in disease surveillance [85].

18.2.8 Carbohydrate Antigen 19-9

An additional marker initially isolated in patients with colorectal and pancreatic carcinomas is carbohydrate antigen 19-9 (CA19-9) [86]. Further investigation of this carbohydrate antigen, also identified as a sialylated Lewis blood group antigen, demonstrated elevated serum concentrations >37 U/mL are associated with gastrointestinal and pancreatic cancer [87]. Increased levels of CA19-9 may also be seen in pancreatitis, cirrhosis, and biliary tract diseases. This antigen was later identified in epithelia of the Müllerian tract, thereby establishing the role of CA19-9 in evaluation in gynecologic diseases [88].

CA19-9 expression has been identified in several benign gynecologic processes. In evaluation of women with pelvic pain, CA19-9 has served as a useful marker in identification of endometriosis and has demonstrated positive correlation with advanced stages of disease [89]. CA19-9 generally is not elevated in cases where uterine leiomyoma or adenomyosis has been identified unlike CA125 [90]. Retrospective analysis of women with mature germ cell teratoma of the ovary identified abnormal elevations in CA19-9 for 37% of patients; however no correlation with presence of squamous cell carcinoma in final pathology has been established [91]. Patients with invasive EOC of the ovary demonstrate histology-specific patterns similar to CEA with propensity for elevated serum levels in mucinous carcinomas. While serum CA19-9 is elevated in 17% of all patients with invasive ovarian carcinoma, 45–52% of patients with borderline serous and mucinous tumors will have abnormally high levels of this marker [80, 81].

18.3 Conclusion

With a multitude of serum assays and commercially available combination biomarker panels, the search for an ideal tumor marker in gynecologic disease is ongoing. The Cancer Genome Atlas (TCGA) and comprehensive genomic analysis of ovarian, endometrial, and cervical cancers has done much for the understanding of the molecular basis of these diseases; however correlation to readily identifiable sensitive and specific biomarker testing is lacking. Growing investigation into elevated circulating microRNAs and their potential role in regulation of oncogenes and tumor-suppressor genes in epithelial ovarian cancer has demonstrated with prospective validation pending [92, 93]. Cell-free DNA has also been identified as a potential target for screening as aberrant mutations or methylation patterns of normal cellular and tumor-derived DNA have been identified in gynecologic cancers via serologic or liquid-based cytologic testing [94]. To date, no single marker has demonstrated greater clinical value or consistency than CA125. With incorporation of newer techniques stemming from better understanding of molecular basis of gynecologic diseases, earlier detection through less invasive testing methods with improved disease survival may soon be accomplished.

Key Points

- Serum tumor markers have a pivotal role in the screening, differential diagnosis, risk stratification, management, and surveillance of gynecologic diseases.
- Ideal screening tests, including use of serum biomarkers, have high sensitivity and high specificity to correctly identify patients with disease and minimize risk of false-positive results that may prompt invasive medical intervention.
- CA125 can be used to identify symptomatic patients with an adnexal mass at increased risk of malignancy but may be artificially elevated by benign gynecologic conditions or medical comorbidities.
- Treatment response and disease surveillance in patients with epithelial ovarian cancers is primarily accomplished by serial assessment of CA125.
- HE4 has demonstrated high sensitivity and specificity for diagnoses of ovarian carcinoma, particularly in combination with serum CA125 assessment.
- Presence and surveillance of germ cell tumors of the ovary may be achieved by serum assessment of AFP, hCG, and LDH.
- Carcinoembryonic antigen and CA19-9 are primary gastrointestinal tumor markers that can help differentiate metastatic disease to the ovary but may also be elevated by borderline ovarian pathology and endometriosis.
- MicroRNAs and cell-free DNA may serve as potential targets for new tumor markers that can aid in detection of gynecologic diseases.
- No perfect serum tumor marker has been identified, and use of tumor markers alone or in conjunction with imaging or combined panel screening requires a comprehensive understanding of processes that lead to spurious results.

References

1. www.who.int/mediacentre/factsheets/fs297/en/. Accessed 13 Mar 2018.
2. Wilson JM, Jungner G. The principles and practice of screening for disease. Geneva: World Health Organization; 1968. p. 66–8.
3. Yin BW, Dnistrian A, Lloyd KO. Ovarian cancer antigen CA125 is encoded by the MUC16 mucin gene. Int J Cancer. 2002;98(5):737–40.
4. Bast RC, Feeney M, Lazarus H, Nadler LM, Colvin RB, Knapp RC. Reactivity of a monoclonal antibody with human ovarian carcinoma. J Clin Invest. 1981;68(5):1331–7.
5. Kabawat SE, Bast RC, Bhan AK, Welch WR, Knapp RC, Colvin RB. Tissue distribution of a coelomic-epithelium-related antigen recognized by the monoclonal antibody OC125. Int J Gynecol Pathol. 1983;2(3):275–85.
6. Grover S, Koh H, Weidemann P, Quinn MA. The effect of menstrual cycle on serum CA125 levels: a population study. Am J Obstet Gynecol. 1992;167:1379–81.
7. Moore RG, Miller MC, Steinhoff MM, Skates SJ, Lu KH, Lambert-Messerlain G, Bast RC Jr. Serum HE4 levels are less frequently elevated than CA125 in women with benign gynecologic disorders. Am J Obstet Gynecol. 2012;206(4):351.e1–8.
8. Jacobs I, Bast RC Jr. The CA 125 tumor-associated antigen: a review of the literature. Hum Reprod. 1989;4(1):1–12.
9. Miralles C, Orea M, España P, Provencio M, Sanchez A, Cantos B, et al. Cancer antigen 125 associated with multiple benign and malignant pathologies. Ann Surg Oncol. 2003;10(2):150–4.
10. Han SN, Lotgerink A, Gziri MM, van Calsteren K, Hanssens M, Amant F. Physiologic variations of serum tumor markers in gynecological malignancies during pregnancy: a systematic review. BMC Med. 2012;10:86.
11. Bast RC, Klug TL, St John E, Jenison E, Niloff JM, Lazarus H, et al. A radioimmunoassay using a monoclonal antibody to monitor the course of epithelial ovarian cancer. N Engl J Med. 1983;309:883–7.
12. Bon GG, Kenemans P, Verstraeten R, van Kamp GJ, Hilgers J. Serum tumor marker immunoassays in gynecologic oncology: establishment of reference values. Am J Obstet Gynecol. 1996;174:107–14.
13. Miller RW, Ueland FR. Risk of malignancy in sonographically confirmed ovarian tumors. Clin Obstet Gynecol. 2012;55:52–64.
14. Moyer VA. Screening for ovarian cancer: U.S. Preventive Services Task Force reaffirmation recommendation statement. U.S. Preventive Services Task Force. Ann Intern Med. 2012;157:900–4.
15. Hirsch M, Duffy J, Davis CJ, Nieves Plana M, Khan KS. Diagnostic accuracy of cancer antigen 125 for endometriosis: a systematic review and meta-analysis. BJOG. 2016;123(11):1761–8.
16. Santulli P, Streuli I, Melonio I, Marcellin L, M'Baye M, Bititi A, et al. Increased serum cancer-antigen 125 is a marker for severity of deep endometriosis. J Minim Invasive Gynecol. 2015;22(2):275–84.
17. Kadan Y, Fiascone S, McCourt C, Raker C, Granai CO, Steinhoff M, et al. Predictive factors for the presence of malignant transformation of pelvic endometriosis. Eur J Obstet Gynecol Reprod Biol. 2015;185:23–7.

18. Dawood MY, Kahn-Dawood FS. Plasma insulin-like growth factor-I, CA-125, estrogen and progesterone in women with leiomyomas. Fertil Steril. 1994;61(4):617–21.
19. Babacan A, Kizilaslan C, Gun I, Muhcu M, Mungen E, Atay V. CA 125 and other tumor markers in uterine leiomyomas and their association with lesion characteristics. Int J Clin Exp Med. 2014;7(4):1078–83.
20. Yilmaz N, Sahin I, Kilic S, Ozgu E, Gungor T, Bilge U. Assessment of the predictivity of preoperative serum CA 125 in the differential diagnosis of uterine leiomyoma and uterine sarcoma in the Turkish female population. Eur J Gynaecol Oncol. 2009;30(4):412–4.
21. Juang CM, Yen MS, Horng HC, Twu NF, Yu HC, Hsu WL. Potential role of preoperative serum CA125 for the differential diagnosis between uterine leiomyoma and uterine leiomyosarcoma. Eur J Gynaecol Oncol. 2006;27(4):370–4.
22. Buys SS, Partridge E, Black A, Johnson CC, Lamerato L, Isaacs C, et al. Effect of screening on ovarian cancer mortality: the Prostate, Lung, Colorectal and Ovarian (PLCO) Cancer Screening Randomized Control Trial. JAMA. 2011;305(22):2295–303.
23. Jacobs IJ, Menon U, Ryan A, Gentry-Maharaj A, Burnell M, Kalski JK, et al. Ovarian cancer screening and mortality in the UK Collaborative Trial of Ovarian Cancer Screening (UKCTOCS): a randomised control trial. Lancet. 2016;387(100022):945–56.
24. Jacobs I, Oram D, Fairbanks J, Turner J, Frost C, Grudzinskas JG. A risk of malignancy index incorporating CA 125, ultrasound and menopausal status for the accurate preoperative diagnosis of ovarian cancer. Br J Obstet Gynaecol. 1990;97(10):922–9.
25. Nagele F, Petru E, Medl M, Kainz C, Graf AH, Sevelda P. Preoperative CA 125: an independent prognostic factor in patients with stage I epithelial ovarian cancer. Obstet Gynecol. 1995;86(2):259–64.
26. Chi DS, Venkatraman ES, Masson V, Hoskins WJ. The ability of preoperative serum CA-125 to predict optimal primary tumor cytoreduction in stage III epithelial ovarian carcinoma. Gynecol Oncol. 2000;77(2):227–31.
27. Nick AM, Coleman RL, Ramirez PT, Sood AK. A framework for personalized surgical approach to ovarian cancer. Nat Rev Clin Oncol. 2015;12(4):239–45.
28. Zivanovic O, Sima CS, Iasonos S, Bell-McGuinn KM, Sabbatini PJ, Leitao MM, et al. Exploratory analysis of serum CA-125 response to surgery and the risk of relapse in patients with FIGO stage IIIC ovarian cancer. Gynecol Oncol. 2009;115(2):209–14.
29. Zwakman N, van de Laar R, van Gorp T, Zusterzeel PL, Snijders MP, Ferreira I, et al. Perioperative changes in serum CA125 levels: a prognostic factor for disease-specific survival in patients with ovarian cancer. J Gynecol Oncol. 2017;28(1):e1–7.
30. Rustin GJ, Marples M, Nelstrop AE, Mahmoudi M, Meyer T. Use of CA-125 to define progression of ovarian cancer in patients with persistently elevated levels. J Clin Oncol. 2001;19:4054–7.
31. Rustin GJ, van der Burg ME, Griffin CL, Guthrie D, Lamont A, Jayson GC, et al. Early versus delayed treatment of relapsed ovarian cancer (MRC OV05/EORTC 55955): a randomized trial. Lancet. 2010;376(9747):1155–63.
32. Sood AK, Buller RE, Burger RA, Dawson JD, Sorosky JI, Berman M. Value of preoperative CA125 level in the management of uterine cancer and prediction of clinical outcome. Obstet Gynecol. 1997;90(3):441–7.
33. Niloff JM, Klug TL, Schaetzl E, Zurawski VR Jr, Knapp RC, Bast RC Jr. Elevation of serum CA125 in carcinomas of the fallopian tube, endometrium and endocervix. Am J Obstet Gynecol. 1984;148(8):1057–8.
34. Rose PG, Sommers RM, Reale FR, Hunter RE, Fournier L, Nelson BE. Serial serum CA 125 measurements for evaluation of recurrence in patients with endometrial carcinoma. Obstet Gynecol. 1994;84(1):12–6.
35. Chung HH, Kim JW, Park NH, Song YS, Kang SB, Lee HP. Use of preoperative serum CA-125 levels for prediction of lymph node metastasis and prognosis in endometrial cancer. Acta Obstet Gynecol Scand. 2006;85(12):1501–5.
36. Drapkin R, von Hortsten HH, Lin Y, Mok SC, Crump CP, Welch WR, et al. Human epididymis protein 4 (HE4) is a secreted glycoprotein that is overexpressed by serous and endometrioid ovarian carcinomas. Cancer Res. 2005;65(6):2162–9.
37. Hellström I, Raycraft J, Hayden-Ledbetter M, Ledbetter JA, Schummer M, McIntosh M, et al. The HE4 (WFDC2) protein is a biomarker for ovarian carcinoma. Cancer Res. 2003;63(13):3695–700.
38. Galgano MT, Hampton GM, Frierson JF Jr. Comprehensive analysis of HE4 expression in normal and malignant human tissues. Mod Pathol. 2006;19:847–53.
39. Moore RG, Miller MC, Eklund EE, Lu KH, Bast RC Jr, Lambert-Messerlain G. Serum levels of the ovarian cancer biomarker HE4 are decreased in pregnancy and increase with age. Am J Obstet Gynecol. 2012;206:349.e1–7.
40. Escudero JM, Auge JM, Filella X, Torne A, Pahisa J, Molina R. Comparison of serum human epididymis protein 4 with cancer antigen 125 as a tumor marker in patients with malignant and nonmalignant diseases. Clin Chem. 2001;57(1):1534–44.
41. Lin J, Qin J, Sangvatanakul V. Human epidiymis protein 4 for differential diagnosis between benign gynecologic disease and ovarian cancer: a systematic review and meta-analysis. Eur J Obstet Gynecol Reprod Biol. 2013;167(1):81–5.
42. Moore RJ, Brown AK, Miller MC, Skates SJ, Allard WJ, Verch T, et al. The use of multiple novel tumor biomarkers for the detection of ovarian carcinoma in patients with a pelvic mass. Gynecol Oncol. 2008;108(2):402–8.
43. Partheen K, Kristjansdottir B, Sundfeldt K. Evaluation of ovarian cancer biomarkers HE4 and CA-125 in

women presenting with a suspicious cystic ovarian mass. J Gynecol Oncol. 2011;22:244–52.
44. Holcomb K, Vucetic Z, Miller MC, Knapp RC. Human epididymis protein 4 offers superior specificity in the differentiation of benign and malignant adnexal masses in premenopausal women. Am J Obstet Gynecol. 2011;205:358.e1–6.
45. Kondalsamy-Chennakesavan S, Hackethal A, Bowtell D, Obermair A, Australian Ovarian Cancer Study Group. Differentiating stage 1 epithelial ovarian cancer from benign ovarian tumours using a combination of tumour markers HE4, CA125 and CEA and patient's age. Gynecol Oncol. 2013;129(3):467–71.
46. Romagnolo C, Leon AE, Fabricio ASC, Taborelli M, Polesel J, del Pup L, et al. HE4, CA125 and risk of ovarian malignancy algorithm (ROMA) as diagnostic tools for ovarian cancer in patients with a pelvic mass: an Italian multicenter study. Gynecol Oncol. 2016;141(2):303–11.
47. Moore RG, McMeekin DS, Brown AK, DiSilvestro P, Miller MC, Allard WJ, et al. A novel multiple marker bioassay utilizing HE4 and CA125 for the prediction of ovarian cancer in patients with a pelvic mass. Gynecol Oncol. 2009;112(1):40–6.
48. van Gorp T, Cadron I, Despierre E, Daemen A, Leunen A, Amant F, et al. HE4 and CA125 as a diagnostic test in ovarian cancer: prospective validation of the Risk of Ovarian Malignancy Algorithm. Br J Cancer. 2011;104(5):863–70.
49. Steffensen KD, Waldstrom M, Brandslund I, Jakobsen A. Prognostic impact of prechemotherapy serum levels of HER2, CA125 and HE4 in ovarian cancer. Int J Gynecol Cancer. 2011;21(6):1040–7.
50. Braicu EI, Fotopoulou C, Van Gorp T, Richter R, Chekerov R, Hall C, et al. Preoperative HE4 expression in plasma predicts surgical outcome in primary ovarian cancer patients: results from the OVCAD study. Gynecol Oncol. 2013;128(2):245–51.
51. Anastasi E, Marchei GG, Viggiani V, Gennarini G, Frati L, Reale MG. HE4: a new potential early biomarker for the recurrence of ovarian cancer. Tumour Biol. 2010;31(2):113–9.
52. Schummer M, Drescher C, Forrest R, Gough S, Thorpe J, Hellström I, et al. Evaluation of ovarian cancer remission markers HE4, MMP7 and mesothelin by comparison to the established marker CA125. Gynecol Oncol. 2012;125:65–9.
53. Simmons AR, Baggerly K, Bast RC Jr. The emerging role of HE4 in the evaluation of advanced epithelial ovarian and endometrial carcinomas. Oncology (Williston Park). 2013;27(6):548–56.
54. Kalogera E, Scholler N, Powless C, Weaver A, Drapkin R, Li J, et al. Correlation of serum HE4 with tumor size and myometrial invasion in endometrial cancer. Gynecol Oncol. 2012;124(2):270–5.
55. Stiekema A, van de Vijver KK, Boot H, Broeks A, Korse CM, van Driel WJ, et al. Human epididymis protein 4 immunostaining of malignant ascites differentiates cancer of Müllerian origin from gastrointestinal cancer. Cancer. 2017;125(3):197–204.
56. Kawai M, Furuhashi Y, Kano T, Misawa T, Nakashima N, Hattori S, et al. Alpha-fetoprotein in malignant germ cell tumors of the ovary. Gynecol Oncol. 1990;39(2):160–6.
57. Gershenson DM. Management of ovarian germ cell tumors. J Clin Oncol. 2007;25(20):2938–43.
58. Murugaesu N, Schmid P, Dancey G, Agarwal R, Holden L, McNeish I, et al. Malignant ovarian germ cell tumors: identification of novel prognostic markers and long-term outcome after multimodality treatment. J Clin Oncol. 2006;24(3):4862–6.
59. Chow SN, Yang JH, Lin YH, Chen YP, Lai JI, Chen RJ, et al. Malignant ovarian germ cell tumors. Int J Gynaecol Obstet. 1996;53(2):151–8.
60. Muller CY, Cole LA. The quagmire of hCG and hCG testing in gynecologic oncology. Gynecol Oncol. 2009;112(3):663–72.
61. FIGO Committee on Gynecologic Oncology. Current FIGO stating for cancer of the vagina, fallopian tube, ovary and gestational trophoblastic neoplasia. Int J Gynaecol Obstet. 2009;105(1):3–4.
62. Cole LA. HCG variants, the growth factors which drive human malignancies. Am J Cancer Res. 2012;2(1):22–35.
63. Skeiko MC, Hart WR. Ovarian germinoma (dysgerminoma) with elevated serum lactic dehydrogenase: case report and review of literature. Cancer. 1982;49(5):944–8.
64. Zondag HA. Enzyme activity in dysgerminoma and seminoma. A study of lactic dehydrogenase isoenzymes in malignant diseases. R I Med J. 1964;47:273–81.
65. Pressley RH, Muntz HG, Falkenberry S, Rice LW. Serum lactate dehydrogenase as a tumor marker in dysterminoma. Gynecol Oncol. 1992;44(3):281–3.
66. Makanji Y, Zhu J, Mishra R, Holmquist C, Wong WPS, Schwartz NB, et al. Inhibin at 90: from discovery to clinical application, a historical review. Endocr Rev. 2014;35(5):747–94.
67. Lappöhn RE, Burger HG, Bouma J, Bangah M, Krans M, de Bruijn HWA. Inhibin as a marker for granulosa-cell tumors. N Engl J Med. 1989;321(12):790–3.
68. Healy DL, Burger HG, Mamers P, Jobling T, Bangah M, Quinn M, et al. Elevated serum inhibin concentration in postmenopausal women with ovarian tumors. N Engl J Med. 1993;329(21):1539–42.
69. Frias AE Jr, Li H, Keeney GL, Podratz KC, Woodruff TK. Preoperative serum level of inhibin A is an independent prognostic factor for the survival of postmenopausal women with epithelial ovarian carcinoma. Cancer. 1999;85(2):465–71.
70. Mangili G, Ottolina J, Gadducci A, Giorda G, Breda E, Savarese A, et al. Long-term follow-up is crucial after treatment for granulosa cell tumours of the ovary. Br J Cancer. 2013;109(1):29–34.
71. Mom CH, Engelen MJ, Willemese PH, Gietema JA, ten Hoor KA, de Vries EG, et al. Granulosa cell tumors of the ovary: the clinical value of serum inhibin A and B levels in a large single center cohort. Gynecol Oncol. 2007;105(2):365–72.

72. Boggess JF, Soules MR, Goff BA, Greer BE, Cain JM, Tamimi HK. Serum inhibin and disease status in women with ovarian granulosa cell tumors. Gynecol Oncol. 1997;64:64–9.
73. Geerts I, Vergoti I, Neven P, Billen J. The role of inhibins B and antimüllerian hormone for the diagnosis and follow-up of granulosa cell tumors. Int J Gynecol Cancer. 2009;19(5):847–55.
74. Hammarström S. The carcinoembryonic antigen (CEA) family: structures, suggested functions and expression in normal and malignant tissues. Semin Cancer Biol. 1999;9(2):67–81.
75. Gold P, Freedman SO. Specific carcinoembryonic antigens of the human digestive system. J Exp Med. 1965;122(3):467–81.
76. Locker GY, Hamilton S, Harris J, Jessup JM, Kemeny N, Macdonald JS, et al. ASCO 2006 update of recommendations for the use of tumor markers in gastrointestinal cancer. J Clin Oncol. 2006;24(33):5313–27.
77. Bast RC Jr, Klug TL, Schaetzl E, Lavin P, Niloff JM, Greber TF, et al. Monitoring human ovarian carcinoma with a combination of CA 125, CA 19-9 and carcinoembryonic antigen. Am J Obstet Gynecol. 1984;149(5):553–9.
78. Panza N, Pacilio G, Campanella L, Peluso G, Battista C, Amoriello A, et al. Cancer antigen 125, tissue polypeptide antigen, carcinoembryonic antigen, and beta-chain human chorionic gonadotropin as serum markers of epithelial ovarian carcinoma. Cancer. 1988;61(1):76–83.
79. Tholander B, Taube A, Lindgren A, Sjöberg O, Stendhal U, Kiviranta A, et al. Pretreatment serum levels of CA-125, carcinoembryonic antigen, tissue polypeptide antigen, and placental alkaline phosphatase, in patients with ovarian carcinoma, borderline tumors, or benign adnexal masses: relevance for differential diagnosis. Gynecol Oncol. 1990;39(1):16–25.
80. Tamakoshi K, Kikkawa F, Shibata K, Tomoda K, Obata NH, Wakahara F, et al. Clinical value of CA125, CA19-9, CEA, CA72-4, and TPA in borderline ovarian tumor. Gynecol Oncol. 1996;62(1):67–72.
81. Engelen MJ, de Bruijn HW, Hollema H, ten Hoor KA, Willemse PH, Aalders JG, et al. Serum CA 125, carcinoembryonic antigen, and CA 19-9 as tumor markers in borderline ovarian tumors. Gynecol Oncol. 2000;78(1):16–20.
82. Fleuren GJ, Nap M. Carcinoembryonic antigen in primary and metastatic ovarian tumors. Gynecol Oncol. 1998;39(3):407–15.
83. Skirnisdottir I, Garmo H, Holmberg L. Non-genital tract metastases to the ovaries presented as ovarian tumors in Sweden 1990-2003: occurrence, origin and survival compared to ovarian cancer. Gynecol Oncol. 2007;105(1):166–71.
84. Miller BE, Pittman B, Wan JY, Fleming M. Colon cancer with metastasis to the ovary at time of initial diagnosis. Gynecol Oncol. 1997;66(3):368–71.
85. Leminen A. Tumor markers CA125, carcinoembryonic antigen and tumor-associated trypsin inhibitor in patients with cervical adenocarcinoma. Gynecol Oncol. 1990;39(3):358–63.
86. Koprowski H, Herlyn M, Steplewski Z, Sears HF. Specific antigen in serum of patients with colon carcinoma. Science. 1981;212(4490):53–5.
87. Steinberg W. The clinical utility of the CA 19-9 tumor-associated antigen. Am J Gastroenterol. 1990;85(4):350–5.
88. Scharl A, Crombach G, Vierbuchen M, Göhring U, Göttert T, Holt JA. Antigen CA 19-9: presence in mucosa of nondiseased müllerian duct derivatives and marker for differentiation in their carcinomas. Obstet Gynecol. 1991;77(4):580–5.
89. Harada T, Kubota T, Aso T. Usefulness of CA19-9 versus CA125 for the diagnosis of endometriosis. Fertil Steril. 2002 Oct;78(4):733–9.
90. Kurdoglu Z, Gursoy R, Kurdoglu M, Erdem M, Erdem O, Erdem A. Comparison of the clinical value of CA19-9 versus CA 125 for the diagnosis of endometriosis. Fertil Steril. 2009;92(5):1761–3.
91. Frimer M, Seagle BL, Chudnoff S, Goldberg GL, Shahabi S. Role of elevated cancer antigen 19-9 in women with mature cystic teratoma. Reprod Sci. 2014 Oct;21(10):1307–11.
92. Zhang B, Cai FF, Zhong XY. An overview of biomarkers for the ovarian cancer diagnosis. Eur J Obstet Gynecol Reprod Biol. 2011;158(2):119–23.
93. Taylor DD, Gercel-Taylor C. MicroRNA signatures of tumor-derived exomes as diagnostic biomarkers of ovarian cancer. Gynecol Oncol. 2008;110(1):13–21.
94. Schwarzenbach H, Hoon DS, Pantel K. Cell-free nucleic acids as biomarkers in cancer patients. Nat Rev Cancer. 2011;11(6):426–37.

19 Screening for Ovarian Cancer

Angelito Magno

19.1 Introduction

There were 239,000 new cases of ovarian cancer and 152,000 deaths from the disease reported worldwide in 2013 [1] with highest rates seen in North America and Eastern and Central Europe with rates of more than 8 per 100,000. In China, the incidence rate showed an ascending trend from 2000 to 2013 with 1.4% annual percentage change. In 2015, 52,000 new cases of ovarian cancer and 22,500 cancer deaths were estimated to occur in China [2].

The lifetime risk of a woman to develop ovarian cancer is 1 in 75 and the risk of death from the disease is 1 in 100. There is only a 2–4% increase in survival rate from 1995 to present even with the advancements in diagnosis and management of ovarian cancer. The overall survival rate of ovarian cancer is 30–40% with 29% of cases diagnosed late [2, 3]. Risk factors for ovarian cancer include family history of breast or ovarian cancer [4], infertility, history of endometriosis, obesity, smoking (for mucinous type) [5], and high-fat diet [6]. Early age of menarche and late menopause, use of hormonal replacement therapy, asbestos and talc exposure, alcohol consumption, and smoking (for other types) have inconsistent data on the risk of ovarian cancer. Lactation [7], tubal ligation [8], and oral contraceptive pills confer protection against ovarian cancer. Aspirin, nonsteroidal anti-inflammatory drugs (NSAIDs) [7], and metformin [5] also give protection against ovarian cancer, but more studies are needed to establish the risk reduction.

Majority of ovarian cancers have epithelial histology with more than 90% of cases followed by sex cord-stromal tumors and germ cell tumors. A huge amount of studies have focused on genetic, diagnosis, and management of epithelial ovarian cancer. A new concept of classification of epithelial ovarian cancer divides all epithelial histologic subtypes into two types, Type 1 and Type 2. Type 1 ovarian cancer is a group of ovarian malignancies where the precursor lesions in the ovary have been identified. This includes mucinous, endometrioid, low-grade serous, clear cell, and transitional carcinomas. Type 2 ovarian cancers, which comprise of high-grade serous carcinomas, undifferentiated carcinomas, and carcinosarcomas, are malignancies where in the precursor lesions have not been yet described and tumors may arise from tubal and/or ovarian surface and/or peritoneal lining [9].

19.2 Ovarian Cancer Screening for General Population

The Prostate, Lung, Colorectal and Ovarian (PLCO) cancer screening trial compared the annual ovarian cancer screening using ultrasound

A. Magno (✉)
Department of Obstetrics and Gynecology, Section of Gynecologic Oncology, De La Salle Health Sciences Institute, De La Salle University Medical Center, Dasmarnas City, Philippines

S. Mehta, A. Singla (eds.), *Preventive Oncology for the Gynecologist*,
https://doi.org/10.1007/978-981-13-3438-2_19

and CA-125 versus the usual care among healthy population (1993–2001) [10]. Of the 39,115 individuals randomized to receive screening, only 29 neoplasms were identified, 20 of which were invasive. The positive predictive value for invasive cancer was 3.7% for abnormal CA-125, 1.0% for abnormal TVU, and 23.5% if both tests are abnormal. The initial report of the study in 2005 recommended long-term follow-up to determine the effect on mortality of ovarian cancer. In 2011, after a median follow-up of 12.4 years (range 10.9–13 years), the PLCO trial did not show reduction in mortality among individuals who have undergone screening with CA-125 and TVU compared to usual care [11]. In addition, the ovarian cancer screening modalities provided high false-positive results (n = 3285) leading to unnecessary surgeries in 1080 subjects with at least 1 serious complication in 15% of subjects. An extended follow-up study on the PLCO subjects with median follow-up period of 14.7 years (maximum 19.3 years) was reported in 2016 [12]. Out of more than 78, 200 subjects, there were 363 deaths (187 from intervention group, screening with TVU and CA-125, and 176 from usual care group) from ovarian cancer for a risk ratio of 1.06. Risk ratios were similar according to length of study years: 0–7 (RR = 10.4), 7–14 (RR = 1.06), and 14+ (RR = 1.09). This extended follow-up study did not show mortality benefit of ovarian cancer screening. The US Preventive Services Task Force recommends against screening for ovarian cancer in general population with D recommendation [13].

Another landmark trial on ovarian cancer screening is the United Kingdom Collaborative Trial of Ovarian Cancer Screening (UKCTOCS) [14]. A total of 202,546 women were randomly allocated to annual multimodal screening (MMS) using serum CA-125 with use of ROCA and annual transvaginal screening (USS) and no screening and analyzed. There were a total of 1282 confirmed ovarian cancer cases (MMS = 338, USS = 314, and no screening = 630), 649 of which died of ovarian cancer (MMS = 148, USS = 154, and no screening = 347). The mortality reduction within 0–14 years using the primary Cox analysis was not significant with 11% (−7 to 27; p = 0.21) in the USS group and 15% (95% CI −3 to 30; p = 0.10) in the MMS group. However, on a secondary analysis excluding prevalent cases (those women with ovarian cancer cases before screening starts), the mortality reduction for MMS was significant [(p = 0.021, 95% CI −2 to 40; 0–7 years after screening = 8% (−27 to 43) and 7–14 years after screening = 28% (−3 to 49)]. This trial showed the delayed mortality reduction after 7 years from screening using TVU and serum CA-125. The summary of PLCO and UKCTOCS trials is in Table 19.1.

19.3 Ovarian Cancer Screening for Women with Increased Risk

Women with increased risk of developing ovarian cancer include those with (1) familial genetic mutation like BRCA 1 and 2 mutation and Lynch syndrome and (2) family history of ovarian cancer.

BRCA 1 and 2 mutation carriers have 11–62% lifetime risk of developing ovarian cancer, whereas patients with hereditary nonpolyposis colorectal cancer (HNPCC or Lynch syndrome) have 10–15% risk [15, 16]. Germline mutation of BRCA 1 and 2 accounts for 5–10% of all ovarian malignancy in the United States, mostly the serous or high-grade histology, which has poor prognosis. Individuals with multiple first- or second-degree blood relatives with ovarian and/or breast cancers are considered high risk for developing the disease.

A group from Massachusetts General Hospital reported a study on the use of Risk of Ovarian Cancer Algorithm (ROCA) with frequent Ca-125 testing in women with increased familial/genetic risk [17]. A new approach on detection of early ovarian cancer among high-risk women includes (1) personalized screening by identifying each woman's baseline Ca-125 and detecting significant rises above the Ca125 baseline, (2) more frequent Ca-125 testing, and (3) transvaginal ultrasound (TVU) only when significant rises in Ca-125 are reached. Ca-125 tests every 3 months

Table 19.1 Summary of PLCO and UKCTOCS trial

	The Prostate, Lung, Colorectal and Ovarian (PLCO) cancer screening trial [11]	UK Collaborative Trial of Ovarian Cancer Screening (UKCTOCS) [14]
Date of accrual	1993–2001	2001–2005
Study design	Randomized controlled trial	Randomized controlled trial
Place	United States (10 screening centers)	United Kingdom (13 centers in National Health Service Trusts in England, Wales, and Northern Ireland)
Age group	55–74 years	50–74 years
Control arm	Usual care	No screening
Intervention arm	Annual screening with CA-125 and TVU	Two arms: 1. Annual TVU screening (USS) 2. Multimodal screening (MMS) (Annual CA-125, ROCA with TVU)
Number of participants	39,105 (intervention group) 39,111 (control group)	USS: 50,623 MMS: 50,624 No screening: 101,299
Primary outcome: Effect on mortality	Intervention: 118 deaths from ovarian cancer (3.1 per 10,000 person-years) Control group: 100 deaths (2.6 per 10,000 person-years) no statistically significant difference	Primary analysis: Mortality reduction, 0–14 years USS = 11% (−7 to 27; $p = 0.21$) MMS = 15% (95% CI −3 to 30; $p = 0.10$) no statistically significant difference Secondary analysis: Mortality reduction with prevalent cases excluded MMS 0–14 years: 20% (95% CI −2 to 40, $p = 0.021$) 0–7 years = 8% (−27 to 43) 7–14 years = 28% (−3 to 49)
Secondary outcome: Ovarian cancer incidence	Intervention: 212 women (5.7 per 10,000 person-years) Control: 176 (4.7 per 10,000 person-years)	
Complication	15% (163/1080) who underwent surgery had at least 1 complication	

were done in 3449 increased familial/genetic risk individuals. ROCA was calculated in every patient with their age and menopausal status and triaged as normal risk (if <1% ROCA), intermediate risk (1–10% ROCA), and elevated risk (>10% ROCA). Transvaginal ultrasound was added to Ca-125 testing to all intermediate-risk individuals, and additional gynecologic oncologist referral was done to all elevated-risk individuals. There were only 19 cases of ovarian cancer detected in this study, 6 of which were diagnosed by long-term screening program (incident cases) and 9 by risk-reducing salpingo-oophorectomy and 4 were prevalent cases (ROCA screen-detected and positive by >35 U/ml rule). Of the 6 incident cases, 3 patients were detected to have ovarian cancer by ROCA even before Ca-125 levels exceed 35 U/ml threshold. Although larger study population is needed, the group recommended the use of ROCA every 3 months for better early-stage sensitivity at high specificity and acceptable positive predictive value compared to Ca-125 > 35 U/ml every 6–12 months.

Another approach for BRCA 1 and 2 mutation carriers is the risk-reducing salpingo-oophorectomy (RRSO). Due to the absence of reliable screening methods for ovarian cancer, the National Comprehensive Cancer Network (NCCN) recommended RRSO after childbearing in increased-risk women [16]. Studies have shown reduction of BRCA 1- and 2-associated ovarian cancer by 80–85% [18, 19]. In a study by Mourits et al., there is a 96% detection of ovarian cancer among women with BRCA 1 or 2 mutation (hazard ratio, 0.21; 95% CI, 0.12–0.39) [20].

For women who did not undergo ovarian cancer risk-reducing surgery, it is recommended to have concurrent transvaginal ultrasound and CA-125 testing every 6 months although newer approach supports for more frequent tumor marker determination (q3 months) starting at age 35 years or 5–10 years earlier than the earliest age of first diagnosis of ovarian cancer in the family [16].

19.4 Risk Assessment in Adnexal Masses

Ovarian masses are a common condition encountered by obstetrician-gynecologists. Most commonly, these masses are incidentally detected on routine physical examination or by ultrasound for other purposes. However, some patients consult for non-specific symptoms like pain and abdominal enlargement. Aside from the absence of effective screening test for ovarian cancer, absence of specific signs and symptoms contribute to its late diagnosis and poor prognosis. The role of obstetrician-gynecologists is to determine if the ovarian mass is benign or malignant to prevent delay in the management and increase the disease prognosis.

19.4.1 Symptoms and Physical Examination

A systematic review by Ebell et al. [21] on symptoms associated with ovarian cancer included 17 case-control and cohort studies for analysis. Symptoms with highest positive likelihood ratios (LR+) include presence of abdominal mass (LR+30), abdominal distention or increased girth (LR+16), abdominal or pelvic pain (LR+10.4), abdominal or pelvic bloating (LR+9.3), loss of appetite (LR+9.2), and family history of ovarian cancer (LR+7.51) with high specificity (range 95–99%) but modest sensitivity for ovarian cancer. Age of >50 years, bowel symptoms, and weight loss only have moderate LR+ (<7). No symptom had a LR of less than 0.5 indicating very little value of ruling out ovarian cancer when the symptom is absent. Goeff and his group developed the Ovarian Cancer Symptom Index (OCSI), a scoring system of symptoms for a period of time. Presence of any of six symptoms (abdominal or pelvic pain, increased abdominal size or bloating, and feeling full or difficulty eating) for less than 1 year and occurring for more than 12 times per month is considered positive. Combining all studies that use the OCSI gives a LR+ of 9. This systematic review relied heavily on case-control and cohort studies which are at risk of biases (i.e., recall bias). Another systematic review was done to determine the accuracy of pelvic examination as a screening test for ovarian cancer and to distinguish benign from malignant ovarian tumor [22]. Eight studies with 36,599 asymptomatic women and 7 studies with 782 symptomatic women were included in the study analysis. The sensitivity and specificity of bimanual examination as screening test for ovarian cancer were 0.44 (95% CI1/40.32, 0.57) and 0.98 (95% CI1/40.97, 0.99), respectively. The positive and negative likelihood ratios were 24.7 (95% CI1/415.8, 37) and 0.57 (95% CI1/40.45, 0.72). This result translates to an increased likelihood of an abnormal pelvic examination to be associated with ovarian cancer, but a negative pelvic examination cannot rule out an ovarian malignancy. With significant heterogeneity in the sensitivity (0.43–0.93), specificity (0.53–0.91), and negative likelihood ratio (0.12–0.62) of studies included, the author concluded that pelvic examination is an unreliable test to differentiate benign ovarian mass from malignant lesions.

19.4.2 Imaging Studies

With symptoms and pelvic examination giving inconclusive results in determining whether an ovarian tumor is benign or malignant, imaging studies aim to help distinguish the two. The International Ovarian Tumor Analysis (IOTA) group has been working on algorithms to calculate risk of malignancy for adnexal masses based on clinical and ultrasound findings. Four algorithms, Simple Rules, Logistic Regression (LR) 1, Logistic Regression (LR) 2, and ADNEX, were developed.

The IOTA Simple Rule relies solely on sonographic descriptions of ovarian masses. It has benign (B) features (unilocular cyst, presence of solid component of maximum diameter of only 7 mm, presence of acoustic shadows, smooth multilocular tumor with largest diameter of <100 mm, and no blood flow on Doppler study) and malignant (M) features (irregular solid tumor, presence of ascites, >4 papillary structures, irregular multilocular solid tumor with largest diameter of >100 mm, and increased blood flow on Doppler study) [23]. Presence of one or more M-features in the absence of any B-feature classified the mass as malignant and warrants gynecologic oncology referral. Presence of one or more B-features in the absence of any M-feature classified the mass a benign thus conservative management by a general gynecologist is an option. But if both B and M-features are present, IOTA finding is inconclusive and warrants referral to an expert sonographer or further evaluation of the tumor. Using this strategy, the reported sensitivity is 95%, specificity 91%, LR+ 10.37, and LR− 0.06. The Royal College of Obstetricians and Gynecologists (RCOG) and American College of Obstetricians and Gynecologists (ACOG) recommended the use of IOTA Simple Rules [24, 25]. The IOTA Simple Rules is easy to use without the need for calculation; however its limitations, aside from being sonographer-dependent, is the absence of estimated risk of malignancy (in %) and presence of inconclusive result.

The IOTA group also developed two Logistic Regression models to calculate % risk of malignancy using both clinical and ultrasound findings [26].

Logistic Regression 1 (LR1) uses 12 variables to calculate the malignant probability. These include:

1. Personal history of ovarian cancer (yes = 1, no = 0)
2. Age of patient (in years)
3. Current hormonal therapy use (yes = 1, no = 0)
4. Presence of ascites (yes = 1, no = 0)
5. Presence of papillations with detectable blood flow (yes = 1, no = 0)
6. Maximal diameter of largest solid component (in mm)
7. Irregular cyst wall (yes = 1, no = 0)
8. Presence of acoustic shadowing (yes = 1, no = 0)
9. Maximum diameter of lesion (in mm)
10. Intratumor color Doppler flow (no flow = 1, minimal = 2, moderate = 3, strong = 4)
11. Presence of abdominal pain during examination (yes = 1, no = 0)
12. Presence of solid tumor (yes = 1, no = 0)

The probability of malignancy can be computed using the equation $y = 1/(1+ e^{-z})$, where $z = -6.7468 + 1.5985\ (1) - 0.9983\ (2) + 0.0326\ (3) + 0.00841\ (4) - 0.8577\ (5) + 1.5513\ (6) + 1.1737\ (7) + 0.9281\ (8) + 0.0496\ (9) + 1.1421\ (10) - 2.3550\ (11) + 0.4916\ (12)$, and e is the mathematical constant and base value of natural logarithms.

The Logistic Regression 2 (LR2) is a simplified LR model using six variables. These variables include (1) age of the patient (in years), (2) presence of ascites (yes = 1, no = 0), (3) presence of papillations with blood flow (yes = 1, no = 0), (4) maximal diameter of largest solid component (in mm), (5) irregular cyst wall (yes = 1, no = 0), and (6) presence of acoustic shadows (yes = 1, no = 0). At a cutoff probability of 10% malignancy, the sensitivity and specificity of M1 and M2 are 92.7% and 74.3% and 89.9% and 70.7%, respectively.

Lastly, the Assessment of Different Neoplasias in the adnexa (ADNEX) model was developed using nine parameters, including:

1. Age of the patient (in years)
2. Presence of oncologic referral center
3. Maximal diameter of the lesion (in mm)
4. Maximal diameter of the largest solid part (in mm)
5. Presence of more than ten locules
6. Presence of acoustic shadow
7. Presence of ascites
8. Number of papillary projections
9. CA-125 value (U/ml)

The ADNEX model detects probability of malignancy in all five main categories, namely, benign, borderline tumor, stage I malignant disease, stage II–IV malignant disease, and metastatic disease. Froyman et al. [27] compared the ADNEX and Simple Rule Risk (SRR/Logistic Regression) models for the diagnosis of early-stage ovarian cancer. Using the 1% risk threshold at 95% CI, the sensitivity of ADNEX and SRR is 100% (98.4–100%) and specificity of 19.4% (17.4–21.5%) and 38% (35.5–40.6%), respectively. Using 30% risk malignancy threshold, the sensitivity and specificity of ADNEX and SRR are 84.5% (80.5–89.6%) and 84.5% (82.6–86.3%) and 88.3% (83.5–91.8%) and 81.1% (79.0–83%), respectively. This study shows that both ADNEX and SRR strategies have good ability to discriminate between stage I–II ovarian cancer and benign adnexal lesion prior to surgery.

Manegold-Brauer reviewed different imaging modalities in characterizing adnexal masses. Magnetic resonance imaging (MRI) is a reliable diagnostic tool for diagnosis of adnexal masses and for tumor staging. Benign MR feature includes high-signal intensity on T1-weighted images and low-signal intensity on T2-weighted images. Malignant morphologic findings on MR include presence of both solid and cystic areas within a mass, necrosis within a solid tumor, septation especially if irregular and thickened, presence of ascites, peritoneal spread, lymph node metastasis, and bilateral adnexal involvement. The sensitivity and specificity of MRI in diagnosing adnexal masses are 91.9% and 88.4%, which is lower than the ultrasound (sensitivity 96% and specificity 90%). The role of computed tomography (CT) scan in ovarian cancer lies on its ability for tumor staging rather than determining the character of adnexal mass. CT scan has sensitivity and specificity of 87.2% and 84.0%, respectively. A more recent imaging tool developed is the F-fluorodeoxyglucose positron emission tomography/CT (FDG-PET/CT) combining metabolic and physical characteristics of the tumor. The principle of FDG-PET lies on the increased glucose (FDG, a glucose analogue) metabolism of most tumor cells combined with the accurate anatomic localization of areas with increased FDG uptake from the CT scan. Limitation of this diagnostic tool is its non-specificity to malignancy. Physiologic uptake of the uterus and ovaries on certain menstrual cycle days and infectious process can have increased FDG uptake causing false-positive result. FDG-PET/CT has a sensitivity of 97.9% and specificity of 73.3%. High cost of this imaging tool also limits its use in gynecologic cancer evaluation [23].

19.4.3 Tumor Markers

Tumor markers are soluble glycoproteins released in the blood in different conditions and detected by monoclonal antibodies during tumor marker testing. Every tumor marker has its own diagnostic, prognostic, and treatment response and recurrence monitoring benefits. In epithelial ovarian cancer, the most common tumor marker used is cancer antigen 125 (CA-125). CA-125 is a glycoprotein expressed in coelomic epithelium during fetal development. Increased CA-125 is associated with epithelial ovarian cancer. However, other malignancies (gynecologic cancers: fallopian tube, primary peritoneal, and advanced endometrial carcinoma; non-gynecologic cancers—breast, lung, gastric, hepatic, and pancreatic cancers) and benign conditions (uterine myoma, pregnancy, menstruation, pelvic inflammatory disease, endometriosis) can increase CA-125 level [28]. A normal value of CA-125 is <35 U/ml, but with the level of >200 U/ml, the likelihood of a benign cause of elevation is unlikely with 80% at this level associated with ovarian cancer and 50% associated with early-stage disease.

Another tumor marker evaluated to differentiate benign from malignant epithelial ovarian tumor is the human epididymal protein 4 (HE4). The normal value threshold for HE4 is 140 pmol/L. Glycosylated HE4 is secreted and detectable in the bloodstream or urine of patients with ovarian carcinoma. However, expression of HE4 has been reported also in pulmonary, endometrial, and breast adenocarcinomas, mesotheliomas, and gastrointestinal and renal carcinomas. Renal failure is a major nonmalignant cause of elevated HE4; thus HE4 results in patients with creatinine concentration more than 1.3 mg/dL (115 umol/L) should be evaluated with caution. CA-125 and HE4 were compared to determine which of the two tumor markers has higher specificity. HE4 was increased in 12.3% of benign diseases and in only 1.3% of gynecologic cases, whereas CA-125 was increased in 37% of benign conditions and in 33.2% of gynecologic conditions. HE4 is less influenced by gender, menopausal status, and presence of liver disease but strongly affected by presence of renal failure [29]. Authors recommended a combination of CA-125 and HE4 testing to increase the detection of malignant ovarian tumor [29, 30]. Comparing CA125 to HE4 in distinguishing benign from malignant tumors, HE4 has higher sensitivity in ruling out benign conditions including endometriosis (97.6 vs. 71.3%), but CA-125 correctly classified a higher percentage of malignant ovarian masses as compared to HE4 (90.7% vs. 71.2%; $p < 0.001$) [31].

19.4.4 Risk of Malignancy Index (RMI) and Risk of Ovarian Malignancy Algorithm (ROMA)

The Risk of Malignancy Index (RMI) utilizes menopausal status, ultrasound findings, and CA-125 level in predicting epithelial ovarian cancer. Ultrasound findings such as multiloculated cyst, solid areas, positive metastasis, positive ascites, and bilateral ovarian lesion each have 1 point. Absence of any of the ultrasound finding gets a score of 0, and presence of 1 finding gives a score of 1 and score of 3 for presence of 2 or more ultrasound findings. Premenopausal status is given a score of 1, whereas menopausal status gets a score of 3. CA-125 level is taken as absolute value (Table 19.2). RMI is computed by multiplying the ultrasound score to menopausal status score and CA-125 level. A score of more than 200 indicates malignancy with sensitivity of 85% and specificity of 97%. The Risk of Ovarian Malignancy Algorithm utilizes menopausal status and CA-125 and HE4 levels in predicting epithelial ovarian cancer. For premenopausal

Table 19.2 Risk of Malignancy Index

Ultrasound (U)	Ultrasound findings
0 = for score of 0	Multiloculated cyst
1 = for score of 1	Solid areas
3 = for score of 2–5	Positive metastasis
	Positive ascites
	Bilateral lesions (1 point for each finding)
Menopausal status	1 = premenopausal
	3 = menopausal
CA-125	Serum level

Computation for RMI = U × M × CA-125
Cut-off is 200; >200 indicates malignancy with sensitivity of 85% and specificity of 97%

women, ROMA value of >7.4% is considered high risk for malignancy and <7.4% is low risk. For postmenopausal women, ROMA value of >25.3% is considered high risk and <25.3% is low risk for malignancy.

A study of 128 subjects was done to determine the accuracy of CA-125, HE4, ROMA, and RMI in distinguishing malignant from benign ovarian masses. The sensitivity of CA-125, HE4, ROMA, and RMI in distinguishing benign from malignant masses (including low malignant potential) is 70.4%, 79.6%, 74.1%, and 63%, respectively. If the low malignant potential tumors are classified as benign, the sensitivities for CA-125, HE4, ROMA, and RMI were increased to 83.8%, 86.5%, 83.8%, and 75.7%, respectively. These sensitivities were further increased to 93.5%, 87.1%, 95.2%, and 87.1% when CA-125, HE4, ROMA, and RMI were used to discriminate among primary ovarian carcinomas. The study reported similar level of accuracy in differentiating adnexal masses. RMI is found to have the lowest sensitivity of the four parameters but with the best numeric accuracy. HE4 demonstrated the best sensitivity in evaluation of malignant ovarian tumor and ruling out endometriosis [32].

Another study of 349 subjects (pre- and postmenopausal women and aged 18 or older) who underwent surgical removal of adnexal mass was done using CA-125 and HE4 and calculated ROMA to determine accuracy of the 3 parameters in discriminating benign from malignant adnexal tumor. The resultant accuracy (using receiver operating characteristics, ROC area) values were all high for CA-125, HE4, and ROMA with values ranging from 84% to 97%. Regardless of the menopausal status, ROMA has higher accuracy than CA-125 (92.9 vs. 89.9%, $p = 0.040$) but not compared to HE4. In postmenopausal women, ROMA also has better accuracy (93.3% vs. 90.3%, $p = 0.0018$) but not for HE4 (91.5%, $p = 0.199$), but comparing CA-125 to HE4, they are statistically similar. For premenopausal women, CA-125, HE4, and ROMA have statistically similar accuracy [31].

Table 19.3 ACOG Guidelines for Gynecologic Oncology Consultation

ACOG Guideline for Gynecologic Oncology Consultation [33]	
Premenopausal women	1. Very elevated CA-125 (>67 U/ml) 2. Ascites 3. Evidence of abdominal or distant metastasis
Postmenopausal women	1. Elevated CA-125 (>35 U/ml) 2. Nodular or fixed pelvic mass 3. Ascites 4. Evidence of abdominal or distant metastasis

19.4.5 Multimodel Marker

A newer concept in diagnosis of ovarian malignancy is the combination of multiple tumor markers and analyzed by multivariate analysis. Multivariate index assay (MIA, commercially available as Ova1) is a US Food and Drug Authority (FDA)-cleared assay that incorporates CA-125 (CA-125-II), transferrin, transthyretin (prealbumin), apolipoprotein A1, and beta-2-microglobulin. The results of this assay is calculated using the OvaCal software (Vermillion, Inc., Austin, TX) using a multivariate algorithm to compute for ovarian cancer risk score (0.0–10.0). MIA score of >5.0 (premenopausal) or >4.4 (postmenopausal) is considered high risk for ovarian malignancy. A study of 770 subjects compared MIA to CA-125, clinical assessment (physical examination, family history, imaging and laboratory test including CA-125 except MIA), and modified-ACOG (Table 19.3) referral guidelines in triaging a patient for gynecologic oncology referral. MIA resulted to a statistically significantly higher sensitivity (90.2%, 95% CI 84.7–93.9) compared with CA125 (68.4%, 95% CI, 60.8–74.9), clinical assessment (73.2%, 95% CI, 65.9–79.4), and modified-ACOG guidelines (79.3%, 95% CI, 72.4–84.8) ($P < 0.0001$). Specificity of MIA is statistically significantly lower compared to the other three parameters. This means that MIA has the highest accuracy of ruling out nonmalignant ovarian tumor compared to CA-125, clinical assessment, and modified-ACOG guidelines [33]. In clinical practice, MIA may change the referral behavior of non-gynecologic oncologists to gynecologic oncologists once MIA determines that a tumor is high risk for malignancy. A Chinese group evaluated CA-125, HE4, progesterone (Prog), and estradiol (E2) for differentiating pelvic masses in postmenopausal women. Progesterone is considered a protective factor against ovarian cancer progression. Its level is inversely correlated with the risk of ovarian cancer. Estradiol, on the other hand, reduces gonadotrophin levels, which is the main culprit in ovarian malignancy. Reduction in gonadotrophin level leads to prevention of ovarian epithelial cell stimulation avoiding ovarian cancer formation. The study was divided into building differentiation model phase and validation model phase. CA-125, HE4, progesterone, and estradiol were detected in 57 patients with benign pelvic mass and 92 patients with epithelial ovarian cancer (EOC). Sixty-six percent (66%) of the samples were used during the building differentiation model phase, and the remaining 33% were used during validation model phase. Combination of HE4 + CA-125 + E2 was chosen to have the best multi-marker model. During the building differentiation model phase, the area under the curve of HE4 + CA-125 + E2 model was 0.97 (0.93–1.00) with sensitivities distinguishing benign pelvic mass from EOC, from early EOC, and from advanced EOC of 90.16, 86.2, and 95.6%, respectively, and specificities of 92.1, 92.1, and 92.1%, respectively. During the validation model phase, the sensitivities and specificities of HE4 + CA-125 + E2 model for distinguishing benign pelvic masses

Table 19.4 Tumor markers for other types of ovarian cancer

Carcinoembryonic antigen (CEA) Cancer antigen (CA) 19–9	Mucinous histology (mucinous ovarian tumor, appendiceal cancer, pancreatic and gastrointestinal cancer)
Lactate dehydrogenase (LDH)	Dysgerminoma, mixed germ cell tumor
Inhibin B	Granulosa cell tumor
Beta-HCG	Choriocarcinoma, mixed germ cell tumor
Alpha-fetoprotein (AFP)	Yolk sac tumor/endodermal sinus tumor, polyembryonal tumor, immature teratoma

from EOC, from early EOC, and from advanced EOC were 96.7 and 84.2%, 100 and 100%, and 87.5 and 84.2%, respectively. This multi-marker model utilizes different tumor markers from what was used by Bristow et al., and the result also showed improvement in differentiation of benign from malignant masses compared to CA-125 or HE4 alone [34].

A second-generation multivariate index assay (MIA) was cleared by FDA to be commercially available (as Overa), and it utilizes individual markers CA125-II, HE4, apolipoprotein A-1, follicle-stimulating hormone, and transferrin. Sensitivity and specificity of Overa were 91% and 69%, respectively [35–37].

Other tumor markers used in other less common types of ovarian cancers are enumerated in Table 19.4.

19.4.6 Intraoperative Frozen Section

Despite all the advancement in imaging studies and tumor markers, there are times that an adnexal mass is difficult to classify as benign or malignant. Utilization of intraoperative frozen section analysis has been studied by many groups, many of which were included in a systemic review published in Cochrane Library [38]. The group aims to assess the diagnostic test accuracy of frozen section to diagnose ovarian cancer in women with suspicious pelvic masses. Thirty-eight studies from 1946 to 2015 with 11,181 participants were included. The review reported an average sensitivity of 90.0% (95% CI 87.6–92.0%; range of 71–100%) and average specificity 99.5% (95% CI 99.2–99.7%; range 96–100%) of frozen section analysis to differentiate invasive tumor from borderline and benign tumor combined. When differentiating invasive and borderline ovarian tumors from benign, the average sensitivity of frozen section analysis is 96.5% (95% CI 95.5–97.3%; range 83–100%) and average specificity of 89.5% (95% CI 86.6–91.9%; range 58–99%). The review also reported that 94% of benign tumors and 99% of invasive tumors were correctly diagnosed as benign and invasive by frozen section compared to the final paraffin report. However, 21% of borderline tumor in frozen section later read as invasive cancer in the final report.

19.5 Conclusion

The lifetime risk of a woman to develop ovarian cancer is 1 in 75 and the risk of death from the disease is 1 in 100. The overall survival rate of ovarian cancer is 30–40% with 29% of cases diagnosed late [39]. Screening for ovarian cancer in general population is not advocated. In the high-risk group, ultrasonography and CA-125 every 6 months starting 35 years or 5–10 years earlier than the age of the first reported ovarian cancer in the family is recommended. Due to the absence of reliable screening methods for ovarian cancer, NCCN recommends risk-reducing salpingo-oophorectomy after childbearing in increased-risk women. Risk assessment of ovarian masses can be done using RMI or ROCA. A summary of recommendations for ovarian cancer screening is shown in Table 19.5.

Key Points

- Risk factors for ovarian cancer include family history of breast or ovarian cancer, infertility, history of endometriosis, obesity, smoking (for mucinous type), and high-fat diet. Early age of menarche and late menopause, use of hormonal replacement therapy, asbestos and talc exposure, alcohol consumption, and

Table 19.5 Summary of recommendations for ovarian cancer screening

General population	Recommend against routine screening [13]
Increased-risk individuals	• TVU + CA-125 every 6 months starting 35 years OR 5–10 years earlier than the age of the first reported ovarian cancer in the family [16] (benefit of more frequent CA-125 q3 month is reported) [17] • Risk-reducing salpingo-oophorectomy [16]
Management of adnexal masses	• TVUTS: IOTA strategies • Tumor markers: CA-125 and HE4 or other more appropriate tumor marker for age and ultrasound picture of the masses • Computation of RMI and ROCA • Utilization of frozen section during surgery

smoking (for other types) have inconsistent data on the risk of ovarian cancer.

- Majority of ovarian cancers have epithelial histology with more than 90% of cases followed by sex cord-stromal tumors and germ cell tumors.
- Screening for ovarian cancer in general population is not advocated.
- In the high-risk group, ultrasonography and CA-125 every 6 months starting 35 years or 5–10 years earlier than the age of the first reported ovarian cancer in the family is recommended.
- In epithelial ovarian cancer, the most common tumor markers used are cancer antigen 125 (CA-125) and human epididymal protein 4 (HE4).
- International ovarian tumor analysis (IOTA) group has given algorithms to calculate risk of malignancy for adnexal masses based on clinical and ultrasound findings. Four algorithms, simple rules, logistic regression (LR)1, logistic regression (LR) 2, and ADNEX, are being used.
- The risk of malignancy index (RMI) utilizes menopausal status, ultrasound findings, and CA-125 level in predicting epithelial ovarian cancer. A score of more than 200 indicates malignancy with sensitivity of 85% and specificity of 97%.
- The risk of ovarian malignancy algorithm (ROMA) utilizes menopausal status and CA-125 and HE4 levels in predicting epithelial ovarian cancer. For premenopausal women, ROMA value of >7.4% is considered high risk for malignancy and < 7.4% is low risk. For postmenopausal women, ROMA value of >25.3% is considered high risk and < 25.3% is low risk for malignancy.
- Multivariate index assay (MIA, commercially available as Ova1) is a multimodel assay that incorporates CA-125, transferrin, transthyretin (prealbumin), apolipoprotein A1, and beta-2-microglobulin and computes for ovarian cancer risk score using a multivariate algorithm.

References

1. Torre LA, Bray F, Siegel RL, Ferlay J, Lortet-Tieulent J, Jemal A. Global cancer statistics, 2012. CA Cancer J Clin. 2015;65(2):87–108.
2. Jiang X, Tang H. Epidemiology of gynecologic cancers in China. J Gynecol Oncol. 2018;29(1):e7.
3. Reid BM, Permuth JB, Sellers TA. Epidemiology of ovarian cancer: a review. Cancer Biol Med. 2017;14(1):9–32.
4. Pal T, Permuth-Wey J, Betts JA, Krischer JP, Fiorica J, Arango H, et al. BRCA1 and BRCA2 mutations account for a large proportion of ovarian carcinoma cases. Cancer. 2005;104(12):2807–16.
5. Viswanathan A, Kim DH, Reid N, Kline DG. Surgical management of the pelvic plexus and lower abdominal nerves. Neurosurgery. 2009;65(4 Suppl):A44–51.
6. Huncharek M, Kupelnick B. Dietary fat intake and risk of epithelial ovarian cancer: a meta-analysis of 6,689 subjects from 8 observational studies. Nutr Cancer. 2001;40(2):87–91.
7. Crew KD, Neugut AI. Aspirin and NSAIDs: effects in breast and ovarian cancers. Curr Opin Obstet Gynecol. 2006;18(1):71–5.
8. Kjaer SK, Mellemkjaer L, Brinton LA, Johansen C, Gridley G, Olsen JH. Tubal sterilization and risk of ovarian, endometrial and cervical cancer. A Danish population-based follow-up study of more than 65 000 sterilized women. Int J Epidemiol. 2004;33(3):596–602.
9. Koshiyama M, Matsumura N. Recent concepts of ovarian carcinogenesis: type I and type II. Biomed Res Int. 2014;2014:934261.

10. Buys SS, Partridge E, Greene MH, Prorok PC, Reding D, Riley TL, et al. Ovarian cancer screening in the Prostate, Lung, Colorectal and Ovarian (PLCO) cancer screening trial: findings from the initial screen of a randomized trial. Am J Obstet Gynecol. 2005;193(5):1630–9.
11. Buys SS, Partridge E, Black A, Johnson CC, Lamerato L, Isaacs C, et al. Effect of screening on ovarian cancer mortality: the Prostate, Lung, Colorectal and Ovarian (PLCO) cancer screening randomized controlled trial. JAMA. 2011;305(22):2295–303.
12. Pinsky PF, Prorok PC, Yu K, Kramer BS, Black A, Gohagan JK, et al. Extended mortality results for prostate cancer screening in the PLCO trial with median follow-up of 15 years. Cancer. 2017;123(4):592–9.
13. Moyer VA. Screening for ovarian cancer: U.S. Preventive Services Task Force reaffirmation recommendation statement. Ann Intern Med. 2012;157(12):900–4.
14. Jacobs IJ, Menon U, Ryan A, Gentry-Maharaj A, Burnell M, Kalsi JK, et al. Ovarian cancer screening and mortality in the UK Collaborative Trial of Ovarian Cancer Screening (UKCTOCS): a randomised controlled trial. Lancet. 2016;387(10022):945–56.
15. Mills K, Fuh K. Recent advances in understanding, diagnosing, and treating ovarian cancer. F1000Res. 2017;6:84.
16. Daly M, Allen J, Axilbund J, Buys S, Crawford B, Farrell C, et al. NCCN clinical practice guidelines in oncology: genetic/familial high-risk assessment: breast and ovarian (version 1/2011). Fort Washington: National Comprehensive Cancer Network; 2011.
17. Skates SJ, Greene MH, Buys SS, Mai PL, Brown P, Piedmonte M, et al. Early detection of ovarian cancer using the risk of ovarian cancer algorithm with frequent CA125 testing in women at increased familial risk - combined results from two screening trials. Clin Cancer Res. 2017;23(14):3628–37.
18. Rebbeck TR, Kauff ND, Domchek SM. Meta-analysis of risk reduction estimates associated with risk-reducing salpingo-oophorectomy in BRCA1 or BRCA2 mutation carriers. J Natl Cancer Inst. 2009;101(2):80–7.
19. Kauff ND, Domchek SM, Friebel TM, Robson ME, Lee J, Garber JE, et al. Risk-reducing salpingo-oophorectomy for the prevention of BRCA1- and BRCA2-associated breast and gynecologic cancer: a multicenter, prospective study. J Clin Oncol. 2008;26(8):1331–7.
20. Mourits MJ, de Bock GH. European/U.S. comparison and contrasts in ovarian cancer screening and prevention in a high-risk population. Am Soc Clin Oncol Educ Book. 2017;37:124–7.
21. Ebell MH, Culp MB, Radke TJ. A systematic review of symptoms for the diagnosis of ovarian cancer. Am J Prev Med. 2016;50(3):384–94.
22. Ebell MH, Culp M, Lastinger K, Dasigi T. A systematic review of the bimanual examination as a test for ovarian cancer. Am J Prev Med. 2015;48(3):350–6.
23. Manegold-Brauer G, Bellin AK, Tercanli S, Lapaire O, Heinzelmann-Schwarz V. The special role of ultrasound for screening, staging and surveillance of malignant ovarian tumors: distinction from other methods of diagnostic imaging. Arch Gynecol Obstet. 2014;289(3):491–8.
24. Kaloo PL, Khazali S, Hoy D, Sadoon S. Management of suspected ovarian masses in premenopausal women. 2011.
25. American College of Obstetricians and Gynecologists' Committee on Practice Bulletins—Gynecology. Practice Bulletin No. 174: evaluation and management of adnexal masses. Obstet Gynecol. 2016;128(5):e210–e26.
26. Timmerman D, Testa AC, Bourne T, Ferrazzi E, Ameye L, Konstantinovic ML, et al. Logistic regression model to distinguish between the benign and malignant adnexal mass before surgery: a multicenter study by the International Ovarian Tumor Analysis Group. J Clin Oncol. 2005;23(34):8794–801.
27. Timmerman D, Van Calster B, Testa A, Savelli L, Fischerova D, Froyman W, et al. Predicting the risk of malignancy in adnexal masses based on the simple rules from the International Ovarian Tumor Analysis group. Am J Obstet Gynecol. 2016;214(4):424–37.
28. Perkins GL, Slater ED, Sanders GK, Prichard JG. Serum tumor markers. Am Fam Physician. 2003;68(6):1075–82.
29. Escudero JM, Auge JM, Filella X, Torne A, Pahisa J, Molina R. Comparison of serum human epididymis protein 4 with cancer antigen 125 as a tumor marker in patients with malignant and nonmalignant diseases. Clin Chem. 2011;57(11):1534–44.
30. Park Y, Lee JH, Hong DJ, Lee EY, Kim HS. Diagnostic performances of HE4 and CA125 for the detection of ovarian cancer from patients with various gynecologic and non-gynecologic diseases. Clin Biochem. 2011;44(10–11):884–8.
31. Sandri MT, Bottari F, Franchi D, Boveri S, Candiani M, Ronzoni S, et al. Comparison of HE4, CA125 and ROMA algorithm in women with a pelvic mass: correlation with pathological outcome. Gynecol Oncol. 2013;128(2):233–8.
32. Anton C, Carvalho FM, Oliveira EI, Maciel GA, Baracat EC, Carvalho JP. A comparison of CA125, HE4, risk ovarian malignancy algorithm (ROMA), and risk malignancy index (RMI) for the classification of ovarian masses. Clinics (Sao Paulo). 2012;67(5):437–41.
33. Bristow RE, Hodeib M, Smith A, Chan DW, Zhang Z, Fung ET, et al. Impact of a multivariate index assay on referral patterns for surgical management of an adnexal mass. Am J Obstet Gynecol. 2013;209(6):581.e1–8.
34. Zhang P, Wang C, Cheng L, Zhang P, Guo L, Liu W, et al. Development of a multi-marker model combining HE4, CA125, progesterone, and estradiol for distinguishing benign from malignant pelvic masses in postmenopausal women. Tumour Biol. 2016;37(2):2183–91.

35. Ueland FR. A perspective on ovarian cancer biomarkers: past, present and yet-to-come. Diagnostics (Basel). 2017;7(1):E14.
36. Coleman RL, Herzog TJ, Chan DW, Munroe DG, Pappas TC, Smith A, et al. Validation of a second-generation multivariate index assay for malignancy risk of adnexal masses. Am J Obstet Gynecol. 2016;215(1):82.e1–e11.
37. Bristow RE, Smith A, Zhang Z, Chan DW, Crutcher G, Fung ET, et al. Ovarian malignancy risk stratification of the adnexal mass using a multivariate index assay. Gynecol Oncol. 2013;128(2):252–9.
38. Ratnavelu ND, Brown AP, Mallett S, Scholten RJ, Patel A, Founta C, et al. Intraoperative frozen section analysis for the diagnosis of early stage ovarian cancer in suspicious pelvic masses. Cochrane Database Syst Rev. 2016;3:Cd010360.
39. Siegel R, Ma J, Zou Z, Jemal A. Cancer statistics, 2014. CA Cancer J Clin. 2014;64(1):9–29.

Prevention of Ovarian Cancer

20

Sarika Gupta, Sarfraz Ahmad, and Lorna A. Brudie

20.1 Introduction

Ovarian cancer is one of the leading causes of cancer-related death in women. As per the American Cancer Society, 22,240 new cases of ovarian cancer will be diagnosed in 2018, and 14,070 women will die of ovarian cancer in the United States [1]. More than 70% of ovarian cancer cases are diagnosed in the advanced stages when cure rates for ovarian cancer are rather dismal despite multimodality treatment modalities. The incidence of ovarian cancer can be reduced by controlling risk factors and detecting the preinvasive disease. However, complex and diverse pathogenesis of ovarian cancer is a major barrier to develop homogeneous prediction models and screening tools. Targeted preventative program appears to be the most effective strategy to reduce the incidence, morbidity, and mortality from this lethal cancer.

20.2 Risk Factors, Precursor Lesions, and Carcinogenesis

Knowledge of the risk factors and precursor lesions is the elemental step in preventing cancer. Older age, nulliparity, null lactation, cigarette smoking, alcohol, obesity, low dietary fat, and relatively long-term hormone replacement therapy (HRT) are among the few important risk factors associated with ovarian cancer [2–4]. These factors have been found to have a modest association with certain non-serous histologies, rather than more aggressive serous carcinoma [5, 6]. Hereditary mutations are the strongest known risk factors for ovarian cancer. It is estimated that around 15% of women with ovarian cancer have family history of two or more relatives with breast or ovarian cancer or breast cancer (BRCA) 1/2 or hereditary nonpolyposis colorectal cancer (HNPCC) germline mutations [7].

Earlier, ovarian carcinoma was considered to arise directly from the ovarian surface epithelium, its intraparenchymal inclusions, or from a preexisting benign ovarian cyst [8]. In 1999, Dubeau et al. proposed that the Müllerian epithelium could have a role in ovarian carcinogenesis [9]. Numerous subsequent studies

S. Gupta (✉)
Department of Gynecology, Indraprastha Apollo Hospital, New Delhi, India

S. Ahmad
Department of Gynecologic Oncology, Florida Hospital (AdventHealth) Cancer Institute, Florida State University, Orlando, FL, USA

Department of Gynecologic Oncology, Colleges of Medicine, University of Central Florida, and Florida State University, Orlando, FL, USA

L. A. Brudie
Department of Gynecologic Oncology, Orlando Health UF Health Cancer Center, Orlando, FL, USA

S. Mehta, A. Singla (eds.), *Preventive Oncology for the Gynecologist*,
https://doi.org/10.1007/978-981-13-3438-2_20

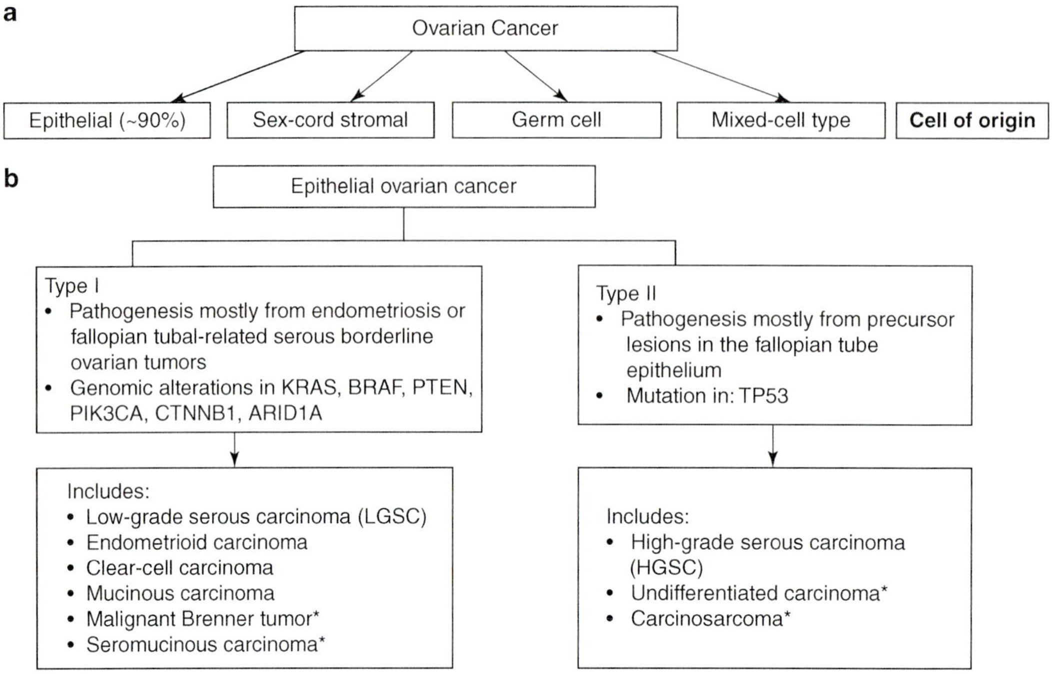

Fig. 20.1 Clinicopathologic and molecular classification of ovarian cancer. (**a**) Classification of ovarian cancer. (**b**) Classification of epithelial ovarian cancer. Adapted from [16]

suggested that the cells of origin of serous, endometrioid, and clear cell carcinomas are derived from the fallopian tube and the endometrium [10–13].

It is notable that the previous subclassification of epithelial ovarian cancer into serous, endometrioid, clear cell, mucinous, and malignant Brenner tumors and mixed histologies has been abandoned after a series of research papers reported on molecular pathology of ovarian cancer [14, 15]. The World Health Organization (WHO) has revised the classification according to the clinical, pathologic precursor, and molecular characteristics (Fig. 20.1). Type I tumors are clinically indolent and detected in the early-stage of the disease. In contrast, Type II tumors are aggressive and detected in the advanced stages of the disease. Type I tumors are thought to originate from benign lesions like endometriosis or borderline tumors. In contrast, most of the Type II tumors are thought to originate from serous tubal intraepithelial carcinoma (Fig. 20.2). Mutations associated with the Type I tumors usually involve *KRAS*, *BRAF*, *PTEN*, *PIK3CA*, *CTNNB1*, *ARID1A*, and *PPP2R1A* genes. Type II tumors mostly have p53 gene mutations. Low-grade serous, low-grade endometrioid, clear cell, mucinous, and malignant Brenner tumors are categorized as Type I. The Type II ovarian tumors comprise of high-grade serous, high-grade endometrioid, and undifferentiated carcinomas as well as malignant mixed mesodermal tumors (carcinosarcoma). This new classification that divides ovarian neoplasm into the two types enables the clinicians to predict accurate prognosis and devise superior prevention and management strategies [16] (Table 20.1).

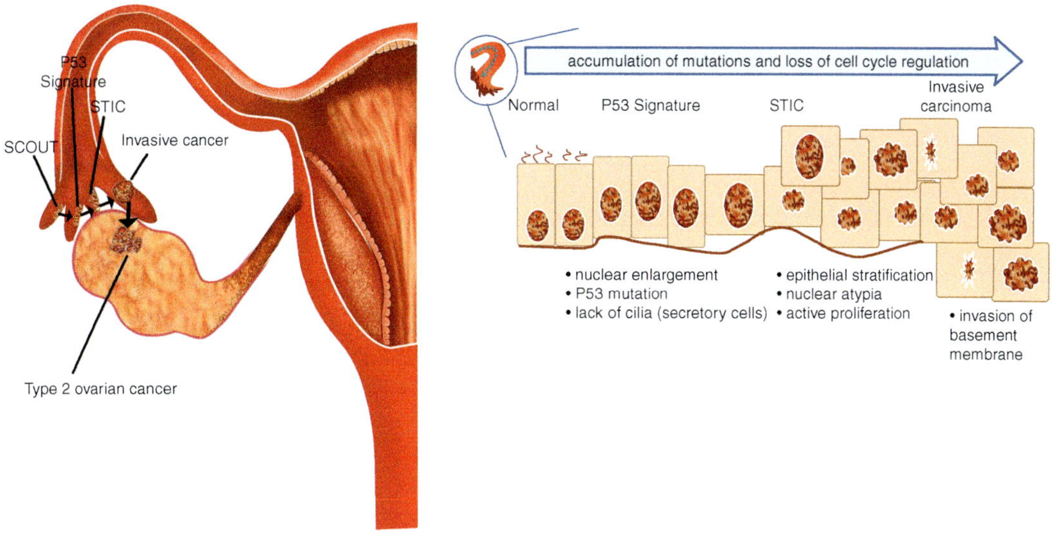

Fig. 20.2 Tubal origin of Type II high-grade serous carcinoma. *SCOUT* secretory cell outgrowths, *P53 signatures* clonal variation in p53 gene in the tubal epithelium, *STIC* serous tubal in situ carcinoma

Table 20.1 Tissue of origin, precursor lesion molecular alteration, and preventive strategies for major types of ovarian cancer

Tumor type	Tissue of origin	Precursor lesion	Molecular alteration	Preventive strategy
High-grade serous	Fallopian tube, fimbria, or cortical inclusion cyst	STIC	BRCA1, BRCA2, BRIP1, PALB2, RAD51C and RAD51D, p53	RRSO, opportunistic salpingectomy, OCP, tubal ligation
Low-grade serous	Endosalpingiosis or papillary tubal hyperplasia	Serous borderline tumor	KRAS, BRAF, PIK3CA, MSI	Opportunistic salpingectomy, OCP, tubal ligation
Endometrioid	Endometriosis	Endometrioid borderline tumor	MLH2, PMS2, MSH2, MSH6	Opportunistic salpingectomy, OCP, tubal ligation
Mucinous	Unknown, tubal, peritoneal junction	Mucinous borderline tumor	KRAS, HER2	Opportunistic salpingectomy, OCP, tubal ligation
AGCT	Granulose cell	Unknown	None	None
SLCT	Granulose cell	Unknown	None	None

STIC serous tubal in situ carcinoma, *RRSO* risk-reducing salpingo-oophorectomy, *OCP* oral contraceptive pills, *AGCT* adult granulosa cell tumor, *SLCT* Sertoli-Leydig cell tumor

20.3 Precise Risk Assessment

Ovarian cancer is a low-prevalence disease. The average lifetime risk of ovarian cancer in the general population is around 1.3% [17]. It implies that primary or secondary preventive practices in general population could impact very few women. Evidence based on the US Preventive Services Task Force (USPSTF) 2018 recommendations re-proclaim that screening for the early detection of ovarian cancer in asymptomatic, average-risk women is not recommended [18]. Hence, identification of high-risk women and targeted primary prevention appears to be the most effective strategy to lower the burden of ovarian cancer in the community.

The BRCA1 and 2 genetic susceptibility is well known; however there is now enough evidence to suggest that ovarian cancer susceptibility is much impacted by other genetic variations and polymorphisms. It is necessary to understand how penetrance and prevalence of gene mutation contribute to the individual's risk for cancer. It is also important to interpret the results of multigene panel testing and then tailor the risk management [19].

20.3.1 High-Penetrance Genetic Susceptibility

The BRCA mutations are discredited for high penetrance. The estimated cumulative ovarian cancer risk with BRCA1 mutation carrier ranges from 39 to 44% and 10–17% for BRCA2 mutations by the age of 70 [20–23]. The population prevalence of BRCA1/2 mutation carriers has been reported to be 0.07–0.22% depending on the specific gene and penetrance function used for the calculation [24]. Prophylactic salpingo-oophorectomy in these high-risk women has been established to reduce the risk of ovarian cancer by about 80% [25, 26].

20.3.2 Moderate-Penetrance Genetic Susceptibility

A number of moderate penetrance genes have been implicated in ovarian cancer. One such moderate penetrance gene is DNA mismatch repair gene, i.e., *MSH6*, *MSH2*, and *MLH*1 [27]. Incidence of ovarian cancer in genetically diagnosed HNPCC syndrome ranges from 6.5% to 13% [28, 29].

Next-generation sequencing technologies have identified more moderate-penetrance germline mutations. A recent study reported the lifetime ovarian cancer risk in RAD51C and RAD51D mutated women to be 11.2% (confidence interval [CI] 5.7–21.3%) [30] and 11.9% (CI 5.7–24.6%), respectively [31, 32]. Similarly, increased frequency of BRIP1 mutations has been found in epithelial ovarian cancer (EOC) patients, relative risk 11.22 for invasive EOC (CI = 3.22–34.10) [33, 34].

20.3.3 Low-Penetrance Genetic Susceptibility

Only 23% of ovarian carcinomas have been found to be associated with the known gene mutations. Consequently, majority of the ovarian cancer burden appears to be contributed by the mutations that are yet to be discovered. More recently, the genome-wide association studies (GWAS) have identified multiple ovarian cancer susceptibility genes [35, 36], and the most common gene variation in population is single nucleotide polymorphism (SNP). There are about 10 million SNPs in the human genome that have been reported to influence the individual's susceptibility to the disease and environmental factors such as toxins [37]. Albeit SNPs have weak penetrance to the development of epithelial ovarian cancer [relative risk (RR) of <1.5], their potential role in the etiology of epithelial ovarian cancer cannot be denied as the frequency of aberrant SNP is much higher than the aberrant BRCA gene mutation. Also, combination of SNP susceptibility may have an additive effect in one's risk of ovarian cancer.

20.4 Influence of Age on Susceptibility

Aging is a critical factor that determines the risk of ovarian cancer. The cumulative lifetime risk of ovarian cancer in BRCA mutation is found to increase with age. In a recent meta-analysis of 6036 BRCA1 carriers and 3828 BRCA2 female carriers, the cumulative risk of ovarian cancer in BRCA1 mutation carriers was determined to be 1–3% in women of age group 30–40 years and 6–12% in the age group 40–50 years. For the BRCA2 mutation carriers, this risk was estimated as 7% in the age group 50–60 years [38]. Finch et al. followed 5783 women with a BRCA1/2 mutation for a period of 5.6 years and estimated that the annual risk of ovarian cancer in BRCA1 mutation carriers was highest in the age group of 50–59 years (1.7%) and for the BRCA2 mutation carriers, it was observed between the ages of 60 and 69 years (0.6%) [26].

20.5 Genetic Testing and Counseling

About 15–23% of all the ovarian cancer cases are caused by hereditary or genetic factors, and in 65–85% of hereditary ovarian cancer, the genetic aberration is BRCA mutation [39]. The EOC in BRCA mutation carrier is associated with a positive family or personal history of breast/ovarian cancer and younger age of diagnoses [40]. However, a family or personal history is often absent and results in poor identification of these high-risk individuals [41–43]. Identification of high-risk women on the basis of history of personal cancer at a relatively younger age and family history has the potential to miss out women who need maximum evaluation.

Genetic testing facilitates preventive strategies for breast and ovarian cancers. Detection of a high risk for cancer mutation in a family can help prevent hereditary cancers in a number of kin women, who may benefit from more intensive screening and risk-reducing surgeries. With the advent of poly ADP-ribose polymerase (PARP) inhibitors, genetic testing additionally has therapeutic value.

The Society of Gynecologic Oncology (SGO) committee recently recommended guidelines that state candidature for genetic counseling and testing in 2015 (Table 20.2). Recently, the American College of Obstetricians and Gynecologists (ACOG) and SGO have endorsed the term "cascade testing" which refers to genetic counseling and testing in blood relatives of individuals with specific genetic mutations [44].

Genetic testing for all women with high-grade epithelial tumors is also globally recommended [45–48]. However, less than 20% of women with a diagnoses of high-grade ovarian cancer are sent for genetic referral [44, 49, 50]. Impediments to genetic testing include the lack of physician knowledge, unavailability of genetic services, relatively high cost of testing, lengthy process of counseling, and often patient refusal [51, 52].

Genetic referral emerges to be a public responsibility to improve the health and quality of life of the patient and her family members. Genetic screening can be improved by educating the

Table 20.2 Criteria for further genetic evaluation for hereditary breast and ovarian cancers[a]

Women affected with one or more of the following have an increased likelihood of having an inherited predisposition to breast[b] and ovarian, tubal, or peritoneal cancer and should receive genetic counseling and be offered genetic testing
Epithelial ovarian, tubal, or peritoneal cancer
Breast cancer at age 45 years or less
Breast cancer and have a close relative[c] with breast cancer at age 50 years or less or close relative[c] with epithelial ovarian, tubal, or peritoneal cancer at any age
Breast cancer at age 50 years or less with a limited or unknown family history[d]
Breast cancer and have two or more close relatives[c] with breast cancer at any age
Breast cancer and have two or more close relatives[c] with pancreatic cancer or aggressive prostate cancer (Gleason score equal to or greater than 7)
Two breast cancer primaries, with the first diagnosed before age 50 years
Triple-negative breast cancer at age 60 years or less
Breast cancer and Ashkenazi Jewish ancestry at any age
Pancreatic cancer and have two or more close relatives[c] with breast cancer; ovarian, tubal, or peritoneal cancer; pancreatic cancer; or aggressive prostate cancer (Gleason score equal to or greater than 7)
Women unaffected with cancer, but with one or more of the following have an increased likelihood of having an inherited predisposition to breast and ovarian, tubal, or peritoneal cancer and should receive genetic counseling and be offered genetic testing
A first-degree or several close relatives[c] that meet one or more of the aforementioned criteria
A close relative[c] carrying a known BRCA1 or BRCA2 mutation[e]
A close relative[c] with male breast cancer

[a]Adapted from Gynecologic Oncology, 136(1), Lancaster JM, Powell CB, Chen LM, Richardson DL, Society of Gynecologic Oncology statement on risk assessment for inherited gynecologic cancer predispositions, 3-7, Copyright 2015, with permission from Elsevier

[b]Invasive and ductal carcinoma in situ breast cancer

[c]Close relative is defined as first-degree (parent, sibling, offspring), second-degree (grandparent, grandchild, uncle, aunt, nephew, niece, half-sibling), or third-degree (first cousin, great-grandparent or greatgrandchild)

[d]Limited family history includes fewer than two first-degree or second-degree female relatives surviving beyond age 45 years

[e]Or carrying another known actionable deleterious mutation associated with hereditary breast and ovarian cancer syndrome

physician about various types of genetic susceptibilities, the type of tests available, and their clinical implications. With the higher referral rates, the test would also become more affordable and accessible. Apart from generating awareness about the referral to genetic counseling and testing, the test process needs to be more streamlined with quicker turnaround time.

20.6 Risk Prediction Models

The risk prediction models are used to calculate the combined risk and utilize it for devising preventive measures and creation of the risk-benefit indices [41]. However, risk prediction for ovarian cancer is problematic as the risk factors are globally diverse and often inconsistent. Various epidemiologic risk factors were mathematically combined by Rosen et al. and Li et al. independently, to identify women for screening and chemoprevention [53, 54]. Pfeiffer et al. predicted absolute risk of breast, ovarian, and endometrial cancers among the women older than 50 years of age through a model combining the reproductive factors and family history of breast and ovarian cancers [55]. An optimal model incorporating parity, breast feeding, tubal ligation, family history, SNPs, and BRCA1/2 mutations was proposed by Giannakeas et al., in order to discriminate the women above and below 5% risk [3]. The Ovarian Cancer Consortium recently published a risk model incorporating 17 epidemiological risk factors and 17 genome-wide single nucleotide polymorphisms. Their data included 5703 invasive epithelial ovarian cancer cases and 9512 controls. The study concluded that the addition of 17 confirmed SNPs improved the predictive ability of the model in women older than 50 years (with SNP/area under the curve [AUC] = 0.664; without SNP: AUC = 0.6490) [56].

These types of risk assessment models eventually help in making decisions regarding the risk-reducing salpingo-oophorectomy, but these models are found to have low discriminatory power, and henceforth, screening and surgical prevention on the basis of these models is not validated yet. It is therefore suggested that improved knowledge of low-penetrance genetic susceptibility will likely improve the risk assessment accuracy. Precise risk assessment will ultimately provide enhanced target of primary and secondary prevention schemes in terms of cost-effectiveness and the risk versus benefit ratio [56]. A clinically applicable accurate predictability can be further achieved by discovery and inclusion of additional novel risk factors.

20.7 Surgical Prevention

Removal of female gonads could be justified in sufficiently high-risk population, where the benefit of surgery outweighs the cost and risk of surgery. Risks of salpingo-oophorectomy include intraoperative injury to the bowel, bladder, ureter, and vessels and long-term morbidity [57, 58].

20.7.1 Risk-Reducing Salpingo-oophorectomy for High-Risk Women

Currently, risk-reducing salpingo-oophorectomy is offered to women with strong family history of breast or ovarian cancers and to BRCA1 or BRCA2 carriers, between the ages of 35 and 40 years, after completion of childbearing [59, 60]. Risk-reducing salpingo-oophorectomy (RRSO) for the management of ovarian cancer risk in BRCA2 mutation carrier can be delayed until the patients' age of 40–45 years [26, 61].

There is strong and consistent evidence that demonstrates the effectiveness of RRSO in reducing risk for ovarian cancer in BRCA mutation carriers. A prospective study of 5783 BRCA mutation carrier women reported that RRSO was associated with an 80% reduction in the risk of ovarian, fallopian tube, or peritoneal cancer in the BRCA1 or BRCA2 carriers and a 77% reduction in all-cause mortality [26]. There was a residual risk for primary peritoneal cancer of approximately 1–4.3% after RRSO [62–64]. A large meta-analysis of ten studies also testified similar reduction in the risk of ovarian cancer [63]. The cost-effectiveness of RRSO (alone or in combination with mastectomy) is also well established for the BRCA mutation carriers [57]. However, recently it is proposed to have lower the risk threshold for surgical prevention and offer risk-reducing salpingo-oophorectomy to intermediate-risk women [65–67].

RRSO is a safe procedure and can be performed laparoscopically. Complications are limited to anesthesia risk; risk of injury to the bladder, bowel, and vessel; and infections. Kenkhuis et al. evaluated short-term surgical outcome and safety of 159 high-risk women who underwent RRSO. A total of 96.9% cases had laparoscopic surgery with an intraoperative complication rate of 1.3%, and the postoperative complication rate was 3.1% [68]. Manchanda et al. reported an intraoperative complication rate of 1.2% and postoperative complication rate of 2.7% in a cohort of 308 women with unknown mutation status [69].

Studies suggest that most women are relieved of ovarian cancer-specific distress and worry after the risk-reducing surgery [70]. In a questionnaire-based study on 846 cases, women who chose RRSO had no measurable adverse effect on the quality of life. RRSO was considered a valued procedure that they would recommend to fellow high-risk woman [71]. Most bothersome symptoms following RRSO are dyspareunia, vaginal dryness, and sexual dysfunction [70, 72]; these symptoms are worse after surgical salpingo-oophorectomy as compared to natural menopause [73]. Hormone replacement therapy (HRT) is debated in BRCA mutation carrier women. Quality of life after RRSO can be improved with HRT [74]. Multiple studies and expert reviews have demonstrated non-inferior oncological outcomes in women who received short-term HRT [75–80]. However, due to the paucity of quality evidence, HRT prescription to BRCA carriers after RRSO should be undertaken with caution (Table 20.3) [59, 90].

20.7.2 Opportunistic Salpingo-oophorectomy in Average-Risk Women

Opportunistic oophorectomy is salpingo-oophorectomy at the time of benign hysterectomy for an average-risk woman. There is evidence that removal of ovaries in premenopausal and postmenopausal women has significant, long-term

Table 20.3 Evidence-based risk-reducing salpingo-oophorectomy (RRSO) recommendations[a]

Women with	Ovarian cancer risk	Recommended age in years for RRSO	Evidence
BRCA1 mutation	40–60%	>35–40	Levy-Lahad and Friedman [22], Domchek [25], Evans et al. [81], Antoniou et al. [82], Mavaddat et al. [83]
BRCA2 mutation	10–30%	>40–45	Levy-Lahad and Friedman [22], Domchek [25], Evans et al. [81]
RAD51C or RAD51D mutation	9–12%	>40–50[b]	Loveday et al. [31], Coulet et al. [84], Evans et al. [81], Pearce et al. [85]
BRIP1 mutation	5.80%	>50[b]	Ramus et al. [34]
HBOC or HOC (untested)	7–10%	>40–45[b]	Sutcliffe et al. [86], Srivastava et al. [87], Hemminki et al. [1], Jervis et al. [88, 89]
Polygenic (SNP) ± epidemiological-based risk	Model-based estimation >4–5% risk	>50[b]	Jervis et al. [89], Pearce et al. [85]
Lynch syndrome: MLH1, MSH2, MSH6 mutations	6–14%	>40[b] (combined with hysterectomy for EC risk)	Pearce et al. [85]

HBC high-risk breast cancer only family, *HBOC* high-risk breast and ovarian cancer family, *HOC* high-risk ovarian cancer only family, *SNP* single nucleotide polymorphism

[a]Adapted from [65]

[b]Limited data

negative effects. A prospective study of 30,117 women participants of the Nurses' Health Study, who underwent hysterectomy for benign conditions, was analyzed by Parker et al. [91]. After a follow-up of 28 years, oophorectomy was associated with the reduced risk of death from ovarian cancer (hazard ratio [HR] = 0.06; 95% CI, 0.02–0.17), but it was unpredictably associated with near twice all-cause mortality as compared to ovarian conservation (HR = 1.13; 95% CI, 1.06–1.21). Women who underwent hysterectomy and oophorectomy before the age 50 and never used hormone therapy had significantly associated high mortality from coronary heart disease (CHD), colorectal cancer, total cancers, and all-causes. Multivariable analyses exhibited that at no age, oophorectomy is associated with increased overall survival [91]. Similar results were presented by Rocca et al. [92], who studied 2390 women with oophorectomy and 2390 referent women. The authors reported a significantly higher all-cause mortality in women who had oophorectomy before the age of 45 years and who were not exposed to hormone replacement therapy. Recently, Evans et al. [93] reviewed 26 peer-reviewed articles comparing the risk versus benefit associated with salpingo-oophorectomy and ovarian conservation. The authors concluded that despite lowering the prevalence of reoperation rates and ovarian cancer, bilateral salpingo-oophorectomy can largely be detrimental to health, especially in women younger than the age of 45 years. It cannot be stressed enough that RRSO is indicated only for the women at high risk for breast and ovarian cancers. Physicians should avoid giving the option of oophorectomy during benign hysterectomy in the general population to evade a small risk of reoperation and ovarian cancer. Women should be educated about the higher mortality associated with oophorectomy as compared to the prevention of a rare cancer for them.

20.7.3 Opportunistic Salpingectomy in Average-Risk Women

The fallopian tube is agreed to be the site of origin for most epithelial ovarian cancer, and thus, salpingectomy seems to have a potential role in the prevention of ovarian cancer in both the average-risk and high-risk women. Only few retrospective studies revealed the role of bilateral salpingectomy in the reduction of ovarian cancer risk; however it is proposed to be beneficial owing to the interrelated evidence on tubal ligation [94, 95]. Falconer et al. studied the risk of ovarian cancer rates in women ($n = 5,251,465$) who underwent tubal ligation, unilateral salpingectomy, bilateral salpingectomy, and hysterectomy for benign conditions and compared it with the risk of ovarian cancer in unexposed population ($n = 55,449,119$).Women with previous salpingectomy were noted to have reduced risk for ovarian cancer (HR = 0.65, 95% CI = 0.52–0.81) when compared with the unexposed population [96].

Known et al. [97] estimated the cost-effectiveness of opportunistic salpingectomy during hysterectomy for benign conditions and sterilization, by Monte Carlo stimulation model in the average-risk hypothetical women. Their model demonstrated salpingectomy to be slightly costlier than the tubal ligation but more effective prevention strategy in the general population. A relative 29.2% risk reduction was noted in ovarian cancer diagnoses with the use of salpingectomy versus tubal ligation. Apart from the cost-effectiveness, opportunistic salpingectomy was associated with an insignificant operative morbidity and short-term preservation of ovarian function [5, 98–103].

20.7.4 Interval Salpingectomy with Delayed Oophorectomy in High-Risk Women

Interval salpingectomy with delayed oophorectomy is a newer risk management option to prevent ovarian cancer in high-risk women. This strategy involves bilateral salpingectomy at the completion of childbearing followed by bilateral oophorectomy at a later date to defer menopausal symptoms at an early age. Risk-reducing salpingectomy comprises of peritoneal washings, removal of the entire fallopian tube, and excision of the ovarian capsule adhered to the fimbria.

The specimen is meticulously processed using detailed sectioning and extensive examination of the fimbriated end is done (SEE-FIM) method [96, 97].

Though this alternative looks promising, its effectiveness should be taken with due caution as there is no actual data available to substantiate this hypothesis. Several studies are in progress, to determine the feasibility and effectiveness of this strategy in the prevention of ovarian cancer in high-risk women [104–108]. A Markov Monte Carlo simulation-based study reported that bilateral salpingo-oophorectomy at the age of 40 years offers the greatest risk reduction for breast and ovarian cancers among the BRCA mutation carriers at minimum cost. However, when quality-of-life years are taken into considerations, salpingectomy at the age of 40 years followed by delayed oophorectomy at the age of 50 years offers the highest quality-adjusted life expectancy with incremental cost-effectiveness ratios of $37,805 and $89,680 per quality-adjusted life-year for BRCA1 and BRCA2, respectively [109].

This approach lacks the best security for both ovarian and breast cancers. The fallopian tube is contemplated as the putative precursor of most serous ovarian cancer, nonetheless for all ovarian cancer. Retaining the ovaries for a few susceptible years may not completely protect against ovarian cancer. Delaying oophorectomy would additionally demand screening, chemoprevention, and bilateral mastectomy at an early age. Other hitches are uncertain compliance for the delayed oophorectomy and the recurring risks of surgery.

20.7.5 Tubal Ligation

Women who undergo permanent sterilization by bilateral tubal ligation are recognized to have relatively lower risk of ovarian cancer since the 1980s [110–114]. A meta-analysis done by Cibula et al. [115] in 2010 analyzed 13 carefully selected studies and reported reduction in the risk of EOC by 34% after tubal ligation (RR = 0.66, 95% CI 0.60–0.73). Tubal ligation was associated with higher reductions for endometrioid invasive cancers (RR = 0.40, 95% CI 0.30–0.53) in comparison with the other histological types. Recent meta-analyses by Rice et al. [116] also observed similar results. It should be noted that tubal ligation as an ovarian cancer prevention strategy in high-risk women is still not recommended [115, 117].

20.8 Nonsurgical Risk Reduction: Chemoprevention

Oral contraceptive pills (OCPs), metformin, and aspirin have been investigated for chemoprevention. However, randomized controlled trials are unavailable. Below we briefly outline some of the key properties and functional roles of these risk-reducing chemopreventive agents.

20.8.1 OCP

OCPs appear to be a promising, nonsurgical primary prevention strategy for ovarian cancer [118]. Several studies have demonstrated a lower overall ovarian cancer risk in OCP users as compared to nonusers [118–120]. Havrilesky et al. published a random effect meta-analysis of 24 case-control and cohort studies, comparing the risk of ovarian cancer risk in "ever-user" with "never-user" of OCPs with average risk. The authors observed that there was a 27% reduction in the ovarian cancer risk in women who have ever used OCPs. The odds ratio (OR) for the ever-use group compared with the never-use of OCPs was 0.73 (95% CI 0.66–0.81). Analysis of ten case-control studies and five cohort studies showed a significant duration-response relationship, with the risk reduction of more than 50% among the women using OCPs for 10 or more years. Furthermore, the relative composition of hormone doses in OCPs was not found to have any effect on the ovarian cancer incidence. Progesterone-only pills were not found to be protective [121]. Similar protection for ovarian cancer is reported in the BRCA1 and BRCA2 mutation carriers [122]. A meta-analysis published in 2013

[123] determined the risks of ovarian cancer and breast cancer associated with oral contraceptive(OC) use among the women at elevated risk for hereditary breast and ovarian cancers. The analysis revealed a significant risk reduction of ovarian cancer (OR 0.58; 95% CI, 0.46–0.73) and a non-statistically significant higher risk of breast cancer (OR, 1.21; 95% CI, 0.93–1.58) in OC users. The association of OC with the higher risk of breast cancer was inconsistent and inconclusive. Based on the aforementioned meta-analysis, OCPs can be advocated as an alternative chemopreventive strategy in the high-risk women but used with discretion.

20.8.2 Metformin

Many studies have discerned a significant antiproliferative and pro-apoptotic effect of metformin on cancer cells. Metformin triggers adenosine monophosphate (AMP)-activated protein kinase (AMPK) that, in turn, inhibits the mammalian target of rapamycin complex 1 (mTORC1), which further inhibits cancer cell proliferation. Metformin also activates *LKB1* (serine/threonine kinase 11), a tumor suppressor gene [124–128]. Metformin has shown to be a chemoprevention strategy in translational studies; however clinical evidence is largely lacking [129].

20.8.3 Aspirin

Aspirin is associated with reduced risk of various malignancies [130]. There are multiple small studies examining the role of aspirin in chemoprevention of ovarian cancer [131–133]. Trabert et al. performed a meta-analysis of 12 case-control studies, comprising of 10,161 ovarian cancer patients and 12,382 control subjects. The analysis reported the risk reduction of EOC by 9% in at least once per week aspirin users and 20% in daily users. Risk reduction was as high as 34% among the women taking daily low-dose aspirin. The risk reduction was seen for serous, endometrioid, and mucinous subtypes. No data specific to the BRCA carriers are available yet. There is inconclusive information on the duration of the use and risk reduction. In the subtype analyses, regular aspirin use was associated with a significant risk reduction in serous cancers (OR = 0.89; 95% CI = 0.80–0.99) [130]. However, further research is mandated before the utilization of aspirin as a chemopreventive agent for ovarian cancer in both the high-risk and average-risk population.

20.8.4 Lifestyle Modification

Like other cancers, one of the most important modifiable risk factors for ovarian cancer are obesity and sedentary lifestyles, particularly in the Western world [134–136]. Pregnancy and lactation are also linked to protection against ovarian cancer. High-risk women should be advised to have early pregnancy and prolonged breast feeding to have some protection against breast cancer [137–139].

20.9 Conclusion

Despite advances in preventative medicine, strategies to curb incidence of ovarian cancer in general population still fall behind. Insights into the dual pathogenesis of ovarian cancer are expected to open doors for new strategies for screening and preventive programs for epithelial ovarian cancer. Continued molecular characterization of epithelial ovarian cancer will allow discovery of more specific tumor markers and susceptibility genes. In the light of accumulated evidence, bilateral salpingo-oophorectomy is the only effective way to reduce the risk of epithelial ovarian cancer in high-risk women. Gynecologists should advise genetic counseling for all women with epithelial ovarian cancer. It is also recommended that physicians advise genetic counseling and BRCA testing if indicated, in women with family history of breast, ovarian, tubal, or peritoneal cancer.

Key Points

- About 15–23% of all the ovarian cancer cases are caused by hereditary or genetic factors.
- Screening for the early detection of ovarian cancer in asymptomatic, average-risk women is not recommended.
- RRSO is indicated only for the women at high risk for breast and ovarian cancers. Prophylactic salpingo-oophorectomy in these high-risk women has been established to reduce the risk of ovarian cancer by about 80%.
- Opportunistic bilateral salpingectomy might have potential role in the prevention of ovarian cancer in the average-risk women.
- Genetic testing for all women with high-grade epithelial tumors is recommended.

References

1. Hemminki K, Sundquist J, Brandt A. Incidence and mortality in epithelial ovarian cancer by family history of any cancer. Cancer. 2011;117(17):3972–80.
2. Whittemore AS, Harris R, Itnyre J. Characteristics relating to ovarian cancer risk: collaborative analysis of 12 US case-control studies. II. Invasive epithelial ovarian cancers in white women. Collaborative Ovarian Cancer Group. Am J Epidemiol. 1992;136(10):1184–203.
3. Giannakeas V, Sopik V, Shestopaloff K, Iqbal J, Rosen B, Akbari M, et al. A model for estimating ovarian cancer risk: application for preventive oophorectomy. Gynecol Oncol. 2015;139(2):242–7.
4. Brekelmans CTM. Risk factors and risk reduction of breast and ovarian cancer: current opinion in obstetrics and gynecology. Curr Opin Obstet Gynecol. 2003;15(1):63–8.
5. McAlpine JN, Hanley GE, Woo MMM, Tone AA, Rozenberg N, Swenerton KD, et al. Opportunistic salpingectomy: uptake, risks, and complications of a regional initiative for ovarian cancer prevention. Am J Obstet Gynecol. 2014;210(5):471.e1.
6. Wentzensen N, Poole EM, Trabert B, White E, Arslan AA, Patel AV, et al. Ovarian cancer risk factors by histologic subtype: an analysis from the ovarian cancer cohort consortium. J Clin Oncol. 2016;34(24):2888–98.
7. Narod SA. Salpingo-oophorectomy and the risk of ovarian, fallopian tube, and peritoneal cancers in women with a BRCA1 or BRCA2 mutation. J Am Med Assoc. 2006;296(2):185–92.
8. Scully RE. Early de novo ovarian cancer and cancer developing in benign ovarian lesions. Int J Gynecol Obstet. 1995;49(suppl):S9–15.
9. Dubeau L. The cell of origin of ovarian epithelial tumors and the ovarian surface epithelium dogma: does the emperor have no clothes? Gynecol Oncol. 1999;72:437–42.
10. Colgan TJ, Murphy J, Cole DEC, Narod S, Rosen B. Occult carcinoma in prophylactic oophorectomy specimens: prevalence and association with BRCA germline mutation status. Am J Surg Pathol. 2001;25(10):1283–9.
11. Piek JMJ, Van Diest PJ, Zweemer RP, Jansen JW, Poort-Keesom RJJ, Menko FH, et al. Dysplastic changes in prophylactically removed Fallopian tubes of women predisposed to developing ovarian cancer. J Pathol. 2001;195(4):451–6.
12. Leeper K, Garcia R, Swisher E, Goff B, Greer B, Paley P. Pathologic findings in prophylactic oophorectomy specimens in high-risk women. Gynecol Oncol. 2002;87(1):52–6.
13. Kindelberger DW, Lee Y, Miron A, Hirsch MS, Feltmate C, Medeiros F, et al. Intraepithelial carcinoma of the fimbria and pelvic serous carcinoma: evidence for a causal relationship. Am J Surg Pathol. 2007;31(2):161–9.
14. McCluggage WG. Morphological subtypes of ovarian carcinoma: a review with emphasis on new developments and pathogenesis. Pathology. 2011;43:420–32.
15. Meinhold-Heerlein I, Fotopoulou C, Harter P, Kurzeder C, Mustea A, Wimberger P, et al. The new WHO classification of ovarian, fallopian tube, and primary peritoneal cancer and its clinical implications. Arch Gynecol Obstet. 2016;293(4):695–700.
16. Kurman RJ, Shih IM. The origin and pathogenesis of epithelial ovarian cancer: a proposed unifying theory. Am J Surg Pathol. 2010;34(3):433–43.
17. Bethesda M. SEER cancer statistics fact sheet: ovary cancer. SEER. 2014. Retrieved from https://seer.cancer.gov/archive/csr/1975_2014/
18. Grossman DC, Curry SJ, Owens DK, Barry MJ, Davidson KW, Doubeni CA, et al. Screening for ovarian cancer. JAMA. 2018;319(6):588.
19. Hall MJ, Forman AD, Pilarski R, Wiesner G, Giri VN. Gene panel testing for inherited cancer risk. J Natl Compr Cancer Netw. 2014;12(9):1339–46.
20. Kuchenbaecker KB, Hopper JLBD. Risk of breast, ovarian and contralateral breast cancer BRCA 1 and BRCA2 mutation carriers. JAMA. 2017;317:2402–16.
21. Rebbeck TR, Mitra N, Wan F, Sinilnikova OM, Healey S, McGuffog L, et al. Association of type and location of BRCA1 and BRCA2 mutations with risk of breast and ovarian cancer. JAMA. 2015;313(13):1347–61.
22. Levy-Lahad E, Friedman E. Cancer risks among BRCA1 and BRCA2 mutation carriers. Br J Cancer. 2007;96:11–5.
23. Chen S, Parmigiani G. Meta-analysis of BRCA1 and BRCA2 penetrance. J Clin Oncol. 2007;25(11):1329–33.

24. Anglian Breast Cancer Study Group. Prevalence and penetrance of BRCA1 and BRCA2 mutations in a population-based series of breast cancer cases. Br J Cancer. 2000;83(10):1301–8.
25. Domchek SM, Friebel TM, Singer CF, Evans DG, Lynch HT, Isaacs C, et al. Association of risk-reducing surgery in BRCA1 or BRCA2 mutation carriers with cancer risk and mortality. JAMA. 2010;304(9):967.
26. Finch APM, Lubinski J, Møller P, Singer CF, Karlan B, Senter L, et al. Impact of oophorectomy on cancer incidence and mortality in women with a BRCA1 or BRCA2 mutation. J Clin Oncol. 2014;32(15):1547–53.
27. Song H, Cicek MS, Dicks E, Harrington P, Ramus SJ, Cunningham JM, et al. The contribution of deleterious germline mutations in BRCA1, BRCA2 and the mismatch repair genes to ovarian cancer in the population. Hum Mol Genet. 2014;23(17):4703–9.
28. Watson P, Vasen HFA, Mecklin JP, Bernstein I, Aarnio M, Järvinen HJ, et al. The risk of extra-colonic, extra-endometrial cancer in the Lynch syndrome. Int J Cancer. 2008;123(2):444–9.
29. Aarnio M, Sankila R, Pukkala E, Salovaara R, Aaltonen LA, de la Chapelle A, et al. Cancer risk in mutation carriers of DNA-mismatch-repair genes. Int J Cancer. 1999;81(2):214–8.
30. Meindl A, Hellebrand H, Wiek C, Erven V, Wappenschmidt B, Niederacher D, et al. Germline mutations in breast and ovarian cancer pedigrees establish RAD51C as a human cancer susceptibility gene. Nat Genet. 2010;42(5):410–4.
31. Loveday C, Turnbull C, Ramsay E, Hughes D, Ruark E, Frankum JR, et al. Germline mutations in RAD51D confer susceptibility to ovarian cancer. Nat Genet. 2011;43(9):879–82.
32. Song H, Dicks E, Ramus SJ, Tyrer JP, Intermaggio MP, Hayward J, et al. Contribution of germline mutations in the RAD51B, RAD51C, and RAD51D genes to ovarian cancer in the population. J Clin Oncol. 2015;33(26):2901–7.
33. Rafnar T, Gudbjartsson DF, Sulem P, Jonasdottir A, Sigurdsson A, Jonasdottir A, et al. Mutations in BRIP1 confer high risk of ovarian cancer. Nat Genet. 2011;43(11):1104–7.
34. Ramus SJ, Song H, Dicks E, Tyrer JP, Rosenthal AN, Intermaggio MP, et al. Germline mutations in the BRIP1, BARD1, PALB2, and NBN genes in women with ovarian cancer. J Natl Cancer Inst. 2015;107(11):djv214.
35. Kuchenbaecker KB, Ramus SJ, Tyrer J, Lee A, Shen HC, Beesley J, et al. Identification of six new susceptibility loci for invasive epithelial ovarian cancer. Nat Genet. 2015;47(2):164–71.
36. Phelan CM, Kuchenbaecker KB, Tyrer JP, Kar SP, Lawrenson K, Winham SJ, et al. Identification of 12 new susceptibility loci for different histotypes of epithelial ovarian cancer. Nat Genet. 2017;49(5):680–91.
37. Thomas D. Gene-environment-wide association studies: emerging approaches. Nat Rev Genet. 2010;11:259–72.
38. Kuchenbaecker KB, Hopper JL, Barnes DR, Phillips K-A, Mooij TM, Roos-Blom M-J, et al. Risks of breast, ovarian, and contralateral breast cancer for BRCA1 and BRCA2 mutation carriers. JAMA. 2017;317(23):2402.
39. Walsh T, Casadei S, Lee MK, Pennil CC, Nord AS, Thornton AM, et al. Mutations in 12 genes for inherited ovarian, fallopian tube, and peritoneal carcinoma identified by massively parallel sequencing. Proc Natl Acad Sci U S A. 2011;108(44):18032–7.
40. Boyd J, Sonoda Y, Federici MG, Bogomolniy F, Rhei E, Maresco DL, et al. Clinicopathologic features of BRCA-linked and sporadic ovarian cancer. JAMA. 2000;283(17):2260.
41. Norquist BM, Pennington KP, Agnew KJ, Harrell MI, Pennil CC, Lee MK, et al. Characteristics of women with ovarian carcinoma who have BRCA1 and BRCA2 mutations not identified by clinical testing. Gynecol Oncol. 2013;128(3):483–7.
42. Kwon JS, Daniels MS, Sun CC, Lu KH. Preventing future cancers by testing women with ovarian cancer for BRCA mutations. J Clin Oncol. 2010;28(4):675–82.
43. Eccles DM, Balmaña J, Clune J, Ehlken B, Gohlke A, Hirst C, et al. Selecting patients with ovarian cancer for germline BRCA mutation testing: findings from guidelines and a systematic literature review. Adv Ther. 2016;33:129–50.
44. Meyer LA, Anderson ME, Lacour RA, Suri A, Daniels MS, Urbauer DL, et al. Evaluating women with ovarian cancer for BRCA1 and BRCA2 mutations: missed opportunities. Obstet Gynecol. 2010;115(5):945–52.
45. Modesitt C, Lu Karen M. Practice bulletin no 182: hereditary breast and ovarian cancer syndrome. Obstet Gynecol. 2017;130(3):e110–26.
46. Moyer VA. Risk assessment, genetic counseling, and genetic testing for BRCA-related cancer in women: U.S. preventive services task force recommendation statement. Ann Intern Med. 2014;160(4):271–81.
47. Hampel H, Bennett RL, Buchanan A, Pearlman R, Wiesner GL. A practice guideline from the American College of Medical Genetics and Genomics and the National Society of Genetic Counselors: referral indications for cancer predisposition assessment. Genet Med. 2015;17:70–87.
48. Lu KH, Wood ME, Daniels M, Burke C, Ford J, Kauff ND, et al. American Society of Clinical Oncology Expert Statement: collection and use of a cancer family history for oncology providers. J Clin Oncol. 2014;32(8):833–40.
49. McGee J, Panabaker K, Leonard S, Ainsworth P, Elit L, Shariff SZ. Genetics consultation rates following a diagnosis of high-grade serous ovarian carcinoma in the Canadian province of Ontario. Int J Gynecol Cancer. 2017;27(3):437–43.

50. Ricci MT, Sciallero S, Mammoliti S, Gismondi V, Franiuk M, Bruzzi P, et al. Referral of ovarian cancer patients for genetic counselling by oncologists: need for improvement. Public Health Genomics. 2015;18(4):225–32.
51. Hoskins PJ, Gotlieb WH. Missed therapeutic and prevention opportunities in women with BRCA-mutated epithelial ovarian cancer and their families due to low referral rates for genetic counseling and BRCA testing: a review of the literature. CA Cancer J Clin. 2017;67(6):493–506.
52. Sussner KM, Jandorf L, Thompson HS, Valdimarsdottir HB. Barriers and facilitators to BRCA genetic counseling among at-risk Latinas in New York City. Psychooncology. 2013;22(7):1594–604.
53. Rosner BA, Colditz GA, Webb PM, Hankinson SE. Mathematical models of ovarian cancer incidence. Epidemiology. 2005;16(4):508–15.
54. Li K, Hüsing A, Fortner RT, Tjønneland A, Hansen L, Dossus L, et al. An epidemiologic risk prediction model for ovarian cancer in Europe: the EPIC study. Br J Cancer. 2015;112(7):1257–65.
55. Pfeiffer RM, Park Y, Kreimer AR, Lacey JV, Pee D, Greenlee RT, et al. risk prediction for breast, endometrial, and ovarian cancer in white women aged 50 y or older: derivation and validation from population-based cohort studies. PLoS Med. 2013;10(7):e1001492.
56. Clyde MA, Palmieri Weber R, Iversen ES, Poole EM, Doherty JA, Goodman MT, et al. Risk prediction for epithelial ovarian cancer in 11 United States-based case-control studies: incorporation of epidemiologic risk factors and 17 confirmed genetic loci. Am J Epidemiol. 2016;184(8):555–69.
57. Anderson K, Jacobson JS, Heitjan DF, Zivin JG, Hershman D, Neugut AI, et al. Cost-effectiveness of preventive strategies for women with a BRCA1 or a BRCA2 mutation. Ann Intern Med. 2006;144(6):397–406.
58. Parker WH, Feskanich D, Broder MS, Chang E, Shoupe D, Farquhar CM, et al. Long-term mortality associated with oophorectomy compared with ovarian conservation in the Nurses' Health Study. Obstet Gynecol. 2013;121(4):709–16.
59. Pilarski R, Buys SS, Farmer M, Khan S, Klein C, Kohlmann W, et al. NCCN guidelines index table of contents discussion NCCN guidelines version 1. 2018 Panel Members Genetic/Familial High-Risk Assessment: Breast and Ovarian. 2018.
60. Walker JL, Powell CB, Chen LM, Carter J, Bae Jump VL, Parker LP, et al. Society of Gynecologic Oncology recommendations for the prevention of ovarian cancer. Cancer. 2015;121:2108–20.
61. Kang S, Yoo HJ, Hwang JH, Lim M-C, Seo S-S, Park S-Y. Sentinel lymph node biopsy in endometrial cancer: meta-analysis of 26 studies. Gynecol Oncol. 2011;123(3):522–7.
62. Finch A, Shaw P, Rosen B, Murphy J, Narod SA, Colgan TJ. Clinical and pathologic findings of prophylactic salpingo-oophorectomies in 159 BRCA1 and BRCA2 carriers. Gynecol Oncol. 2006;100(1):58–64.
63. Rebbeck TR, Kauff ND, Domchek SM. Meta-analysis of risk reduction estimates associated with risk-reducing salpingo-oophorectomy in BRCA1 or BRCA2 mutation carriers. J Natl Cancer Inst. 2009;101(2):80–7.
64. Finch A, Beiner M, Lubinski J, Lynch HT, Moller P, Rosen B, et al. Salpingo-oophorectomy and the risk of ovarian, fallopian tube, and peritoneal cancers in women with a BRCA1 or BRCA2 mutation. JAMA. 2006;296(2):185.
65. Manchanda R, Menon U. Setting the threshold for surgical prevention in women at increased risk of ovarian cancer. Int J Gynecol Cancer. 2017;28(1):1.
66. Manchanda R, Legood R, Pearce L, Menon U. Defining the risk threshold for risk reducing salpingo-oophorectomy for ovarian cancer prevention in low risk postmenopausal women. Gynecol Oncol. 2015;139(3):487–94.
67. Manchanda R, Legood R, Antoniou AC, Gordeev VS, Menon U. Specifying the ovarian cancer risk threshold of "premenopausal risk-reducing salpingooophorectomy" for ovarian cancer prevention: a cost-effectiveness analysis. J Med Genet. 2016;53(9):591–9.
68. Kenkhuis MJA, de Bock GH, Oude Elferink P, Arts HJG, Oosterwijk JC, Jansen L, et al. Short-term surgical outcome and safety of risk reducing salpingo-oophorectomy in BRCA1/2 mutation carriers. Maturitas. 2010;66(3):310–4.
69. Manchanda R, Abdelraheim A, Johnson M, Rosenthal AN, Benjamin E, Brunell C, et al. Outcome of risk-reducing salpingo-oophorectomy in BRCA carriers and women of unknown mutation status. BJOG. 2011;118(7):814–24.
70. Finch A, Metcalfe KA, Chiang J, Elit L, McLaughlin J, Springate C, et al. The impact of prophylactic salpingo-oophorectomy on quality of life and psychological distress in women with a BRCA mutation. Psychooncology. 2013;22(1):212–9.
71. Madalinska JE, Hollenstein J, Bleiker E, Van Beurden M, Valdimarsdottir HB, Massuger LF, et al. Quality-of-life effects of prophylactic salpingo-oophorectomy versus gynecologic screening among women at increased risk of hereditary ovarian cancer. J Clin Oncol. 2005;23(28):6890–8.
72. Robson M, Hensley M, Barakat R, Brown C, Chi D, Poynor E, et al. Quality of life in women at risk for ovarian cancer who have undergone risk-reducing oophorectomy. Gynecol Oncol. 2003;89(2):281–7.
73. Benshushan A, Rojansky N, Chaviv M, Arbel-Alon S, Benmeir A, Imbar T, et al. Climacteric symptoms in women undergoing risk-reducing bilateral salpingo-oophorectomy. Climacteric. 2009;12(5):404–9.
74. Limouzin-Lamothe MA, Mairon N, Joyce CRB, Le Gal M. Quality of life after the menopause: influence of hormonal replacement therapy. Am J Obstet Gynecol. 1994;170(2):618–24.

75. Rebbeck TR, Friebel T, Wagner T, Lynch HT, Garber JE, Daly MB, et al. Effect of short-term hormone replacement therapy on breast cancer risk reduction after bilateral prophylactic oophorectomy in BRCA1 and BRCA2 mutation carriers: the PROSE Study Group. J Clin Oncol. 2005;23(31):7804–10.
76. Eisen A, Lubinski J, Gronwald J, Moller P, Lynch HT, Klijn J, et al. Hormone therapy and the risk of breast cancer in BRCA1 mutation carriers. J Natl Cancer Inst. 2008;100(19):1361–7.
77. Armstrong K, Schwartz JS, Randall T, Rubin SC, Weber B. Hormone replacement therapy and life expectancy after prophylactic oophorectomy in women with BRCA1/2 mutations: a decision analysis. J Clin Oncol. 2004;22(6):1045–54.
78. Marchetti C, Iadarola R, Palaia I, di Donato V, Perniola G, Muzii L, et al. Hormone therapy in oophorectomized BRCA1/2 mutation carriers. Menopause. 2014;21(7):763–8.
79. Birrer N, Chinchilla C, Del Carmen M, Dizon DS. Is hormone replacement therapy safe in women with a BRCA mutation? Am J Clin Oncol. 2016;41(3):313–5.
80. Madalinska JB, Van Beurden M, Bleiker EMA, Valdimarsdottir HB, Hollenstein J, Massuger LF, et al. The impact of hormone replacement therapy on menopausal symptoms in younger high-risk women after prophylactic salpingo-oophorectomy. J Clin Oncol. 2006;24(22):3576–82.
81. Evans DG, Shenton A, Woodward E, Lalloo F, Howell A, Maher ER. Penetrance estimates for BRCA1 and BRCA2 based on genetic testing in a clinical cancer genetics service setting: risks of breast/ovarian cancer quoted should reflect the cancer burden in the family. BMC Cancer. 2008;8(1):155.
82. Antoniou A, Pharoah PD, Narod S, et al. Average risks of breast and ovarian cancer associated with BRCA1 or BRCA2 mutations detected in case Series unselected for family history: a combined analysis of 22 studies. Am J Hum Genet. 2003;72(5):1117–30.
83. Mavaddat N, Peock S, Frost D, Ellis S, Platte R, Fineberg E, Gareth Evans D, Izatt L, Eeles RA, Adlard J, Davidson R, Eccles D, Cole T, Cook J, Brewer C, Tischkowitz M, Douglas F, Hodgson S, Walker L, Porteous ME, Morrison PJ, Side LE, John Kennedy M, Houghton C, Donaldson A, Rogers MT, Dorkins H, Miedzybrodzka Z, Gregory H, Eason J, Barwell J, McCann E, Murray A, Antoniou AC, Easton DF, EMBRACE. Cancer risks for BRCA1 and BRCA2 mutation carriers: results from prospective analysis of EMBRACE. J Natl Cancer Inst. 2013;105(11):812–22. https://doi.org/10.1093/jnci/djt095.
84. Coulet F, Fajac A, Colas C, Eyries M, Dion-Minière A, Rouzier R, et al. Germline RAD51C mutations in ovarian cancer susceptibility. Clin Genet. 2013;83(4):332–6.
85. Pearce CL, Stram DO, Ness RB, Stram DA, Roman LD, Templeman C, et al. Population distribution of lifetime risk of ovarian cancer in the United States. Cancer Epidemiol Biomark Prev. 2015;24(4):671–6.
86. Sutcliffe S, Pharoah PD, Easton DF, Ponder BA. Ovarian and breast cancer risks to women in families with two or more cases of ovarian cancer. Int J Cancer. 2000;87(1):110–7.
87. Srivastava A, McKinnon W, Wood ME. Risk of breast and ovarian cancer in women with strong family histories. Oncology. 2001;15(7):889–902.
88. Jervis S, Song H, Lee A, Dicks E, Tyrer J, Harrington P, et al. Ovarian cancer familial relative risks by tumour subtypes and by known ovarian cancer genetic susceptibility variants. J Med Genet. 2014;51(2):108–13.
89. Jervis S, Song H, Lee A, Dicks E, Harrington P, Baynes C, et al. A risk prediction algorithm for ovarian cancer incorporating BRCA1, BRCA2, common alleles and other familial effects. J Med Genet. 2015;52(7):465–75.
90. Siyam T, Ross S, Campbell S, Eurich DT, Yuksel N. The effect of hormone therapy on quality of life and breast cancer risk after risk-reducing salpingo-oophorectomy: a systematic review. BMC Womens Health. 2017;17:22.
91. Parker WH, Feskanich D, Broder M, Chang E, Shoupe D, Farquhar C, et al. Long-term mortalilty associated with oophorectomy versus ovarian conservation in the Nurses' Health Study. Obstet Gynecol. 2013;121(4):709–16.
92. Rocca WA, Grossardt BR, de Andrade M, Malkasian GD, Melton LJ. Survival patterns after oophorectomy in premenopausal women: a population-based cohort study. Lancet Oncol. 2006;7(10):821–8.
93. Evans EC, Matteson KA, Orejuela FJ, Alperin M, Balk EM, El-Nashar S, et al. Salpingo-oophorectomy at the time of benign hysterectomy: a systematic review. Obstet Gynecol. 2016;128:476–85.
94. Lancaster JM, Powell CB, Chen LM, Richardson DL. Society of gynecologic oncology statement on risk assessment for inherited gynecologic cancer predispositions. Gynecol Oncol. 2015;136(1):3–7.
95. Committee on Gynecologic Practice. Committee opinion no. 620: salpingectomy for ovarian cancer prevention. Obstet Gynecol. 2015;125(1):279–81.
96. Falconer H, Yin L, Grönberg H, Altman D. Ovarian cancer risk after salpingectomy: a nationwide population-based study. J Natl Cancer Inst. 2015;107(2):dju410.
97. Kwon JS, Mcalpine JN, Hanley GE, Finlayson SJ, Cohen T, Miller DM, et al. Costs and benefits of opportunistic salpingectomy as an ovarian cancer prevention strategy. Obstet Gynecol. 2015;125(2):338–45.
98. Minig L, Chuang L, Patrono MG, Cárdenas-Rebollo JM, García-Donas J. Surgical outcomes and complications of prophylactic salpingectomy at the time of benign hysterectomy in premenopausal women. J Minim Invasive Gynecol. 2015;22(4):653–7.

99. Morelli M, Venturella R, Mocciaro R, Di Cello A, Rania E, Lico D, et al. Prophylactic salpingectomy in premenopausal low-risk women for ovarian cancer: primum non nocere. Gynecol Oncol. 2013;129(3):448–51.
100. Findley AD, Siedhoff MT, Hobbs KA, Steege JF, Carey ET, McCall CA, et al. Short-term effects of salpingectomy during laparoscopic hysterectomy on ovarian reserve: a pilot randomized controlled trial. Fertil Steril. 2013;100(6):1704–8.
101. Ni L, Sadiq S, Mao Y, Cui Y, Wang W, Liu J. Influence of various tubal surgeries to serum antimullerian hormone level and outcome of the subsequent IVF-ET treatment. Gynecol Endocrinol. 2013;29(4):345–9.
102. Ye X, Yang Y, Sun X. A retrospective analysis of the effect of salpingectomy on serum antiMüllerian hormone level and ovarian reserve. Am J Obstet Gynecol. 2015;212(1):e53.e1–e53.e10.
103. Vorwergk J, Radosa MP, Nicolaus K, Baus N, Jimenez Cruz J, Rengsberger M, et al. Prophylactic bilateral salpingectomy (PBS) to reduce ovarian cancer risk incorporated in standard premenopausal hysterectomy: complications and re-operation rate. J Cancer Res Clin Oncol. 2014;140(5):859–65.
104. ClinicalTrials.gov identifier (NCT number): NCT01907789. Prophylactic salpingectomy with delayed oophorectomy, risk-reducing salpingo-oophorectomy, and ovarian cancer screening among BRCA mutation carriers: a proof-of-concept study.
105. M.D. Anderson Cancer Center. The women choosing surgical prevention (WISP) trial - Full Text View - ClinicalTrials.gov. ClinicalTrials.gov Identifier: NCT02760849.
106. Harmsen MG, Arts-de Jong M, Hoogerbrugge N, Maas AHEM, Prins JB, Bulten J, et al. Early salpingectomy (TUbectomy) with delayed oophorectomy to improve quality of life as alternative for risk-reducing salpingo-oophorectomy in BRCA1/2 mutation carriers (TUBA study): a prospective non-randomised multicentre study. BMC Cancer. 2015;15(1):593.
107. Leblanc E, Narducci F, Farre I, Peyrat J-P, Taieb S, Adenis C, et al. Radical fimbriectomy: a reasonable temporary risk-reducing surgery for selected women with a germ line mutation of BRCA 1 or 2 genes? Rationale and preliminary development. Gynecol Oncol. 2011;121(3):472–6.
108. Centre Oscar Lambret. Radical fimbriectomy for young BRCA mutation carriers - FullText View - ClinicalTrials.gov. ClinicalTrials.gov Identifier: NCT01608074.
109. Kwon JS, Tinker A, Pansegrau G, McAlpine J, Housty M, McCullum M, et al. Prophylactic salpingectomy and delayed oophorectomy as an alternative for BRCA mutation carriers. Obstet Gynecol. 2013;121(1):14–24.
110. Rice MS, Murphy MA, Vitonis AF, Cramer DW, Titus LJ, Tworoger SS, et al. Tubal ligation, hysterectomy and epithelial ovarian cancer in the New England Case-Control Study. Acta Obstet Gynecol Scand. 2013;133(10):86–94.
111. Rice MS, Hankinson SE, Tworoger SS. Tubal ligation, hysterectomy, unilateral oophorectomy, and risk of ovarian cancer in the Nurses' Health Studies. Fertil Steril. 2014;102(1):192.e3–8.e3.
112. Lessard-Anderson CR, Handlogten KS, Molitor RJ, Dowdy SC, Cliby WA, Weaver AL, et al. Effect of tubal sterilization technique on risk of serous epithelial ovarian and primary peritoneal carcinoma. Gynecol Oncol. 2014;135:423–7.
113. Madsen C, Baandrup L, Dehlendorff C, Kjaer SK. Tubal ligation and salpingectomy and the risk of epithelial ovarian cancer and borderline ovarian tumors: a nationwide case-control study. Acta Obstet Gynecol Scand. 2015;94(1):86–94.
114. Gaitskell K, Green J, Pirie K, Reeves G. Tubal ligation and ovarian cancer risk in a large cohort: substantial variation by histological type. Int J Cancer. 2016;138(5):1076–84.
115. Cibula D, Widschwendter M, Májek O, Dusek L. Tubal ligation and the risk of ovarian cancer: review and meta-analysis. Hum Reprod Update. 2011;17:55–67.
116. Rice MS, Murphy MA, Tworoger SS. Tubal ligation, hysterectomy and ovarian cancer: a meta-analysis. J Ovarian Res. 2012;5(1):13.
117. Chan J, Sammel MD, Friebel TM, Gracia C, Rebbeck TR. Tubal ligation does not modify ovarian cancer risk in BRCA mutation carriers. Fertil Steril. 2015;104(3):e259.
118. Beral V, Doll R, Hermon C, Peto R, Reeves G, Collaborative Group on Epidemiological Studies of Ovarian Cancer. Ovarian cancer and oral contraceptives: collaborative reanalysis of data from 45 epidemiological studies including 23,257 women with ovarian cancer and 87,303 controls. Lancet. 2008;371(9609):303–14.
119. Franceschi S, Parazzini F, Negri E, Booth M, La Vecchia C, Beral V, et al. Pooled analysis of 3 european case-control studies of epithelial ovarian cancer: III. Oral contraceptive use. Int J Cancer. 1991;49(1):61–5.
120. Bosetti C, Negri E, Trichopoulos D, Franceschi S, Beral V, Tzonou A, et al. Long-term effects of oral contraceptives on ovarian cancer risk. Int J Cancer. 2002;102(3):262–5.
121. Havrilesky LJ, Moorman PG, Lowery WJ, Gierisch JM, Coeytaux RR, Urrutia RP, et al. Oral contraceptive pills as primary prevention for ovarian cancer: a systematic review and meta-analysis. Obstet Gynecol. 2013;122:139–47.
122. Cibula D, Zikan M, Dusek L, Majek O. Oral contraceptives and risk of ovarian and breast cancers in BRCA mutation carriers: a meta-analysis. Expert Rev Anticancer Ther. 2011;11(8):1197–207.
123. Moorman PG, Havrilesky LJ, Gierisch JM, Coeytaux RR, Lowery WJ, Peragallo Urrutia R, et al. Oral contraceptives and risk of ovarian cancer and breast can-

cer among high-risk women: a systematic review and meta-analysis. J Clin Oncol. 2013;31(33):4188–98.
124. Stine JE, Bae-Jump V. Metformin and gynecologic cancers. Obstet Gynecol Surv. 2014;69(8):477–89.
125. Gadducci A, Biglia N, Tana R, Cosio S, Gallo M. Metformin use and gynecological cancers: a novel treatment option emerging from drug repositioning. Crit Rev Oncol Hematol. 2016;105:73–83.
126. Rattan R, Giri S, Hartmann LC, Shridhar V. Metformin attenuates ovarian cancer cell growth in an AMP-kinase dispensable manner. J Cell Mol Med. 2011;15(1):166–78.
127. Li C, Liu VWS, Chan DW, Yao KM, Ngan HYS. LY294002 and metformin cooperatively enhance the inhibition of growth and the induction of apoptosis of ovarian cancer cells. Int J Gynecol Cancer. 2012;22(1):15–22.
128. Al-Wahab Z, Mert I, Tebbe C, Chhina J, Hijaz M, Morris RT, et al. Metformin prevents aggressive ovarian cancer growth driven by high-energy diet: similarity with calorie restriction. Oncotarget. 2015;6(13):10908–23.
129. Algire C, Amrein L, Bazile M, David S, Zakikhani M, Pollak M. Diet and tumor LKB1 expression interact to determine sensitivity to anti-neoplastic effects of metformin in vivo. Oncogene. 2011;30(10):174–82.
130. Trabert B, Ness RB, Lo-Ciganic W-H, Murphy MA, Goode EL, Poole EM, et al. Aspirin, nonaspirin nonsteroidal anti-inflammatory drug, and acetaminophen use and risk of invasive epithelial ovarian cancer: a pooled analysis in the Ovarian Cancer Association Consortium. J Natl Cancer Inst. 2014;106(2):djt431.
131. Baandrup L, Faber MT, Christensen J, Jensen A, Andersen KK, Friis S, et al. Nonsteroidal anti-inflammatory drugs and risk of ovarian cancer: systematic review and meta-analysis of observational studies. Acta Obstet Gynecol Scand. 2013;92(3):245–55.
132. Baandrup L. Drugs with potential chemopreventive properties in relation to epithelial ovarian cancer-DOUBLEHYPHENa nationwide case-control study. Dan Med J. 2015;62(7):B5117.
133. Tsoref D, Panzarella T, Oza A. Aspirin in prevention of ovarian cancer: are we at the tipping point? J Natl Cancer Inst. 2014;106(2):djt453.
134. Olsen CM, Green AC, Whiteman DC, Sadeghi S, Kolahdooz F, Webb PM. Obesity and the risk of epithelial ovarian cancer: a systematic review and meta-analysis. Eur J Cancer. 2007;43(4):690–709.
135. Zhang M, Xie X, Lee AH, Binns CW. Sedentary behaviours and epithelial ovarian cancer risk. Cancer Causes Control. 2004;15(1):83–9.
136. Poorolajal J, Jenabi E, Masoumi SZ. Body mass index effects on risk of ovarian cancer: a meta- analysis. Asian Pac J Cancer Prev. 2014;15(18):7665–71.
137. Gwinn ML, Lee NC, Rhodes PH, Layde PM, Rubin GL. Pregnancy, breast feeding, and oral contraceptives and the risk of epithelial ovarian cancer. J Clin Epidemiol. 1990;43(6):559–68.
138. Whiteman DC, Siskind V, Purdie DM, Green AC. Timing of pregnancy and the risk of epithelial ovarian cancer. Cancer Epidemiol Biomark Prev. 2003;12(1):42–6.
139. Jordan SJ, Cushing-Haugen KL, Wicklund KG, Doherty JA, Rossing MA. Breast-feeding and risk of epithelial ovarian cancer. Cancer Causes Control. 2012;23(6):919–27.

Part IV

Vulva and Vagina

21 Risk Factors and Classification of Vulvar Intraepithelial Lesions

Kiran Abhijit Kulkarni, Geeta Acharya, and G. Sumangala

21.1 Introduction

Over the last few decades, an increasing trend in the incidence of high-grade preinvasive vulvar lesions, also at a younger age, has been reported [1]. The incidence of invasive vulvar cancer is also on the rise, though less compared to the rise in preinvasive lesions [2]. The Surveillance, Epidemiology, and End Results (SEER) data reported and estimated 6020 new cases in 2017 with an incidence of 2.5 per 100,000 women per year. The number of deaths was 0.5 per 100,000 women per year. Approximately 0.3% of women will be diagnosed with vulvar cancer at some point during their lifetime, based on 2012–2014 data [3].

Though almost 85% of high-grade vulvar intraepithelial neoplasia (VIN) lesions are related to human papilloma virus (HPV), HPV DNA is detectable only in 40% of the invasive cancers [4]. In elderly women, many of the HPV-negative vulvar malignancies are associated with chronic dermatologic conditions such as lichen sclerosus [5].

K. A. Kulkarni (✉) · G. Acharya · G. Sumangala
Department of Gynaecological Oncology, St. John's Medical College and Hospital,
Bangalore, Karnataka, India

21.2 Classification of VIN

VIN and vulvar squamous cell carcinoma (VSCC) represent neoplastic changes in the epithelium of the vulva. The causes of VIN and VSCC can be broadly categorized into two categories: (1) HPV-related and (2) non-HPV-related inflammatory skin conditions such as lichen sclerosus. The earlier terminology of vulvar lesions did not distinguish the etiopathogenic pathways [6] nor the different malignant potential of these lesions. Over the years, classification and terminology for VIN have been revised to be able to do so. The latest revision was recommended by the International Society for the Study of Vulvovaginal Disease (ISSVD) in 2015 [7].

21.3 Evolution of Nomenclature

The first description of squamous preinvasive lesions of the vulva was around a century ago.

In 1912, J. T. Bowen, a dermatologist, noted hyperplasia of the epidermis of the vulva with absence of the stratum granulosum along with increased mitoses and clumping of the nuclei. There was no evidence of dermal invasion; however, he did speculate that these lesions may be precancerous [8].

S. Mehta, A. Singla (eds.), *Preventive Oncology for the Gynecologist*,
https://doi.org/10.1007/978-981-13-3438-2_21

After a decade, Hudelo et al. coined the term 'erythroplasiform dyskeratosis of the vulvar mucosa' to describe the histological features of Bowen's disease [9].

More such cases were reported in the 1940s with one case being associated with vulvar squamous cell carcinoma highlighting the possibility of progression to malignancy [10].

The term 'carcinoma in situ' (CIS) was proposed by Woodruff et al. in 1958, to reduce the variability in the terminology used to describe the precursor lesions [11].

Based on their observations in 1961 on a relatively large number of carcinomas of the vulva, Abell and Gosling [12] reported that intraepithelial squamous cell carcinoma of the vulva exists in three forms:

- Intraepithelial carcinoma simplex, associated with leukoplakic vulvitis
- Intraepithelial carcinoma of Bowen's type
- Intraepithelial carcinoma of Paget's type

Kaufman in 1965 classified the premalignant lesions of the vulva as Queyrat erythroplasia, bowenoid carcinoma in situ and carcinoma simplex [13].

Some studies reported spontaneous regression of lesions similar to CIS, especially in young pregnant women [14, 15]. This made it evident that there was a difference in the natural history of some lesions.

The term 'intraepithelial neoplasia' was first proposed by Richart in 1967 and subsequently by Crum in 1982. The terminology was instituted initially for lesions of the cervix and, later, the vulva [16].

The term bowenoid papulosis of the genitalia was described by Wade et al. in 1979, with many giving a history of preceding viral infection. These lesions on histopathological examination revealed features of carcinoma in situ and stated that bowenoid papulosis was a new entity whose clinical behaviour was unknown if left untreated [17].

21.4 Role of the International Society for the Study of Vulvovaginal Disease (ISSVD)

A society composed of dermatologists, pathologists, and gynaecologists has contributed significantly in determining the terminology used for vulvar lesions over the years since its inception in 1970.

21.4.1 ISSVD (1976)

In 1976, ISSVD came up with a new terminology with the idea of reducing the confusing array of terms. They proposed the term 'squamous cell carcinoma in situ' and 'hyperplastic dystrophy'. Hyperplastic dystrophy was further qualified as mild, moderate or severe atypia [18].

In 1982, the term 'VIN' was first introduced [19], and the ISSVD adopted it as a general category of intraepithelial squamous neoplasms in 1986.

21.4.2 ISSVD (1986)

The ISSVD subdivided the terminology into the following categories:

- Squamous (may include HPV change):
  - VIN 1—mild atypia
  - VIN 2—moderate atypia
  - VIN 3—severe atypia, carcinoma in situ
- Non-squamous: Paget's disease and melanoma in situ.
- The additional category, 'VIN III, differentiated type', was also introduced to include cases associated with dermatologic conditions such as lichen sclerosus [20].

21.4.3 ISSVD (2004)

Over the ensuing years, it was quite evident that VIN 1, 2 and 3 did not exist on a biological continuum, as earlier thought. VIN 1 composed of condyloma acuminatum and was associated with low-risk HPV types 6 and 11. It did not carry a risk of progression to invasive lesion. However, VIN 2 and 3 were associated with high-risk HPV types and carried a risk of progression to squamous cell carcinoma.

Inclusion of VIN 1 in the earlier classification led to overdiagnosis and unnecessary interventions in low-grade disease and misunderstanding the HPV effect on vulvar lesions [6].

Considering the difference in risk of progression and prognosis, VIN 1 was dropped, and ISSVD proposed a two-tier classification system in 2004 [21]:

- Usual VIN (uVIN): It includes lesions previously classified as VIN 2 and VIN 3. It is subdivided into warty, basaloid, and mixed types and is associated with HPV infection.
- Differentiated VIN (dVIN): It is associated with dermatologic conditions such as lichen sclerosus, not associated with HPV infection.

21.5 Other Classifications

21.5.1 World Health Organization (WHO) Classification

In 2003 WHO had come up with a similar classification and continued to use the VIN 1 as a small proportion of VIN 1 cases were associated with high-risk HPV [22]. WHO revised this classification in 2014.

21.5.2 Bethesda System-Like Classification (2005)

In 2005, Medeiros et al. [23] proposed a classification scheme similar to the Bethesda system for cervical precursor lesions:

- Low-grade vulvar intraepithelial lesion (LG-VIL) category which encompassed several variants of condyloma
- High-grade VIL category (HG-VIL) which included uVIN and dVIN

21.5.3 Recent Classification Systems

21.5.3.1 Lower Anogenital Squamous Terminology (LAST) 2012

After almost 100 years of evolution, there was some consensus among multiple committees, all supporting the terminology 'squamous intraepithelial lesion' (SIL). The College of American Pathologists (CAP) and American Society for Colposcopy and Cervical Pathology (ASCCP) jointly published the Lower Anogenital Squamous Terminology (LAST) guidelines in 2012 [24], unifying the terminology in consensus with ISSVD. It applied to all HPV lesions involving the cervix, vulva, vagina, anus, perineum and penis, under two headings:

- Low-grade squamous intraepithelial lesion (LSIL), equivalent to uVIN 1
- High-grade squamous intraepithelial lesion (HSIL) encompassing uVIN 2 and uVIN 3

The intraepithelial neoplasia (IN) grade could be included in parentheses, if so desired. The LAST terminology was thought to be more reproducible and biologically relevant compared to the earlier systems; however, it was not applicable to the non-HPV-related lesions. Another fallacy of the LAST terminology was that it reintroduced the concept of VIN 1 as LSIL.

21.5.3.2 The WHO 2014 Classification

WHO accepted the SIL terminology but in addition included dVIN as a separate category [25].

The WHO currently classifies vulvar lesions into two different lesions of the squamous epithelium based on the pathogenesis (HPV-induced or HPV-negative).

Squamous intraepithelial lesion (SIL): SIL includes HPV-associated intraepithelial lesions and is further categorized into LSIL and HSIL similar to cervical and vaginal lesions.

Differentiated VIN (dVIN): dVIN refers to HPV-negative lesions which arise in the context of dermatoses (lichen sclerosus and lichen planus). In contrast to HPV-associated lesions (SIL), severity of dVIN is not graded.

While vulvar LSIL has a high rate of spontaneous remission, HSIL and dVIN have a significant risk of progression to invasive carcinoma. dVIN, though less common than HSIL, progresses faster to invasive carcinoma [26].

21.5.3.3 ISSVD 2015

The rationale for changing the terminology in 2015 by ISSVD was to address two major concerns of the LAST terminology: (1) it did not include dVIN lesions, and (2) it had reintroduced the concept of LSIL corresponding to VIN 1 with a potential increase in overdiagnosis and overtreatment [7].

The ISSVD 2015 recommends the following terms:

- Low-grade squamous intraepithelial lesion of the vulva (vulvar LSIL) which includes external genital warts corresponding to VIN 1 lesions (Fig. 21.1)
- High-grade squamous intraepithelial lesion of the vulva (vulvar HSIL) (Fig. 21.2)
- DVIN: vulvar intraepithelial neoplasia, differentiated

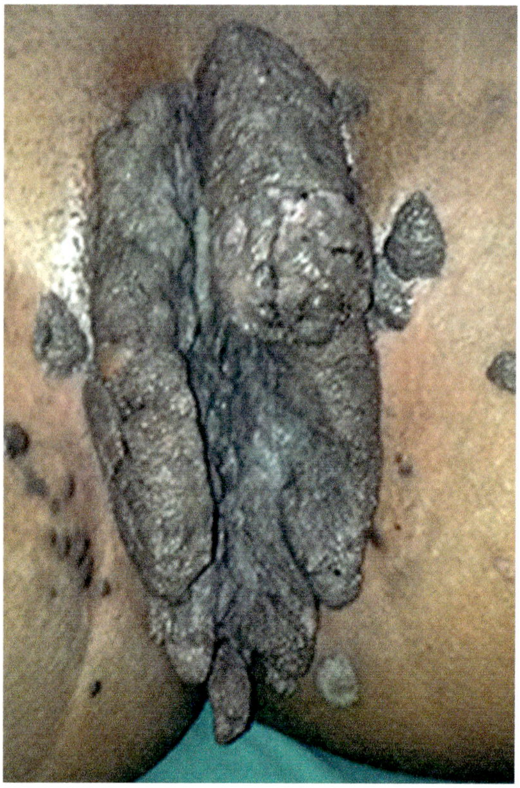

Fig. 21.1 Genital wart. Low-grade squamous intraepithelial lesion

The committee came to a conclusion that a modified form of the WHO 2014 classification would address both the concerns regarding the LAST terminology. The version that was finally adopted by the ISSVD does contain LSIL. However, the word 'neoplasia' is replaced by 'lesion', and in parentheses, it needs to be stated whether the meaning of this term is a flat condyloma or HPV effect. This expresses the approach of the ISSVD that LSIL is not precancerous and does not need to be treated, unless symptomatic.

The term HSIL is used, maintaining in parentheses the previous term of usual VIN. Table 21.1 shows comparison between dVIN and HSIL.

'Vulvar intraepithelial neoplasia differentiated' is the third category, just as in the previous ISSVD terminologies.

This terminology was presented, discussed and accepted by a majority vote at the ISSVD World Congress on 28 July 2015. The ISSVD executive council recommends that the present terminology replace all previous versions of terminology of VIN.

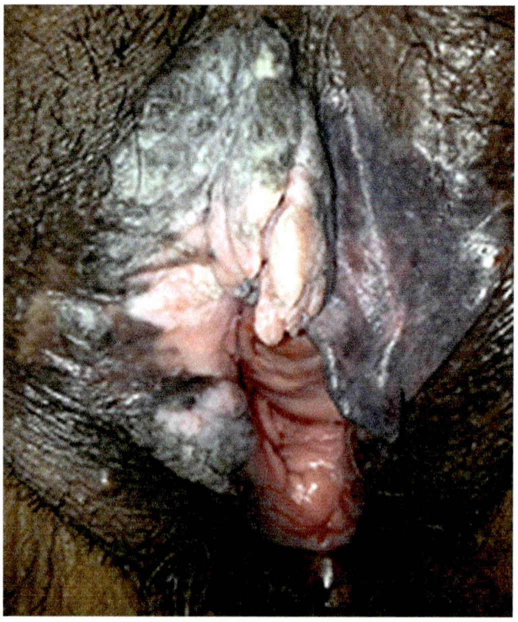

Fig. 21.2 High-grade squamous intraepithelial lesion

Table 21.1 Comparison between dVIN and HSIL[a]

	dVIN	HSIL
Age	Sixth to eighth decade	Third to fifth decade
Percentage of all vulvar preinvasive diagnosis	5	95
Multifocality	Unusual	>50%
Smoking	Not associated	Associated in 60%
Associated conditions	Chronic inflammatory dermatosis, most commonly lichen sclerosus Only 1.5% dVIN HPV+	>80% HPV+
Pigmented clinically	Unknown	10%
Progression to carcinoma	35%	5%
Time from biopsy to invasion	23 months	41 months
Recurrence	Common	less common than dVIN but significant at 15–50%
Immunohistochemistry	Commonly p53+, basal and suprabasal layers	p16 block positivity
Adnexal extension (follicles and sebaceous glands)	Rare	Common
Most common invasion histology if progresses	Keratinizing SCC	Warty/basaloid SCC

dVIN differentiated vulvar intraepithelial neoplasia, *HSIL* high-grade squamous intraepithelial lesion, *SCC* squamous cell carcinoma

[a]Reprinted from Obstetrics and Gynecology Clinics of North America, 44(3), Allbritton JI, Vulvar neoplasms, benign and malignant, 339-352, Copyright 2017, with permission from Elsevier

Table 21.2 Evolution of nomenclature for vulvar pre invasive lesions[a]

ISSVD 1976	ISSVD 1986	ISSVD 2004, WHO 2003	Bethesda-like (2005)	LAST 2012 WHO 2014 ISSVD 2015
Mild atypia	VIN I	[b]	LG-VIL – Condyloma – VIN 1	LSIL—VIN 1, condyloma, mild dysplasia, koilocytic atypia
Moderate/severe atypia, CIS	VIN II, VIN III, CIS	uVIN – VIN 2, 3	HG-VIL—VIN 2, 3	HSIL—VIN 2, 3 Moderate/severe dysplasia, CIS
	VIN III, differentiated type	dVIN	dVIN	dVIN[c]

CIS carcinoma in situ, *dVIN* differentiated type VIN, *HG-VIL* high-grade vulvar intraepithelial lesion, *HSIL* high-grade squamous intraepithelial lesion, *ISSVD* International Society for the Study of Vulvovaginal Disease, *LAST* lower anogenital squamous terminology, *LG-VIL* low-grade vulvar intraepithelial lesion, *LSIL* low-grade squamous intraepithelial lesion, *uVIN* usual-type VIN, *VIN* vulvar intraepithelial neoplasia, *WHO* World Health Organization

[a]Reprinted from Pathology, 48(4), Hoang LN, Park KJ, Soslow RA, Murali R, Squamous precursor lesions of the vulva: current classification and diagnostic challenges, Pathology, 291-302, Copyright 2016, with permission from Elsevier

[b]The 2004 ISSVD no longer recognized VIN, but the 2003 WHO retained the designation

[c]dVIN not included in the LAST guidelines

A brief summary stating the various nomenclature classifications is depicted in Table 21.2.

Table 21.3 depicts the latest classification system proposed by the ISSVD 2015.

Table 21.3 Squamous intraepithelial neoplasia—ISSVD 2015 terminology[a]

ISSVD 2015 terminology	Significance	Alias terminology
Low-grade squamous intraepithelial lesion of the vulva	Infection with low-risk HPV causing viral cytopathic effect, atypia in less than or equal to lower third of the vulvar epithelium without cytopathic effect	Flat condyloma Condyloma accuminatum VIN 1 Mild dysplasia
High-grade squamous intraepithelial lesion of the vulva	Premalignant change in more than a third of the epithelium with basaloid/warty appearance, signifies infection with high-risk HPV	Usual VIN, VIN 2, 3 Moderate/severe dysplasia Intraepithelial carcinoma, Bowen type
Differentiated VIN	Premalignant change often associated with an inflammatory dermatosis (e.g. lichen sclerosus), rather than HPV, more aggressive than high-grade squamous intraepithelial lesion	Simplex-type VIN Intraepithelial carcinoma, simplex type Squamous cell hyperplasia with atypia

HPV human papilloma virus, *VIN* vulvar intraepithelial neoplasia
[a]Data from [7]

21.6 Risk Factors for Vulvar Intraepithelial Lesions

Women with vulvar dermatological problems visit various healthcare professionals such as gynaecologists, dermatologists, primary-care physicians and nursing personnel. With the incidence of VIN on the rise and with a potential to progress to malignancy, early diagnosis of VIN is important.

The incidence of both uVIN and dVIN has increased over the last few decades, while the incidence of VSCC has remained relatively unaltered [1].

21.6.1 Race

The incidence of VIN is reported to be higher among white women compared to black, Asian/Pacific Islander or Hispanic women [27].

21.6.2 Age

VIN, usual type, is regarded as a disease of primarily younger women, 3rd to 5th decade of life. Several studies report that the mean age of women diagnosed with VIN 3 has reduced over the years which coincided with an increased incidence of VIN 3 [28].

There is often a second peak in incidence of VIN in the 60- to 80-year range, which may reflect the peak incidence of differentiated-type VIN. Differentiated VIN comprises less than 5–30% of all VIN [29]. Older women with VIN have a higher risk of progression to malignancy.

21.6.3 Behaviour

The increased incidence of VIN is probably a result of certain behavioural changes such as increased sexual promiscuity, HPV, smoking and improved awareness of the disease [30], which also correlate with presence of intraepithelial lesions in the rest of the lower genital tract such as the cervix and vagina.

21.6.4 Risk Factors for Progression to Invasive Carcinoma

Studies have reported presence of dVIN adjacent to VSCC in approximately 40% of the cases. These findings implied that dVIN was more likely to progress to VSCC than uVIN (32.8% vs. 5.7%) and in a shorter time (22.8 months vs. 41.4 months) than uVIN [31, 32]. A history of prior, synchronous or subsequent VSCC is more often found in dVIN than uVIN (85.7% vs. 25.7% for uVIN) [30].

dVIN are less prevalent, probably because they are transient and/or underreported or underdiagnosed; however, they carry a higher malignant potential than uVIN.

Risk factors for malignant progression in uVIN included advanced age, radiotherapy and immunocompromised status [33].

Human papilloma virus and VIN: Prior to the understanding of the role of HPV as the causative agent of cervical carcinoma, multiple etiological agents were implicated such as herpes simplex virus (HSV), arsenic and even granulomas [11].

Subsequently research revealed that HPV was found to be responsible for the vast majority of anogenital squamous carcinomas and was also detected in VIN [34, 35].

HPV infection is strongly associated with uVIN. Many studies have reported a HPV positivity of >80% [36–38].

HPV16 was the most common type (77.2%), followed by HPV33 (10.6%) and HPV18 (2.6%). Over 90% of LSIL were attributed to low-risk HPV types 6 and 11 [39].

The rate of positivity of high-risk HPV in uVIN is disproportionately higher than that seen in vulvar squamous cell carcinoma. In a study of 1709 VSCC, only 28.6% of cases harboured HPV [40]. This discrepancy led investigators to explore alternative HPV-independent pathways to VSCC, leading to the identification of dVIN as a separate oncogenic pathway to VSCC. A cumulative 134 cases of dVIN have been tested for HPV in the literature, of which only 2 (1.5%) were positive [41].

Failure of the immune system to produce an effective response to high-risk HPV is related to virus persistence and host factors such as age, smoking and sexual behaviour. With the persistence of high-risk HPV infection, viral oncoproteins E6 and E7 can interfere with important control mechanisms of the cell cycle leading to malignancy.

Immunization with the quadrivalent or 9-valent human papillomavirus vaccine, which is effective against human papillomavirus genotypes, has been shown to decrease the risk of vulvar high-grade squamous intraepithelial lesion (HSIL) (VIN usual type) [42].

21.6.5 Smoking and VIN

It has been found that there is a strong association between cigarette smoking and various neoplasms, including vulvar intraepithelial neoplasia. These women present with VIN at a younger age. The percentage of cigarette smokers within the study cohort was similar to that of cervical cancer [43] and had multicentric disease. Smokers are more likely to have microinvasion at the first excision and were not cured in a single session, needing multiple sessions of therapy [44]. Women who continued to smoke after treatment were 30 times more likely to have persistent vulvar disease. A complete assessment of these cases should include proctoscopy in addition to the colposcopic examination of the cervix and vagina [44].

21.6.6 Immunosuppression

Immunosuppression has been reported to increase the incidence of intraepithelial lesions and also the risk of progression to invasive disease. Therefore, the need for follow-up is heightened among these women.

- Iatrogenic immunosuppression: Women who have had renal transplants have been shown to be up to 40 times more at risk of vaginal or vulvar cancers and more likely to develop genital tract dysplasia [45].
- Chronic steroid use with autoimmune disorders and post chemotherapy is also associated with increased incidence of VIN [46].
- Human immunodeficiency virus (HIV): A meta-analysis of 50,000 women with human immunodeficiency virus (HIV) reported a relative risk for VIN of 4.6 and 5.8 for invasive cancer of the vulva and vagina, respectively [47].

HIV-positive women frequently present at a younger age with multifocal and multicentric disease. Close surveillance of the lower genital tract is mandatory to enable early recognition and treatment of any suspicious lesions. Close follow-up after treatment of VIN is essential to exclude early recurrence or progression [48].

21.6.7 Chronic Dermatologic Conditions

- Lichen sclerosus (LS): Lichen sclerosus (LS) is a chronic non-neoplastic, non-infectious, inflammatory skin disorder with a predilection for the genital area with a chronic relapsing remitting course. The condition is currently considered as an autoimmune disorder occurring in genetically predisposed patients. LS predisposes to infections such as candidiasis, herpes or HPV-related lesions due to long-term usage of topical steroids.

  LS is frequently seen in association with dVIN. Long-term studies have shown that LS has 1–3% of progression to VSCC [49, 50] (Fig. 21.3).

  LS has been referred to as atypical LS when there is basal nuclear atypia. Atypical LS may show increased p53 staining and may represent a very early form of dVIN [31].

  LS with hyperplasia, dyskeratosis and parakeratosis, referred to as hypertrophic LS, may or may not have increased risk of progression to VSCC [51].

  It has been proposed that dVIN can develop from lichen sclerosus and that the presence of both strongly increases the cancer risk, especially in women >70 years of age. Women with lichen sclerosus with concurrent VIN had a 10-year VSCC risk of 18% compared with 3% in lichen sclerosus women without VIN [52].

  As a supporting observation, several authors have found both dVIN and lichen sclerosus adjacent to VSCC in 25–65% of the cancer cases [53]. dVIN should be suspected if there is any circumscribed lesion resistant to ultra-potent topical corticosteroids.

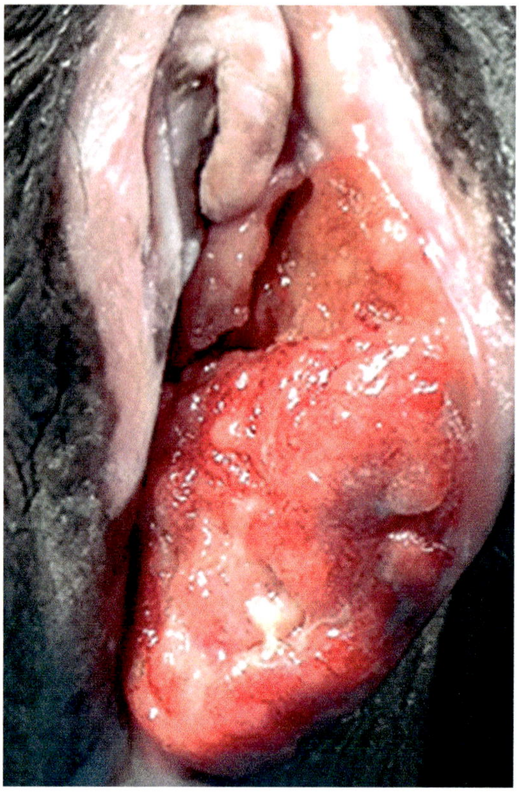

Fig. 21.3 Vulvar squamous cell carcinoma with a backdrop of lichen sclerosus

  Further studies with long-term follow-up are needed to clarify the natural history of LS, atypical LS and hypertrophic LS.
- Lichen planus (LP): Vulvar LP is a chronic condition, with an unpredictable relapsing and remitting course. Transformation into squamous cell carcinoma is rare but documented, especially with erosive LP. It is likely that LP, like LS, has a precursor stage which is resistant to steroids (differentiated VIN, acanthotic LP or usual VIN) before progressing into malignancy [54].

21.6.8 Other Preinvasive Conditions

21.6.8.1 Vulvar Paget's Disease (VPD)

The World Health Organization (WHO) defines VPD as 'an intraepithelial neoplasm of epithelial origin expressing apocrine or eccrine glandular-like features and characterized by distinctive large cells with prominent cytoplasm, referred to as Paget cells'. It is further classified as primary (cutaneous) and secondary (non-cutaneous) VPD [55].

Primary (cutaneous) VPD:

- Type 1a: Intraepithelial lesion without dermal invasion
- Type 1b: Dermal invasion of Paget's cells
- Type 1c: Cutaneous vulvar disease as a manifestation of an underlying vulvar adenocarcinoma

Secondary (non-cutaneous VPD):

- Type 2: VPD originates from rectal or anal adenocarcinoma
- Type 3: VPD originates from urogenital neoplasia

In approximately 25% of the cases, VPD is invasive; in these cases, the prognosis is worse than in non-invasive cases. Recurrence rates in invasive VPD are high, 33% in cases with clear margins, and even higher when surgical margins are not clear, regardless of invasion.

21.6.8.2 Melanoma In Situ

Melanoma in situ is an uncommon pigmented nonepithelial vulvar preinvasive lesion. The lesion may be clinically similar to more common benign pigmented lesions such as melanosis. Biopsy is a must for diagnosis. The risk of progression to malignancy is unknown, though documented [56]. The in situ phase may extend over a long period of time.

21.7 Conclusion

The incidence of high-grade preinvasive disease of the vulva is increasing and that too in the younger age group. Majority of VIN is associated with HPV infection though in elderly women many of the vulvar malignancies are HPV-negative and are associated with chronic dermatologic conditions. The common risk factors for VIN are persistent high-risk HPV infection, smoking, immunosuppression, promiscuous sexual behaviour and presence of chronic dermatologic conditions such as lichen sclerosus and lichen planus. A high index of suspicion for VIN in women with these risk factors can help in diagnosing the disease early.

Key Points

- Increasing trend in the incidence of high-grade preinvasive vulvar lesions at a younger age has been reported with a relatively stable incidence of invasive cancer.
- The terminology for vulvar epithelial lesions has been modified many times over the years. The present recommended terminology is the one proposed by ISSVD in 2015.
- VIN has dual oncogenic pathways: HPV-related and non-HPV-related, reflected in the present classification systems as LSIL, HSIL for HPV-related lesions and dVIN for non-HPV-related lesions.
- dVIN, though less common, has a higher risk of progression to malignancy, especially with advanced age.
- The common risk factors for VIN are persistent high-risk HPV infection, smoking, immunosuppression, promiscuous sexual behaviour and presence of chronic dermatologic conditions such as lichen sclerosus and lichen planus.
- Non-squamous intraepithelial lesions are extramammary Paget's disease and melanoma in situ.

Acknowledgement and Consent The authors acknowledge the patients who gave an informed consent to the publication of the images.

References

1. Judson PL, Habermann EB, Baxter NN, Durham SB, Virnig BA. Trends in the incidence of invasive and in situ vulvar carcinoma. Obstet Gynecol. 2006;107:1018–22.
2. Bodelon C, Madeleine MM, Voigt LF, Weiss NS. Is the incidence of invasive vulvar cancer increasing

in the United States? Cancer Causes Control. 2009;20(9):1779–82.
3. SEER Cancer Stat Facts 2017: Vulvar Cancer. National Cancer Institute. Bethesda, MD. http://seer.cancer.gov/statfacts/html/vulva.html.
4. De Yust H, Clifford GM, Nascimento MC, Madeleine MM, Franceschi S. Prevalence and type distribution of human papillomavirus in carcinoma and intraepithelial neoplasia of the vulva, vagina and anus: a meta-analysis. Int J Cancer. 2009;124(7):1626–36. https://doi.org/10.1002/ijc.24116.
5. Trimble CL, Hildesheim A, Brinton LA, Shah KV, Kurman RJ. Heterogeneous etiology of squamous carcinoma of the vulva. Obstet Gynecol. 1996;87(1):59–64.
6. Preti M, Scurry J, Marchitelli CE, Micheletti L. Vulvar intraepithelial neoplasia. Best Pract Res Clin Obstet Gynaecol. 2014;28:1051–62.
7. Bornstein J, Bogliatto F, Haefner HK, Stockdale CK, Preti M, Bohl TG, et al. The 2015 International Society for the Study of Vulvovaginal Disease (ISSVD) terminology of vulvar squamous intraepithelial lesions. J Low Genit Tract Dis. 2016;20:11–4.
8. Bowen JT. Centennial paper. May 1912 (J Cutan Dis Syph 1912;30:241-255). Precancerous dermatoses: a study of two cases of chronic atypical epithelial proliferation. Arch Dermatol. 1983;119:243–60.
9. Hudelo ML, Cailliau O. Dyskeratose erythroplasiforme de la muqueuse vulvaire. Bull Soc Franc Dermatol Syph. 1922;29:139–42.
10. Knight RVD. Bowen's disease of the vulva. Am J Obstet Gynecol. 1943;undefined:514–24.
11. Woodruff JD, Hildebrandt EE. Carcinoma in situ of the vulva. Obstet Gynecol. 1958;12(4):414–24.
12. Abell MR, Gosling JR. Intraepithelial and infiltrative carcinoma of vulva: Bowen's type. Cancer. 1961;14:318–29.
13. Preti M, Van Seters M, Sideri M, Van Beurden M. Squamous vulvar intraepithelial neoplasia. Clin Obstet Gynecol. 2005;48:845–61.
14. Berger BW, Hori Y. Multicentric Bowen's disease of the genitalia: spontaneous regression of lesions. Arch Dermatol. 1978;114:1698–9.
15. Friedrich EG. Reversible vulvar atypia. A case report. Obstet Gynecol. 1972;39:173–81.
16. Richart RM. Natural history of cervical intraepithelial neoplasia. Clin Obstet Gynecol. 1967;10:748–84.
17. Wade TR, Kopf AW, Ackerman AB. Bowenoid papulosis of the genitalia. Arch Dermatol. 1979;115:306–8.
18. Kaufman R, DiPaola G, Friedrich E, et al. New nomenclature for vulvar disease. Obstet Gynecol. 1976;47:122–4.
19. Crum CP, Fu YS, Levine RU, Richart RM, Townsend DE, Fenoglio CM. Intraepithelial squamous lesions of the vulva: biologic and histologic criteria for the distinction of condylomas from vulvar intraepithelial neoplasia. Am J Obstet Gynecol. 1982;144:77–83.
20. Wilkinson EJ, Kneale B, Lynch PJ. Report of the ISSVD terminology committee. Reprod Med. 1986;31:973–4.
21. Sideri M, Jones RW, Wilkinson EJ, Preti M, Heller DS, Scurry J, et al. Squamous vulvar intraepithelial neoplasia: 2004 modified terminology, ISSVD Vulvar Oncology Subcommittee. J Reprod Med. 2005;50:807–10.
22. Scurry J, Wilkinson EJ. Review of terminology of precursors of vulvar squamous cell carcinoma. J Low Genit Tract Dis. 2006;10:161–9.
23. Medeiros F, Nascimento AF, Crum CP. Early vulvar squamous neoplasia: advances in classification, diagnosis, and differential diagnosis. Adv Anat Pathol. 2005;12:20–6.
24. Darragh TM, Colgan TJ, Thomas Cox J, Heller DS, Henry MR, Luff RD, McCalmont T, Members of the LAST Project Work Groups, et al. The lower anogenital squamous terminology standardization project for HPV associated lesions: background and consensus recommendations from the College of American Pathologists and the American Society for Colposcopy and Cervical Pathology. Int J Gynecol Pathol. 2013;32(1):76–115.
25. Kurman RJ, Carcangiu ML, Herrington CS, editors. WHO classification of tumours of female reproductive organs. 4th ed. Lyon: International Agency for Research on Cancer; 2014. p. 229–53.
26. Van de Nieuwenhof HP, van der Avoort IA, de Hullu JA. Review of squamous premalignant vulvar lesions. Crit Rev Oncol Hematol. 2008;68:131–56.
27. Saraiya M, Watson M, Wu X, King JB, Chen VW, Smith JS, et al. Incidence of in situ and invasive vulvar cancer in the US,1998 - 2003. Cancer. 2008;113:2865–72.
28. Committee opinion no. 675 summary: management of vulvar intraepithelial neoplasia. Obstet Gynecol 2016;128:937–8.
29. Eva LJ, Ganesan R, Chan KK, Honest H, Luesley DM. Differentiated-type vulval intraepithelial neoplasia has a high-risk association with vulval squamous cell carcinoma. Int J Gynecol Cancer. 2009;19:741–4.
30. Preti M, Bucchi L, Ghiringhello B, Privitera S, Frau V, Corvetto E, et al. Risk factors for unrecognized invasive carcinoma in patients with vulvar high-grade squamous intraepithelial lesion at vulvoscopy-directed biopsy. J Gynecol Oncol. 2017;28(4):e27. https://doi.org/10.3802/jgo.2017.28.e27.
31. Chiesa-Vottero A, Dvoretsky PM, Hart WR. Histopathologic study of thin vulvar squamous cell carcinomas and associated cutaneous lesions: a correlative study of 48 tumors in 44 patients with analysis of adjacent vulvar intraepithelial neoplasia types and lichen sclerosus. Am J Surg Pathol. 2006;30:310–8.
32. Van de Nieuwenhof HP, Massuger LF, van der Avoort IA, Bekkers RL, Casparie M, Abma W, et al. Vulvar squamous cell carcinoma development after diagnosis of VIN increases with age. Eur J Cancer. 2009;45:851–6.
33. Jones RW, Rowan DM, Stewart AW. Vulvar intraepithelial neoplasia: aspects of the natural history

and outcome in 405 women. Obstet Gynecol. 2005;106:319–1326.
34. Zur Hausen H. Papillomaviruses in the causation of human cancers – a brief historical account. Virology. 2009;384:260–5.
35. Zachow KR, Ostrow RS, Bender M, Watts S, Okagaki T, Pass F, et al. Detection of human papillomavirus DNA in anogenital neoplasias. Nature. 1982;300:771–3.
36. Haefner HK, Tate JE, McLachlin CM, Crum CP. Vulvar intraepithelial neoplasia: age, morphological phenotype, papillomavirus DNA, and coexisting invasive carcinoma. Hum Pathol. 1995;26:147–54.
37. Park JS, Jones RW, McLean MR, Currie JL, Woodruff JD, Shah KV, et al. Possible etiologic heterogeneity of vulvar intraepithelial neoplasia. A correlation of pathologic characteristics with human papillomavirus detection by in situ hybridization and polymerase chain reaction. Cancer. 1991;67:1599–607.
38. Del Pino M, Rodriguez-Carunchio L, Ordi J. Pathways of vulvar intraepithelial neoplasia and squamous cell carcinoma. Histopathology. 2013;62:161–75.
39. Léonard B, Kridelka F, Delbecque K, Goffin F, Demoulin S, Doyen J, et al. A clinical and pathological overview of vulvar condyloma acuminatum, intraepithelial neoplasia, and squamous cell carcinoma. Biomed Res Int. 2014;2014:480573.
40. De Sanjosé S, Alemany L, Ordi J, Tous S, Alejo M, Bigby SM, et al. Worldwide human papillomavirus genotype attribution in over 2000 cases of intraepithelial and invasive lesions of the vulva. Eur J Cancer. 1990;49:3450–61.
41. Santos M, Landolfi S, Olivella A, Lloveras B, Klaustermeier J, Suárez H, et al. p16 overexpression identifies HPV-positive vulvar squamous cell carcinomas. Am J Surg Pathol. 2006;30:1347–56.
42. Committee opinion no. 675 summary: management of vulvar intraepithelial neoplasia. Obstet Gynecol. 2016;128(4):937–8. https://doi.org/10.1097/AOG.0000000000001704.
43. Wilkinson EJ, Cook JC, Friedrich EG Jr, Massey J. Vulvar intraepithelial neoplasia: association with cigarette smoking. J Gynecol Surg. 2009;4(3):153–9. https://doi.org/10.1089/gyn.1988.4.153.
44. Khan AM, Freeman-Wang T, Pisal N, Singer A. Smoking and multicentric vulval intraepithelial neoplasia. J Obstet Gynaecol. 2009;29(2):123–5. https://doi.org/10.1080/01443610802668938.
45. MacLean AB, Lynn KL, Bailey RR, Swainson CP, Walker RJ. Colposcopic assessment of the lower genital tract in female renal transplant recipients. Clin Nephrol. 1986;26:45–7.
46. Wallbillich JJ, Rhodes HE, Milbourne AM, Munsell MF, Frumovitz M, Brown J, et al. Vulvar intraepithelial neoplasia (VIN2/3): comparing clinical outcomes and evaluating risk factors for recurrence. Gynecol Oncol. 2012;127(2):312–5. https://doi.org/10.1016/j.ygyno.2012.07.118.
47. Ferenczy C, Coutlée F, Franco E, Hankins C. Human papilloma virus and HIV confection and the risk of neoplasias of the lower genital tract: a review of recent developments. CMAJ. 2003;169:431–4.
48. Bradbury M, Cabrera S, García-Jiménez A, Franco-Camps S, Sánchez-Iglesias JL, Díaz-Feijoo B, et al. Vulvar intraepithelial neoplasia: clinical presentation, management and outcomes in women infected with HIV. AIDS. 2016;30(6):859–68. https://doi.org/10.1097/QAD.0000000000000984.
49. Hart WR, Norris HJ, Helwig EB. Relation of lichen sclerosus et atrophicus of the vulva to development of carcinoma. Obstet Gynecol. 1975;45:369–77.
50. Lee A, Bradford J, Fischer G. Long-term management of adult vulvar lichen sclerosus: a prospective cohort study of 507 women. JAMA Dermatol. 2015;151:1061–7.
51. Weyers W. Hypertrophic lichen sclerosus with dyskeratosis and parakeratosis—a common presentation of vulvar lichen sclerosus not associated with a significant risk of malignancy. Am J Dermatopathol. 2013;35:713–21.
52. Bleeker MC, Visser PJ, Overbeek LI, van Beurden M, Berkhof J. Lichen sclerosus: incidence and risk of vulvar squamous cell carcinoma. Epidemiol Biomarkers Prev. 2016;25(8):1224–30. https://doi.org/10.1158/1055-9965.EPI-16-0019.
53. Bigby SM, Eva LJ, Fong KL, Jones RW. The natural history of vulvar intraepithelial neoplasia, differentiated type: evidence for progression and diagnostic challenges. Gynecol Pathol. 2016;35(6):574–84.
54. Simpson RC, Littlewood SM, Cooper SM, Cruickshank ME, Green CM, Derrick E, et al. Real-life experience of managing vulval erosive lichen planus: a case-based review and U.K. multicentre case note audit. Br J Dermatol. 2012;167:85e91.
55. Crum CP, Herrington CS, McCluggage WG, et al. Tumours of the vulva: epithelial tumours. In: Kurman JR, Carcangiu ML, Herrington CS, Young RH, editors. World Health Organization classification of tumours of the female reproductive organs. 4th ed. Lyon: IARC Press; 2014. p. 232–41.
56. Kingston NJ, Jones RW, Baranyai J. Recurrent primary vulvovaginal malignant melanoma arising in melanoma in situ—the natural history of lesions followed for 23 years. Int J Gynecol Cancer. 2004;14:628–32.

22 Detection of Precancerous Lesions of the Vulva

T. S. Premalatha, Vishakha Chandrakant Bidkar, T. Parvathi, and Elizabeth Vallikad

22.1 Introduction

Vulvar squamous cell carcinoma (SCC) has two different causal pathways, a HPV-related and a non-HPV-related pathway with two well-defined precursor lesions, namely, the vulvar high-grade squamous intraepithelial lesion (HSIL) or uVIN (Figs. 22.1, 22.2, and 22.3) and the differentiated (simplex) vulvar intraepithelial neoplasia (dVIN). The HSIL arises from infection from high-grade human papilloma virus (HPV), whereas the dVIN arises from chronic dermatosis such as lichen sclerosus (LS) and lichen planus of the vulva [1, 2]. The lower anogenital squamous terminology (LAST) unified all the HPV-related disease of the lower anogenital tract in 2012. The LAST terminology did not address the differences in the malignant potential between the two disease pathways of vulvar intraepithelial neoplasia (VIN). The World Health Organization modified the terminology in 2014, which was accepted by the International Society for the Study of Vulvovaginal Disease (ISSVD) in 2015, and dVIN is included as a lesion of malignant potential distinct from HSIL [3] (Table 22.1). More than 80% of VIN are HPV-related, whereas 80% of the squamous cancers of the vulva are non-HPV associated and are found to have a coexisting inflammatory skin disease like LS. LS is not a premalignant disease but the dVIN which is seen in the background of LS has a higher rate of progression in a shorter

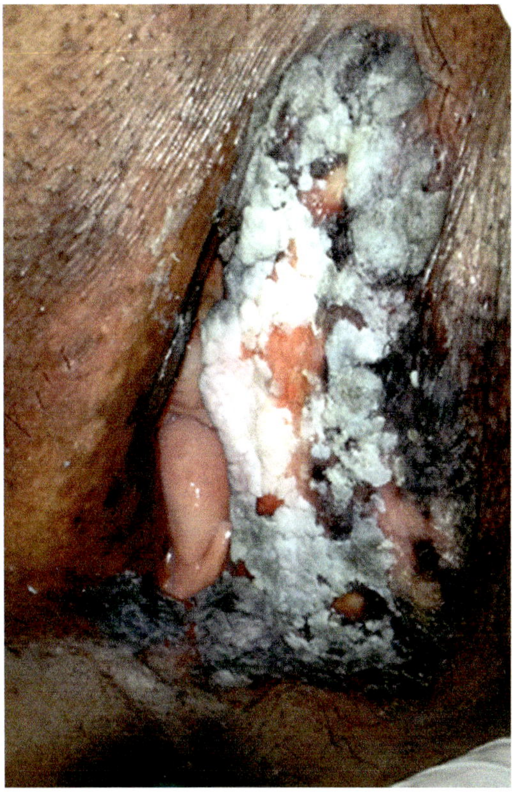

Fig. 22.1 Single, large, white-pink-gray-black plaque of HSIL of the left labia majora and minora

T. S. Premalatha (✉) · V. C. Bidkar · T. Parvathi
E. Vallikad
Department of Gynaecological Oncology, St. John's Medical College and Hospital, St. John's National Academy of Health Sciences, Bangalore, Karnataka, India

S. Mehta, A. Singla (eds.), *Preventive Oncology for the Gynecologist*, https://doi.org/10.1007/978-981-13-3438-2_22

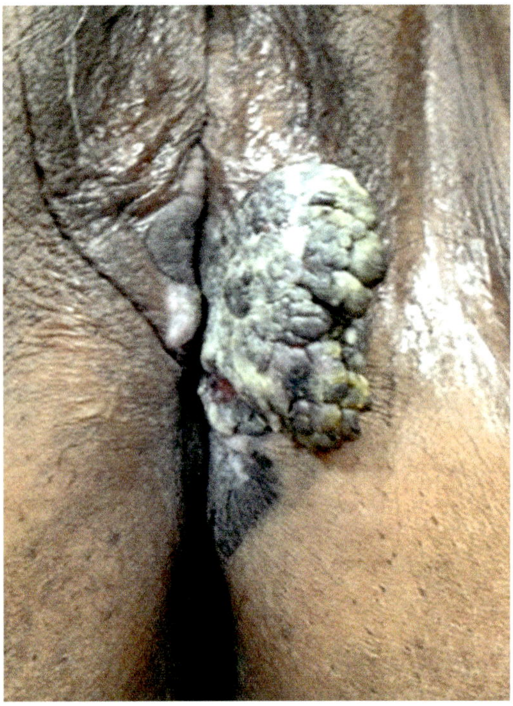

Fig. 22.2 HSIL and invasive SCC in HIV-positive patient

time interval [1, 4, 5]. Nearly 20% of SCC are said to progress from HSIL [1, 6].

The non-squamous vulvar intraepithelial lesions include the extramammary Paget disease (EMPD) and melanoma in situ (MIS).

- Vulvar Paget disease is a rare intraepithelial adenocarcinoma arising from apocrine, eccrine, or mammary-like glands in the vulva and accounts for about 1% of vulvar malignancies, and 80% of EMPD arises in the vulva [7]. It is classified into primary cutaneous and secondary non-cutaneous forms. Secondary EMPD arises from an underlying non-cutaneous adenocarcinoma with the primary from the breast, pancreas, endometrium, bladder, stomach, and rectum. Dermal invasion is seen in 16% [8].
- Dysplastic nevi or melanoma in situ (MIS) is a rare pigmented vulvar premalignant lesion. This is known to have a slow progression to invasive melanoma [9]. Dysplastic nevi are considered as a risk factor for melanoma rather than a premalignant lesion [10].

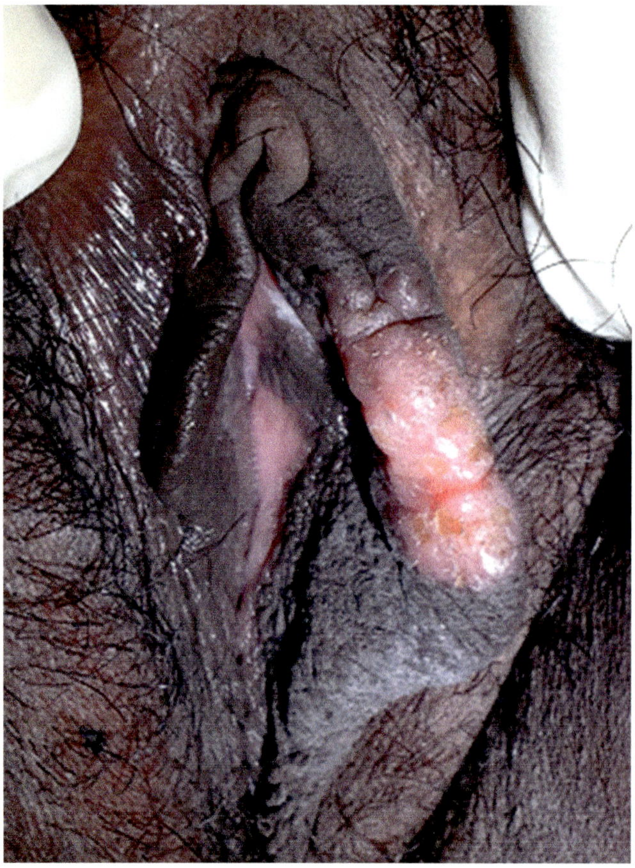

Fig. 22.3 HSIL and invasive SCC (patient had HSIL of cervix-multicentric HPV infection)

Table 22.1 Classification systems for VIN

ISSVD 1986	WHO 1994	ISSVD 2004	LAST 2013	WHO 2014	ISSD 2015
VIN 1	LISL	Flat condyloma, HPV effect	LISL	LSIL	LSIL (vulvar LSIL, flat condyloma, or HPV effect)
VIN 2, 3	HSIL	VIN, usual type (a) warty (b) basaloid (c) mixed	HSIL	HSIL	HSIL (vulvar HSIL, VIN usual type)
VIN 3, differentiated type		VIN, differentiated type		VIN, differentiated	DVIN

22.2 Detection of Precancerous Lesions of the Vulva

22.2.1 High-Grade Squamous Intraepithelial Lesion

HSIL of the vulva is usually asymptomatic, but women may present with pruritis, irritation, burning, and pain. They sometimes present with problems with urination, defecation, or sexual intercourse. Few women may complain of a definitive vulvar lesion [11]. HSIL is often diagnosed in younger women, and as in cervical dysplasia, it is associated with smoking and immunosuppression. As nearly 40% of women can be asymptomatic, routine vulvar inspection during gynecologic examination is important. Commonest affected sites are the labia majora and minora and the fourchette [11]. The perianal area and the anal canal may also be involved. The lesions can be flat or raised, with or without fissures, erosions, or ulcers. The color can vary from red to brown to black or from white to gray. The lesions can be multifocal and multicentric in HSIL [12]. Hence, a careful examination of the lower anogenital tract (cervix, vagina, vulva, perineum, and perianal areas) is mandatory. Warts or condyloma acuminatum is benign squamoproliferative lesions caused by low-grade HPV and is not a cancer precursor lesion. Hence, all warty lesions need not be biopsied, but warts in postmenopausal women, human immunodeficiency virus (HIV)-seropositive patients, and patients on immunosuppression after organ transplant may need a biopsy even when the level of suspicion is low [13].

Differentiated VIN is reported less frequently than HISL and occurs in older women as compared to those with HSIL. Patients are symptomatic and complain of long-lasting itching and/or burning due to the underlying dermatosis. dVIN is often misinterpreted clinically due to extremely subtle changes of white and pink patches in the background of benign dermatosis. Sometimes this can even be mistaken in histopathology [14]. Lichen sclerosis and its associated changes can be seen adjacent to invasive SCC rather than dVIN (Fig. 22.4). It is proposed that dVIN is not often diagnosed as it has a relatively short intraepithelial phase before it progresses to

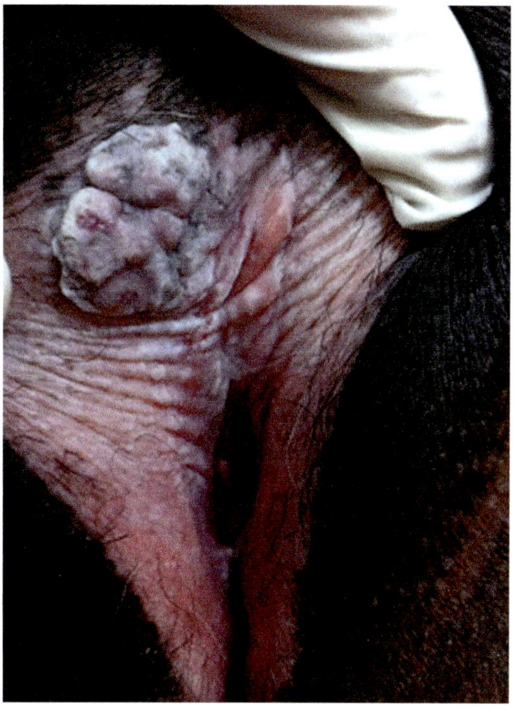

Fig. 22.4 Severe LS showing thin wrinkled skin with SCC. Note the distinction between labia majora and minora is lost and the clitoris is buried with fused prepuce due to chronic LS

Table 22.2 Comparison between dVIN and HSIL [1, 6]

Comparison between differentiated vulvar intraepithelial neoplasia and HSIL		
	dVIN	HSIL
Age	Sixth to eighth decade	Third to fifth decade
Precancer diagnosis	5–10%	80–95%
Multifocality	Uncommon	>50%
Smoking	Not associated	Associated
Associated conditions	Chronic inflammatory dermatoses like lichen sclerosis	>80% HPV
Progression to carcinoma	High Keratinizing SCC	Low Warty, basaloid SCC
Immunohistochemistry	p53+ in basal and suprabasal layers	p16+

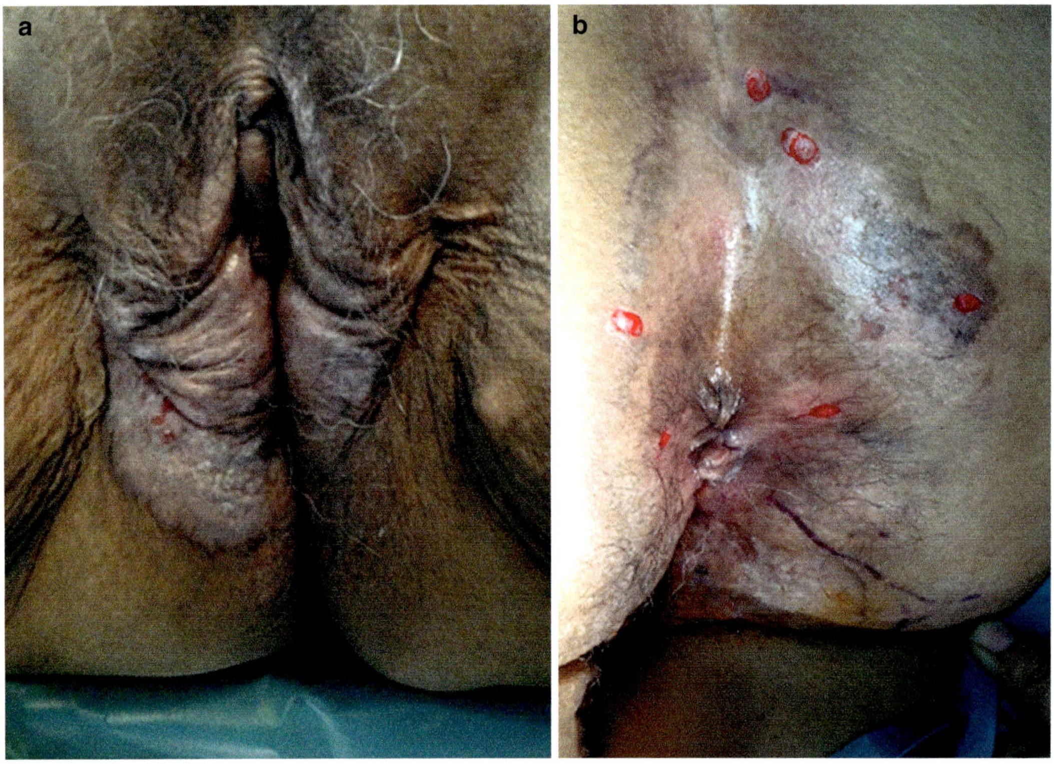

Fig. 22.5 (**a**) Extramammary Paget disease of the vulva showing extensive erythematous plaque involving the vulva, perineum, and perianal region. (**b**) Paget disease of the vulva showing large erythematous plaque involving the perineum and perianal skin, with scouting biopsies to rule out invasive disease

cancer [15]. Careful inspection and biopsy of irregular, rough areas, surface with hyperkeratosis, and ulceration are warranted. Comparison of HSIL and dVIN is discussed in Table 22.2.

22.2.2 Vulvar Paget Disease

Vulvar Paget disease is frequently seen in postmenopausal elderly white women. They present with intense pruritis, burning, moistening, and bleeding, and the symptoms may be incorrectly attributed to infection, and so the diagnosis is often delayed [16]. The size at presentation is often large and can be multifocal [17]. The lesion is typically an erythematous plaque with hyperkeratotic white scales [18] (Figs. 22.5a, b and 22.6). Any nonresolving erythematous hyperkeratotic plaque requires biopsy. Multiple scouting biopsies are needed to exclude invasive disease. A thorough

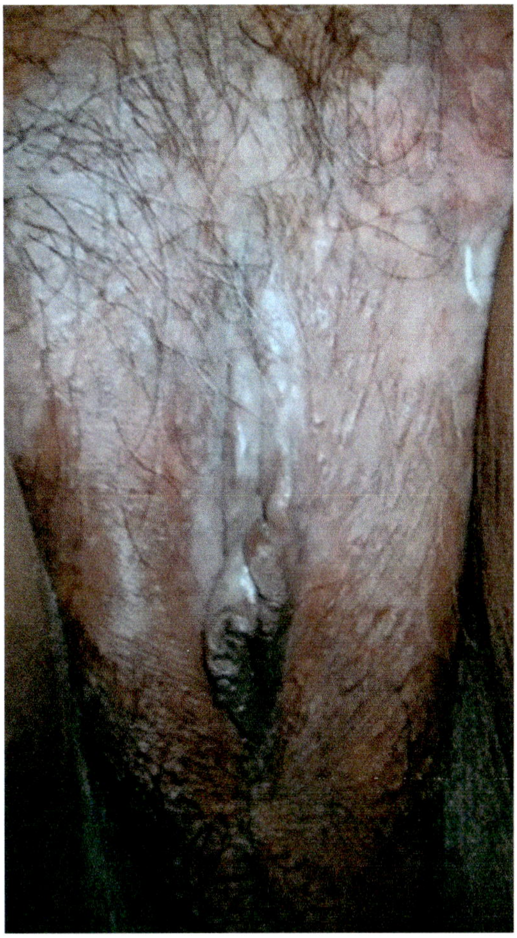

Fig. 22.6 Vulvar Paget disease showing extensive erythematous plaque with hyperkeratotic white scale

history of genitourinary, gastrointestinal, and gynecologic symptoms should be elicited to evaluate for an underlying carcinoma [19]. A complete gynecologic examination with evaluation of the cervix and vagina with additional investigations like cystoscopy, proctoscopy, etc. depending on the pertinent symptoms should be performed. Complete vulvar mapping is recommended in primary Paget disease. The depth of invasion in millimeters should be requested to plan further management.

22.2.3 Melanoma In Situ/ Dysplastic Nevi

Melanoma in situ can be mistaken for benign melanosis as both lesions appear similar with variegated color, indistinct border, and asymmetry. They commonly arise on the hair-bearing genital skin and often larger than 6 mm with an erythematous to tan center and hyperpigmented periphery. The ABCDE scheme for recognition of melanoma should be applied in all pigmented lesions (*a*symmetry, *b*order irregularities, *c*olor variation, *d*iameter >6 mm, *e*nlargement, or *e*volution of color change, shape, or symptoms) to decide on biopsy [20]. Vulvar melanoma more often arises de novo rather than in a preexisting nevus [21].

22.3 Evaluation and Work-up

Vulvar lesions are diagnostically challenging due to nonspecific clinical morphology and hence a variety of differential diagnosis. It is often complicated by secondary changes due to over-the-counter medication and excoriation due to scratching (Table 22.5). Hence, a thorough history including allergies, drugs, immune status, and systemic disease and a detailed physical examination are mandatory. Diagnosis cannot be based on visual assessment. Vulvoscopy can help in localizing the lesion but cannot predict the histological nature of the lesion. Therefore, the diagnosis of a vulvar lesion always requires biopsy.

22.3.1 Vulvoscopy

Vulvoscopy or role of colposcope for examination of the vulva is debated [22, 23]. Examination of the vulva under magnification is useful in localizing the lesion especially in women with persistent focal pruritis and pain with no gross lesions [22]. The entire vulva should be inspected with separation of the labia majora and minora and exploration of the entire vestibule to look for redness, hyperkeratinization, pigmentations, ulcerations, and atrophy. Application of acetic acid has less prominent effect on the vulva due to the keratinized skin and hence should be applied frequently with more concentration (5%). Acetowhite lesions can be made out, but punctuation and mosaic may be appreciated only on the mucosal surface of the labia minora. The International

Table 22.3 The 2011 IFCPC clinical/colposcopic terminology of the vulva[a]

Section	Pattern
Basic definitions	Various structures Urethra, Skene duct openings, clitoris, prepuce, frenulum, pubis, labia majora, labia minora, interlabial sulci, vestibule, vestibular duct openings, Bartholin duct openings, hymen, fourchette, perineum, anus, anal squamocolumnar junction (dentate line) Composition Squamous epithelium: hairy/nonhairy, mucosa
Normal findings	Micropapillomatosis, sebaceous glands (Fordyce spots), vestibular redness
Abnormal findings General principles Size in centimeters, location	Primary Lesion type Macule and patch Papule Plaque Nodule Cyst Vesicle Bulla Pustule Lesion color Skin colored red White Dark Secondary morphology Eczema Lichenification Excoriation Purpura Scarring Ulcer Erosion Fissure Wart
Miscellaneous findings	Trauma and malformation
Suspicion of malignancy	Gross neoplasm, ulceration, necrosis, bleeding, exophytic lesion, hyperkeratosis with or without white, gray, red, or brown discoloration
Abnormal colposcopic/other magnification findings	Acetowhite epithelium, punctuation, atypical vessels, surface irregularities, abnormal anal squamocolumnar junction (note location about the dentate line)

[a]Reprinted with permission from Bornstein J, Sideri M, Tatti S, Walker P, Preniville W, et al. 2011 Terminology of the Vulva of the International Federation for Cervical Pathology and Colposcopy. J Low Genit Tract Dis 2012 Nov 3; 16: 290-295
https://journals.lww.com/jlgtd/Abstract/2012/07000/2011_Terminology_of_the_Vulva_of_the_International.15.aspx

Federation of Cervical Pathology and Colposcopy has finalized a clinical and colposcopy terminology for the vulva in March 2012. The terminology is part of a comprehensive terminology of the lower genital tract, standardized for colposcopists and clinicians taking care of women with lesions in these areas. The terminology includes basic definitions, normal findings, abnormal findings, and patterns to identify malignancy [24] (Tables 22.3, 22.4, and 22.5).

The Collins test is performed by applying 1% aqueous solution of toluidine blue to the vulvar skin for 2 min and rinsing with 1% acetic acid. Toluidine blue is a nuclear stain which fixes to the surface cell nuclei. The normal surface epithelium, which does not contain nuclei, will not be stained. All foci of nuclear activity will retain the color and will be visible as fine blue spots. False-positive results can be seen in ulcerations, lacerations, reparative changes, and parakeratosis. It's a simple test which can help to choose a biopsy site [25].

Table 22.4 Definitions of primary lesion types[a]

Macule	Small (<1.5 cm) area of color change; no elevation and no substance on palpation
Patch	Large (>1.5 cm) area of color change; no elevation and no substance on palpation
Papule	Small (<1.5 cm) elevated and palpable lesion
Plaque	Large (>1.5 cm) elevated, palpable, and flat-topped lesion
Nodule	A large papule (>1.5 cm); often hemispherical or poorly marginated; may be located on the surface, within, or below the skin; nodules may be cystic or solid
Vesicle	Small (<0.5 cm) fluid-filled blister; the fluid is clear (blister: a compartmentalized, fluid-filled elevation of the skin or mucosa)
Bulla	A large (>0.5 cm) fluid-filled blister; the fluid is clear
Pustule	Pus-filled blister; the fluid is white or yellow

[a]Reprinted with permission from Bornstein J, Sideri M, Tatti S, Walker P, Preniville W, et al. 2011 Terminology of the Vulva of the International Federation for Cervical Pathology and Colposcopy. J Low Genit Tract Dis 2012 Nov 3; 16: 290-295
https://journals.lww.com/jlgtd/Abstract/2012/07000/2011_Terminology_of_the_Vulva_of_the_International.15.aspx

Table 22.5 Definitions of secondary morphology presentation[a]

Eczema	A group of inflammatory diseases that are clinically characterized by the presence of itchy, poorly marginated red plaques with minor evidence of microvesiculation and/or, more frequently, subsequent surface disruption
Lichenification	Thickening of the tissue and increased prominence of skin markings Scale may or may not be detectable in vulvar lichenification. It may be bright-red, dusky-red, white, or skin colored in appearance
Excoriation	Surface disruption (notably excoriations) occurring as a result of the "itch-scratch cycle"
Fissure	A thin, linear erosion of the skin surface
Ulcer	Deeper defect; absence of the epidermis and some, or all, of the dermis

[a]Reprinted with permission from Bornstein J, Sideri M, Tatti S, Walker P, Preniville W, et al. 2011 Terminology of the Vulva of the International Federation for Cervical Pathology and Colposcopy. J Low Genit Tract Dis 2012 Nov 3; 16: 290-295
https://journals.lww.com/jlgtd/Abstract/2012/07000/2011_Terminology_of_the_Vulva_of_the_International.15.aspx

The dermoscope, a handheld light source and magnifying device, is commonly used by dermatologists for evaluation of vulvar lesions.

22.3.2 Biopsy

Vulvoscopy/magnification or naked eye examination can localize the lesion for biopsy. Large lesions and multicentric lesions will require multiple biopsies. Vulvar biopsy can be performed using a variety of instruments under local anesthesia. The type of biopsy depends on the type of lesion and its anatomic location. The various kinds of biopsies are:

- Lesions closer to the vagina can be biopsied using cervical biopsy forceps.
- Suture tenting and removal with a curved iris scissors can be used for sampling mucus membranes of the labia minora or introitus.

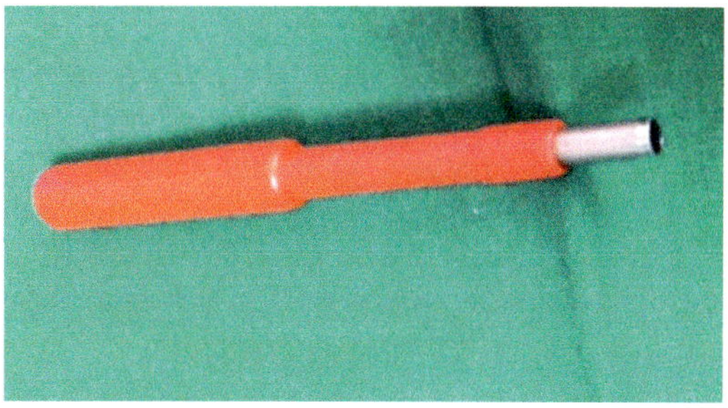

Fig. 22.7 Keyes punch biopsy forceps

- Shave sampling especially for a melanocytic lesion can lead to misdiagnosis and inaccurate micro staging [26, 27].

The Keyes punch biopsy forceps can be used to obtain a punch biopsy of the vulva by firmly pushing the punch into the skin with a rotatory action (Fig. 22.7). It will remove a round skin area of desired diameter. It is an excellent tool for evaluating melanocytic lesions and tumors with deep involvement [26]. A fine tissue forceps or scissors should be used to detach the specimen from the dermal tissue. The defect that remains after the biopsy can be left open to heal spontaneously. Monsel's solution (ferric subsulfate) can be used to control the bleeding.

While biopsying an ulcer, a better yield is obtained at the edge where the ulcer bed abuts the intact epithelium as the ulcer base may yield only necrotic tissue. Tissue manipulation can result in artifacts. A needle can be used to lift the tissues from a punch biopsy rather than forceps to reduce crush injury of the biopsy specimen.

22.3.2.1 Documentation of the Vulvar Findings

The findings should be precisely documented, preferably with a schematic drawing depicting the various structures and the location of the lesions.

Clinical photographs may be a more objective way of documentation.

22.3.2.2 Histology

There is loss of maturation with increased nuclear density and nuclear atypia involving both the upper and lower epithelial layers in HSIL. Histopathologically, HSIL is classified into different subtypes, warty, basaloid, and mixed, depending on the architecture and the cytological appearance of the neoplastic cells [28].

Atypia is confined to the basal and parabasal layers of the epithelium in dVIN. The diagnosis of dVIN may be mistaken for an epithelial hyperplasia or a benign inflammatory dermatosis due to high degree of cellular differentiation [29].

Biochemical and viral markers may be used as adjunct to morphologic diagnosis.

22.3.3 Biochemical and Viral Markers

22.3.3.1 Biochemical Markers

- p16 protein is overexpressed when there is a dysfunction in the progression of the cell cycle and in cell proliferation. p16 protein is positive in HPV-associated VIN but negative in dVIN [30].
- Ki-67 is a nuclear antigen present in human proliferating cells in all stages of the cell cycle except in the G0 phase. MIB-1, a monoclonal antibody against the Ki-67 antigen, is a proliferation marker. MIB-1 expression is confined to the basal layers in dVIN. This helps to distinguish dVIN from normal epithelium where the basal cell layer is often negative for MIB-1 [30, 31].
- p53 protein is involved in apoptosis regulation. The basal cell layer in dVIN often has more than 90% p53 labeling index and may help to distinguish dVIN from normal squamous epithelium [32].

22.3.3.2 Viral Markers

Low-risk HPV is associated with anogenital warts or flat condyloma, and high-risk HPV is associated with HSIL as seen in cervical high-grade squamous intraepithelial lesions (HSIL); the majority of vulvar HSIL lesions contain HPV 16 [33, 34]; dVIN is not related with HPV.

22.4 Conclusion

Vulvar lesions are diagnostically challenging. Though the diagnosis of many vulvar conditions is clinical, lesions have to be biopsied, when they do not resolve after standard therapy or when precancer/malignancy is suspected. The evaluation of vulvar premalignancies must be included in training programs and patient care especially in centers caring for immunocompromised patients. Patients with LS should be on a long-term follow-up. Collaboration clinicians and pathologists are required to care for women with precancerous lesions of the vulva.

Key Points

- Precancers of the vulva include squamous vulvar intraepithelial neoplasia, vulvar Paget disease, and melanoma in situ.
- Vulvar squamous cell carcinoma (SCC) has two different causal pathways, a HPV-related and a non-HPV-related pathway with two well-defined precursor lesions, namely, the vulvar high-grade squamous intraepithelial lesion (HSIL) or uVIN and the differentiated (simplex) vulvar intraepithelial neoplasia (dVIN).
- An appropriate examination of the vulva and biopsy, occasionally immunoprofile in difficult cases, are essential for the diagnosis of precancerous vulvar lesions.
- Differentiated VIN (dVIN) is often missed clinically and histologically. Although dVIN represents a small proportion of VIN lesions, it has higher risk of progression to invasive cancer than HSIL.
- Patients with LS should be on a long-term surveillance.
- The ABCDE scheme for recognition of melanoma should be applied in all pigmented lesions (asymmetry, border irregularities, color variation, diameter >6 mm, enlargement, or evolution of color change, shape, or symptoms) to decide on site of biopsy.

References

1. Hoang LN, Park KJ, Soslow RA, Murali R. Squamous precursor lesions of the vulva: current classification and diagnostic challenges. Pathology. 2016;48(4):291–302. https://doi.org/10.1016/j.pathol.2016.02.015.
2. Van de Nieuwenhof HP, van der Avoort IAM, de Hullu JA. Review of squamous premalignant vulvar lesions. Crit Rev Oncol Hematol. 2008;68:131–56.
3. Bornstein J, Bogliatto F, Haefner HK, Stockdale CK, Preti M, Bohl TG, et al. The 2015 ISSVD terminology of vulvar squamous intraepithelial lesions. J Low Genit Tract Dis. 2016;20(2):190.
4. Van de Nieuwenhof HP, Bulten J, Hollema H, Dommerholt RG, Massuger LF, van der Zee AG, et al. Differentiated vulvar intraepithelial neoplasia is often found in lesions, previously diagnosed as lichen sclerosus, which have progressed to vulvar squamous cell carcinoma. Mod Pathol. 2010;24(2):297–305.
5. Eva LJ, Ganesan R, Chan KK, Honest H, Luesley DM. Differentiated-type vulval intraepithelial neoplasia has a high-risk association with vulval squamous cell carcinoma. Int J Gynecol Cancer. 2009;19:741–4.
6. Preti M, Scurry J, Marchitelli CE, Micheletti L. Vulvar intraepithelial neoplasia. Best Pract Res Clin Obstet Gynaecol. 2014;28(7):1051–62.
7. Chanda JJ. Extramammary Paget's disease: prognosis and relationship to internal malignancy. J Am Acad Dermatol. 1985;13(6):1009–14.
8. Iacoponi S, Zalewski K, Fruscio R, Diaz-De la Noval B, De Iaco P, Ceccaroni M, et al. Prognostic factors for recurrence and survival among patients with invasive vulvar Paget disease included in the VULCAN study. Int J Gynaecol Obstet. 2016;133(1):76–9.
9. Kingston NJ, Jones RW, Baranyai J. Recurrent primary vulvovaginal malignant melanoma arising in melanoma in situ–the natural history of lesions followed for 23 years. Int J Gynecol Cancer. 2004;14:628–32.
10. Duffy K, Grossman D. The dysplastic nevus: from historical perspective to management in the modern era. J Am Acad Dermatol. 2012;67(1):19.e1–12.
11. McNally OM, Mulvany NJ, Pagano R, Quinn MA, Rome RM. VIN 3: a clinicopathologic review. Int J Gynecol Cancer. 2002;12:490–5.
12. van Beurden M, ten Kate FJ, Smits HL, Berkhout RJ, de Craen AJ, van der Vange N, et al. Multifocal vulvar intraepithelial neoplasia grade III and multicentric lower genital tract neoplasia is associated with transcriptionally active human papillomavirus. Cancer. 1995;75:2879–84.
13. Spitzer M. Lower genital tract neoplasia in HIV-infected women: guidelines for evaluation and management. Obstet Gynecol Surv. 1999;54:131Y7.
14. Yang B, Hart WR. Vulvar intraepithelial neoplasia of the simplex (differentiated) type: a clinicopathologic study including analysis of HPV and p53 expression. Am J Surg Pathol. 2000;24:429–41.
15. Hart WR. Vulvar intraepithelial neoplasia: historical aspects and current status. Int J Gynecol Pathol. 2001;20:16e30.
16. Niikura H, Yoshida H, Ito K, Takano T, Watanabe H, Aiba S, et al. Paget's disease of the vulva: clinicopathologic study of type 1 cases treated at a single institution. Int J Gynecol Cancer. 2006;16:1212–5.
17. Shaco-Levy R, Bean SM, Vollmer RT, Papalas JA, Bentley RC, Selim MA, et al. Paget disease of the vulva: a histologic study of 56 cases correlating pathologic features and disease course. Int J Gynecol Pathol. 2010;29:69–78.
18. Delport ES. Extramammary Paget's disease of the vulva: an annotated review of the current literature. Austral J Dermatol. 2013;54(1):9–21, 2013.
19. van der Linden M, Meeuwis KAP, Bulten J, et al. Paget disease of the vulva. Crit Rev Oncol Hematol. 2016;101:60–74.
20. Tran KT, Wright NA, Cockerell CJ. Biopsy of the pigmented lesion–when and how. J Am Acad Dermatol. 2008;59:852–71.
21. Murzaku EC, Penn LA, Hale CS, Pomeranz MK, Polsky D. Vulvar nevi, melanosis, and melanoma: an epidemiologic, clinical, and histopathologic review. J Am Acad Dermatol. 2014;71(6):1241–9.
22. Sacher BC. The normal vulva, vulvar examination, and evaluation tools. Clin Obstet Gynecol. 2015;58(3):442–52.
23. Micheletti L, Bogliatto F, Lynch PJ. Vulvoscopy: review of a diagnostic approach requiring clarification. J Reprod Med. 2008;53:179–82.
24. Bornstein J, Sideri M, Tatti S, Walker P, Preniville W, et al. 2011 terminology of the vulva of the international federation for cervical pathology and colposcopy. J Low Genit Tract Dis. 2012;16(3):290–5.
25. Collins CG, Hansen LH, Theriot E. A clinical stain for use in selecting biopsy sites in patients with vulvar disease. Obstet Gynecol. 1966;28:158.
26. Ng JC, Swain S, Dowling JP, Wolfe R, Simpson P, Kelly JW. The impact of partial biopsy on histopathologic diagnosis of cutaneous melanoma: experience of an Australian tertiary referral service. Arch Dermatol. 2010;146(3):234–9.
27. Mir M, Chan CS, Khan F, Krishnan B, Orengo I, Rosen T. The rate of melanoma transection with various biopsy techniques and the influence of tumor transection on patient survival. J Am Acad Dermatol. 2013;68(3):452–8.
28. Kurman RJ, Toki T, Schiffman MH. Basaloid and warty carcinomas of the vulva: distinctive types of squamous cell carcinoma frequently associated with human papillomaviruses. Am J Surg Pathol. 1993;17:133e45.
29. Scurry J, Wilkinson EJ. Review of terminology of precursors of vulvar squamous cell carcinoma. J Lower Gen Tract Dis. 2006;10:161Y9.
30. Hoevenaars BM, van der Avoort IA, de Wilde PC, Massuger LF, Melchers WJ, de Hullu JA, et al.

A panel of p16(INK4A), MIB1 and p53 proteins can distinguish between the 2 pathways leading to vulvar squamous cell carcinoma. Int J Cancer. 2008;123:2767Y73.
31. van der Avoort IA, van der Laak JA, Paffen A, Grefte JM, Massuger LF, de Wilde PC, et al. MIB1 expression in basal cell layer: a diagnostic tool to identify premalignancies of the vulva. Mod Pathol. 2007;20:770Y8.
32. Yang B, Hart WR. Vulvar intraepithelial neoplasia of the simplex (differentiated) type: a clinicopathologic study including analysis of HPV and p53 expression. Am J Surg Pathol. 2000;24:429Y41.
33. Buscema J, Naghashfar Z, Sawada E, Daniel R, Woodruff JD, Shah K. The predominance of human papillomavirus type 16 in vulvar neoplasia. Obstet Gynecol. 1988;71:601–6.
34. Garland SM, Insinga RP, Sings HL, Haupt RM, Joura EA. Human papillomavirus infections and vulvar disease development. Cancer Epidemiol Biomark Prev. 2009;18:1777–84.

Management of Vulvar Intraepithelial Neoplasia

23

Divya Pandey and Sumita Mehta

23.1 Introduction

Vulvar intraepithelial neoplasia (VIN) is a premalignant condition of the vulva, which is increasingly becoming common especially during the fifth decade of life. The cause of this increase is the rise in anogenital HPV infections, increased prevalence of smoking among women and more liberal use of vulvar biopsy for confirming the diagnosis. Women in their mid-40s are at highest risk, and then there is a second increase seen in women in 60–80 years age group. This is due to the increase in differentiated VIN which follows chronic vulvar dermatoses in elderly women [1].

As per the latest ISSVD (International Society for the Study of Vulvovaginal Disease) terminology, HSIL (high-grade squamous intraepithelial lesion) and dVIN (differentiated vulvar intraepithelial neoplasia) can progress to invasive cancer. These two entities are fairly different in terms of aetiology, treatment and malignant potential.

D. Pandey (✉)
Department of Obstetrics and Gynecology, Vardhman Mahavir Medical College and Safdarjung Hospital, New Delhi, India

S. Mehta
Department of Obstetrics and Gynecology, Babu Jagjivan Ram Memorial Hospital, New Delhi, India

23.2 Terminology

In 1976, Friedrich described vulvar lesions into vulvar atypia (with and without dystrophy) and squamous vulvar carcinoma in situ [2]. Later in 1986, the ISSVD classified VIN into three grades: VIN1 (LSIL), VIN2 (HSIL) and VIN3 (HSIL) [3]. VIN1 was considered as a cancer precursor which needed treatment. Later in 2004, VIN has been classified into two main classes:

1. VIN, usual type (uVIN)—Lesions associated with human papillomavirus. This included the former subclassification of VIN:
   (a) VIN, warty type
   (b) VIN, basaloid type
   (c) VIN, mixed (warty, basaloid type)
2. VIN, differentiated type (dVIN)—These intraepithelial lesions are not associated with HPV infection but are associated with vulvar dermatoses mainly lichen sclerosus. This category included VIN, simplex type.

In 2004, the ISSVD recommended the term VIN to be limited to HSIL (formerly termed VIN2 and VIN3). Lesions formerly called VIN1 were recommended to be referred to as condyloma acuminatum [4]. In 2012, the Lower Anogenital Squamous Terminology (LAST) project of the College of American Pathologists and American Society for Colposcopy and Cervical Pathology (ASCCP) suggested changes

S. Mehta, A. Singla (eds.), *Preventive Oncology for the Gynecologist*,
https://doi.org/10.1007/978-981-13-3438-2_23

Table 23.1 Shows the development of current (2015) and previous (2004) ISSVD nomenclature

2015 terminology	2004 terminology
Low-grade squamous intraepithelial lesion of the vulva (vulvar LSIL, flat condyloma or HPV effect)	Condyloma, HPV effect
High-grade squamous intraepithelial lesion of the vulva (vulvar HSIL; VIN usual type, uVIN)	Usual-type VIN(uVIN) subdivided into: (a) VIN, warty type (b) VIN, basaloid type (c) VIN, mixed type
Differentiated-type VIN(dVIN)	Differentiated-type VIN(dVIN)

in the terms used to describe HPV-associated squamous lesions of the anogenital tract. According to the LAST classification, VIN2 and VIN3 are referred to as HSIL [5, 6].

It was seen that differentiated VIN was the precursor lesion in 80% of vulvar cancers, while HPV-associated vulvar HSIL was noted to be a precursor lesion in the rest 20% of squamous cell carcinoma type of vulvar cancer [7].

Two concerns were raised about the LAST terminology. First, it included vulvar LSIL which was eliminated as per 2004 ISSVD classification, and, secondly, the differentiated-type VIN, which accounts for majority of VIN cases that progress to invasive cancer, was not included [2].

Finally, the 2015 ISSVD terminology for vulvar intraepithelial lesions was based on the review of previous ISSVD, LAST and WHO terminologies [8] (Table 23.1).

The latest ISSVD terminology includes:

- LSIL of vulva (synonyms are vulvar LSIL, flat condyloma or HPV effect)
- HSIL of vulva (vulvar HSIL, VIN usual type)
- VIN, differentiated type (dVIN)

23.3 Signs and Symptoms

More than half of women with vulval intraepithelial lesions have no symptoms. In the rest of the cases, pruritus is the major symptom. The presence of a mass or discharge raises suspicion of invasive cancer. The early stages of VIN appear as pale areas, while later stages may present as papules, macules and discrete or confluent, single or multiple lesions. Hyperpigmentation can be found in 10–15% of VIN. While lesions on the cutaneous surface may appear as white, hyperkeratotic or lichenified, those on mucosal surface are usually pink or red.

23.3.1 Vulvar HSIL

Patients present with itching, burning, irritation, pain or psychosexual symptoms. They may even be asymptomatic and may harbour the disease in the form of vulvar lesion. The clinical appearance of the vulvar lesion is highly variable ranging from multifocal lesions to whitish, erythematous, pigmented lesions or sometimes plaques.

23.3.2 Differentiated VIN (dVIN)

Here the symptoms are due to underlying lichen sclerosus or lichen planus. These may also be associated with psychosexual symptoms. The lesions are mostly unifocal in contrast to HSIL lesions. They range from grey white to red lesions with rough or ulcerated surface.

23.4 Diagnosis

Till date there are *no screening strategies* for early detection of vulvar HSIL (VIN, usual type).

The various modalities used for diagnosis of VIN include visual examination, vulvoscopy and biopsy. These methods have been discussed in detail in Chap. 22. A brief mention of the modalities is mentioned here.

23.4.1 Visual Assessment

Can raise index of suspicion for malignancy depending on appearance, colour and pattern of the lesion; hence, careful vulvar inspection in good light at the time of routine pelvic examination is recommended. However, tissue biopsy from suspicious lesions followed by histopathological confirmation remains the gold standard test.

23.4.2 Role of Vulvoscopy

Vulvoscopy is done after application of 3–5% acetic acid (owing to keratinized squamous epithelium of vulva). It is indicated in:

(a) Women with persistent focal vulvar pruritus and pain with no apparent lesion
(b) Women where disease extent is not clearly demarcated
(c) Women in whom symptoms of vulvovaginitis persist even after appropriate treatment

Evaluation of the whole vulva, perineum and perianal area is a must to avoid missing any multifocal lesion. Using a higher concentration (5%) of acetic acid can help in identifying subtle lesions. The lesions on the skin (keratinized stratified squamous epithelium) require longer duration of acetic acid application. After diagnosing a lesion, colposcopy of the entire vulva and perineum and the perianal skin must follow to delineate all the multifocal lesions, more common in the premenopausal age group. After application of 5% acetic acid, the lesions appear as dense acetowhite areas with well-defined margins. Vascular patterns are often unremarkable even in high-grade vulvar preinvasive lesions especially in the presence of hyperkeratosis, but macular lesions on the mucous membrane may reveal capillary punctation pattern. Marked vascular abnormalities like varicose pattern, widely spaced punctations and mosaicism are signs of invasive cancer, and thus lesions with such findings must always be excised. Colposcopy of the vulva should always be followed by colposcopy of the vagina and cervix as intraepithelial lesions often coexist.

Collins Test 1% aqueous toluidine blue solution application for 2–3 min followed by washing with 1–2% acetic acid can also help to localise areas of increased nuclear activity which stain royal blue. It is more helpful in diagnosing vaginal lesions than vulvar HSIL. The visible lesions can be flat or elevated, white to grey or red to brown to black. Malignancy should be suspected in lesions with atypical vascular patterns, rapidly changing lesions in terms of colour, border or size and the lesions not responding to usual therapy.

23.4.3 Biopsy

After identifying suspicious lesions, biopsy is done under local anaesthesia (lignocaine or bupivacaine) using Keyes dermatologic punch (4–6 mm) which allows adequate sampling of the tissue. Haemostasis can be achieved with silver nitrate, Monsel's paste or suturing if required. Biopsy is warranted in lesions indicative of malignancy as mentioned above. These are different schools of thought regarding whether to biopsy warty lesions. ACOG (2015) recommends that postmenopausal females with genital warts and women of all ages with suspected condyloma with failed topical treatment must be biopsied. Even in immunocompromised females like HIV-seropositive patients and patients after organ transplant, all genital lesions need to be biopsied. In the case of multifocal lesions, mapping of all lesions should be done and multiple biopsies taken.

23.5 Treatment

Studies have reported occult carcinomas in 15–22% of cases with VIN. Regression is seen in only 1% and is generally associated with a younger age, multifocal disease and pregnancy [9]. Because of low regression rates and propensity for progression to invasive carcinoma if left untreated, all cases of VIN need to be treated. The treatment for VIN depends upon the characteristics of the lesions and the patient. The important points to be kept in mind when formulating treatment plans include:

- Lesion size and location
- Presence of multifocal disease
- Patient's characteristics—Age, symptoms and comorbidities
- Patient's compliance for follow-up after treatment
- Availability of equipment and medical resources

The goals of treatment in VIN are:

1. To prevent the development of vulvar squamous carcinoma
2. To relieve the symptoms
3. To preserve the normal vulvar functions and anatomy

dVIN: As this is strongly associated with invasive cancer, so women with dVIN are treated surgically. Biopsy specimens should be carefully evaluated to ascertain the degree of stromal invasion. Medical therapies should be avoided in dVIN.

uVIN/vulvar HSIL: Treatment is recommended for all women with vulvar HSIL (VIN, usual type) (Fig. 23.1). Conservative modalities are advocated as it is usually seen in younger age group with low progression rates. Extensive surgery is associated with negative body image and causes sexual dysfunction.

In women with vulvar HSIL without suspicion of cancer (absence of high-risk factors), the choice of treatment depends on location, extent and patient's preference. Available options are excision, ablative therapy and topical immune-modulator application (the last two options can help in maintaining vulvar anatomy). Although, surgical excision is the mainstay of treatment of VIN, laser ablation is also a frequently used technique, especially, for multifocal disease. Recently a promising medical treatment is the application of immune response modulators like imiquimod which has indirect antiviral and antitumour properties.

When carcinoma is suspected (raised, ulcerative surface or/and irregular borders) or there are associated high-risk factors for invasive disease like previous VIN or vulvar carcinoma, immunosuppression, tobacco use, age > 45 years or lichen sclerosus, even if biopsy shows vulvar HSIL, wide local excision should be done due to high potential for occult invasion [3]. Historically, vulvar CIS has been managed by simple vulvectomy, which in today's era is not justified, especially in young women as it is associated with scarring, dyspareunia, urinary difficulties and fibrosis. There is a need for individualized approach towards treating VIN, pertaining to its broad age range and marked variation in its extent, symptoms and distribution.

The various treatment options for VIN are shown in Fig. 23.1.

23.6 Surgical Therapy

23.6.1 Wide Local Excision (WLE)

WLE, as initial intervention, is preferred as it provides specimen for histopathology which is especially helpful in cases where invasive cancer cannot be ruled out from their clinico-pathological findings despite a biopsy diagnosis of only vulvar HSIL (VIN, usual type). During wide excision, it is important to include a margin of 0.5–1 cm around the visible lesion, but this is not always possible to avoid injury to the clitoris, urethra or anus. The depth of excision should be at least 2 mm in non-hair-bearing area and 4 mm in hair-bearing areas.

Wide, local excision is also best suited for high-grade intraepithelial neoplasia seen in haemorrhoids. The wound can be managed by primary closure which gives satisfactory cosmetic and functional results. WLE with adequate disease-free margin provides a cure rate of 90% for localized disease and 50% if margins are involved. One prospective study showed a recurrence rate of 46% post excision with positive histological margins and 17% recurrence if the margins were negative at 7 months follow-up.

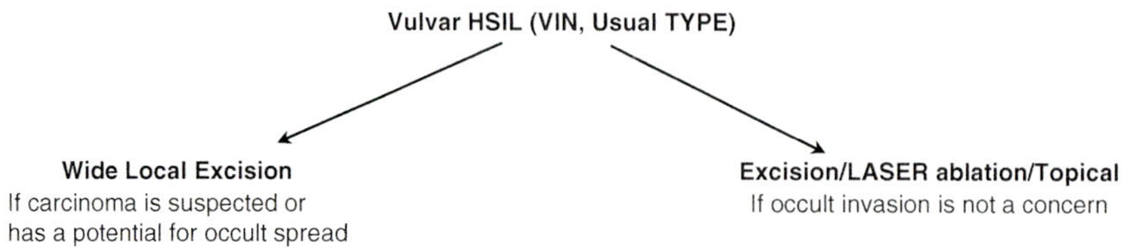

Fig. 23.1 Treatment options

23.6.2 Skinning Vulvectomy

Skinning vulvectomy involves removal of the epidermis and the underlying dermis while preserving the subcutaneous tissues of the vulva. It is useful for the cases with confluent multifocal lesions or recurrent VIN, as found in immunocompromised women. In these multicentric lesions, the involved skin is excised, and the defect should be primarily closed or replaced by split-thickness skin graft taken from the buttocks or inner aspect of the thigh. Rutledge and Sinclair in 1968 had first introduced skinning vulvectomy and skin graft procedure with ectopic epidermis from donor site [10]. This technique was particularly introduced for extensive VIN lesions involving hair-bearing areas where the skin appendages could be involved. After carefully mapping the lesions, a shallow layer of the vulvar skin is excised in order to preserve the subcutaneous tissue of the vulva for better functional and cosmetic results. Care should be taken to preserve vulvar anatomy and avoid excision of the anterior vulva and clitoris, if possible.

23.6.3 Simple Vulvectomy

It involves removal of the entire vulva including the epidermis, dermis and the underlying subcutaneous tissue to a depth of about 4–5 mm. Though not routinely used for treatment of VIN, the indications for its use include:

- Widespread VIN where invasive cancer cannot be ruled out. Though CO_2 laser can be used in these situations, but since a specimen for histopathological review cannot be obtained, so simple vulvectomy is better [11]
- Extensive Paget's disease [12]
- VIN in elderly women—As the risk of invasive cancer increases with age and the desire for cosmesis is less in elderly, so surgical excision is preferred
- In recurrent VIN following previous failed treatments.

While planning the incision during the procedure, maximum skin of the vestibule around the urethera is left so as to avoid distortion of the meatus. The outer incision is carried down from the mons to the lateral aspect of labia on both sides and across the perineum. If the labia minora, clitoris and vestibule are not involved, they should be preserved. The skin edges are held and the skin is dissected off the subcutaneous tissues. The dissection progresses from above downward and lateral to medial; it is done superficially preserving the deep fascia and muscles of urogenital diaphragm. The incision can be carried almost up to the anal mucosa, but care should be taken to avoid damage to the external anal sphincter. Haemostasis is achieved by clamping and ligating the vessels, the main being dorsal vein of the clitoris and branches of the pudendal vessels. Primary closure is done if it can be easily accomplished without excessive tension on the suture line; otherwise, a split-thickness graft is used.

The complications of vulvectomy (skinning and simple) include:

- Wound infections
- Failure of graft to take over
- Hematoma formation
- Urinary infection
- Sexual dysfunction—This is a long-term sequelae related to disturbance in body image, depression and hypoactive sexual state. It is seen more commonly with simple vulvectomy [13].

23.7 Laser Ablation

Laser ablation is used for treatment of single or confluent vulvar HSIL (VIN, usual type) in whom invasion is not suspected. This is particularly useful for extensive VIN, affecting young women where anatomic distortion following wide excision is of concern. It is performed with a CO_2 laser which is controlled using a micromanipulator through a colposcope or an operating microscope, with appropriate power density of 600–1000 W/cm^2. Colposcopy helps in defining the lesion margins, and the use of a micromanipulator with a depth gauge allows application of high power density without inadvertent defocusing. The CO_2 laser is the only laser proven to be both safe and effective for treating high-grade VIN.

To avoid deep coagulation injury, as with excision, a 0.5–1 cm margin of normal-appearing skin must be treated. It is recommended that destruction of 1 mm depth of non-hair-bearing epithelium (through the dermis) and if the skin appendages are involved, destruction of 2.5–3 mm distance is to be done. Laser ablation must extend for more than 3 mm in hair-bearing area and up to 2 mm in non-hair-bearing area. The newer ultra-pulse technology or the rapid super pulse temporal mode causes precise vaporisation of the diseased tissue with minimal heat propagation to adjacent tissues, thus decreasing the morbidity of laser procedures. It is done under general anaesthesia.

Postoperative pain is a major concern for which application of local anaesthetics and oral pain medications like narcotics may be needed. Postoperative sitz bath, topical local anaesthetic and rinsing with water after each act of urination and defecation followed by drying (using a hair dryer) are very important.

The disadvantages of this procedure are that it can be painful and costly and does not provide tissue for histopathological diagnosis. Thermal injury can be minimized by cooling the vulvar skin before and after the procedure with ice packs which will reduce postoperative pain and promote healing.

23.7.1 Cavitron Ultrasonic Surgical Aspirator (CUSA)

CUSA has dual advantage of removal of the superficial dermal layers with laser without scars and resection of lesion with specimen for pathological evaluation [14]. CUSA is an acceptable ablative option with similar recurrence rates as seen with laser. Recurrences are seen more frequently if VIN is present in the hair-bearing areas in comparison to if it is localized to labia minora and introitus. No statistically significant difference is seen in disease recurrence after 1 year, pain, scarring, dysuria, adhesions or infection between women who undergo CO_2 laser surgery and those who receive CUSA. According to the Cochrane Review 2014, as not many trials have been done comparing the two interventions with respect to their effectiveness and safety, so any definitive recommendations for clinical practice cannot be given [15].

23.8 Medical Therapy

23.8.1 Imiquimod

Imiquimod is an immune response modulator with indirect antitumour and antiviral properties. It helps in the release of interferon α and cytokines from macrophages and dendritic cells. Although not FDA approved, 5% imiquimod has been effective in the treatment of vulvar HSIL (VIN, usual type) in many RCTs [9, 16]. The recommended regime is three times weekly application over lesions for 12–20 weeks, followed by colposcopic assessment at 4–6-week intervals during treatment [2]. Local side effects may necessitate dose reductions. Residual lesions require surgical treatment [17]. Because of its immune-mediated function, it is not recommended in immunocompromised patients.

It has demonstrated response rates ranging from 26 to 100%. In a large prospective RCT with 52 patients, complete response was seen in 35% women, and a partial response was observed in 46% women. The disease recurred in only one patient during the follow-up period of 7 years, thereby suggesting the role of imiquimod in long-term sustained response [18].

23.8.2 Cidofovir (CDV)

CDV is an acyclic nucleoside phosphonate with broad spectrum antiviral activity. It causes apoptosis induction, S-phase accumulation and increased levels of tumour-suppressor proteins. It has been earlier used in the treatment of high-grade intraepithelial disease of the cervix. It is used as topical formulation of 1%. The initial study to assess its efficacy in the management of high-grade VIN was done by Tristram et al. in 2005. During the trial period, 40% women had complete response, while 30% had partial response to topical cidofovir. He concluded that cidofovir had a place in the therapeutic armamentarium of high-grade VIN [19]. Stier et al. studied the safety and efficacy of topical CDV to treat high-grade perianal and vulvar intraepithelial lesions in HIV-positive men and women. He concluded that topical CDV had an efficacy of 51% in the short-term treatment of high-grade perianal intraepithelial neoplasia (PaIN) and VIN with acceptable toxicity in HIV-positive individuals but longer follow-up was required to assess whether the effect was sustained [20].

Tristram et al. studied the efficacy and feasibility of CDV and imiquimod for the treatment of VIN. 180 women from 32 centres were recruited to receive either of the 2 drugs. At post-treatment assessment, a complete response had been achieved by 46% (90% CI, 37–55.3) women in the CDV group and 46% (37.2–55.3) in the imiquimod group. Adverse events in the form of pain in vulva, pruritus, fatigue and headache were reported in 37% and 46% of women, respectively. They concluded that both the drugs were safe, active and feasible for VIN treatment [21].

Sustained effect with topical treatment of uVIN for 16 weeks with imiquimod or cidofovir is limited. It has been seen that smaller lesions are more responsive. Topical treatment is opted by some women over primary surgery, but long-term data is still not clear to assess any effect on sustained benefit and progression to vulval cancer [22].

The Cochrane review 2016 lacks data on comparison of medical treatment with surgical treatment. Whether a woman undergoes surgical excision or laser vaporisation for uVIN, the chances for recurrence are about 50% at 1 year, and this is especially more for multifocal lesions. The management should be tailored according to the site and extent of disease. The combination of treatment modalities may be required in some complex cases. If suspicion of malignancy is high, surgical excision is preferred [17].

23.8.3 Photodynamic Therapy

Photodynamic therapy (PDT) requiring special equipment and training has been seen to be effective in some studies [23]. The PDT technique involves the topical application of a photosensitizer, 5-aminolevulinic acid (ALA) or its methyl ester (MAL) followed by illumination of the skin area with light of the appropriate wavelength. PDT produces an immune response and causes suppression of antitumour responses. It is a useful alternative especially at VIN sites that are cosmetically sensitive or prone to impaired wound healing [24].

Evidence on PDT is varied depending on the type of photosensitizer used, route of its administration, type and wavelength of light used and number of treatment cycles [25–27]. Martin-Hirsch was the first one to study PDT in 1998 followed by various other studies. They all concluded that PDT is an effective and safe treatment for VIN with favourable cosmetic results with response rates ranging from 20 to 67% for histological response and 52–89% for symptom response [28].

Advantages of PDT therapy:

- Multifocal disease can be treated without tissue loss
- Healing time is less
- Tissue destruction is minimal
- Preservation of vulval anatomy
- Good cosmetic results.

Disadvantages of PDT therapy:

- Painful procedure—Pain at times leads to early termination of treatment and decreases therapeutic efficacy [29].
- Requires analgesia or anaesthesia—Though about 50%–60% of women can be treated without analgesia, others require either intravenous opioids or spinal/general anaesthesia during the procedure [30].

23.8.4 Topical 5-Fluorouracil (5-FU)

5-FU targets thymidylate synthetase in tumour cells. The target cells incorporate 5-FU, thereby increasing its selectivity for neoplastic and dysplastic cells. Topical 5-FU cream causes a chemical desquamation of the VIN lesion and response rates as high as 75% have been reported, but it is poorly tolerated due to burning, pain, inflammation, oedema and painful ulcers. Thus, 5-FU has a limited role in the treatment of VIN. Downs AM et al. studied the sequential effect of topical 5-FU on imiquimod-treated patients, and they concluded that there was no improvement in cure rates if both the topical treatments were used sequentially. This was due to the severe inflammation caused by imiquimod around the dysplastic cells which interferes with the uptake of 5-FU later. 5-FU therefore fails to reach the target sites of DNA or RNA within the dysplastic cells [31].

23.9 Investigational Therapies

Topical indole-3-carbinol, sinectechins and the use of chemoprotective agents like retinyl acetate gel are still under investigation.

23.10 Management of VIN in Pregnancy

Any vulvar lesion noted during pregnancy must be biopsied as in non-pregnant women because about 15% of vulvar carcinomas have been reported in women under the age of 40. During pregnancy, gestational age is the most important factor in determining further treatment, whether to continue with expectant management or to surgically intervene [32].

1. *Surgical treatment* with local excision or ablative therapy should follow same principles as in non-pregnant population. This is done for patient with VIN during pregnancy that is remote from delivery.
2. *Expectant treatment until after delivery*. If invasive carcinoma has been ruled out, treatment of VIN can be deferred to the postpartum period, especially in cases where detection is done in the third trimester.

Medical treatment is generally not recommended. Imiquimod is category C drug by USFDA, and the use is limited to cases where potential benefit justifies the potential risk to foetus, while 5-FU is a category D drug and should not be used during pregnancy.

23.11 Follow-Up

Higher recurrence rates have been seen with multiple lesions and positive excision margins [33, 34]. The recurrence rate is even higher in those with HPV infection, and despite treatment, invasive cancer will still develop in 3–5% of women [35]. This recurrence risk is high for high-grade VIN, multifocal intraepithelial neoplasia and high-risk HPV infection.

If follow-up visits at 6 months and 12 months show no new lesions, then the women should be monitored by visual inspection of the vulva annually thereafter (ACOG 2016) [36]. In a study on 445 cases of VIN (HSIL) to study the natural history, a high recurrence rate of 50% was seen in those with positive surgical margins [37]. In a systematic analysis of 3322 patients with VIN3, 6.5% patients progressed to invasive cancer. Recurrences were lower in women with free surgical margins after local excision and vulvectomy. Occult carcinoma was diagnosed in 3.2% of patients, and 3.3% cancers were diagnosed during follow-up. Only 1.2% of 3222 patients showed complete regression [38].

23.12 Primary Prevention

The proportion of women with VIN who are current smokers has been reported as 32–84%, and even a higher number have a history of smoking [39–41]. The association with smoking is seen more frequently with usual VIN rather than dVIN. Cessation of smoking would help in preventing vulvar HSIL. As dVIN is associated with vulvar dermatoses, treatment of vulvar dermatologic disorders especially of lichen sclerosus decreases the risk of vulvar carcinoma [42].

Quadrivalent or nonavalent HPV vaccines which are effective against HPV genotypes 6, 11, 16 and 18 and 6, 11, 16, 18, 31, 33, 45, 52 and 58, respectively, are now available. Large studies assessing the efficacy of these vaccines have reported seroconversion in approximately 98% of women, antibody titres raised for at least 5 years and prevention of warts, VIN and VaIN [43, 44].

23.13 Conclusion

Surgical excision remains the mainstay of treatment of VIN in the majority of women. Conservative management is generally not preferred as the risk of occult carcinoma at presentation is high. But in young women in whom cosmesis is important, ablative (Laser or CUSA) or topical therapies in the form of imiquimod, CDV ointment or PDT are an attractive alternative. With the advent of vaccines against HPV, a decrease in the incidence of HPV-associated VIN is expected, and management of VIN in elderly group may become more important and challenging.

Key Points

- The ISSVD 2015 terminology for VIN is vulvar LSIL (not premalignant, equivalent to condyloma acuminate and not associated with HPV), vulvar HSIL (associated with HPV) and dVIN (not associated with HPV).
- VIN is more common in premenopausal than in postmenopausal women. While postmenopausal women have more non-HPV-associated VIN and unifocal lesions, those in premenopausal women are multifocal and associated with HPV, immunosuppression and smoking.
- Squamous intraepithelial neoplasia is multifocal, i.e. involves more than one site (vulva, vagina, cervix or perianal skin).
- There are no screening strategies for VIN.
- Tissue biopsy is mandatory for diagnosis. Site of biopsy is decided by physical examination and vulvoscopy.
- Treatment goal is to prevent disease progression to invasive carcinoma and relief of symptoms while preserving normal vulvar anatomy and function.
- In vulvar HSIL with significant risk factors (previous VIN or vulvar carcinoma, immunocompromised state, smoking, age > 45 years, lichen sclerosus) and clinical suspicion of malignancy (raised, ulcerative growth with irregular borders), surgical excision is done.
- Vulvar HSIL with no suspicion of HSIL is excised. In young women, multifocal disease, involving the urethra, anus, clitoris and vaginal introitus (where excision can lead to adverse effect), ablative therapy is preferred.
- Ablative treatment is done with Laser or topical CDV and imiquimod.
- For dVIN, surgical excision rather than ablation or pharmacologic therapy is done.
- If there are no new lesions at 6 months and 12 months follow-up visits, the woman should be monitored by visual inspection of the vulva annually thereafter.

References

1. Judson PL, Habermann EB, Baxter NN, Durham SB, Virnig BA. Trends in the incidence of invasive and in situ vulvar carcinoma. Obstet Gynecol. 2006;107:1018–22.
2. Friedrich EG. Report of the committee on terminology. New nomenclature for vulvar disease. Obstet Gynecol. 1976;49:122–4.
3. Bornstein J, Bogliatto F, Haefner HK, et al. The 2015 International Society for the study of vulvovaginal disease (ISSVD) terminology of vulvar squamous intraepithelial lesion. J Low Genit Tract Dis. 2016;20:11–4.
4. Committee on Gynecologic Practice of American College of Obstetricians and Gynecologista. ACOG Committee opinion no. 509. Management of vulvar intraepithelial neoplasia. Obstet Gynecol. 2011;118:1192.
5. Waxman AG, Chelmow D, Darragh TH, et al. Revised terminology foe cervical histopathology and its implications for management of high grade squamous intraepithelial lesions of the cervix. Obstet Gynecol. 2012;120:1465.
6. Darragh TM, Colgan TJ, Thomas Cox J, et al. The Lower Anogenital Squamous terminology standardization project for HPV-associated lesion: background and consequence recommendations from the College of American Pathologists and the American Society for colposcopy and Cervical Pathology. Int J Gynecol Pathol. 2013;32:76.

7. Wilkinson E. The histopathology of vulvar neoplasia. Global Library of women's medicine (ISSN:175-2228). 2002. https://doi.org/10.3843/GLOWM.10256. Accessed 8 Feb 2016.
8. Crum CP, Herrington CS, McCluggage WG, et al. Tumours of the vulva; epithelial tumours. In: Kurman RJ, Carcangiu ML, Herrington CS, et al., editors. WHO classification of tumours of female reproductive organs. 4th ed. Lyon: IARC Press; 2014.
9. Cullis P, Mudzamiri T, Millan D, Siddiqui N. Vulval intraepithelial neoplasia: making sense of the literature. Obstet Gynecol. 2011;13:73–8.
10. Rutledge F, Sinclair M. Treatment of intraepithelial carcinoma of the vulva by skin excision and graft. Am J Obstet Gynecol. 1968;102:807.
11. Podczaski E, Sexton M, Kaminski P, et al. Recurrent carcinoma of the vulva after conservative treatment for microinvasive disease. Gynecol Oncol. 1990;39:65–8.
12. Baachi CE, Goldfogel GA, Greer BE, et al. Paget's disease and melanoma of the vulv. Gynecol Oncol. 1992;46:216.
13. Hacker NF. Surgery for malignant tumours of the vulva. In: Gershansen DM, Dc Cherney AH, Curry SL, Brubaker L, editors. Operative gynecology oncology. 2nd ed. Philadelphia: WB Saunders; 2001. p. 237–63.
14. Brigitte E, Miller MD. VIN treated with Cavitron ultrasonic surgical aspirator. Gynecol Oncol. 2002;85:114–8.
15. Kaushik S, Pepas L, Nordin A, Bryant A, Dickinson HO. Surgical interventions for high-grade vulval intraepithelial neoplasia. Cochrane Database Syst Rev. 2014;3:CD007928. https://doi.org/10.1002/14651858.CD007928.pub3.
16. Mathiesen O, Buus SK, Cramers M. Topical imiquimod can reverse vulvar intraepithelial neoplasia: a randomised, double-blinded study. Gynecol Oncol. 2007;107:219–22.
17. Lawrie TA, Nordin A, Chakrabarti M, Bryant A, Kaushik S, Pepas L. Medical and surgical interventions for the treatment of usual-type vulval intraepithelial neoplasia. Cochrane Database Syst Rev. 2016;1:CD011837. https://doi.org/10.1002/14651858.CD011837.pub2.
18. Terlou A, van Seters M, Ewing PC, Aaronson NK, Gundy CM, Heijmans-Antonissen C, Quint WG, Blok LJ, van Beurden M, Helmerhorst TJ. Treatment of vulvar intraepithelial neoplasia with topical imiquimod: seven years median follow-up of a randomized clinical trial. Gynecol Oncol. 2011;121:157–62. https://doi.org/10.1016/j.ygyno.2010.12.340.
19. Tristam A, Flander A. Clinical responses to Cidofovir applied topically to women with high grade vulval intraepithelial neoplasia. Gynecol Oncol. 2005;99(3):652–5.
20. Stier EA, Goldstone SE, Einstein MH, Jay N, Berry JM, et al. Safety and efficacy of topical cidofovir to treat high-grade perianal and vulvar intraepithelial neoplasia in HIV-positive men and women. AIDS. 2013;27(4):545–51.
21. Tristram T, Hurt CN, Madden T, Powell N, Man S, et al. Activity, safety, and feasibility of cidofovir and imiquimod for treatment of vulval intraepithelial neoplasia (RT[3]VIN): a multicentre, open-label, randomised, phase 2 trial. Lancet Oncol. 2014;15(12):1361–8. https://doi.org/10.1016/S1470-2045(14)70456-5.
22. Pepas L, Kaushik S, Nordin A, Bryant A, Lawrie TA. Medical interventions for high-grade vulval intraepithelial neoplasia. Cochrane Database Syst Rev. 2015;8:CD007924. https://doi.org/10.1002/14651858.CD007924.pub3.
23. Hillemanns P, Wnag X, Staehle S, Michels W, Dannecker C. Evaluation of different treatment modalities for vulvar intra epithelial neoplasia: CO_2 laser vaporization, photodynamic therapy, excision and vulvectomy. Gynecol Oncol. 2006;100:271–5.
24. Morton CA, McKenna KE, Rhodes LE, British Association of Dermatologists Therapy Guidelines and Audit Subcommittee and the British Photodermatology Group. Guidelines for topical photodynamic therapy: update. Br J Dermatol. 2008;159:1245–66. https://doi.org/10.1111/j.1365-2133.2008.08882.x.
25. Kurwa HA, Barlow RJ, Neill S. Single-episode photodynamic therapy and vulval intraepithelial neoplasia type III resistant to conventional therapy. Br J Dermatol. 2000;143:1040–2. https://doi.org/10.1046/j.1365-2133.2000.03785.x.
26. Hillemanns P, Untch M, Dannecker C, Baumgartner R, Stepp H, Diebold J, Weingandt H, Pröve F, Korell M. Photodynamic therapy of vulvar intraepithelial neoplasia using 5-aminolevulinic acid. Int J Cancer. 2000;85:649–53. https://doi.org/10.1002/(SICI)1097-0215(20000301)85:5<649:AID-IJC9>3.0.CO;2-E.
27. Fehr MK, Hornung R, Schwarz VA, Simeon R, Haller U, Wyss P. Photodynamic therapy of vulvar intraepithelial neoplasia III using topically applied 5-aminolevulinic acid. Gynecol Oncol. 2001;80:62–6. https://doi.org/10.1006/gyno.2000.6028.
28. Martin-Hirsch PL, Whitehurst C, Buckley CH, Moore JV, Kitchener HC. Photodynamic treatment for lower genital tract intraepithelial neoplasia. Lancet. 1998;351:1403. https://doi.org/10.1016/S0140-6736(98)24019-0.
29. Ang JM, Riaz IB, Kamal MU, Paragh G, Zeitouni NC. Photodynamic therapy and pain: a systematic review. Photodiagn Photodyn Ther. 2017;19:308–44. https://doi.org/10.1016/j.pdpdt.2017.07.002.
30. Soergel P, Hillemanns P. Photodynamic therapy for intraepithelial neoplasia of the lower genital tract. Photodiagn Photodyn Ther. 2010;7:10–4. https://doi.org/10.1016/j.pdpdt.2009.12.007.
31. Downs AM, Geraghty JM, Jones C. Fluorouracil does not improve the outcome of imiquimoid treatment of vulvar intraepithelial lesions. Acta Derm Venereol. 2005;85:368–70.
32. Tseng J-Y, Baster E, Gungor UF. Management of precancerous lesions prior to conception and during

pregnancy: a narrative review of the literature. Eur J Cancer Care. 2012;21(6):703–11.
33. Van Esch EM, Dam MC, Osse ME, Putter H, Trimbos BJ, Fleuren G, et al. Clinical characteristics associated with development of recurrence and progression in usual type vulvar intra-epithelial neoplasia. Int J Gynecol Cancer. 2013;23:1476–83.
34. Modesitt SC, Waters AB, Walton L, Fowler WC Jr, Van Le L. Vulvar Intraepithelial neoplasia III: occult cancer and the impact of margin status on recurrence. Obstet Gynecol. 1998;92:962–6.
35. Hillemanns P, Wang X, Stachle S, Michels W, Dannecker C. Evaluation of different treatment modalities for vulva intraepithelial neoplasia (VIN):CO2 laser vaporization, photodynamic therapy, excision and vulvectomy. Gynecol Oncol. 2006;100(2):271–5.
36. Management of Vulvar Intraepithelial Neoplasia, ACOG and ASCCP Committee opinion no. 675. 2016.
37. Jones RW, Rowan DM, Stewart AW. Vulvar Intra epithelial neoplasia: aspects of natural history and outcome in 405 women. Obstet Gynecol. 2005;106(6):1319–26.
38. Van seters M, Van Buerden M, de Craen AJ. Is the assumed natural history of vulvar intraepithelial neoplasia III based on enough evidence? A systematic review of 3322 published patients. Gynecol Oncol. 2005;97(2):645–51.
39. van Beurden M, ten Kate FJ, Smits HL, Berkhout RJ, de Craen AJ, van der Vange N, et al. Multifocal vulvar intraepithelial neoplasia grade III and multicentric lower genital tract neoplasia is associated with transcriptionally active human papillomavirus. Cancer. 1995;75:2879–84. https://doi.org/10.1002/1097-0142(19950615)75:123.0.CO;2-W.
40. McNally OM, Mulvany NJ, Pagano R, Quinn MA, Rome RM. VIN 3: a clinicopathologic review. Int J Gynecol Cancer. 2002;12:490–5. https://doi.org/10.1046/j.1525-1438.2002.01140.x.
41. Pilotti S, Rotola A, D'Amato L, Di Luca D, Shah KV, Cassai E, et al. Vulvar carcinomas: search for sequences homologous to human papillomavirus and herpes simplex virus DNA. Mol Pathol. 1990;3:442–8.
42. Lee A, Bradford J, Fischer G. Long term management of adult vulvar lichen sclerosus: a prospective cohort study of 507 women. JAMA Dermatol. 2015;151:1061–7.
43. Villa LL, Costa RL, Petta CA, Andrade RP, Ault KA, Giuliano AR, et al. Prophylactic quadrivalent human papillomavirus (types 6, 11, 16, and 18) L1 virus-like particle vaccine in young women: a randomised double-blind placebo-controlled multicentre phase II efficacy trial. Lancet Oncol. 2005;6:271–8. https://doi.org/10.1016/S1470-2045(05)70101-7.
44. Davidson EJ, Boswell CM, Sell P, Pawlita M, Tomlinson AC, McVey RJ, et al. Immunological and clinical responses in women with vulval intraepithelial neoplasia vaccinated with a vaccinia virus encoding human papillomavirus 16/18 oncoproteins. Cancer Res. 2003;63:6032–41.

24 Vaginal Cancer: Epidemiology and Risk Factors

Rani Bhat

24.1 Introduction

A rare cancer, primary vaginal malignancy, constitutes only 1–2% of all malignant gynecologic tumors ranking fifth in frequency behind cancer in the cervix, uterus, ovary, and vulva. The age-adjusted incidence is 0.2–0.8 per 100,000 women per year in India. According to the International Federation of Gynaecology and Obstetrics (FIGO), a vaginal lesion involving the cervix should be managed as a cervical cancer; a tumor involving both the vulva and the vagina should be considered as a primary vulvar cancer. About 80% of vaginal cancers are metastatic with primaries being the cervix or the endometrium and less common sites being the vulva, ovaries, choriocarcinoma, rectosigmoid, and bladder. Metastasis through the blood or lymphatic system can also occur from colon cancer, renal cell carcinoma, melanoma, and breast cancer.

The strict criteria used to define vaginal cancer may have contributed to its low incidence. Squamous cell carcinoma (85%) and adenocarcinoma (15%) are the two different histological types varying in pathogenesis and natural history. Clear cell adenocarcinoma is rare and occurs most often in young patients with an in utero exposure to diethylstilbestrol (DES). Rarely, melanoma, sarcoma, and adenosquamous carcinoma may occur as primary vaginal cancers. Cervical and vulvar carcinomas need to be ruled out by biopsy and clinical examination. Early-stage vaginal cancer is often curable, and the role of imaging cannot be underestimated.

R. Bhat (✉)
Department of Gynaecological Oncology, Healthcare Global Enterprises Ltd., Bangalore, Karnataka, India

24.2 Epidemiology

Vaginal cancer accounts for 2% of all gynecologic cancers with a lifetime risk of 1 in 1100 women. As it is extremely rare, there are only a limited number of reports regarding its epidemiological analysis. The American Cancer Society estimates for the United States in 2018 are that 5170 new cases will be diagnosed with the death of 1330 women among them [1]. In 2015, 232 new cases were detected in the United Kingdom which accounted for <1% of all cancer cases with an age incidence of 80–84 years, and overall the trend has remained the same. There were 110 deaths from vaginal cancer in 2014, and mortality rates have decreased by 44% since the 1970s [2].

According to the Cancer Registry and Statistics, National Cancer Center, Japan, the crude incidence rate during 2008–2014 was about 0.7 cases per lakh women. According to Yagi et al., the age-adjusted incidence rate was 0.25 per lakh women which is lower than the US population, 0.69 per lakh women. They also found a significant increase in number of vaginal

S. Mehta, A. Singla (eds.), *Preventive Oncology for the Gynecologist*,
https://doi.org/10.1007/978-981-13-3438-2_24

cancers registered per 5-year increment in the Japanese population. This could be because of the increase in the elderly population of the country.

Using the Japanese model population of 1985, the age-adjusted incidence rate per lakh women has significantly dropped from 1976 to 2010 and is comparable to the European age-standardized incidence of cancer in vagina which has also decreased by 14% during 1975–2013 [3].

In accordance with cervical cancer, most of the vaginal cancers (68%) occur in the developing countries. The ratio of carcinoma of vagina to cervix was found to be 1:32 at the Gujarat Cancer and Research Institute, Ahmedabad, India [4].

Table 24.1 shows the Indian Cancer Registry incidences of vaginal cancer.

Studies have shown that vaginal squamous cell carcinoma (SCC) (the main histopathological type) may have many risk factors similar to cervical cancer, especially an association with persistent human papillomavirus (HPV) infection which accounts for almost 40% of the vaginal cancers [5–12]. Of this HPV, type 16 (HPV-16) is detected in 50–64% of high-grade vaginal intraepithelial lesions [13–15]. The main types are squamous cell carcinoma (90%), followed by clear cell adenocarcinomas and melanoma. Metastatic cervical cancer may be misclassified as vaginal cancers.

The median age of invasive cancer is more in comparison with in situ lesions (68 vs. 58 years). The age-adjusted incidence of vaginal cancer is also significantly higher among black and Hispanic women than white women.

Figure 24.1 shows incidence rates of vaginal cancer by age group in India. Invasive vaginal cancer is diagnosed primarily in old women (≥65 years), and the diagnosis is rare in women under 45 years, whereas the peak incidence of carcinoma in situ is observed between ages 55 and 70.

Table 24.1 Vaginal cancer incidence in India by cancer registry

Cancer registry	Period	N cases[a]	Crude rate[b]	ASR[b]
Ahmedabad[c]	1993–1997	65	0.7	1.1
Bangalore[d]	2005–2007	54	0.6	0.8
Barshi[e]	1988–1992	3	0.3	0.3
Barshi, Paranda, and Bhum[d]	2003–2007	6	0.5	0.5
Chennai[d]	2003–2007	79	0.7	0.8
Delhi[c]	1993–1996	58	0.3	0.5
Dindigul[c], Ambilikkai[d]	2003–2007	39	0.8	0.8
Karunagappally[d]	2003–2007	2	0.2	0.2
Mizoram[d]	2003–2007	4	0.2	0.3
Mumbai[d]	2003–2007	160	0.6	0.7
Nagpur[f]	1998–2002	0	0.0	0.0
New Delhi[d]	2003–2007	97	0.3	0.4
Poona[d]	2003–2007	44	0.4	0.6
Sikkim State[d]	2003–2007	4	0.3	0.6
Trivandrum[d]	2005–2007	8	0.5	0.4

Data accessed on May 5, 2015

ASR: age-standardized rate. Standardized rates have been estimated using the direct method and the world population as the reference

Please refer to original source (available at http://c15.iarc.fr/CI5i-ix.htm)

[a]Accumulated number of cases during the period in the population covered by the corresponding registry

[b]Rates per 100,00 women per year

[c]Parkin DM, Whelan SL, Ferlay J, Teppo L, Thomas DB, editors. Cancer incidence in five continents, vol. VIII. Lyon: IARC Scientific Publications No. 55; 2002

[d]Forman D, Bray F, Brewster DH, Gombe Mbalawa C, Kohler B, Pineros M, et al., editors. Cancer incidence in five continents, vol. X (electronic version). Lyon: IARC http://ci5.iarc.fr

[e]Parkin DM, Whelan SL, Ferlay J, Raymond L, Young J, editors. Cancer incidence in five continents, vol. VII. Lyon: IARC Scientific Publications No. 143; 1997

[f]Curado MP, Edwards B, Shin HR, Storm H, Ferlay J, Heanue M, Boyle P, editors. Cancer incidence in five continents, vol. IX. Lyon; IARC Scientific Publications No. 160; 2007

24.3 Types of Vaginal Cancer

- *Squamous cell carcinoma:* Squamous cell carcinoma accounts for 85–90% of all the subtypes, progressive developing from precancerous conditions called vaginal intraepithelial neoplasia or VaIN.
- *Adenocarcinoma*: Adenocarcinoma arises from vaginal glands and accounts for 5–10% of all cases. The four main subtypes of adenocarcinoma of the vagina are:
  - Clear cell adenocarcinoma: Exposure to DES in utero is the main causative factor with 1 in 1000 exposed, developing a vaginal cancer. Clear cell cancers of the vagina usually develop in women in their

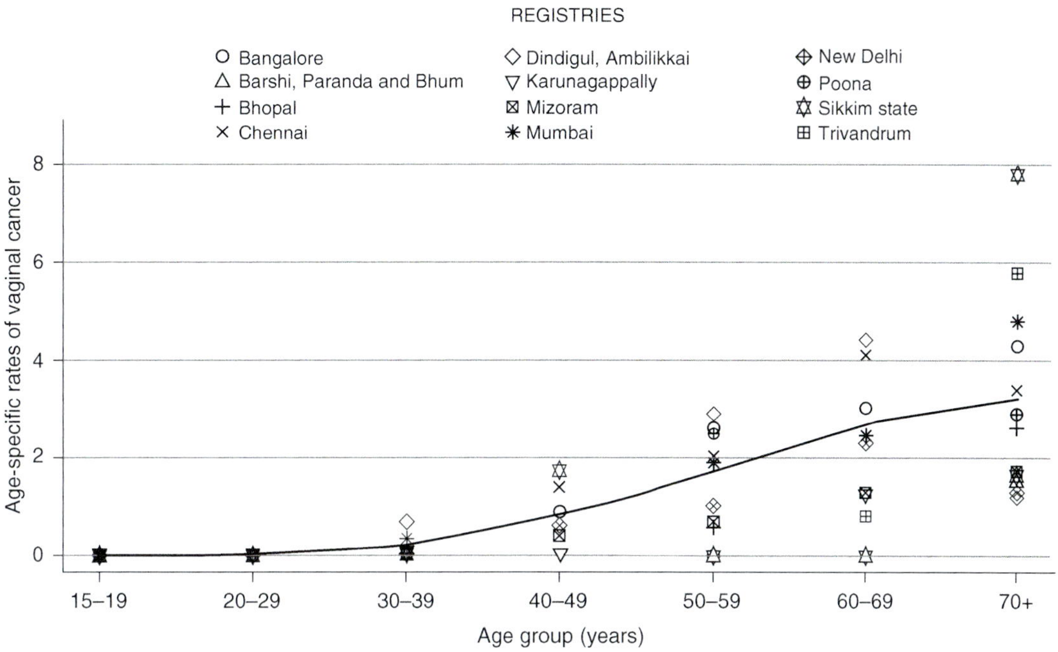

Fig. 24.1 Incidence rates of vaginal cancer by age group in India

teens or twenties, but there are reports of women being diagnosed in their early forties. As it's now more than 40 years since DES was used in pregnancy, these cancers are becoming even rarer.

- Papillary adenocarcinoma: Papillary cancers can grow throughout the connective tissues that surround the vagina.
- Mucinous adenocarcinoma: Primary mucinous adenocarcinoma of the vagina is one of the rarest subtypes.
- Adenosquamous cancers: Adenosquamous carcinoma of the vagina is a rare form of cancer having malignant squamous cells and malignant glandular cells. They are also called mixed epithelial tumors. They are often quickly growing tumors.

• *Melanoma*: Although it is rare, melanoma can begin in the vagina. Melanomas are usually found in some exposed body areas rarely developed without sun exposure also. Melanomas appear as dark-colored lesions with irregular borders (Fig. 24.2a, b).

• *Sarcomas:* Sarcomas are cancers that start in the body's connective tissues and tend to grow quite quickly. Different types of sarcoma can start in the vagina, including leiomyosarcoma and rhabdomyosarcoma. These are both muscle tumors. About two thirds of vaginal sarcomas are leiomyosarcomas. It's possible to have other types of sarcoma, such as mixed mullerian sarcoma, but these are extremely rare.

24.4 Vaginal Cancer: Risk Factors

The exact etiology of vaginal cancer is yet to be established. Since different histological subtypes exist with different characteristics, age predilection, aggressiveness, and prognosis, a multifactorial etiology is more likely. A variety of agents have been implicated, but so far no clear cause-and-effect relationship has been proved.

24.4.1 HPV and Other Infectious Agents

Since HPV deoxyribonucleic acid (DNA) has been detected in squamous cancer cells by in situ hybridization (21%) and Southern blot hybridiza-

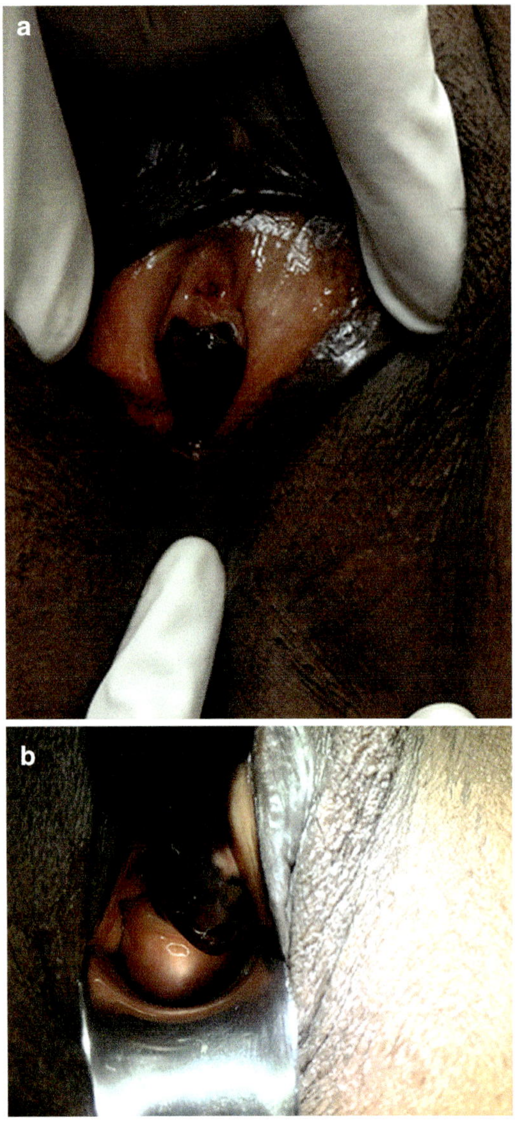

Fig. 24.2 (a, b) Vaginal melanomas

tion (56%), a possible role for HPV in the pathogenesis of squamous cell vaginal cancers cannot be overemphasized [16, 17].

HPV subtypes 16 and 18 with the highest oncogenic potential have been associated with dysplastic changes in the female genital tract. Since HPV is sexually transmitted, whether women who engage in high-risk sexual behaviors may be at a higher than average risk of developing vaginal malignancy.

Though persistent oncogenic HPV infections are of similar occurrence in the cervix and vagina [18], the incidence of cervical cancer is much more than cancer of the vagina across the globe. The most probable reason is that the cervical transformation zone is more susceptible to persistent oncogenic HPV infection [15, 19]. Also the premalignant lesions of the vagina, i.e., VaIN, are associated with HPV infection.

Other associated infectious agents are herpes simplex virus (HSV) and *Trichomonas vaginalis*. Lee and colleagues reported a rapidly progressive vaginal squamous cell carcinoma in HIV-positive young woman, suggesting that coinfection with both HIV and HPV increased the risk of more aggressive and less responsive vaginal cancer [20].

24.4.2 History of Carcinoma

Co-association of cervical intraepithelial neoplasia (CIN) and invasive cervical and vulval carcinoma has been noted with vaginal cancer. As high as 30% women with primary vaginal cancer have a history of in situ or invasive cervical cancer treatment done in the past 5 years [21–23].

24.4.3 Diethylstilbestrol Exposure

Diethylstilbestrol (DES), in the late 1940s, was used to prevent miscarriage and has been implicated as a causative factor for clear cell adenocarcinoma of the vagina [24]. These women are at higher risk of developing adenocarcinoma than the general population with an estimated risk of 1 in 1000.

24.4.4 Prior Hysterectomy

Hysterectomy per se is not a risk factor, but by virtue of these women being poorly screened, as high as 59% hysterectomized women develop vaginal cancer. Herman and colleagues demonstrated that when the effect of age and prior cervical cancer is nullified, the risk of vaginal cancer is not increased following hysterectomy done for benign disease [25]. Brinton et al. noted that the risk was highest in women who had hysterectomy at the age <40 years [9]. Women with prior hysterectomy were significantly younger at the diagnosis of primary carcinoma of the vagina, and if the hysterectomy was done for a premalignant cervical disease, vaginal carcinoma developed earlier in comparison to hysterectomy done for other reasons. The association noted between Primary cancers of vagina (PCV) and hysterectomy could be due to incompletely resected and screened residual CIN or occult disease. Despite clear surgical margins, the multicentric nature of the disease hampers the total resection of the involved areas [26]. The author noticed that the majority of non-hysterectomized patients with prior CIN developed the vaginal carcinoma in the lower part of the vagina. Since the vagina has a dual embryological origin, the response of the upper and lower one third of vaginal tissue is different to various carcinogenic reasons [27, 28].

24.4.5 Age

The relationship of age with PCV was explored by Hellman et al. in 341 cases. HPV dependence and relation to cervical neoplasia seem more prudent in young women, though in older counterparts, hormonal factors and vaginal trauma may account for a number of cases [26].

Vaginal cancer is mainly seen in elderly postmenopausal women. In a review done by Dixit et al., mean age of women with vaginal cancer was 47 years with a range from 24 to 72 years. It has been noted that 60% of women who presented with vaginal cancer were below 50 years of age with a preponderance of younger age distribution in Indian population [4].

24.4.6 Additional Factors

Chronic irritation as in cases of procidentia and long-term pessary use has been associated with vaginal cancer.

Estrogen deficiency as in postmenopausal women might play a role in the pathogenesis of PCV. Panhysterectomy and irradiation done to the ovary are some examples. Almost 10% of women diagnosed with primary vaginal carcinoma have a lifetime history of irradiation to the pelvis [26]. Low lifetime estrogen exposure includes late menarche, early menopause, and nulliparity, but a high estrogen lifetime exposure (e.g., multiparity, intake of exogenous estrogens, and obesity) might exert a protective effect. Grand multiparity imposes an increased risk due to the repetitive trauma to the vagina.

Other predisposing factors include low socioeconomic conditions, cigarette smoking, and immunosuppressive therapy. According to a cross-sectional study, VaIN risk is higher in women with genital warts, indicating an association with HPV [29].

24.4.7 Autoimmune Conditions

Meta-analysis done by Cao et al. showed vaginal or vulval cancer risk is more than three times as high in women with systemic lupus erythematosus as compared with the general population [30].

24.5 Conclusion

Primary vaginal cancers are rare and comprise 1–2% of all gynecological malignancies. Resistance of the vagina to carcinogenic change and the stricter criteria used for diagnosis is essentially responsible for the low incidence. Cancer found in the vagina is more likely to be metastatic disease than primary disease. Of these, cancers from the cervix, endometrium, and colon/rectum are the most frequent. The commonest histologic type is squamous cell carcinoma, followed by adenocarcinoma. There are some known causes such as HPV infection, age, history of carcinoma, diethylstilbestrol (DES) exposure, autoimmune conditions such as systemic lupus erythematosus, social background, and chronic conditions as well as unknown causes.

References

1. Yagi A, Ueda Y, Kakuda M, Tanaka Y, Egawa-Takata T, Morimoto A, et al. Descriptive epidemiological study of vaginal cancer using data from the Osaka Japan population-based cancer registry: long-term analysis from a clinical viewpoint. Medicine (Baltimore). 2017;96(32):e7751. https://doi.org/10.1097/MD.0000000000007751.
2. American Cancer Society. Key statistics for vaginal cancer. Available from: https://www.cancer.org/cancer/vaginal-cancer/about/key-statistics.html. Accessed 20 Apr 2018.
3. Cancer Research UK. Vaginal cancer statistics. Available for: http://www.cancerresearchuk.org/health-professional/cancer-statistics/statistics-by-cancer-type/vaginal-cancer. Accessed 20 Apr 2018.
4. Dixit S, Singhal S, Baboo HA. Squamous cell carcinoma of the vagina: a review of 70 cases. Gynecol Oncol. 1993;48:80–7.
5. Hellman K, Silfversward C, Nilsson B, Hellstrom AC, Frankendal B, Pettersson F. Primary carcinoma of the vagina: factors influencing the age at diagnosis. The Radiumhemmet series 1956-96. Int J Gynecol Cancer. 2004;14:491–501.
6. Carter JJ, Madeleine MM, Shera K, Schwartz SM, Cushing-Haugen KL, Wipf GC, et al. Human papillomavirus 16 and 18 L1 serology compared across anogenital cancer sites. Cancer Res. 2001;61:1934–40.
7. Daling J, Madeleine M, Schwartz S, et al. A population-based study of squamous cell vaginal cancer: HPV and cofactors. Gynecol Oncol. 2002;84:263–70.
8. Daling JR, Sherman KJ. Relationship between human papillomavirus infection and tumours of anogenital sites other than the cervix. In: Munoz N, Bosch FX, Shah KV, Meheus A, editors. The epidemiology of human papillomavirus and cervical cancer (IARC scientific publication no. 119). Lyon: IARC; 1992. p. 223–41.
9. Brinton LA, Nasca PC, Mallin K, Schairer C, Rosenthal J, Rothenberg R, et al. Case-control study of in situ and invasive carcinoma of the vagina. Gynecol Oncol. 1990;38:49–54.
10. McFarlane MJ, Feinstein AR, Horwitz RI. Diethylstilbestrol and clear cell vaginal carcinoma. Reappraisal of the epidemiologic evidence. Am J Med. 1986;81:855–63.
11. Franco EL. Epidemiology of anogenital warts and cancer. Obstet Gynecol Clin N Am. 1996;23:597–623.
12. Merino MJ. Vaginal cancer: the role of infectious and environmental factors. Am J Obstet Gynecol. 1991;165(4 pt 2):1255–62.
13. Srodon M, Stoler MH, Baber GB, Kurman RJ. The distribution of low and high-risk HPV types in vulvar and vaginal intraepithelial neoplasia (VIN and VaIN). Am J Surg Pathol. 2006;30:1513–8.
14. Hampl M, Sarajuuri H, Wentzensen N, Bender H, Kueppers V. Effect of human papillomavirus vaccines on vulvar, vaginal, and anal intraepithelial lesions and vulvar cancer. Obstet Gynecol. 2006;108:1361–8.
15. Parkin D, Bray F. The burden of HPV-related cancers. Vaccine. 2006;24(suppl 3):S11–25.
16. Ikenberg H, Runge M, Goppinger A. Human papillomavirus DNA in invasive carcinoma of the vagina. Obstet Gynecol. 1990;76(3 Pt 1):432–8.
17. Ostrow RS, Manias DA, Clark BA. The analysis of carcinomas of the vagina for human papillomavirus DNA. Int J Gynecol Pathol. 1988;7(4):308–14.
18. Castle PE, Schiffman M, Bratti MC, Hildesheim A, Herrero R, Hutchinson ML, et al. A population- based study of vaginal human papillomavirus infection in hysterectomized women. J Infect Dis. 2004;190:458–67.
19. Schiffman M, Castle PE, Jeronimo J, Rodriguez AC, Wacholder S. Human papillomavirus and cervical cancer. Lancet. 2007;370:890–907.
20. Lee YC, Holcomb K, Buhl A. Rapid progression of primary vaginal squamous cell carcinoma in a young HIV-infected woman. Gynecol Oncol. 2000;78(3 Pt 1):380–2.
21. Benedet JL, Murphy KJ, Fairey RN, Boyes DA. Primary invasive carcinoma of the vagina. Obstet Gynecol. 1983;62:715–9.
22. Peters WA III, Kumar NB, Morley GW. Carcinoma of the vagina. Cancer. 1985;55:892–7.
23. Rubin SC, Young J, Mikuta JJ. Squamous carcinoma of the vagina: treatment, complications, and long-term follow-up. Gynecol Oncol. 1985;20:346–53.
24. Cogliano VJ, Baan R, Straif K, Grosse Y, Lauby-Secretan B, El Ghissassi F, et al. Preventable exposures associated with human cancers. J Natl Cancer Inst. 2011;103(24):1827–39.
25. Herman JM, Homesley HD, Dignan MB. Is hysterectomy a risk factor for vaginal cancer? JAMA. 1986;256(5):601–3.
26. Hellman K, Silfversward C, Nilsson B. Primary carcinoma of the vagina: factors influencing the age at diagnosis. The Radiumhemmet series 1956-96. Int J Gynecol Cancer. 2004;14(3):491–501.
27. Sillman FH, Fruchter RG, Chen YS, Camilien L, Sedlis A, McTigue E. Vaginal intraepithelial neoplasia: risk factors for persistence, recurrence, and invasion and its management. Am J Obstet Gynecol. 1997;176:93–9.
28. Cunha GR. The dual origin of vaginal epithelium. Am J Anat. 1975;143:387–92.
29. Blomberg M, Friis S, Munk C, Bautz A, Kjaer SK. Genital warts and risk of cancer: a Danish study of nearly 50 000 patients with genital warts. J Infect Dis. 2012;205(10):1544–53.
30. Cao L, Tong H, Xu G, Liu P, Meng H, Wang J, et al. Systemic lupus erythematous and malignancy risk: a meta-analysis. PLoS One. 2015;10(4):e0122964.

25 Vaginal Intraepithelial Neoplasia (VaIN): Diagnosis and Management

Xingnan Zhou, Tien Anh Nguyen Tran, and Robert W. Holloway

25.1 Introduction

Vaginal intraepithelial neoplasia (VaIN) is a premalignant lesion characterized by the presence of dysplastic squamous cells confined to the lining squamous epithelium of the vaginal mucosa without invasion into the underlying stroma of the submucosa. The disease is classified according to the level of epithelial involvement by the dysplastic squamous cells: VaIN 1 (Figs. 25.1 and 25.2) and 2 (Fig. 25.3) involve the lower one-third and two-thirds of the epithelium, respectively, whereas in VaIN 3 (Fig. 25.4), the dysplastic keratinocytes extend into the upper third of the epithelium. Carcinoma in situ (Fig. 25.5) involves the full thickness of the epithelium and is included in the VaIN 3 category. VaIN, just as cervical intraepithelial neoplasia (CIN) and vulvar intraepithelial neoplasia (VIN), is also classified into low-grade (mild dysplasia or grade 1) and high-grade squamous intraepithelial lesions [moderate and severe dysplasia, grades 2–3, and carcinoma in situ (CIS)].

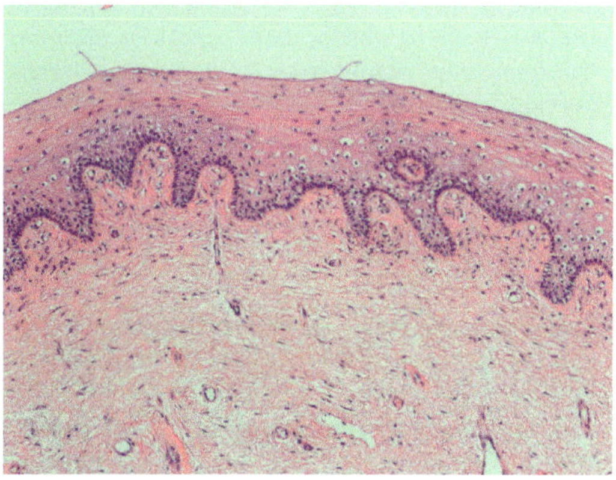

Fig. 25.1 Benign squamous mucosa with a layer of basal cells at the mucosal-submucosal junction and overlying sheets of benign keratinocytes with abundant cytoplasm, indicating normal maturation

The incidence of VaIN has been estimated from an epidemiologic study, the Third National Cancer Survey in the United States in 1977, at 0.2–0.3 cases per 100,000 women, and accounts for 0.4–1.0% of all intraepithelial neoplasia of the lower genital tract [1]. Another epidemiologic study that combined data from two federal cancer surveillance programs, CDC's National Program of Cancer Registries and NCI's Surveillance, Epidemiology, and End Results (SEER) Program, covering 92% of the US population from 1999 to 2004, estimated that the incidence of vaginal carci-

X. Zhou
Department of Obstetrics and Gynecology, Peking Union Medical College Hospital, Peking Union Medical College, Chinese Academy of Medical Sciences, Beijing, China

T. A. N. Tran
Department of Pathology, Florida Hospital Orlando, Orlando, FL, USA

R. W. Holloway (✉)
Florida Hospital Gynecologic Oncology, Orlando, FL, USA

S. Mehta, A. Singla (eds.), *Preventive Oncology for the Gynecologist*,
https://doi.org/10.1007/978-981-13-3438-2_25

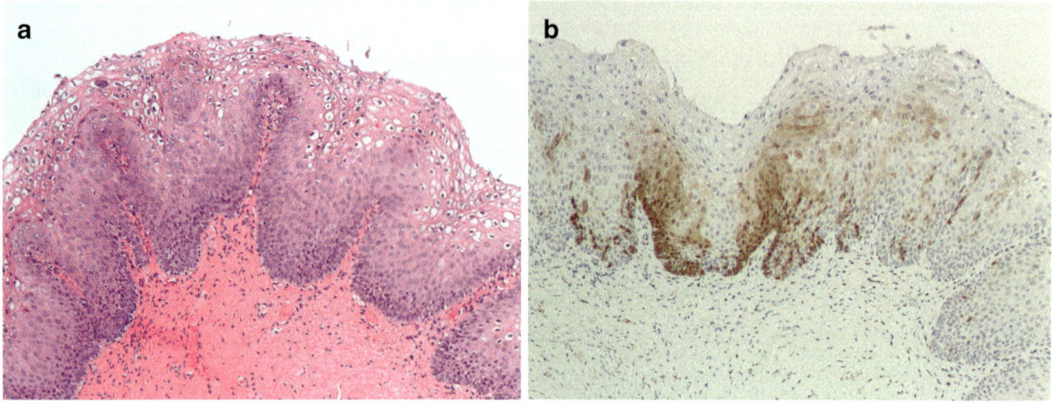

Fig. 25.2 (**a**) Low-grade SIL/VaIN-2 characterized by expansion of the lower third of the squamous mucosa by immature basal cells with increased cellularity, imparting a darker appearance of the lower third of the epithelium. Note the presence of squamous cells on the surface showing irregular nuclei and perinuclear halo. These squamous cells display cytologic features of HPV effects and are coined koilocytes. (**b**) Patchy, weak immunopositivity of a low-grade SIL/VaIN-1 for p16

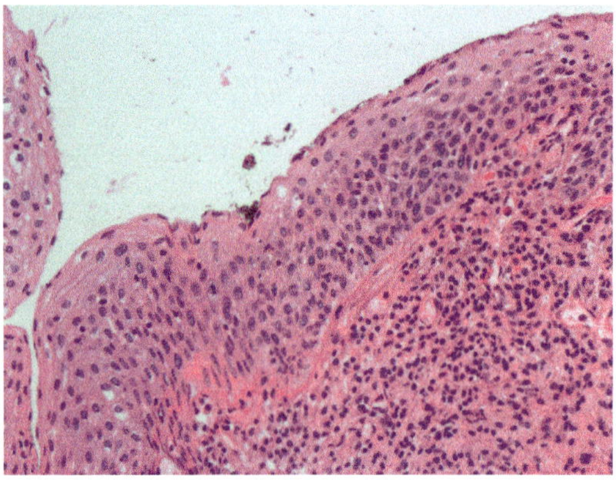

Fig. 25.3 High-grade SIL/VaIN 2 characterized by atypical squamous cells involving the mid third of the squamous epithelium

noma in situ in the United States was 0.1 cases per 100,000 women [2]. In a retrospective analysis of 16,732 cases of lower genital intraepithelial neoplasia from Shanghai, China, CIN, VaIN and VIN accounted for 83.99%, 11.49%, and 4.52% of the total lower genital intraepithelial neoplasia, respectively [3]. This study also showed an increasing annual proportion of VaIN possibly secondary to improved screening and increasing attention to colposcopic inspection of the entire vaginal wall [3]. The average age at diagnosis is about 50 years [4, 5], and the mean age is related to the degree of VaIN. The incidence of VaIN 1–2, VaIN 3, and vaginal CIS peaks at age of 45, 60, and 70–79, respectively [2, 6]. The increasing practice of HPV vaccination should make VaIN an even more uncommon condition in the near future [7].

VaIN is frequently associated with CIN and VIN. VaIN has been diagnosed in patients with histories of CIN and VIN in 65% and 10% of cases, respectively [8]. Kim et al. reported that 52.6% of patients with VaIN had either prior or concurrent CIN [5]. Among women who underwent hysterectomy for cervical cancer, VaIN was identified in 5–15% of cases [9–12]. In contrast, the incidence of VaIN in women following hysterectomy for benign uterine diseases is approximately 1.3% in the subsequent 10 years [13].

Similar to CIN and VIN, HPV is considered pivotal in the pathogenesis of VaIN. Summarizing 22 US studies, a systematic review identified the most common HPV types associated with VaIN 3 and vaginal cancer are HPV 16 and HPV 18, with prevalences of 65.1% and 72.7%, respectively [14]. In another systematic review of summarizing 232 cases of VaIN, Smith et al. reported that 92.6% of VaIN 2-3 and 98.5% VaIN 1 cases had HPV detected by either polymerase chain reaction or hybrid capture assays [15]. The prevalence for any carcinogenic HPV type in vaginal and cervical specimens is similar ($P = 0.3$), indicating that carcinogenic HPV types have equal affinity for vaginal and cervical epithelium [16]. Most CIN occurs

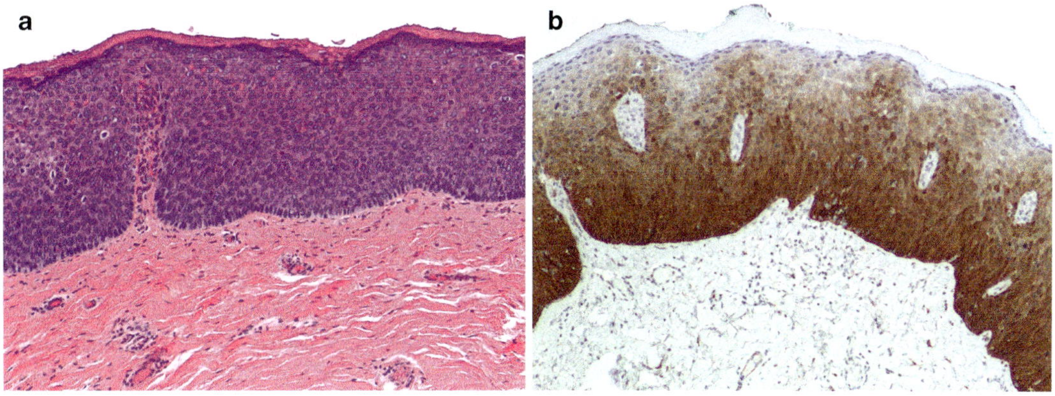

Fig. 25.4 (a) High-grade SIL/VaIN 3 showing involvement of the full thickness of the squamous epithelium by dark atypical basaloid cells. (b) High-grade SIL/VaIN 3 displays strong, diffuse, block-like immunopositivity for p16. Strong immunopositivity for p16 is a surrogate marker for oncogenic HPV infection in the lower genital tract

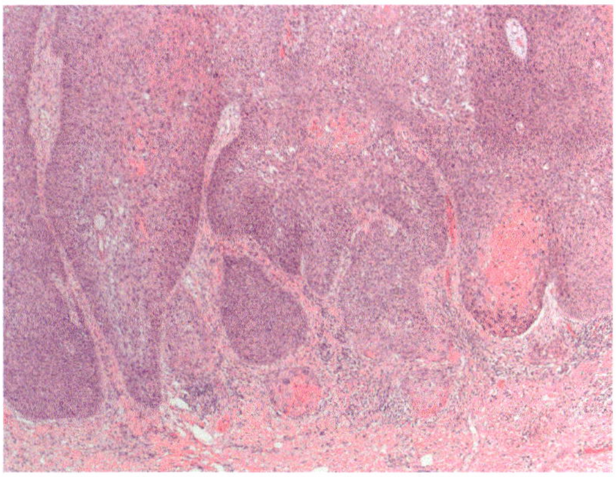

Fig. 25.5 Vaginal squamous mucosa demonstrating full-thickness involvement by dysplastic cells characteristic for squamous cell carcinoma in situ. Note three small nests of malignant keratinocytes in the submucosa separate from the dominant overlying carcinoma in situ consistent with early invasion. The neoplastic cells in the invasive component display abundant eosinophilic cytoplasm which is commonly seen in mature squamous epithelium, a phenomenon known as paradoxical maturation which serves as a clue for early invasion

in the transformation zone of the uterine cervix. It is believed that the columnar epithelium of the cervix undergoes squamous metaplasia at the beginning of the premalignant process and becomes susceptible to the oncogenic HPV effects. Since a transformation zone does not exist in the vagina, the prevalence of VaIN is significantly lower than CIN although the entire lower genital tract is infected by the virus with equal affinity.

In addition to HPV infection, other risk factors for VaIN include radiation therapy, immunosuppression, prenatal exposure to diethylstilbestrol (DES), and smoking. Women who have had pelvic radiation for malignant as well as benign diseases have been reported at an increased risk for development of VaIN [17]. Radiation might induce changes in the vaginal squamous cells on the cellular levels that render already affected or newly infected cells with HPV more susceptible to the oncogenic effects of the viruses. In women with iatrogenic immunosuppression [18] or affected by the human immunodeficiency virus (HIV) infection, the incidence of VaIN rises to approximately 5% [19]. An increased relative risk for CIN 2-3 and VaIN 2-3 has been identified in women exposed to DES in utero [20]. A cohort comprising 3899 DES-exposed and 1374 unexposed daughters was followed for 13 years. The relative risk among DES-exposed women for development of high-grade dysplasia of the lower genital tract is 2.1 [21]. In patients with high-risk (HR) HPV genotypes, smokers are at an increased risk for high-grade VaIN in comparison to patients who have never smoked [22].

The natural history of VaIN is not completely understood. There have been no prospective studies evaluating the potential for disease progression from low-grade VaIN. Several retrospective observational studies have suggested that 90% of low-grade VaIN probably regresses spontaneously as the immune system mounts a response [23, 24]. VaIN 3 lesions have greater malignant potential, and there are no data regarding the spontaneous regression of VaIN 2–3. Observational studies have suggested that 2–8% of patients with VaIN may progress to invasive vaginal carcinoma (see Fig. 25.5) [8, 23, 25, 26]. The estimated mean interval of progression from VaIN 1 to VaIN 2-3 is about 15 years [27]. Furthermore, VaIN 3 biopsies show initial invasion (see Fig. 25.5) in approximately 10–28% of cases [23, 28–30]. The subsequent progression to invasive vaginal carcinoma after appropriate treatment of VaIN ranges from 2% to 5% [8, 31–33]. The scar of the vaginal vault following hysterectomy may represent a site for increased risk of progression from high-grade VaIN to invasive cancer, especially when performed for CIN [34]. This association may be due to incorporation of VaIN into the vaginal cuff closure during hysterectomy, potentially hiding the lesion from cytology screening.

25.2 Diagnosis

VaIN is usually asymptomatic. Although patients can present with postcoital spotting or vaginal discharge, most are diagnosed through colposcopy-guided biopsies performed for evaluation of an abnormal Pap test.

25.2.1 Pap Test

Many studies have demonstrated a correlation between abnormal Pap smears and high-grade VaIN, with one reporting a high-grade cytology including HSIL (high-grade squamous intraepithelial lesions) and ASC-H (atypical squamous cells cannot rule out high-grade SIL) in 89% of VaIN 2-3 [4]. In another study, the referral Pap smears in a cohort of 87 women with a histologic diagnosis of high-grade VaIN were reviewed. When the Pap results were categorized as either low- (defined as atypical squamous cells of undetermined significance/ASCUS and low-grade squamous intraepithelial lesions/LSIL) or high-grade (HSIL and ASC-H), the authors found significantly higher numbers of the referral Pap smears in the high-grade category, particularly if the patients were postmenopausal or had a previous diagnosis of HPV-related cervical diseases. However, the authors also emphasized that a diagnosis of ASCUS or LSIL in the previous referral Pap smear does not exclude high-grade VaIN, especially VaIN 2 [35]. Another study showed a significantly increased detection rate of VaIN in the high-risk (HR) HPV-positive group, suggesting that vaginal cytology and high-risk HPV DNA co-testing might be the preferred method for surveillance in patients with invasive cervical carcinoma after hysterectomy [12]. In patients who have not undergone hysterectomy, an abnormal cytology requires a thorough colposcopic assessment of not only the cervix but also the entire vagina. In postmenopausal patients with urogenital atrophy, a few weeks of topical estrogen treatment will often accentuate visualization and improve detection of VaIN. VaIN should be excluded in all women with an abnormal Pap smear who underwent a previous hysterectomy due to CIN or cervical squamous cancer, and annual vaginal cytology screening should be performed regularly [9, 36] for at least 4–10 years [37]. The sensitivity of vaginal smear cytologic examinations after hysterectomy is more than 80%, similar to cervical screening with the Pap test [38].

25.2.2 Colposcopy of VaIN

Approximately 80% of VaIN lesions are located in the upper one-third of the vagina and 60% of cases are multifocal [8]. After insertion of the speculum and application of 5% acetic acid, VaIN usually appears as acetowhite areas, often with a raised border and a micropapillary appearance in low-grade lesions similar to condyloma acuminata (Fig. 25.6). VaIN 2-3 usually appears more flattened and opaque with punctuation and occasionally mosaicism (Figs. 25.7 and 25.8). The presence of a markedly irregular surface or severe vascular abnormalities with

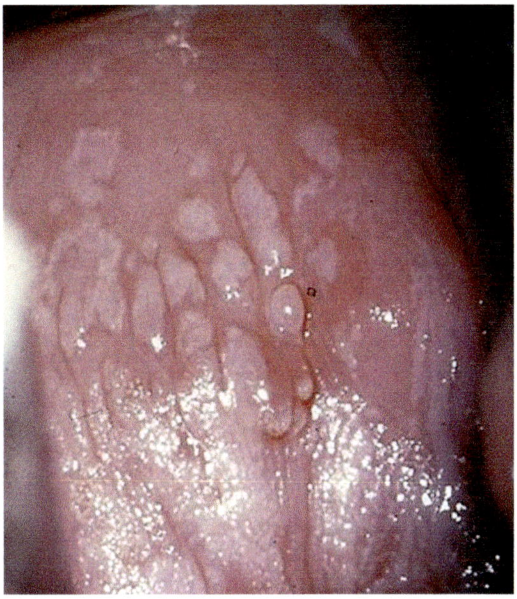

Fig. 25.6 VaIN 1 colposcopy photographs showing acetowhite epithelial changes that are multifocal and slightly raised, in some areas probably representing resolving condylomata

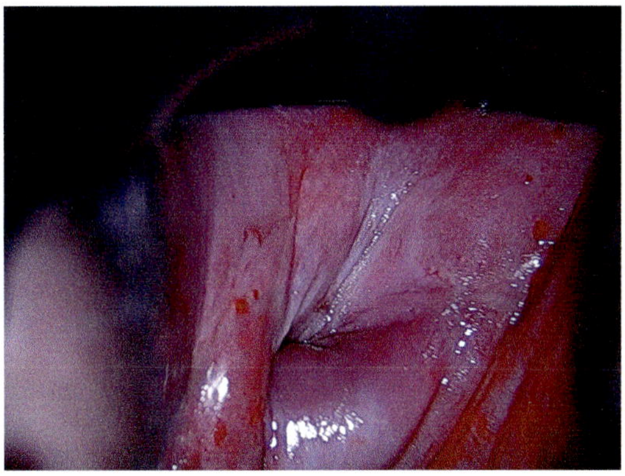

Fig. 25.7 VaIN 2 with surrounding atrophic epithelial changes in menopause. The acetowhite epithelium is less raised and more punctate than VaIN 1 and usually not mosaic as in CIN. Vaginal estrogen should be applied to improve colposcopy and treatment results prior to laser therapy

unusual branching suggests an invasive process. Irrespective of the colposcopic appearance, biopsies are usually warranted prior to ablative therapy for documentation of histology and to assure the lack of invasive disease (see Fig. 25.5). Schiller's or Lugol's iodine solution can be used to detect lesions and confirm boundaries prior to excisional biopsies. In patients with atrophy related to menopause (Fig. 25.9), vaginal estrogen applied for 6 weeks will improve the accuracy of colposcopy and aid in the healing from surgical, ablative, and topical therapies.

In 2011, the International Federation of Cervical Pathology and Colposcopy (IFCPC) agreed on an international revised colposcopic nomenclature of the vagina [39] (Table 25.1). Findings should be described including a general assessment, normal and abnormal colposcopic findings, and other miscellaneous findings such as traumatic lesions, polyps, or endometriosis.

In a recent study of 466 patients with a histopathological diagnosis of vaginal squamous intraepithelial lesions (SIL), Sopracordevole et al. evaluated colposcopic patterns of VaIN and attempted to correlate colposcopy with histopathology [40]. The authors considered thin acetowhite epithelium, fine punctuation, and fine mosaicism as grade I abnormal colposcopic patterns, while dense acetowhite epithelium, coarse punctuation, and coarse mosaicism were considered grade II patterns. In contrast to the 2011 IFCPC terminology (see Table 25.1), in which Lugol's nonstaining areas were considered "nonspecific," the acetonegative Lugol's nonstaining areas were categorized as a grade I abnormality in their study. Furthermore, the colposcopic description of the micropapillary pattern was characterized "as an acetowhite area with an irregular micropapillary surface." The authors concluded that grade I abnormal colposcopic findings and the micropapillary pattern were more commonly observed in low-grade VaIN, while grade II abnormal findings and the presence of vascular patterns were more frequently observed in high-grade VaIN.

25.2.3 Biopsy Technique

A biopsy should be taken from the most colposcopically suspicious area of the vagina, for

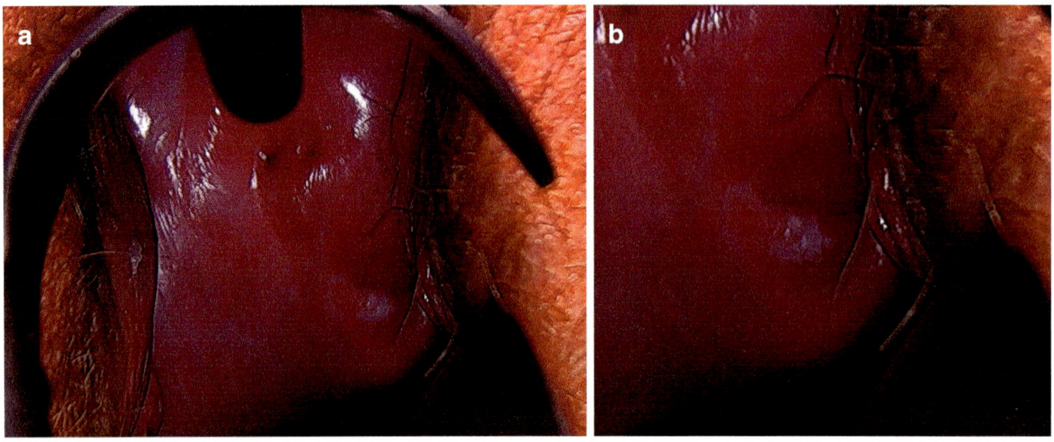

Fig. 25.8 VaIN 2–3 in the posterior fornix. Notice the more acetowhite portion of the lesion is more characteristic for VaIN 1–2, and the more opaque and less acetowhite area is characteristic of VaIN 3. Lugol's solution can help identify areas of VaIN that may be missed with colposcopy but is nonspecific and requires both colposcopic and histopathologic interpretation

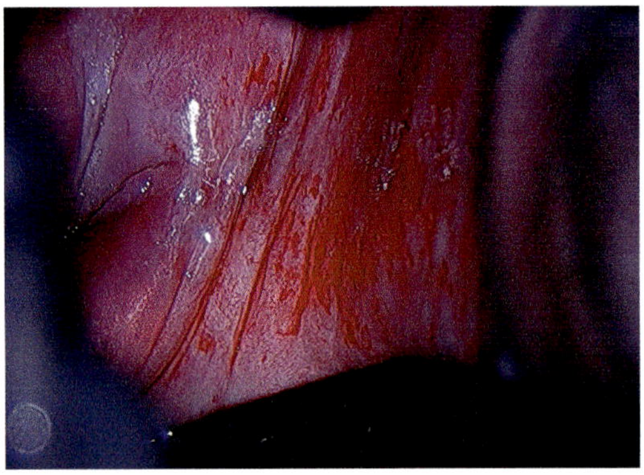

Fig. 25.9 VaIN 2–3 with severe atrophy, magnified colposcopic view

the purpose of defining the degree of dysplasia and to rule out invasive carcinoma. In some cases of multifocal or extremely wide lesions, multiple biopsies may be required. When performing a Tischler-Kevorkian® punch biopsy, it is helpful to partially close the speculum to allow the vagina to fold in on itself. Keeping the vagina taut makes performing a biopsy difficult. Local anesthetic (e.g., 1% lidocaine) can be helpful to reduce pain. Hemostasis is usually obtained with application of Monsel's solution or the use of silver nitrate. If bleeding persists, a suture may be necessary.

Table 25.1 2011 International Federation of Cervical Pathology and Colposcopy (IFCPC) clinical and colposcopic terminology of the vagina [39]

Section	Pattern
General assessment	Adequate or inadequate for the reason (e.g., inflammation, bleeding, scar) transformation zone
Normal colposcopic findings	Squamous epithelium: mature or atrophic
Abnormal colposcopic findings	*General principles*: • Upper third or lower two-thirds • Anterior, posterior, or lateral (right or left) *Grade 1 (minor)*: thin acetowhite epithelium, fine punctation, fine mosaic *Grade 2 (major)*: dense acetowhite epithelium, coarse punctation, coarse mosaic *Suspicious for invasion:* • Atypical vessels • Additional signs: fragile vessels, irregular surface, exophytic lesion, necrosis ulceration (necrotic) tumor, or gross neoplasm *Nonspecific*: Columnar epithelium (adenosis) Lesion staining by Lugol's solution (Schiller's test): stained or nonstained, leukoplakia
Miscellaneous findings	Erosion (traumatic), condyloma, polyp, cyst, endometriosis, inflammation, vaginal stenosis, congenital transformation zone

25.3 Treatment of VaIN

Several treatment options are available for the treatment of VaIN including surgical excision, ablation, topical therapy, and radiation therapy. Each treatment option is associated with potential advantages as well as unique side effects. Therefore, treatment requires individualization according to the patient's characteristics, disease extension, and previous therapeutic procedures. Treatment also varies according to the grade, age, and location of lesions.

VaIN 1 often regresses spontaneously and has very low if not insignificant malignant potential. VaIN 1 lesions typically are multifocal and tend to recur frequently after treatment, although this may actually be persistence of unrecognized lesions or progression of subclinical disease that was not initially recognized. Generally, women with asymptomatic VaIN 1 can be managed by close surveillance rather than treatment, recognizing that acute HPV infection usually resolves over a period of 6–12 months as the immune system responds. For young women with persistent visible lesions, the treatment of choice is CO_2 laser vaporization with an excisional procedure for confirmation of diagnosis. Multifocal lesions and VaIN involving the lower third of the vagina are commonly treated either with laser vaporization or topical 5-FU (Table 25.2). Surgical excision with partial upper vaginectomy is the treatment of choice for apical VaIN 3 or VaIN in the vaginal cuff scar in women post-hysterectomy for cervical neoplasia. Surgical excision of the apex hysterectomy scar containing VaIN 3 is especially recommended to rule out underlying invasive disease and to reduce the incidence of treatment failure.

25.3.1 Surgical Therapy

Surgical excision is the mainstay of VaIN therapy and has the advantage of permitting histologic diagnosis since invasive foci have been detected in up to 28% of resected specimens [41]. Surgical approaches include loop electrosurgical excision procedure (LEEP), partial vaginectomy, total vaginectomy (Table 25.3), and cavitational ultrasonic surgical aspiration (CUSA) (Table 25.4).

Table 25.2 Treatment modalities of vaginal intraepithelial neoplasia (VaIN)

Surgical therapy	Ablation	Topical therapy	Radiation therapy
Vaginectomy, partial vaginectomy	CO_2 laser	Imiquimod	Brachytherapy
Cavitational ultrasonic surgical aspiration (CUSA)	Photodynamic therapy	Topical 5-FU (Efudex®)	
LEEP		Trichloroacetic acid (TCA)	

Table 25.3 Surgical treatment of vaginal intraepithelial neoplasia (VaIN)

Study	Year	Number	Recurrence (%)	Surgical modality	Complications	Follow-up
Hoffman et al. [29]	1992	23	17	Partial vaginectomy (upper vaginectomy)	None	6–73 months
Cheng et al. [75]	1999	40	34	Partial vaginectomy (wide local excision)	4 vaginal bleeding, 4 fever, 4 urinary tract infection	1–124 months
Dodge et al. [8]	2001	13	0	Partial vaginectomy	None	>7 months
Gunderson et al. [4]	2013	44	27	Partial vaginectomy	1 vaginal stump bleeding, 1 vesicovaginal fistula	1–194 months
Choi et al. [76]	2013	3	0	Laparoscopic upper vaginectomy	None	11–29 months
Luyten et al. [77]	2014	33	13	Colposcopic-guided laser-skinning colpectomy	2 moderate shortening of the vagina, 2 required reconstruction of vaginal strictures	12–104 months

Table 25.4 CUSA treatment of vaginal intraepithelial neoplasia (VaIN)

Study	Year	Number	Recurrence (%)	Complications	Follow-up
Robinson et al. [47]	2000	29	34	None	4–94 months
Matsuo et al. [48]	2009	92	19.6	None	54 months (median)
von Gruenigen et al. [49]	2007	45	24.4	Infections, dysuria, adhesions, vaginal discharge	12 months (checkpoint of RCT)

Most excisions are performed transvaginally, although some are done laparoscopically or open, particularly when the upper vaginal cuff is involved.

25.3.1.1 Vaginectomy

Vaginectomy can be total or partial (see Table 25.3). Partial upper vaginectomy is considered treatment of choice for apical VaIN 3 or VaIN in the region of the vaginal cuff scar, especially in women after hysterectomy for cervical neoplasia, since these lesions are frequently buried in suture recesses [28]. Total vaginectomy is rarely indicated and associated with significant risk for morbidity including blood loss, fistula, and loss of sexual function.

Partial upper colpectomy with removal of isolated lesions not involving the vaginal cuff scar can be accomplished with LEEP in histologically confirmed unifocal or clustered of VaIN 2-3 [24]. Excision consists of the vaginal mucosa and a portion of the submucosal tissue. The procedure results in minimal lateral tissue damage, similar to the effects of a laser; however it may be more difficult to control the depth of excision compared to laser. The recurrence rate in 23 patients treated for VaIN with LEEP was 13% at 12 months and 25% at 24 months [42]. LEEP for partial upper vaginectomy can be performed quickly, with minimal blood loss [43], provides an interpretable specimen, needs a short training period, and is associated with low cost [44]. Complications are relatively uncommon; however, they can be significant including sigmoid or rectal perforation [45] and formation of vesicovaginal fistula [46]. Therefore, LEEP requires great care and precision to control depth of penetration in the vaginal wall.

VaIN is often multifocal, and it is necessary to obtain free margins during partial vaginectomy in order to reduce the risk of disease recurrence. In cases with multifocal VaIN that involves both the upper and lower third of the vagina, excision of upper apical lesions (especially when possible microinvasion is suspected) can be combined with laser vaporization of the lower vagina [28].

25.3.1.2 Cavitational Ultrasonic Surgical Aspiration (CUSA)

The use of CUSA in VaIN allows selective removal of tissue while preserving the surrounding normal tissue (see Table 25.4). CUSA is considered relatively easy to perform. However, similar to other ablative therapies, tissue is not preserved for pathologic examination. Therefore, it is also recommended that excisional biopsies be obtained prior to CUSA excisions. In 2000, Robinson et al. retrospectively compared the efficacy of CUSA against other methods (laser vaporization, loop excision, partial vaginectomy, 5-fluorouracil, and surveillance by Pap smear) in the treatment of 46 patients with a spectrum of low- to high-grade VaIN. Although more patients with VaIN 3 underwent therapy with CUSA, a significantly higher number of patients initially treated with CUSA experienced no recurrence (66%) during a mean follow-up of 21 months compared to patients initially treated by other methods [47]. Another retrospective study of 92 women treated for VaIN with CUSA reported a 19.6% recurrence rate with a median follow-up of 4.5 years [48]. Of note, both studies reported no postoperative complications associated with CUSA.

A randomized controlled trial comparing CUSA versus CO_2 laser ablation in the treatment of vaginal and vulvar dysplasia in a cohort of 110 patients (52 VaIN and 44 VIN patients) demonstrated no difference in recurrence during a 1-year follow-up period (24.4% versus 25.5%, respectively) [49]. In the opinion of the authors, there was less postoperative pain and scarring with CUSA, especially when the introitus or adjacent vulva was treated [49].

25.3.2 Ablative Therapies

25.3.2.1 CO_2 Laser

It is commonly used as an ablation method but can also be used as an excisional tool with tissue for histologic evaluation. CO_2 ablation and excisions are generally well tolerated, heal satisfactorily, result in minimal sexual dysfunction, associated with relatively few immediate or long-term side effects, and result in minimal blood loss. Therefore, CO_2 laser is considered the treatment of choice by several authors [24, 31, 50]. However, CO_2 laser also has limitations including high cost for the equipment and maintenance, a relatively long learning curve for excisional techniques, and the potential for missed detection of some VaIN lesions [33] that may require repeated treatment over time.

Because the thickness of the epithelium affected by VaIN varies from 0.1 to 0.3 cm, CO_2 laser vaporization with its properties of limited lateral heat spread is ideally suited to treat this disease without significant damage to the surrounding or underlying normal tissues (Fig. 25.10) [51]. Margins should be obtained 0.5–1 cm around the VaIN, and the depth of laser is usually less than 1 mm and perhaps deeper in the vaginal cuff. Laser ablation is a useful option for women with multifocal VaIN lesions and for women who refuse excisional surgery procedures for lesions confirmed as noninvasive. However, ablative therapy should not be performed if the entire area of abnormal epithelium cannot be visualized or if there is any suspicion of invasion during thorough colposcopy. Careful attention to power density and depth of penetration of the laser beam is required to avoid injury of the underlying bladder or rectum.

Numerous case series have documented the recurrence rates of VaIN following CO_2 laser ranging from 0% to 67% (Table 25.5). Younger age (<48 years) and VaIN 3 involvement of the upper vaginal vault are reported as risk factors for recurrence after laser vaporization [52]. Pain and bleeding are the most frequent complications, requiring intervention in 20% of patients in one series [53]. CO_2 laser ablation is the most commonly performed ablative therapy in modern practice given the wide availability of laser units, quick healing, favorable side-effect profile, and ease of repeat treatment when necessary.

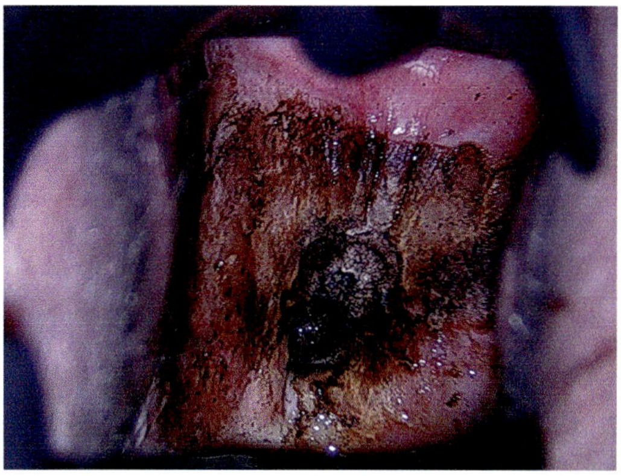

Fig. 25.10 Appearance of the vagina immediately post CO_2 laser ablation for VaIN 3. The mucosa is lasered to the submucosa. Typical vaginal mucosa is 0.1 to 0.3 cm depending on menopausal status, and laser depths are usually no more than 1 mm below the surface of adjacent normal vagina. The appearance of the submucosa after laser is described as "chamois cloth"

25.3.2.2 Photodynamic Therapy (PDT)

Photodynamic therapy is performed by a laser beam with a wavelength of 635 nm and an output of 80–125 J/cm^2 following the application of a photosensitizer (e.g., 10% 5-aminolevulinic acid (ALA) gel) that selectively targets dysplastic cells. ALA is approved by the US Food and Drug Administration (FDA) and commercially available under the name of Levulan® for actinic keratoses (AK) [54]. PDT has only been used experimentally for VaIN and is not currently FDA-approved for treatment of genital lesions [55]. One study of patients with vulvar or vaginal intraepithelial neoplasia grade 2/3 (n = 22) showed a complete clearance rate for intraepithelial neoplasia in 57% (determined by biopsy) and shorter healing time compared to conventional treatments including CO_2 laser and surgical exci-

Table 25.5 Laser treatment of vaginal intraepithelial neoplasia (VaIN)

Study	Year	Number	Recurrence (%)	Follow-up
Krebs et al. [78]	1989	22	27	12–84 months
Audet-LaPointe et al. [27]	1990	32	28	7–85 months
Hoffman et al. [79]	1991	26	42	11–56 months
Diakomanolis et al. [80]	1996	25	32	35–82 months
Sopracordevole et al. [50]	1998	24	33	3–12 months
Campagnutta et al. [81]	1999	39	67	13–90 months
Dodge et al. [8]	2001	42	38	> 7 months
Perrotta et al. [82]	2013	21	14	12–78 months
Gunderson et al. [4]	2013	34	47	1–194 months
Wang et al. [83]	2014	39	0	12–39 months
Piovano et al. [84]	2015	285	25	1–28 months

sion [56]. In another study of 15 patients with a spectrum of vulvar and vaginal premalignant lesions (VIN 2, $n = 3$; VIN 3, $n = 4$; VaIN 2, $n = 2$; VaIN 3, $n = 3$; Paget's disease, $n = 3$), the authors reported a complete response rate of 80% at the 3-month follow-up and 71.4% at the 1-year follow-up. However, recurrence was observed at the 1-year follow-up in two cases of complete response. Adverse events such as photosensitivity reactions including facial edema and urticaria occurred in 13.3% of the patients, and perineal pain occurred in one patient. In the opinion of the authors, PDT may be an effective alternative treatment for premalignant lesions of the female lower genital tract that preserves normal anatomy and sexual function with less short-term side effects. However, there have been no direct comparative studies of photodynamic therapy versus CO_2 laser for safety and efficacy, and this technique remains investigational [57].

25.3.2.3 Topical Therapies

Topical application of therapeutic agents has the advantage of treating the entire vaginal mucosa with good coverage of multifocal disease as well as disease in folds and recesses of the vagina. There are no guidelines clearly defining the ideal treatment for multifocal high-grade VaIN. Topical therapy appears to be an appropriate first-line therapy in women with low-grade VaIN and multifocal disease or those patients who are poor surgical candidates with biopsy-proven VaIN 3. Before starting topical treatment, invasion must be excluded by thorough colposcopic examination and biopsy.

Imiquimod

Imiquimod is an immune response modifier that induces the secretion of interferon-alpha, interleukin-12, and tumor necrosis factor-alpha (TNF-α), locally stimulates natural killer cell activity, promotes the maturation and activity of Langerhans cells, and increases the effectiveness of the T cell-mediated response [58]. Imiquimod is FDA-approved for treatment of actinic keratosis and for external genital/perianal warts.

There are several case series on the off-label use of topical application of 5% imiquimod cream for the treatment of VaIN. In these reports, variable imiquimod treatment regimens have been described. The cream was applied at least three times a week for 8 weeks under colposcopic guidance in one study [59], which had a poor compliance by patients and required a significant time commitment by health providers. Buck et al. in 2003 used imiquimod for the treatment of VaIN 1 with great success; however we now know that spontaneous regression of low-grade VaIN is common [60]. A recent systematic review and meta-analysis of the literature on the efficacy of 5% imiquimod in the treatment of all degrees of VaIN included six studies with a combined 94 patients [61]. With some limitations due to the nature of their study, the authors found that the complete response rate of imiquimod in VaIN treatment was 76.5%, a success rate comparable to laser vaporization. According to their analysis, the HPV clearance with imiquimod was 52.5%, superior to the 11% clearance rate for CO_2 laser. Lastly, the proportion of women with recurrence appeared to be low at 5.6%. According to this

Table 25.6 5-FU treatment of vaginal intraepithelial neoplasia (VaIN)

Study	Year	Number	Recurrence/persistence (%)	Treatment schedule	Follow-up
Caglar et al. [62]	1981	27	15	Once daily × 5–10 days	3–48 months
Kirwan et al. [85]	1985	14	7	Once weekly × 10 weeks	4–42 months
Krebs et al. [78]	1989	37	19	Once weekly × 10 weeks	12–84 months
Audet-LaPointe et al. [27]	1990	12	17	Daily × 5 days	9–42 months
Dodge et al. [8]	2001	22	59	NR	>7 months
Murta et al. [86]	2005	16	38	Once weekly × 10 weeks	NR
Fiascone et al. [87]	2017	47	25.5	Once weekly × 8 weeks	4–92 months

NR not reported

review, 5% imiquimod cream is potentially an effective and safe noninvasive alternative treatment for VaIN, especially among young women with multifocal lesions or postmenopausal women wishing to avoid surgical modalities. However, great care must be exercised prescribing imiquimod off-label, and application should be performed by an experienced practitioner as there are potential toxicities of systemic absorption. A prospective randomized trial comparing imiquimod to expectant management observation or laser for low-grade VaIN is warranted.

5-Fluorouracil (5-FU)

Topical 5-FU has varying rates of reported success for treatment of VaIN and is not FDA-approved for intracavitary applications (Table 25.6). Therefore topical 5-FU cream should be prescribed with caution by those familiar with its intravaginal use, potential toxicities, and informed consent.

Several dosing protocols have been suggested, ranging from twice daily application for 14 days to once weekly for 10 weeks (see Table 25.6). Failure rates are comparable to other techniques for treatment of VaIN. Complications of topical 5-FU include vaginal irritation or burning with prolonged application leading to vaginal ulcerations that can be quite symptomatic [62, 63], even requiring surgical excision [64]. Krebs et al. conducted a retrospective study of 220 patients treated with 5-FU cream, including 104 VaIN patients, reporting 41.8% patients that had clinical signs of acute chemical mucositis of vagina and/or cervix 2–4 weeks after the last 5-FU application [64]. Compared with the continuous regimen, weekly application of 5-FU had similar response rates and similar incidence of chronic vaginal ulceration, about 8% [64]. External zinc oxide cream or petroleum jelly can be used as a barrier to help protect against ulceration in adjacent areas. Topical estrogen also may reduce patient discomfort. However, in the study by Krebs et al., estrogen creams and cauterizing agents failed to accelerate healing of vaginal ulcers [64]. Interestingly, columnar metaplasia of the vaginal mucosa can occur after topical 5-FU, the clinical significance of which is uncertain [65]. Topical 5-FU can be effective for multifocal low- and high-grade VaIN but is associated with short-term side effects including vaginal irritation, discharge, and the potential for vaginal ulceration if therapy is not discontinued when vaginitis symptoms develop.

Trichloroacetic Acid (TCA)

TCA is a powerful keratolytic agent that can coagulate proteins of the skin, destroying all cutaneous structures to the level of the reticular dermis. It has also been shown to have a therapeutic effect on HPV-induced genital warts [66] and HPV infection of the cervix without associated dysplasia [67]. Treatment with intravaginal 50% TCA with a weekly application for 1–4 weeks resulted in regression of VaIN of various grades in 71.4% of cases [68]. Although all VaIN 1 patients demonstrated remission, likely in part related to the known spontaneous regression of low-grade VaIN, the study also showed that VaIN 2–3 may also benefit from repeated TCA treatment [68]. The adverse effects include temporary vaginal discomfort following the application. Because of the potential for significant tissue injury, TCA should only be carefully applied by knowledgeable practitioners using the minimum of TCA on the wooden end of a cotton applicator (not the cotton itself) to prevent surrounding tissue necrosis.

Estrogen

The role of vaginal estrogen in the treatment of VaIN has been evaluated in a single observational retrospective study of 83 patients [69] that had VaIN 2–3 and underwent various treatment modalities including vaginal estrogen, CO_2 laser ablation, topical 5-FU, wide local excision, LEEP, and partial vaginectomy. The authors reported a 90% regression or cure of high-grade disease in the patients treated with vaginal estrogen alone ($n = 40$). Patients treated with vaginal estrogen together with one or more other treatment modalities ($n = 32$) experienced an 81.3% regression or cure rate. In contrast, regression or cure of high-grade disease was documented in 71.4% of patients undergoing treatment without vaginal estrogen ($n = 5$). Of note, a regression or cure of VaIN 2–3 was recorded in all four patients who were followed up without any treatment intervention. Interpretation of the results from this study is limited given the retrospective observational design and lack of biopsies confirming regression or cure (only cytology and colposcopic visual appearance). Furthermore, the authors failed to specify the criteria for triage into the treatment groups. Lastly, the study did not show any statistical significance in terms of treatment response or recurrence between the treatment groups.

The role of vaginal estrogen in the active treatment of high-grade VaIN remains doubtful. Nevertheless, vaginal estrogen therapy may improve the colposcopic accuracy in patients with atrophic vaginitis and may aid the cytologic interpretation of Pap tests by eliminating inflammation and atrophic cells. Furthermore, estrogen may improve healing following ablative and surgical therapies.

25.3.2.4 Radiation Therapy

Brachytherapy is intracavitary radiotherapy whereby the radiation source is placed directly inside the vagina by an applicator, delivering ionizing radiation directly to the surface of the VaIN lesions. Brachytherapy is rarely used because surgical or ablative therapies are usually successful, and brachytherapy is associated with more costs and side effects. Radiation therapy is reserved for patients who (1) failed previous treatments, (2) are poor surgical candidates, (3) have extensive, multifocal disease not easily treated by other methods, or (4) have VaIN 3 lesions that are suspicious for invasive carcinoma despite biopsies showing only VaIN 3. The optimum radiation dose is uncertain. The majority of studies on vaginal brachytherapy for high-grade VaIN reported a recurrence rate in the range of 0–14%, seemingly lower than, or at least comparable to that of other treatment approaches (Table 25.7). Annual colposcopy with Pap or HPV screening is advised considering the risk of both early and late recurrences.

Vaginal complications following brachytherapy include urogenital atrophy, stenosis, and shortening. Bowel and bladder side effects are infrequent given the low level of tissue penetration characteristic of brachytherapy. Poor wound healing of irradiated tissue is a concern for patients who may subsequently require future gynecological vaginal procedures [70]. Other limitations of brachytherapy in the management of high-grade VaIN include the long-term inherent risk of ionizing radiation of inducing a second neoplasm including VaIN and vaginal cancer [71]. Furthermore, the resultant atrophy and sclerosis can compromise the quality of screening of colposcopy during follow-up. The reported cure rates achieved by brachytherapy are some of the highest for VaIN; however it is difficult to draw firm conclusions regarding complications and long-term adverse effects given that most studies are retrospective observations of relatively short follow-up. Clinical experience suggests the potential for significant alteration in the vaginal tissues that may lead to difficulty with intercourse. The early use of vaginal dilators and vaginal estrogen may help prevent or alleviate some of these side effects.

Table 25.7 Brachytherapy studies for vaginal intraepithelial neoplasia (VaIN)

Study (year)	Methods	Dose/fraction (depth in cm)	Number	Histology	Follow-up (median)	Success rate (%)
Woodman et al. 1988 [88]	LDR	27–51 Gy (1)	11	VaIN 3	25 months	100
MacLeod et al. 1997 [89]	HDR	34–45 Gy/4–10 fx (0.5–1)	14	VaIN 3	46 months	85.7
Ogino et al. 1998 [70]	HDR	20–30 Gy/3–6 fx (A point) 15–30 Gy/3–6 fx (1)	6	VaIN 3	90.5 months	100
Teruya et al. 2002 [90]	HDR	30–36 Gy (1) 30–40 Gy (0.5)	13	CIS	127 months	100
Graham et al. 2007 [91]	MDR	48 Gy/2 fx (0.5)	22	VaIN 3	77 months	86.4
Blanchard et al. 2011 [92]	LDR	60 Gy (0.5)	28	VaIN 3	41 months	93
Song et al. 2014 [93]	HDR	30–50 Gy (0–1)	34	VaIN	48 months	88
Zolciak-Siwinska et al. 2015 [94]	HDR	28.0–37.5 Gy (0–1)	20	VaIN 2–3	39 months	90

LDR low-dose rate, *MDR* middle-dose rate, *HDR* high-dose rate, *CIS* carcinoma in situ;depth (cm) to the vagina surface at which radiation dose was prescribed

25.4 Prevention: HPV Vaccines

Similar to CIN, primary prevention through vaccination against the high-risk (HR) HPV sub-types 16 and 18 can be very efficient against the development of high-grade vaginal precancerous lesions. A combined analysis of three trials showed a 100% efficacy of the quadrivalent vaccine (HPV types 6, 11, 16, and 18) against HPV 16- and 18-associated VaIN 2–3 in women naive to these two HR-HPV types. The efficacy against both VaIN and VIN 2–3 caused by HPV 16 and 18 in all enrolled women (n = 18,174) including women with possible HPV exposure at enrollment was 71%. The overall efficacy against any kind of VaIN or VIN 2–3 was 49% at a mean follow-up of 3 years [72]. In another analysis of two randomized controlled trials that enrolled 17,622 women aged 16–26 years and tested the efficacy of quadrivalent HPV vaccine through 42 months of follow-up, the vaccine efficacy against lesions related to the HPV types in the vaccine was 100% for VaIN grade 1 [73]. The current nonavalent HPV vaccine (HPV types 6, 11, 16, 18, 31, 33, 45, 52, and 58) should improve coverage and efficacy for VaIN. Smoking cessation and complete and proper treatment of CIN, VIN, and adenocarcinoma in situ are other interventions recommended to decrease the likelihood of VaIN [74]. Lastly, barrier contraception with condoms may also reduce the incidence of VaIN.

25.5 Conclusion

VaIN is usually asymptomatic and identified from screening cytology or HPV testing and should be considered in women with CIN, VIN, and post-hysterectomy with abnormal Pap tests. Multiple therapeutic options are available for its management including surgical and ablative techniques. The choice of therapy depends on the patient's general health, surgical risks, desire for vaginal sexual function, the presence of multifocal disease, and the certainty with which invasive disease has been excluded.

Key Points

- Vaginal intraepithelial neoplasia (VaIN) is defined by the presence of squamous cell dysplasia confined to the lining squamous mucosa without invasion. The disease is classified according to the level of epithelial involvement.
- The true incidence of VaIN is unknown but is estimated at 0.2–0.3 cases per 100,000 women in the United States. The average patient is between 43 and 60 years of age.

- VaIN is a histologic diagnosis, typically made based upon colposcopically directed biopsy of the vagina.
- Once high-grade VaIN is diagnosed, invasive disease must be excluded by colposcopy and biopsy, especially before undertaking any ablative or topical therapy that does not permit definitive histologic confirmation of the lesion.
- Surgical excision, laser ablation, topical therapy, and intracavitary radiation successfully eliminate the lesion in approximately 70% to 80% of women; there is a 20% to 30% recurrence rate.
- Following therapy, gynecologic examination and vaginal cytology should be performed every 6 months for 1–2 years and annually thereafter to evaluate for persistent or progressive disease. Thereafter, patients can be followed at annual intervals. Human papillomavirus (HPV) testing may be useful as part of posttreatment surveillance.

References

1. Henson D, Tarone R. An epidemiologic study of cancer of the cervix, vagina, and vulva based on the Third National Cancer Survey in the United States. Am J Obstet Gynecol. 1977;129(5):525–32.
2. Watson M, Saraiya M, Wu X. Update of HPV-associated female genital cancers in the United States, 1999-2004. J Women Health (Larchmt). 2009;18(11):1731–8. https://doi.org/10.1089/jwh.2009.1570.
3. Cong Q, Wang Q, Gao SJ, Zhang HW, Du M, Xie F, et al. Detection trend of vaginal intraepithelial neoplasia diagnosed by colposcopy guided biopsy from 2013 to 2015. Zhonghua Fu Chan Ke Za Zhi. 2017;52(4):239–43. https://doi.org/10.3760/cma.j.issn.0529-567X.2017.04.005.
4. Gunderson CC, Nugent EK, Elfrink SH, Gold MA, Moore KN. A contemporary analysis of epidemiology and management of vaginal intraepithelial neoplasia. Am J Obstet Gynecol. 2013;208(5):410.e1–6. https://doi.org/10.1016/j.ajog.2013.01.047.
5. Kim MK, Lee IH, Lee KH. Clinical outcomes and risk of recurrence among patients with vaginal intraepithelial neoplasia: a comprehensive analysis of 576 cases. J Gynecol Oncol. 2018;29(1):e6. https://doi.org/10.3802/jgo.2018.29.e6.
6. Diakomanolis E, Stefanidis K, Rodolakis A, Haidopoulos D, Sindos M, Chatzipappas I, et al. Vaginal intraepithelial neoplasia: report of 102 cases. Eur J Gynaecol Oncol. 2002;23(5):457–9.
7. Dunne EF, Markowitz LE, Saraiya M, Stokley S, Middleman A, Unger ER, et al. CDC grand rounds: reducing the burden of HPV-associated cancer and disease. MMWR Morb Mortal Wkly Rep. 2014;63(4):69–72.
8. Dodge JA, Eltabbakh GH, Mount SL, Walker RP, Morgan A. Clinical features and risk of recurrence among patients with vaginal intraepithelial neoplasia. Gynecol Oncol. 2001;83(2):363–9. https://doi.org/10.1006/gyno.2001.6401.
9. Kalogirou D, Antoniou G, Karakitsos P, Botsis D, Papadimitriou A, Giannikos L. Vaginal intraepithelial neoplasia (VAIN) following hysterectomy in patients treated for carcinoma in situ of the cervix. Eur J Gynaecol Oncol. 1997;18(3):188–91.
10. Coronel-Brizio P, Olivares Nowak J, Palafox SF. Recurrence of high-grade squamous intraepithelial lesions following hysterectomy. Ginecol Obstet Mex. 1999;67:415–8.
11. Schockaert S, Poppe W, Arbyn M, Verguts T, Verguts J. Incidence of vaginal intraepithelial neoplasia after hysterectomy for cervical intraepithelial neoplasia: a retrospective study. Am J Obstet Gynecol. 2008;199(2):113.e1–5. https://doi.org/10.1016/j.ajog.2008.02.026.
12. Li Z, Barron S, Hong W, Karunamurthy A, Zhao C. Surveillance for recurrent cancers and vaginal epithelial lesions in patients with invasive cervical cancer after hysterectomy: are vaginal cytology and high-risk human papillomavirus testing useful? Am J Clin Pathol. 2013;140(5):708–14. https://doi.org/10.1309/ajcph4afszhu8ekk.
13. Piscitelli JT, Bastian LA, Wilkes A, Simel DL. Cytologic screening after hysterectomy for benign disease. Am J Obstet Gynecol. 1995;173(2):424–30. Discussion 30–2
14. Insinga RP, Liaw KL, Johnson LG, Madeleine MM. A systematic review of the prevalence and attribution of human papillomavirus types among cervical, vaginal, and vulvar precancers and cancers in the United States. Cancer Epidemiol Biomarkers Prev. 2008;17(7):1611–22. https://doi.org/10.1158/1055-9965.epi-07-2922.
15. Smith JS, Backes DM, Hoots BE, Kurman RJ, Pimenta JM. Human papillomavirus type-distribution in vulvar and vaginal cancers and their associated precursors. Obstet Gynecol. 2009;113(4):917–24. https://doi.org/10.1097/AOG.0b013e31819bd6e0.
16. Castle PE, Rodriguez AC, Porras C, Herrero R, Schiffman M, Gonzalez P, et al. A comparison of cervical and vaginal human papillomavirus. Sex Transm Dis. 2007;34(11):849–55. https://doi.org/10.1097/OLQ.0b013e318064c8c5.
17. Zaino RJ, Nucci M, Kurman RJ. Diseases of the vagina. In: Kurman RJ, Ellenson LH, Ronnett BM,

editors. Blaustein's pathology of the female genital tract. 6th ed. New York: Springer; 2011. p. 105–54.
18. Bowen-Simpkins P, Hull MG. Intraepithelial vaginal neoplasia following immunosuppressive therapy treated with topical 5-Fu. Obstet Gynecol. 1975;46(3):360–2.
19. Jamieson DJ, Paramsothy P, Cu-Uvin S, Duerr A. Vulvar, vaginal, and perianal intraepithelial neoplasia in women with or at risk for human immunodeficiency virus. Obstet Gynecol. 2006;107(5):1023–8. https://doi.org/10.1097/01.AOG.0000210237.80211.ff.
20. Robboy SJ, Noller KL, O'Brien P, Kaufman RH, Townsend D, Barnes AB, et al. Increased incidence of cervical and vaginal dysplasia in 3,980 diethylstilbestrol-exposed young women. Experience of the National Collaborative Diethylstilbestrol Adenosis Project. JAMA. 1984;252(21):2979–83.
21. Hatch EE, Herbst AL, Hoover RN, Noller KL, Adam E, Kaufman RH, et al. Incidence of squamous neoplasia of the cervix and vagina in women exposed prenatally to diethylstilbestrol (United States). Cancer Causes Control. 2001;12(9):837–45.
22. Sherman JF, Mount SL, Evans MF, Skelly J, Simmons-Arnold L, Eltabbakh GH. Smoking increases the risk of high-grade vaginal intraepithelial neoplasia in women with oncogenic human papillomavirus. Gynecol Oncol. 2008;110(3):396–401. https://doi.org/10.1016/j.ygyno.2008.05.015.
23. Rome RM, England PG. Management of vaginal intraepithelial neoplasia: a series of 132 cases with long-term follow-up. Int J Gynecol Cancer. 2000;10(5):382–90.
24. Massad LS. Outcomes after diagnosis of vaginal intraepithelial neoplasia. J Low Genit Tract Dis. 2008;12(1):16–9. https://doi.org/10.1097/LGT.0b013e318074f968.
25. Jentschke M, Hoffmeister V, Soergel P, Hillemanns P. Clinical presentation, treatment and outcome of vaginal intraepithelial neoplasia. Arch Gynecol Obstet. 2016;293(2):415–9. https://doi.org/10.1007/s00404-015-3835-6.
26. Fehr MK, Baumann M, Mueller M, Fink D, Heinzl S, Imesch P, et al. Disease progression and recurrence in women treated for vulvovaginal intraepithelial neoplasia. J Gynecol Oncol. 2013;24(3):236–41. https://doi.org/10.3802/jgo.2013.24.3.236.
27. Audet-Lapointe P, Body G, Vauclair R, Drouin P, Ayoub J. Vaginal intraepithelial neoplasia. Gynecol Oncol. 1990;36(2):232–9.
28. Indermaur MD, Martino MA, Fiorica JV, Roberts WS, Hoffman MS. Upper vaginectomy for the treatment of vaginal intraepithelial neoplasia. Am J Obstet Gynecol. 2005;193(2):577–80. https://doi.org/10.1016/j.ajog.2005.03.055. Discussion 80–1
29. Hoffman MS, DeCesare SL, Roberts WS, Fiorica JV, Finan MA, Cavanagh D. Upper vaginectomy for in situ and occult, superficially invasive carcinoma of the vagina. Am J Obstet Gynecol. 1992;166(1 Pt 1):30–3.
30. Sopracordevole F, De Piero G, Clemente N, Buttignol M, Mancioli F, Di Giuseppe J, et al. Vaginal intraepithelial neoplasia: histopathological upgrading of lesions and evidence of occult vaginal cancer. J Low Genit Tract Dis. 2016;20(1):70–4. https://doi.org/10.1097/lgt.0000000000000150.
31. Sillman FH, Fruchter RG, Chen YS, Camilien L, Sedlis A, McTigue E. Vaginal intraepithelial neoplasia: risk factors for persistence, recurrence, and invasion and its management. Am J Obstet Gynecol. 1997;176(1 Pt 1):93–9.
32. Gonzalez Sanchez JL, Flores Murrieta G, Chavez Brambila J, Deolarte Manzano JM, Andrade Manzano AF. Topical 5-fluorouracil for treatment of vaginal intraepithelial neoplasms. Ginecol Obstet Mex. 2002;70:244–7.
33. Yalcin OT, Rutherford TJ, Chambers SK, Chambers JT, Schwartz PE. Vaginal intraepithelial neoplasia: treatment by carbon dioxide laser and risk factors for failure. Eur J Obstet Gynecol Reprod Biol. 2003;106(1):64–8.
34. Hoffman MS, Roberts WS, LaPolla JP, Sterghos S Jr, Cavanagh D. Neoplasia in vaginal cuff epithelial inclusion cysts after hysterectomy. J Reprod Med. 1989;34(6):412–4.
35. Sopracordevole F, Mancioli F, Clemente N, De Piero G, Buttignol M, Giorda G, et al. Abnormal Pap smear and diagnosis of high-grade vaginal intraepithelial neoplasia: a retrospective cohort study. Medicine. 2015;94(42):e1827. https://doi.org/10.1097/md.0000000000001827.
36. Mouithys P, Papadopoulos C, Allier G, Lanta S, Delpierre C, Najas S, et al. Is it necessary to make screening Pap smears after hysterectomy? Gynecol Obstet Fertil. 2003;31(7–8):620–3.
37. Frega A, Sopracordevole F, Assorgi C, Lombardi D, DES V, Catalano A, et al. Vaginal intraepithelial neoplasia: a therapeutical dilemma. Anticancer Res. 2013;33(1):29–38.
38. Davila RM, Miranda MC. Vaginal intraepithelial neoplasia and the Pap smear. Acta Cytol. 2000;44(2):137–40.
39. Bornstein J, Bentley J, Bosze P, Girardi F, Haefner H, Menton M, et al. 2011 colposcopic terminology of the International Federation for Cervical Pathology and Colposcopy. Obstet Gynecol. 2012;120(1):166–72. https://doi.org/10.1097/AOG.0b013e318254f90c.
40. Sopracordevole F, Clemente N, Barbero M, Agarossi A, Cattani P, Garutti P, et al. Colposcopic patterns of vaginal intraepithelial neoplasia: a focus on low-grade lesions. Eur Rev Med Pharmacol Sci. 2017;21(12):2823–8.
41. Ireland D, Monaghan JM. The management of the patient with abnormal vaginal cytology following hysterectomy. Br J Obstet Gynaecol. 1988;95(10):973–5.
42. Terzakis E, Androutsopoulos G, Zygouris D, Grigoriadis C, Derdelis G, Arnogiannaki N. Loop electrosurgical excision procedure in Greek patients with vaginal intraepithelial neoplasia. Eur J Gynaecol Oncol. 2010;31(4):392–4.

43. Patsner B. Treatment of vaginal dysplasia with loop excision: report of five cases. Am J Obstet Gynecol. 1993;169(1):179–80.
44. Terzakis E, Androutsopoulos G, Zygouris D, Grigoriadis C, Arnogiannaki N. Loop electrosurgical excision procedure in Greek patients with vaginal intraepithelial neoplasia and history of cervical cancer. Eur J Gynaecol Oncol. 2011;32(5):530–3.
45. Powell JL, Asbery DS. Treatment of vaginal dysplasia: just a simple loop electrosurgical excision procedure? Am J Obstet Gynecol. 2000;182(3):731–2.
46. Harroch J, Siegler E, Bornstein J. Vesicovaginal fistula resulting from loop electrosurgical excision in a woman with intraepithelial neoplasia of the cervix and vagina: a case report. J Low Genit Tract Dis. 2004;8(3):205–6.
47. Robinson JB, Sun CC, Bodurka-Bevers D, Im DD, Rosenshein NB. Cavitational ultrasonic surgical aspiration for the treatment of vaginal intraepithelial neoplasia. Gynecol Oncol. 2000;78(2):235–41. https://doi.org/10.1006/gyno.2000.5881.
48. Matsuo K, Chi DS, Walker LD, Rosenshein NB, Im DD. Ultrasonic surgical aspiration for vaginal intraepithelial neoplasia. Int J Gynaecol Obstet. 2009;105(1):71–3. https://doi.org/10.1016/j.ijgo.2008.11.040.
49. von Gruenigen VE, Gibbons HE, Gibbins K, Jenison EL, Hopkins MP. Surgical treatments for vulvar and vaginal dysplasia: a randomized controlled trial. Obstet Gynecol. 2007;109(4):942–7. https://doi.org/10.1097/01.AOG.0000258783.49564.5c.
50. Sopracordevole F, Parin A, Scarabelli C, Guaschino S. Laser surgery in the conservative management of vaginal intraepithelial neoplasms. Minerva Ginecologica. 1998;50(12):507–12.
51. Benedet JL, Wilson PS, Matisic JP. Epidermal thickness measurements in vaginal intraepithelial neoplasia. A basis for optimal CO_2 laser vaporization. J Reprod Med. 1992;37(9):809–12.
52. Kim HS, Park NH, Park IA, Park JH, Chung HH, Kim JW, et al. Risk factors for recurrence of vaginal intraepithelial neoplasia in the vaginal vault after laser vaporization. Lasers Surg Med. 2009;41(3):196–202. https://doi.org/10.1002/lsm.20741.
53. Sherman AI. Laser therapy for vaginal intraepithelial neoplasia after hysterectomy. J Reprod Med. 1990;35(10):941–4.
54. Allison RR, Mota HC, Sibata CH. Clinical PD/PDT in North America: an historical review. Photodiagnosis Photodyn Ther. 2004;1(4):263–77. https://doi.org/10.1016/s1572-1000(04)00084-5.
55. Allison RR, Cuenca R, Downie GH, Randall ME, Bagnato VS, Sibata CH. PD/PDT for gynecological disease: a clinical review. Photodiagnosis Photodyn Ther. 2005;2(1):51–63. https://doi.org/10.1016/s1572-1000(05)00033-5.
56. Fehr MK, Hornung R, Degen A, Schwarz VA, Fink D, Haller U, et al. Photodynamic therapy of vulvar and vaginal condyloma and intraepithelial neoplasia using topically applied 5-aminolevulinic acid. Lasers Surg Med. 2002;30(4):273–9.
57. Choi MC, Kim MS, Lee GH, Jung SG, Park H, Joo WD, et al. Photodynamic therapy for premalignant lesions of the vulva and vagina: a long-term follow-up study. Lasers Surg Med. 2015; https://doi.org/10.1002/lsm.22384.
58. Miller RL, Gerster JF, Owens ML, Slade HB, Tomai MA. Imiquimod applied topically: a novel immune response modifier and new class of drug. Int J Immunopharmacol. 1999;21(1):1–14.
59. Diakomanolis E, Haidopoulos D, Stefanidis K. Treatment of high-grade vaginal intraepithelial neoplasia with imiquimod cream. N Engl J Med. 2002;347(5):374. https://doi.org/10.1056/nejm200208013470521.
60. Buck HW, Guth KJ. Treatment of vaginal intraepithelial neoplasia (primarily low grade) with imiquimod 5% cream. J Low Genit Tract Dis. 2003;7(4):290–3.
61. Tranoulis A, Laios A, Mitsopoulos V, Lutchman-Singh K, Thomakos N. Efficacy of 5% imiquimod for the treatment of Vaginal intraepithelial neoplasia-A systematic review of the literature and a meta-analysis. Eur J Obstet Gynecol Reprod Biol. 2017;218:129–36. https://doi.org/10.1016/j.ejogrb.2017.09.020.
62. Caglar H, Hertzog RW, Hreshchyshyn MM. Topical 5-fluorouracil treatment of vaginal intraepithelial neoplasia. Obstet Gynecol. 1981;58(5):580–3.
63. Woodruff JD, Parmley TH, Julian CG. Topical 5-fluorouracil in the treatment of vaginal carcinoma-in-situ. Gynecol Oncol. 1975;3(2):124–32.
64. Krebs HB, Helmkamp BF. Chronic ulcerations following topical therapy with 5-fluorouracil for vaginal human papillomavirus-associated lesions. Obstet Gynecol. 1991;78(2):205–8.
65. Dungar CF, Wilkinson EJ. Vaginal columnar cell metaplasia. An acquired adenosis associated with topical 5-fluorouracil therapy. J Reprod Med. 1995;40(5):361–6.
66. Godley MJ, Bradbeer CS, Gellan M, Thin RN. Cryotherapy compared with trichloroacetic acid in treating genital warts. Genitourin Med. 1987;63(6):390–2.
67. Malviya VK, Deppe G, Pluszczynski R, Boike G. Trichloroacetic acid in the treatment of human papillomavirus infection of the cervix without associated dysplasia. Obstet Gynecol. 1987;70(1):72–4.
68. Lin H, Huang EY, Chang HY, ChangChien CC. Therapeutic effect of topical applications of trichloroacetic acid for vaginal intraepithelial neoplasia after hysterectomy. Jpn J Clin Oncol. 2005;35(11):651–4. https://doi.org/10.1093/jjco/hyi176.
69. Rhodes HE, Chenevert L, Munsell M. Vaginal intraepithelial neoplasia (VaIN 2/3): comparing clinical outcomes of treatment with intravaginal estrogen. J Low Genit Tract Dis. 2014;18(2):115–21. https://doi.org/10.1097/LGT.0b013e31829f52f4.
70. Ogino I, Kitamura T, Okajima H, Matsubara S. High-dose-rate intracavitary brachytherapy in the management of cervical and vaginal intraepithelial neoplasia. Int J Radiat Oncol Biol Phys. 1998;40(4):881–7.

71. Liao JB, Jean S, Wilkinson-Ryan I, Ford AE, Tanyi JL, Hagemann AR, et al. Vaginal intraepithelial neoplasia (VAIN) after radiation therapy for gynecologic malignancies: a clinically recalcitrant entity. Gynecol Oncol. 2011;120(1):108–12. https://doi.org/10.1016/j.ygyno.2010.09.005.
72. Joura EA, Leodolter S, Hernandez-Avila M, Wheeler CM, Perez G, Koutsky LA, et al. Efficacy of a quadrivalent prophylactic human papillomavirus (types 6, 11, 16, and 18) L1 virus-like-particle vaccine against high-grade vulval and vaginal lesions: a combined analysis of three randomised clinical trials. Lancet. 2007;369(9574):1693–702. https://doi.org/10.1016/s0140-6736(07)60777-6.
73. Dillner J, Kjaer SK, Wheeler CM, Sigurdsson K, Iversen OE, Hernandez-Avila M, et al. Four year efficacy of prophylactic human papillomavirus quadrivalent vaccine against low grade cervical, vulvar, and vaginal intraepithelial neoplasia and anogenital warts: randomised controlled trial. BMJ. 2010;341:c3493. https://doi.org/10.1136/bmj.c3493.
74. Nelson EL, Stockdale CK. Vulvar and vaginal HPV disease. Obstet Gynecol Clin North Am. 2013;40(2):359–76. https://doi.org/10.1016/j.ogc.2013.03.003.
75. Cheng D, Ng TY, Ngan HY, Wong LC. Wide local excision (WLE) for vaginal intraepithelial neoplasia (VAIN). Acta Obstet Gynecol Scand. 1999;78(7):648–52.
76. Choi YJ, Hur SY, Park JS, Lee KH. Laparoscopic upper vaginectomy for post-hysterectomy high risk vaginal intraepithelial neoplasia and superficially invasive vaginal carcinoma. World J Surg Oncol. 2013;11:126. https://doi.org/10.1186/1477-7819-11-126.
77. Luyten A, Hastor H, Vasileva T, Zander M, Petry KU. Laser-skinning colpectomy for extended vaginal intraepithelial neoplasia and microinvasive cancer. Gynecol Oncol. 2014;135(2):217–22. https://doi.org/10.1016/j.ygyno.2014.08.019.
78. Krebs HB. Treatment of vaginal intraepithelial neoplasia with laser and topical 5-fluorouracil. Obstet Gynecol. 1989;73(4):657–60.
79. Hoffman MS, Roberts WS, LaPolla JP, Fiorica JV, Cavanagh D. Laser vaporization of grade 3 vaginal intraepithelial neoplasia. Am J Obstet Gynecol. 1991;165(5 Pt 1):1342–4.
80. Diakomanolis E, Rodolakis A, Sakellaropoulos G, Kalpaktsoglou K, Aravantinos D. Conservative management of vaginal intraepithelial neoplasia (VAIN) by laser CO_2. Eur J Gynaecol Oncol. 1996;17(5):389–92.
81. Campagnutta E, Parin A, De Piero G, Giorda G, Gallo A, Scarabelli C. Treatment of vaginal intraepithelial neoplasia (VAIN) with the carbon dioxide laser. Clin Exp Obstet Gynecol. 1999;26(2):127–30.
82. Perrotta M, Marchitelli CE, Velazco AF, Tauscher P, Lopez G, Perematеu MS. Use of CO_2 laser vaporization for the treatment of high-grade vaginal intraepithelial neoplasia. J Low Genit Tract Dis. 2013;17(1):23–7. https://doi.org/10.1097/LGT.0b013e318259a3ec.
83. Wang Y, Kong WM, Wu YM, Wang JD, Zhang WY. Therapeutic effect of laser vaporization for vaginal intraepithelial neoplasia following hysterectomy due to premalignant and malignant lesions. J Obstet Gynaecol Res. 2014;40(6):1740–7. https://doi.org/10.1111/jog.12383.
84. Piovano E, Macchi C, Attamante L, Fuso L, Maina G, Pasero L, et al. CO_2 laser vaporization for the treatment of vaginal intraepithelial neoplasia: effectiveness and predictive factors for recurrence. Eur J Gynaecol Oncol. 2015;36(4):383–8.
85. Kirwan P, Naftalin NJ. Topical 5-fluorouracil in the treatment of vaginal intraepithelial neoplasia. Br J Obstet Gynaecol. 1985;92(3):287–91.
86. Murta EF, Neves Junior MA, Sempionato LR, Costa MC, Maluf PJ. Vaginal intraepithelial neoplasia: clinical-therapeutic analysis of 33 cases. Arch Gynecol Obstet. 2005;272(4):261–4. https://doi.org/10.1007/s00404-005-0022-1.
87. Fiascone S, Vitonis AF, Feldman S. Topical 5-fluorouracil for women with high-grade vaginal intraepithelial neoplasia. Obstet Gynecol. 2017;130(6):1237–43. https://doi.org/10.1097/aog.0000000000002311.
88. Woodman CB, Mould JJ, Jordan JA. Radiotherapy in the management of vaginal intraepithelial neoplasia after hysterectomy. Br J Obstet Gynaecol. 1988;95(10):976–9.
89. MacLeod C, Fowler A, Dalrymple C, Atkinson K, Elliott P, Carter J. High-dose-rate brachytherapy in the management of high-grade intraepithelial neoplasia of the vagina. Gynecol Oncol. 1997;65(1):74–7. https://doi.org/10.1006/gyno.1996.4608.
90. Teruya Y, Sakumoto K, Moromizato H, Toita T, Ogawa K, Murayama S, et al. High dose-rate intracavitary brachytherapy for carcinoma in situ of the vagina occurring after hysterectomy: a rational prescription of radiation dose. Am J Obstet Gynecol. 2002;187(2):360–4.
91. Graham K, Wright K, Cadwallader B, Reed NS, Symonds RP. 20-year retrospective review of medium dose rate intracavitary brachytherapy in VAIN3. Gynecol Oncol. 2007;106(1):105–11. https://doi.org/10.1016/j.ygyno.2007.03.005.
92. Blanchard P, Monnier L, Dumas I, Morice P, Pautier P, Duvillard P, et al. Low-dose-rate definitive brachytherapy for high-grade vaginal intraepithelial neoplasia. Oncologist. 2011;16(2):182–8. https://doi.org/10.1634/theoncologist.2010-0326.
93. Song JH, Lee JH, Lee JH, Park JS, Hong SH, Jang HS, et al. High-dose-rate brachytherapy for the treatment of vaginal intraepithelial neoplasia. Cancer Res Treat. 2014;46(1):74–80. https://doi.org/10.4143/crt.2014.46.1.74.
94. Zolciak-Siwinska A, Gruszczynska E, Jonska-Gmyrek J, Kulik A, Michalski W. Brachytherapy for vaginal intraepithelial neoplasia. Eur J Obstet Gynecol Reprod Biol. 2015;194:73–7. https://doi.org/10.1016/j.ejogrb.2015.08.018.

Part V

Breast

Epidemiology of Breast Cancer: Current Figures and Trends

26

Anshuman Kumar and Anshuja Singla

26.1 Introduction

Noncommunicable diseases are fast- and ever-growing health problems, probably due to the westernized lifestyle, increased life expectancy, and increased lifetime exposure to the known risk factors for that particular disease [1]. As a consequence, the incidence of majority types of cancers has increased, may be due to increased access to better screening strategies. According to GLOBOCAN 2012, 14.1 million new cases of cancer were detected with 8.2 million cancer deaths worldwide. Lung cancer accounted for the most number of cases as well as deaths from the same [2]. Breast cancer is a major public health problem for women throughout the world. Breast cancer is the second most common cancer overall and by far the most common cancer in women with slightly more cases estimated to have occurred in developing regions than in developed regions.

A. Kumar
Department of Surgical Oncology, Dharamshila Narayana Superspeciality Hospital, New Delhi, India

A. Singla (✉)
Department of Obstetrics and Gynecology, University College of Medical Sciences and Guru Teg Bahadur Hospital, New Delhi, India

26.2 Epidemiology

On an average, women over 60 years of age are more likely to be diagnosed with breast cancer. Only about 10% to 15% of breast cancers occur in women younger than 45 years. However, this may vary for different races or ethnicities. The incidence of breast cancer increases with age, doubling about every 10 years until the menopause, when the rate of increase slows dramatically.

Breast cancer is the most common cancer with 1.7 million cases but ranks fifth as the cause of mortality (522,000, 6.4%). In 2012, 14.1 million new cases were detected which is expected to rise to 22 million new cases by the next two decades [3].

Breast cancer accounted for almost 11.1% of all cancers in more developed nations compared to 13% in less developed nations. It is the most frequent cause of cancer deaths in females in less developed regions (14.3% of total) and second most common cause of cancer death in developed regions after lung cancer (15.4%).

There is a wide variation in incidence rates of breast cancer ranging from 19.4 per lakh in Eastern Africa to 89.7 per lakh in Western Europe [4].

S. Mehta, A. Singla (eds.), *Preventive Oncology for the Gynecologist*,
https://doi.org/10.1007/978-981-13-3438-2_26

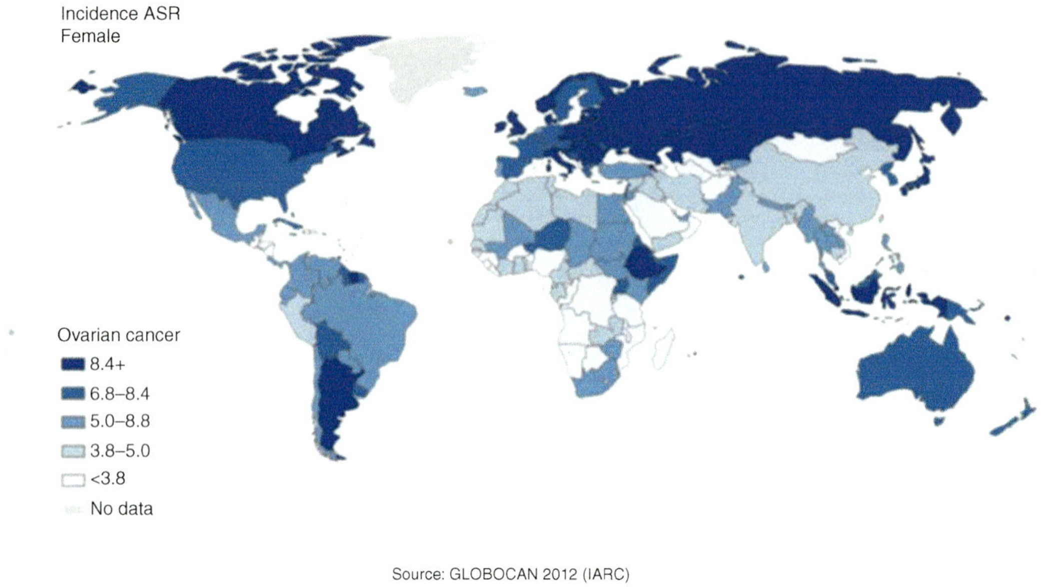

Fig. 26.1 Standardized incidence rate of breast cancer in world in 2012. Adapted with permission from Ferlay J., Soerjomataram I., Ervik M., Dikshit R., Eser S., Mathers C., Rebelo M., Parkin D.M., Forman D., Bray, F. GLOBOCAN 2012 v1.0, Cancer Incidence and Mortality Worldwide: IARC Cancer Base No. 11 [Internet]. Lyon, France: International Agency for Research on Cancer; 2013. Available from: http://gco.iarc.fr/today/home. Source: GLOBOCAN 2012 (IARC)

26.2.1 Incidence Rates (Fig. 26.1)

It was estimated that 1,671,149 new cases of breast cancer occurred in the world in 2012, of which 882.9 (per 100,000) were from less developed countries, while 793.7 (per 100,000) of them occurred in the developed nations. GLOBOCAN 2012 estimated it to be the most common cancer in women with the standardized incidence rate of 43.1 per lakh [2].

Among the six regions of WHO, the highest incidence was observed in PAHO (Pan American Health Organization) and the lowest incidence was noted from SEARO, 66.6 and 27.8, respectively (Southeast Asia Region). Belgium had the highest incidence rate of 111.9, whereas Mongolia and Lesotho had the lowest rate of 9. Belgium, Denmark, Bahamas, and the Netherlands had the highest standardized incidence rates. Northern America and Western Europe had the maximum incidence rates of 91.6 and 91.9, respectively, and middle Africa and Eastern Europe had the lowest incidence rates of 26.8 and 27.0, respectively. In India, the estimated incidence is 1,45,000 cases per year, and the estimated mortality rate is 70,000 deaths per year [5].

26.2.2 Mortality Rates (Fig. 26.2)

521,907 deaths were reported due to breast cancer in 2012. The age-specific standardized mortality rate (ASMR) was 12.9 per lakh after lung cancer in the world. The Eastern Mediterranean Region (EMRO) had the highest standardized mortality rate of 18.6, and the Western Pacific Regional Office of WHO (WPRO) which includes 37 countries had the lowest rate of 7. Africa had the highest mortality rate of 17, whereas Eastern Asia had the lowest mortality rate of 6.9. Fiji (28.4), the Bahamas (26.3), Nigeria (25.9), FYR Macedonia (25.6), and Pakistan (25.2) had the highest standardized mortality rates per lakh [5].

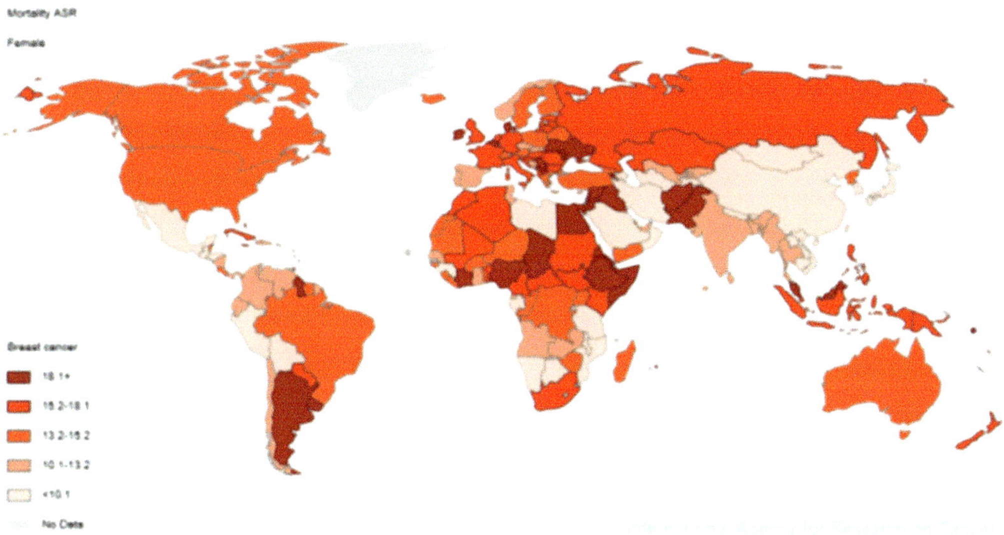

Fig. 26.2 Standardized breast cancer mortality rates in world in 2012. Adapted with permission from Ferlay J., Soerjomataram I., Ervik M., Dikshit R., Eser S., Mathers C., Rebelo M., Parkin D.M., Forman D., Bray, F. GLOBOCAN 2012 v1.0, Cancer Incidence and Mortality Worldwide: IARC Cancer Base No. 11 [Internet]. Lyon, France: International Agency for Research on Cancer; 2013. Available from: http://gco.iarc.fr/today/home

26.2.3 Human Development Index (HDI)

Very high HDI countries had the highest age-specific incidence rates (ASR) of 78 but the lowest mortality rate of 14.1, while low HDI countries had the lowest ASR of 32.6 but the higher mortality rate of 17. The lowest incidence and mortality was seen in countries with medium HDI [6]. In a study by Ghoncheh, increased HDI was associated with increased incidence of cancer though it did not significantly relate to death [7].

The reasons for these fluctuating trends in incidence and mortality rates observed across the globe are partially due to the difference in the risk factors across different geographical boundaries and also due to the differing trends in breast cancer diagnosis.

Factors like obesity and sedentary lifestyle are the primary reasons for higher incidence noted in the developed nations and for ever-increasing rates in Asian and Asian American women [8]. Delayed childbearing has been particularly associated with large increases observed among Hispanic and Hispanic American females [9].

Michelle et al. in their analysis found that western countries had the highest rates ranging from 49.7 per lakh in Puerto Rico to approximately 97 per lakh in countries like America and Australia. These were 3–4 times the rates found in Asia (27.2–36.2). They concluded that though breast cancer incidence rates increased in the 18 countries they studied, still no clear geographic location or ethnicity emerged. The incidence and mortality varied to up to fourfold globally between 1993 and 1997. North America had the maximum incidence followed by Western Europe, Oceania, Scandinavia, and Israel. Eastern Europe, Southern and Latin America, and Asia had the lowest rates [10].

In the date shown by GLOBOCAN 2012, North America and Western Europe still top the list, though the incidence rates have shown a marginal decrease for middle Africa and Eastern Asia from the previous analysis done by Michelle et al. (26.8 and 27.0, respectively) [2].

Japan has registered a 6% increase per year from 1999 to 2008. In South Korea the rates have shown an increase [11], whereas Hong Kong has registered a decline of the same [12]. Highest death rates due to breast cancer have been seen from Malaysia and Thailand [13].

Though race and hereditary are strong predictors for the risk of breast cancer, studies on migrant women from low- to high-income areas reveal that social and environmental issues too play a major role.

Younger age at menarche, late menopause, delayed first birth, and postmenopausal obesity all increase the lifetime exposure to estrogen and are possible explanations for the varying rates observed in American women versus Asian (97/lakh vs 27/lakh) [14, 15]. Shimizu et al. demonstrated that women from low-income countries had lower estrogen levels, in turn a lower risk. An Indian study showed that rural lifestyle decreased the risk of breast cancer [15].

Early detection improves the outcome of treatment and thus 5-year survival which is >80% in North America and <40% in low-resource countries [4]. Socioeconomic status directly correlates with the disease stage and survival [16]. Education goes a long way to help women in choosing the screening at the earliest. Yip et al. showed that cancer mortality was way higher in low-income countries especially Africa where treatment is sought late in the course of the disease [17]. Similar is the case with Kenya and Uganda [18].

Breast cancer care has to be a multimodal approach with the availability of both screening and treatment options, all available to the women in need.

Maybe different strategies have to be planned for both developed and developing nations. Breast self-examination (BSE) first followed by a mammography if required would be a better option in resource-constrained areas. BSE does not decrease death rates but increases awareness as mammography is not cost-effective here [14, 19].

Screening mammography is a better option for developed countries. In western countries, breast cancer incidence rose by ~30% when screening programs were implemented in the late 1980s, whereas in the Asian world, it was not the case as most breast tumors are detected by BSE with the exception of Japan where population screening was started in 1987 [20].

Increase was noted from Latin America and the Caribbean probably due to the increased use of mammography as well as the delayed first birth, but what contributed more is still largely unknown [9, 21].

Finally to contain this issue and the associated morbidity and mortality, a robust and an accessible health system has to be in place so that effective population-based strategies can be planned and implemented to ensure better coverage. Underreporting and failure of diagnosis could be the cause of bias in cancer registration, especially in less developed countries, so population-based cancer registries (PBCR) should be put into place. Among Denmark, the Netherlands, the Bahamas, and Belgium, which have high incidence, all except Bahamas have a PBCR. Countries like Fiji, Nigeria, the Bahamas, and Pakistan, which have the highest death rates from breast cancer, have no PBCR [5].

26.3 Conclusion

GLOBOCAN estimates provide an impetus for regional and national prioritization of cancer control of the predicted 22 million new cases by 2025. The greatest increases are anticipated in low-income countries, so long-term planning is the need of the hour to decrease the future cancer burden by utilizing the available resources appropriately. Though there is a global increase in breast cancer incidence, still the mortality from the same has either plateaued or decreased. The reasons are multiple, from early detection to mass implementation of screening programs to improved and advanced treatment, but still the divide between the rich and the poor is intangible.

Key Points

- Worldwide, breast cancer is the most frequently diagnosed cancer and the leading cause of cancer death among females.
- It is still the most common cause of cancer death in women in developing regions, but the second most common cause of cancer death (after lung cancer) in women in developed regions.
- The incidence of breast cancer increases with age, doubling about every 10 years until the menopause.
- Very high HDI countries had the highest age-specific incidence rates (ASR).
- The fluctuating trends in incidence and mortality rates observed across the globe are partially due to the difference in the risk factors across different geographical boundaries and also due to the differing trends in breast cancer diagnosis.

References

1. Zahedi A, Rafiemanesh H, Enayatrad M, Ghoncheh M, Salehiniya H. Incidence, trends and epidemiology of cancers in North West of Iran. Asian Pac J Cancer Prev. 2015;16:7189–93.
2. Ferlay J, Soerjomataram I, Ervik M, Dikshit R, Eser S, Mathers C, et al. GLOBOCAN 2012 v1.0, cancer incidence and mortality worldwide: IARC cancer base no. 11. Lyon: International Agency for Research on Cancer; 2013.
3. Ferlay J, Soerjomataram I, Dikshit R, Eser S, Mathers C, Rebelo M, et al. Cancer incidence and mortality worldwide: sources, methods and major patterns in GLOBOCAN 2012. Int J Cancer. 2015;136:E359–86.
4. WHO. Breast cancer: prevention and control [Online]. 2015. http://www.who.int/cancer/detection/breast-cancer/en/index1.html. Accessed 5 Apr 2018.
5. World Health Organization (WHO). Noncommunicable diseases (NCD) country profiles. 2014. [Online]. WHO. http://www.who.int/nmh/countries/fji_en.pdf?ua=1. Accessed 7 Apr 2018.
6. Ghoncheh M, Mirzaei M, Salehiniya H. Incidence and mortality of breast cancer and their relationship with the human development index (HDI) in the world in 2012. Asian Pac J Cancer Prev. 2015;16(18):8439–43.
7. Ghoncheh M, Mohammadian-Hafshejani A, Salehiniya H. Incidence and mortality of breast cancer and their relationship to development in Asia. Asian Pac J Cancer Prev. 2014;16:6081–7.
8. Ziegler RG, Hoover RN, Pike MC, Hildesheim A, Nomura AM, West DW, et al. Migration patterns and breast cancer risk in Asian-American women. J Natl Cancer Inst. 1993;85:1819–27.
9. Robles SC, Galanis E. Breast cancer in Latin America and the Caribbean. Rev Panam Salud Publica. 2002;11:178–85.
10. Althuis MD, Dozier JM, Anderson WF, Devesa SS, Brinton LA. Global trends in breast cancer incidence and mortality 1973-1997. Int J Epidemiol. 2005;34(2):405–12.
11. Choi Y, Kim Y, Park SK, Shin HR, Yoo KY. Age-period-cohort analysis of female breast cancer mortality in Korea. Breast Cancer. 2006;13:266–71.
12. Hoerger TJ, Ekwueme DU, Miller JW, Uzunangelov V, Hall IJ, Segel J, et al. Estimated effects of the national breast and cervical cancer early detection program on breast cancer mortality. Am J Prev Med. 2011;40:397–404.
13. Youlden DR, Cramb SM, Yip CH, Baade PD. Incidence and mortality of female breast cancer in the Asia-Pacific region. Cancer Biol Med. 2014;11:101–15.
14. Albert US, Schulz KD. Clinical breast examination: what can be recommended for its use to detect breast cancer in countries with limited resources? Breast J. 2003;9:90–3.
15. Nagrani RT, Budukh A, Koyande S, Panse NS, Mhatre SS, Badwe R. Rural urban differences in breast cancer in India. Indian J Cancer. 2014;51:277–81.
16. Clegg LX, Reichman ME, Miller BA, Hankey BF, Singh GK, Lin YD, et al. Impact of socioeconomic status on cancer incidence and stage at diagnosis: selected findings from the surveillance, epidemiology, and end results: National Longitudinal Mortality Study. Cancer Causes Control. 2009;20:417–35.
17. Yip CH, Buccimazza I, Hartman M, Deo SV, Cheung PS. Improving outcomes in breast cancer for low and middle income countries. World J Surg. 2015;39:686–92.
18. Munzone E. Highlights from the ninth European breast cancer conference, Glasgow, 19–21 March 2014. Ecancermedicalscience. 2014;8:426–32.
19. Harford JB. Breast-cancer early detection in low-income and middle-income countries: do what you can versus one size fits all. Lancet Oncol. 2011;12:306–12.
20. Shapiro S, Coleman EA, Broeders M, Codd M, de Koning H, Fracheboud J, et al. Breast cancer screening programmes in 22 countries: current policies, administration and guidelines. International Breast Cancer Screening Network (IBSN) and the European Network of Pilot Projects for Breast Cancer Screening. Int J Epidemiol. 1998;27:735–42.
21. Nazario CM, Figueroa-Valles N, Rosario RV. Breast cancer patterns and lifetime risk of developing breast cancer among Puerto Rican females. P R Health Sci J. 2000;19:7–13.

Breast Cancer: Role of Imaging

27

Harnoor Singh

27.1 Introduction

Breast cancer mortality for women is only exceeded by lung cancer and its incidence is only second to skin cancer among women in the United States. Invasive cancer development occurs in approximately one in every eight women [1].

The incidence of breast cancer worldwide is about 1.8 million cases with greater than 460,000 deaths from breast cancer, with about 252,710 new diagnoses of invasive breast cancer on an annual basis in the United States and with about 63,410 new cases of noninvasive (in situ) breast cancer. Approximately 40,610 patients will succumb to breast cancer.

The incidence of breast cancer in men is far less, estimated to be about 1 per 1000. On an annual basis, it is estimated that approximately 2470 new cases of male breast cancer will be diagnosed. Male breast cancer is only 0.7% of all breast cancers [2].

The mortality rates from breast cancer have been on the decline since 1989 with women less than 50 years of age demonstrating the most significant change. Women under 50 have experienced the greatest decrease. This is suggested to be primarily due to the result of improvement in the treatment of breast cancer, its early detection by means of screening mammography [3], and better knowledge and education of the population in general.

27.2 Risk Factors Associated with Breast Cancer

- Female gender and increasing age are two major risk factors.
- For women in the postmenopausal age group, obesity has been associated with more risk.
- Early menarche or late menopause, first pregnancy at age greater than 30, absence of breastfeeding, and nulliparity increase the risk, likely due to increase exposure to estrogen.
- Alcohol consumption demonstrates a dose-response relationship to breast cancer risk.
- Current smoking is a risk factor with a complex interaction of smoking with alcohol. Smoking also interacts with endogenous hormones in a detrimental way increasing risk for the development of breast cancer.
- Physical exercise on a regular basis seems to have been associated with a decreased risk pertaining to breast cancer among other things. A healthy diet including fish, fruits, and vegetables, as well as olive oil, may result in a lower risk of breast cancer also [4].
- High Risk: The female population which is at a higher than average risk for breast cancer (i.e., lifetime risk ≥20 to 25%) benefit

H. Singh (✉)
Department of Radiology, Texas Oncology, Amarillo, TX, USA

S. Mehta, A. Singla (eds.), *Preventive Oncology for the Gynecologist*,
https://doi.org/10.1007/978-981-13-3438-2_27

from extra testing including genetic counseling. Thereby, BRCA and other gene mutations can be discovered, and adjunctive breast cancer surveillance may also be performed from an imaging perspective which may include contrast-enhanced breast MRI in addition to mammography and breast ultrasound.

27.3 Normal Breast Anatomy

Terminal ductal lobular unit (TDLU) is the fundamental unit of the breast tissue. Each breast, or mammary gland, contains 15–20 lobes [5], and each lobe is comprised of 20–40 terminal ductal lobular units. They consist of extralobar terminal duct (ETD) which attaches the lobule to the ductal system.

Most of the breast cancer arises within the lobules of the breast or in the ductal connections from these lobules to the nipple. Breast milk is produced within the glands in the breast lobules. The remainder of the breast consists of lymphatic and connective tissue interspersed with fat.

27.4 Role of Imaging

- Screening
- Diagnosis including breast intervention
- Treatment planning including staging of breast cancer and monitoring therapy

27.4.1 Screening for Breast Cancer

Different imaging modalities can be utilized as a screening tool for breast cancer.

These include mammogram (2D and 3D), ultrasonography (USG), and MRI.

27.4.1.1 Mammography

The screening mammogram is performed in a woman with no history of symptoms or complaints [6]. The purpose of the study is to decrease morbidity and mortality by detecting breast cancer in its earliest stages, thereby rendering it treatable. Screening mammography is estimated to reduce breast cancer mortality by almost 40% if performed on an annual basis rather than less frequently [7–13].

Although earlier detection does not necessarily ensure cure, screening mammography is the *best* modality currently available to detect breast cancer that cannot be discovered by clinical examination.

The screening mammogram consists of two standard views. Additional views may be obtained which may include views such as anterior compression, cleavage view, exaggerated craniocaudal (XCCL) view, etc. to maximize the amount of breast tissue that is visualized at the time of screening (Fig. 27.1).

Age of Initiation: The American College of Radiology (ACR), Society of Breast Imaging (SBI), and the National Comprehensive Cancer Network (NCCN) recommendation are as follows: Initiate annual screening mammography at the age of 40.

Age to discontinue screening mammography:

ACR: Continue annual screening mammogram till the life expectancy is less than 5 to 7 years, based upon age or comorbidities.

ACOG: Recommend annual screening mammogram up to the age of 74. Thereafter, they advise women who are 75 years of age and older to consult with their primary care providers to discuss the risks/benefits of annual screening mammograms.

ACS: Annual screening mammogram recommended if a woman is in good health and her life expectancy is 10 years or longer.

SBI: No established age for women to stop screening. According to them women should continue annual screening mammography if they are healthy.

Screening mammography can be performed using a 2D (two-dimensional) mammogram or a 3D (three-dimensional) mammogram.

27.4.1.2 Ultrasonography

Ultrasound (USG) may also be used as an adjunctive imaging modality to screen for breast cancer.

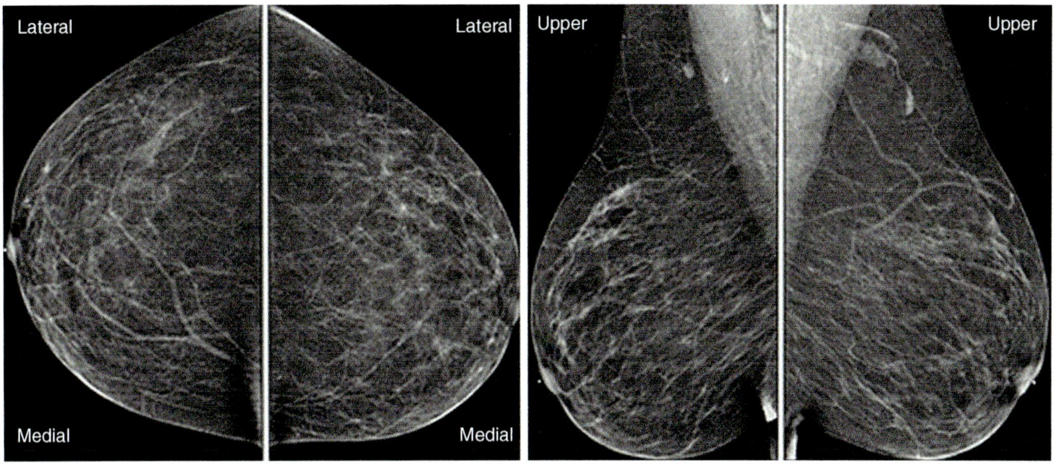

Fig. 27.1 Screening mammogram CC (craniocaudal) and MLO (mediolateral oblique) views of the right and left breast

USG is the diagnostic imaging of choice in a pregnant patient or a female patient less than 30 years of age with specific signs/symptoms or findings.

A retrospective review of ultrasounds performed in one center for the evaluation of focal breast signs or symptoms in women less than 30 years found that the NPV (negative predictive value) and sensitivity of breast ultrasound are 100 percent.

The incidence of breast cancer is on the rise worldwide. However, mammography is not always available to the general population as a screening modality in the developing world even though almost half of the worldwide breast cancer cases are found in these areas of the globe. Ultrasound may be used as an alternative screening tool in such cases [14].

An additional 4.3 cancers per 1000 women screened will be discovered with screening ultrasound when used as an adjunctive tool for screening in addition to mammography. However, the false-positive results also increase since the specificity of ultrasound is not as good (positive predictive value (PPV): mammogram without ultrasound = 22.6 % and it falls to only 11.2% for ultrasound done in addition to mammogram). This translates into an additional 354 biopsies performed per thousand women who have had bilateral screening done every other year for 25 years. Supplemental ultrasound is predicted to prevent about 0.36 additional cancer deaths in these women.

Screening for Breast Cancer: Comparison of Adjunctive Breast Ultrasound with Mammograms

"The recall rate for women undergoing breast ultrasound is comparable to the recall rate with mammography even though the false positive rate is higher with ultrasound"—*American College of Radiology Imaging Network (ACRIN) 6666 trial* study data.

Berg and colleagues collected data from 2662 women in three different countries including the United States, Canada, and Argentina from 20 sites. A total of 7473 exams were performed which included 3 annual rounds of screening with mammography and whole breast. These were interpreted by physicians who also performed the exams. The participants then had a biopsy or were given a 12-month clinical follow-up (*JNCI*, December 28, 2015). One hundred eleven breast cancers were diagnosed among 2662 women, out of which 80.2% were diagnosed with invasive breast cancer and 81% had node-negative breast cancer. The performance of ultrasound and mammography was comparable with ultrasound diagnosis of 52.3% cancers and mammography diagnosis of 53.2%. The recall rate for ultrasound was minimally higher at 10.7% as compared to 9.4% with mammography; similarly, the short interval follow-up rate and biopsy rates were slightly higher for ultrasound, estimated to be 3.9% vs 1.6% and 5.5% vs 2%, respectively. The PPV for ultrasound was lower at 11.7% for ultrasound as compared to 38% for mammography.

Invasive cancer detection percentage was 91.4% for ultrasound vs 69.5% for mammography. Also, the ultrasound-detected cancer was node negative in about 64.2% vs 43.9% with mammography. So, the ultrasound-detected cancer had a better prognosis considering a node-negative status.

27.4.1.3 Breast MRI (Contrast Enhanced)

Breast MRI is another imaging modality used for adjunctive breast cancer surveillance in asymptomatic women.

Recommendations for annual breast MRI are as follows (based on high risk of breast cancer and high sensitivity of MRI):

- BRCA mutation
- First-degree family member (untested) of BRCA carrier
- Higher than average lifetime risk (estimated to be 20–25% or greater), as defined by BRCAPRO or other models based primarily on family history
- Chest radiation between the age of 10 and 30 (generally for lymphoma patients)
- Syndromes: Li-Fraumeni, Cowden, and Bannayan-Riley-Ruvalcaba syndromes and first-degree family member

Not enough evidence to recommend for or against MRI screening:

- Estimated lifetime risk of 15–20%, as per breast cancer models relying primarily on family history including BRCAPRO
- Biopsy results with atypia including ADH (atypical ductal hyperplasia), ALH (atypical lobular hyperplasia), or lobular carcinoma in situ (LCIS)
- Dense breast tissue
- Personal history of breast cancer, including ductal carcinoma in situ (DCIS)

Thermography

The basic principle of thermography is that a metabolically active tissue generates more heat than the surrounding tissue. Cancer is metabolically active due to rapid group supported by neo-angiogenesis taking place within the cancer tissue [15]. Infrared radiation is emitted by this tissue at a wavelength of 0.8 micrometer to 1 micrometer which is detected using an infrared camera [15]. This can then be converted into an energy signal to calculate the actual temperature of the object of interest. These signals can generate a visual map.

Breast thermography is based upon the above principle with the proposed theory behind the process being that this technique may be able to detect cancer earlier than can be seen using mammography or clinical examination [16]. However, despite the high sensitivity of this technique, it displays a significant lack of specificity with a high false-positive rate. In addition, the detected area cannot be localized to the point of interest, and this mechanism fails in metabolically less active tumors.

Therefore, there is no evidence to suggest that thermography may be used as a screening tool.

Molecular Imaging

This is a nuclear medicine technique in which either gamma rays or positrons (PEM, positron emission mammography) may be used to image the patient [17]. The radiopharmaceutical is administered to the patient intravenously, and then the imaging is performed using either a gamma camera or a PEM scanner. These radiotracers accumulate in breast cancer and are then detected as "hot spots" on the images.

The technique has good sensitivity (overall 90% and 82% for lesions smaller than 10 mm). This technique is useful as a problem-solving tool, especially in women with dense breast tissue. It demonstrates a cancer detection rate of about 3.2 per 1000 in dense breast tissue and 12 per 1000 for a combination of mammography and molecular imaging [18].

27.4.2 Diagnostic Imaging

27.4.2.1 Diagnostic Mammography

Diagnostic imaging is performed for women or men who report breast complaints or have had an abnormal clinical examination, and in women who have abnormal screening mammography. Patients with specific symptoms, like a palpable lump, nipple discharge, or focal pain should undergo diagnostic mammography.

The most common findings resulting in an abnormal screening mammogram are suspicious calcifications, masses, architectural distortion, or an asymmetry. In addition, technical factors can require a repeat of a mammogram, for example, an artifact (like hair), motion, and/or improper positioning. These finding may represent benign or malignant breast disease.

27.4.2.2 Ultrasound and MRI

Ultrasound and MRI are also employed as part of diagnostic imaging. Ultrasound is used in the evaluation of every mass to determine internal characteristics, flow, margins, etc. MRI is the imaging modality of choice to evaluate the extent of the disease process, especially in cancer. It is crucial that the images from the abnormal screening mammogram are available during a diagnostic workup, especially if a different provider is doing the diagnostic workup so as to accurately evaluate the reported abnormality.

Images on a diagnostic mammogram include magnification and spot compression views.

Ultrasound is then done to further investigate the mammogram findings.

See Figs. 27.2, 27.3, 27.4, 27.5, 27.6, and 27.7.

27.4.2.3 The BI-RADS Categories

The BI-RADS final assessment categories are used to standardize the reporting of the findings on the mammogram. They include recommendations for further management, such as routine screening, short interval follow-up, or biopsy.

Assessments are either incomplete (category 0) or final assessment categories (categories 1 through 6). These categories refer only to the imaging findings and recommendation and are not based upon the clinical picture even though an attempt is always made to correlate findings with the clinical complaint. For instance, if the patient has negative imaging evaluation but has a clinically suspicious lump, a biopsy may still be indicated even though the BI-RADS category is 1 or 2.

These categories are designated as follows:

- BI-RADS 0: Incomplete assessment; need additional imaging evaluation and/or prior mammograms for comparison.
- This category is used when there is not enough information from the views available to derive a conclusion. This is more commonly used in screening studies, which are interpreted as abnormal when the radiologist is not providing immediate reads. Causes for an incomplete evaluation include technical factors such as suboptimal images due to either improper positioning or motion; a questionable lesion not fully evaluated on the standard screening views; or unavailability of prior mammograms to confirm stability of a possible focal or diffuse abnormality. A recommendation is made regarding the reason for the incomplete report, which may entail additional or repeat imaging and/or comparison to the prior reports.
- BI-RADS 1: Negative.

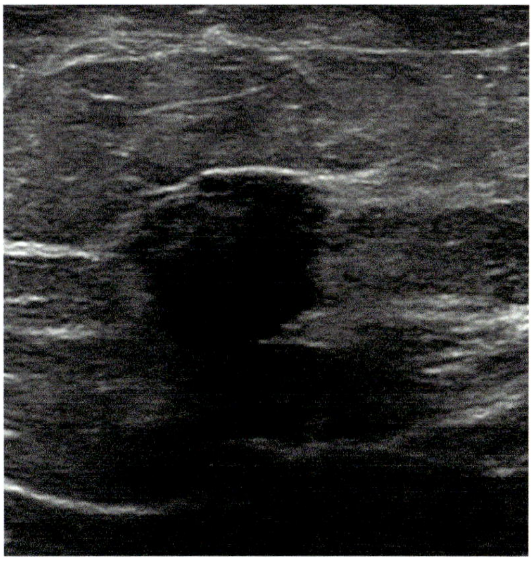

Fig. 27.2 Spiculated breast mass on ultrasound highly suggestive of cancer

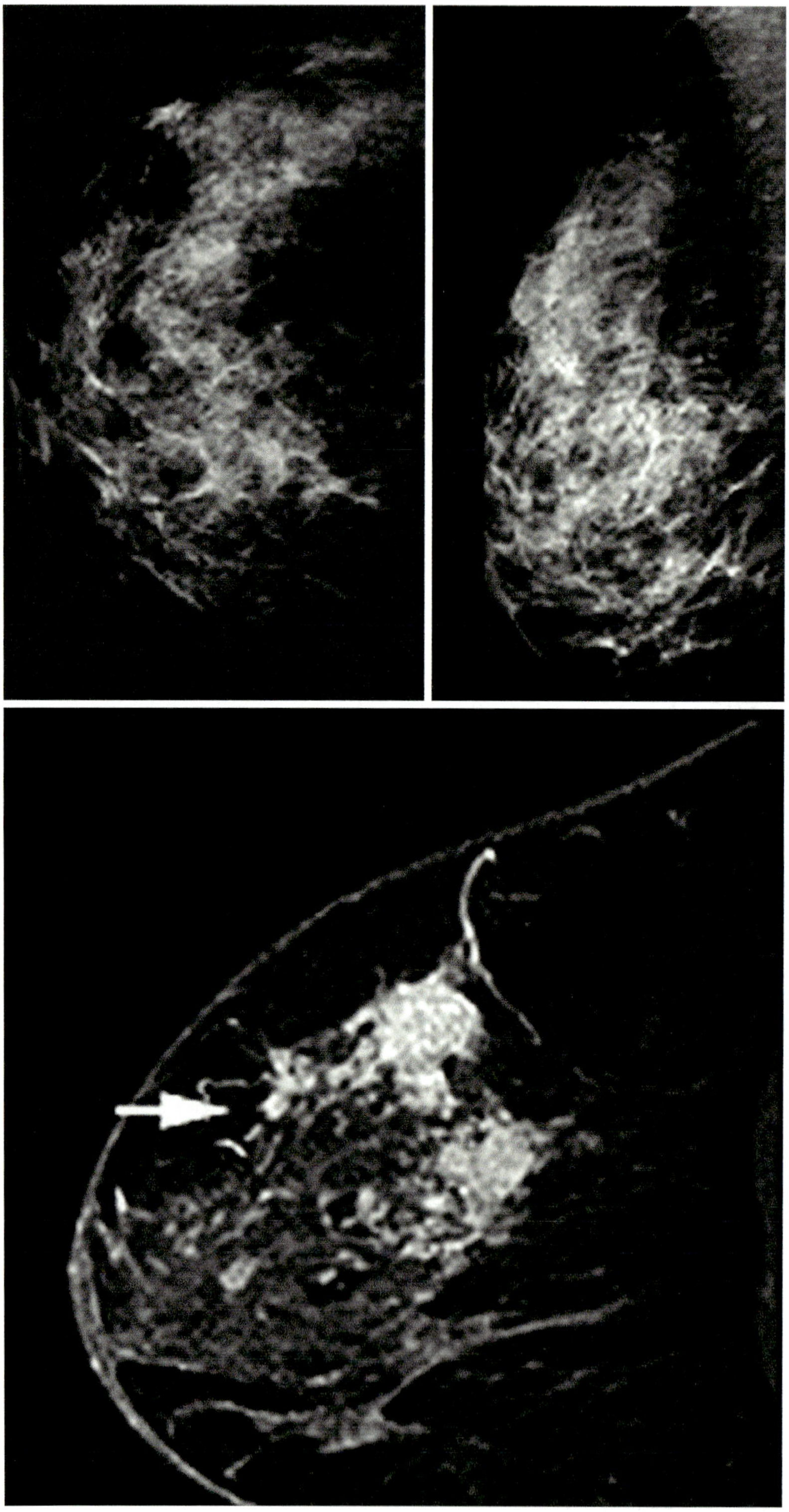

Fig. 27.3 MRI detection of breast cancer (the cancer was not seen on the mammogram)

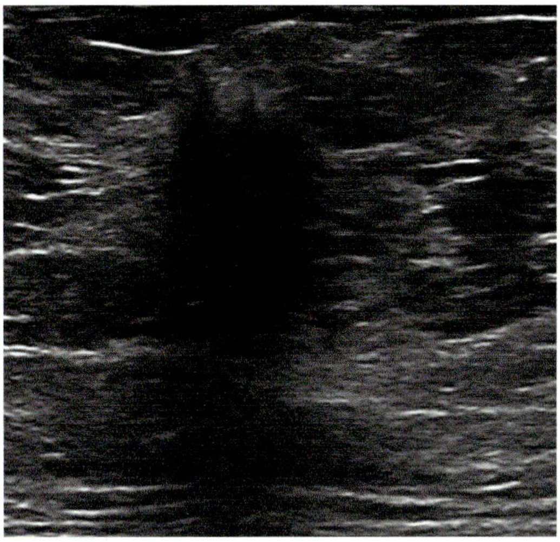

Fig. 27.4 Ultrasound image of biopsy proven malignancy (irregular hypoechoic mass with spiculated margins and posterior shadowing)

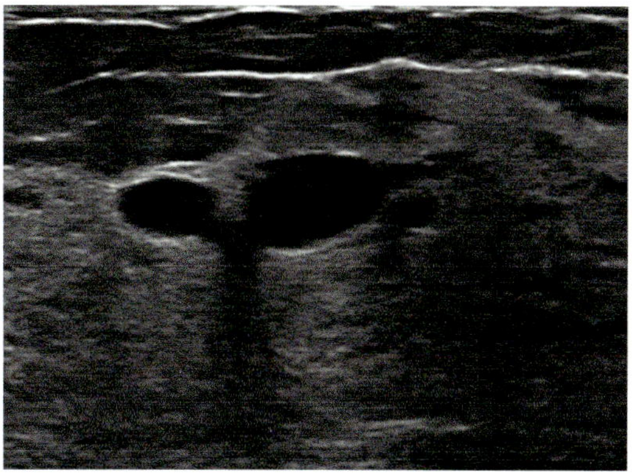

Fig. 27.5 Ultrasound image of breast cysts with characteristic features (anechoic, well-defined back wall and posterior acoustic enhancement)

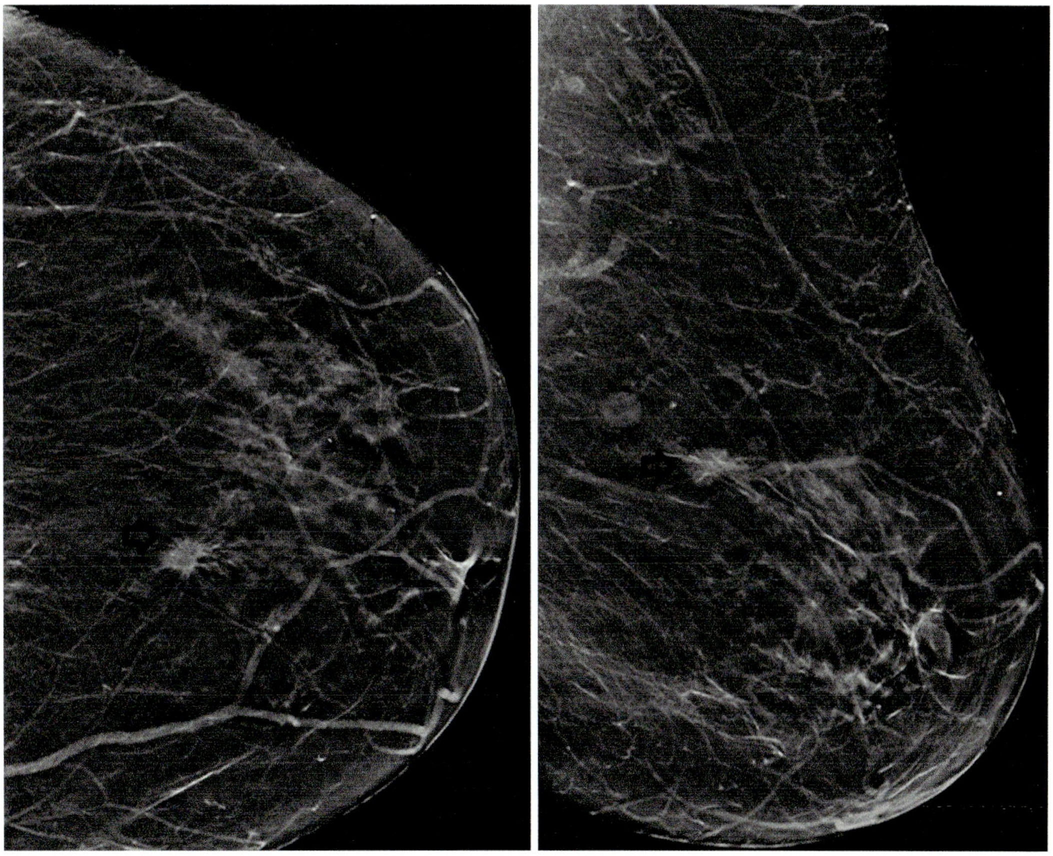

Fig. 27.6 Mammogram images (CC and MLO) of a biopsy proven malignancy showing characteristic features of a BIRADS 5 mass (irregular mass with spiculated margins)

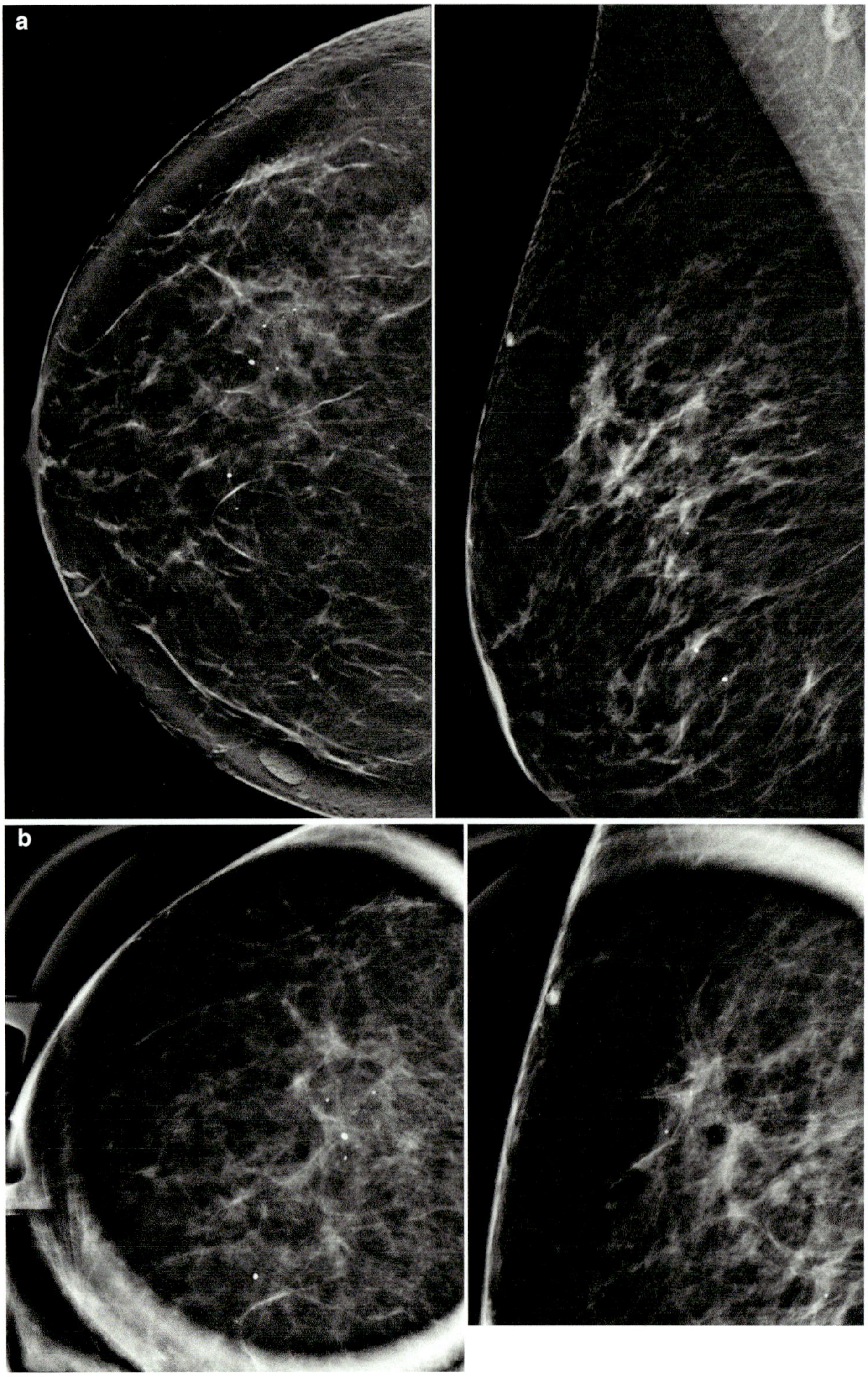

Fig. 27.7 Diagnostic mammogram images of biopsy proven DCIS. (**a**) CC and ML views. (**b**) Spot mag CC and ML images

- No imaging findings are detected. Routine annual screening mammography is recommended along with clinical breast examination as per current guidelines.
- BI-RADS 2: Benign findings.
- There is no concern for malignancy and no further action needs to be taken. Benign findings are noted which may include a fibroadenoma, cyst, or benign calcifications like vascular calcifications, etc. The rationale in reporting these findings is to document benignity and to prevent unnecessary evaluation. Routine follow-up is recommended.
- BI-RADS 3: Probably benign finding.
- This category is used when the likelihood of malignancy is less than 2%, and a definite benign finding is not seen. Examples of things that fall into this category may include an asymmetry, a benign-appearing mass, or other findings that do not have a categorically benign imaging feature.
- The findings in this category are followed at shorter intervals less than 1 year to assess for stability. Most commonly, diagnostic mammography and/or ultrasound at 6-month intervals for 1 year and then annually for an additional 2 years or every 6 months for a total of 2 years is routinely done. Follow-up at shorter intervals may be requested for close surveillance of a lesion that is not clearly benign. At any of these interval follow-ups, the lesion could be downgraded (BI-RADS 2) if it declares itself as clearly benign, or upgraded (BI-RADS 4 or 5) if there is a change with sufficient concern for malignancy.
- BI-RADS 4: Suspicious abnormality; biopsy should be considered.
- A lesion in this category has suspicious features of malignancy. The chance that the imaging finding is a cancer ranges between 2 and 94%. The degree of suspicion for malignancy varies both with the lesion and with the interpreter.
- The BI-RADS 4 category is very broad, and the findings are compatible with both DCIS and invasive breast cancer. Subdivisions of this category were introduced to convey the level of concern to the patient and her clinician. This enables them to make an informed decision for further management.
- These subcategories are:
- 4A (chance of malignancy 2 to 9%)
- 4B (chance of malignancy 10 to 49%)
- 4C (chance of malignancy 50 to 94%)
- BI-RADS 5: Highly suggestive of malignancy; appropriate action should be taken.
- The findings in this category have imaging features characteristic of a malignancy, for example, pleomorphic calcifications, masses with spiculation, and skin retraction. The suspicion for malignancy is between 95 and 100%.
- BI-RADS 6: Biopsy-proven malignancy; appropriate action should be taken.
- This category designates patients with a biopsy-proven malignancy before surgical excision, including patients for the evaluation of response to chemotherapy or evaluation of the contralateral breast. The patients with biopsy-proven cancer who present for a second opinion on prior images also fall under this category.

27.4.2.4 Breast Intervention

- US-guided biopsy: Ultrasound-guided biopsies are performed using ultrasound guidance to localize and target a lesion for biopsy. Generally, a 14-gauge biopsy needle is used to obtain core samples.
- Ultrasound can sometimes be used to biopsy calcifications also, and a needle up to 9-gauge caliber may be used.
- Stereotactic-guided biopsy: A special paddle is used to compress the breast within a central window in a CC (craniocaudal) or lateral projection. If the targeted lesion is identified within the window, then two additional images are obtained called stereotactic images, at +15 and −15°. Thereafter, the area for biopsy is targeted and spatial coordinates obtained in the X, Y, and Z projections.
- The skin entry point is then located and the needle introduced to the desired biopsy spot, verified with additional images and multiple biopsies are then obtained.
- Tomosynthesis guided biopsy: It is similar to stereotactic-guided biopsy in terms of guidance

using mammograms. However, this technique incorporates the use of 3D imaging where lesions seen in only one projection or only on 3D images may be biopsied.
- MRI-guided biopsy: These biopsies are performed using MRI guidance. A prebiopsy breast MRI is performed after intravenous contrast. The suspicious area/mass is then targeted and core biopsy samples obtained. This is generally performed with a vacuum-assisted 9-gauge device. A MRI compatible marker is then placed, with the position of the marker confirmed at post biopsy craniocaudal and lateral light pressure mammogram images.

The above image-guided biopsies may be performed with different type and caliber biopsy devices including vacuum-assisted devices.

27.4.3 Staging Breast Cancer and Monitoring Therapy

A diagnosis of cancer is established, and then imaging is utilized in treatment planning by staging the patient. The staging at diagnosis is performed using mammography, ultrasound, MRI (locoregional staging), and PET/CT (systemic staging).

The staging system used is the AJCC (American Joint Committee on Cancer) 8th edition of breast cancer.

The staging system incorporates not only the anatomic stage based on size of the tumor (T), status of the lymph nodes (N), and metastatic areas (M) but also incorporates various biomarkers including receptor status (estrogen/progesterone hormone receptor status), histologic grade, human epidermal growth factor-2 (HER2), maker for proliferation (such as Ki-67 or a mitotic count), and, for appropriate subgroups of tumor, a genomic panel (such as Oncotype DX, MammaPrint, EndoPredict, Breast Cancer Index, etc.).

Imaging plays a role in deciphering not only the anatomic stage but also helps with other prognostic indicator by providing core samples.

Monitoring of therapy is most accurately performed by comparing a prior chemotherapy baseline MRI to a MRI performed after a few cycles of neoadjuvant chemotherapy. However, mammogram and ultrasound may also be used to assess for response.

This is generally performed after at least two to three cycles of chemotherapy. The results are then utilized to modify or continue treatment.

Prognosis and treatment are currently determined largely on the basis of breast cancer stage. Breast cancer survival varies by stage at diagnosis. Overall 5-year survival rate is calculated to be about 27% for distant-stage disease, 85% for regional disease, and 99% for localized disease. Survival within each stage varies by the size of the tumor (T), calculated as a 5-year relative survival rate. So, the best prognosis is for women with smaller tumors, with survival rate estimated to be about 95% for tumor size less than or equal to 2 cm, and it decreases with increase in size with a rate of 85% for tumor size between 2 and 5 cm and 72% for tumors that are larger than 5 cm in size.

27.5 Conclusion

Imaging is the cornerstone in the detection of early breast cancer and thereby helps in reducing the morbidity and mortality associated with breast cancer. It plays a role not only in the screening and diagnosis of breast cancer but also helps in treatment planning and monitoring of therapy. The different imaging modalities used include mammography, ultrasound, and MRI in addition to PET/CT which are used in staging and monitoring of the disease.

27.5.1 Staging Breast Cancer and Monitoring Therapy

A diagnosis of cancer is established, and imaging is also utilized in treatment planning by staging the patient. The staging at diagnosis is performed using mammography, ultrasound, MRI (locoregional staging), and PET/CT (systemic staging). The staging used is the TNM staging (AJCC, American Joint Committee on Cancer) of breast cancer.

Prognosis and treatment are currently determined largely on the basis of breast cancer stage. Breast cancer survival varies by stage at diagnosis. The overall 5-year relative survival rate is 99% for localized disease, 85% for regional disease, and 27% for distant-stage disease. Survival within each stage varies by tumor size. For example, among women with regional disease, the 5-year relative survival is 95% for tumors less than or equal to 2.0 cm, 85% for tumors 2.1–5.0 cm, and 72% for tumors greater than 5.0 cm.

Key Points

- Reduction in breast cancer mortality by approximately 40% with initiation of annual screening mammography at age 40.
- Breast cancer surveillance can be performed using different imaging modalities including mammography (gold standard), ultrasound, and MRI.
- Women at higher than average risk of breast cancer may require a breast MRI in addition to conventional screening mammogram.
- Ultrasound is the best imaging modality to assess patients less than 30 years of age.
- Breast MRI (with contrast) is the most sensitive imaging modality and best estimates the extent of disease. It may also detect mammogram/ultrasound occult breast cancer.
- Breast MRI (with contrast) has the best sensitivity for the detection of breast cancer.
- Staging of breast cancer is helpful in treatment planning and assessment of prognosis.
- Staging of breast cancer is performed using mammogram, ultrasound, and MRI for locoregional staging and PET/CT for systemic staging depending on the stage of breast cancer.

References

1. Lee SC, Jain PA, Jethwa SC, Tripathy D, Yamashita MW. Radiologist's role in breast cancer staging: providing key information for clinicians. Radiographics. 2014;34(2):330–42.
2. Chen L, Chantra PK, Larsen LH, Barton P, Rohitopakarn M, Zhu EQ, et al. Imaging characteristics of malignant lesions of the male breast. Radiographics. 2006;26(4):993–1006.
3. Broeders M, Moss S, Nyström L, Njor S, Jonsson H, Paap E, et al. The impact of mammographic screening on breast cancer mortality in Europe: a review of observational studies. J Med Screen. 2012;19(Suppl 1):14–25.
4. Chen W. Patient education: factors that modify breast cancer risk in women (beyond the basics). https://www.uptodate.com.
5. Nicholson BT, Harvey JA, Cohen MA. Nipple-areolar complex: normal anatomy and benign and malignant processes. Radiographics. 2009;29(2):509–23.
6. American College of Radiology. Benefits and limitations of mammography. Digest of Council Action 2015-2016: 2002, amended 2012 (Res. 23-c).
7. Coldman A, Phillips N, Wilson C, Decker K, Chiarelli AM, Brisson J, et al. Pan-Canadian study of mammography screening and mortality from breast cancer. J Natl Cancer Inst. 2014;106(11)
8. Helquist BN, Duffy SW, Abdsaleh S, Björneld L, Bordás P, Tabár L, et al. Effectiveness of population-based service screening with mammography for women ages 40-49 years. Cancer. 2010;117(4):714–22.
9. Helvie MA, Chang JT, Hendrick RE, Banerjee M. Reduction in late-stage breast cancer incidence in the mammography era. Cancer. 2014;120(17):2649–56.
10. Koroukian SM, Bakaki PM, Htoo PT, Han X, Schluchter M, Owusu C, et al. The breast and cervical cancer early detection program, medicaid, and breast cancer outcomes among Ohio's underserved women. Cancer. 2017;123(16):3097–106.
11. Hendrick RE, Helvie MA. Mammography screening: a new estimate of number needed to screen to prevent one breast cancer death. AJR Am J Roentgenol. 2012;198:723–8.
12. Howlader N, Noone AM, Krapcho M, et al. SEER cancer statistics review, 1975-2014. https://seer.cancer.gov/csr/1975_2014/, based on November 2016 SEER data submission, posted to the SEER web site, April 2017. Bethesda, MD: National Cancer Institute; 2017.
13. Grady D, Redberg R. Physician adherence to breast cancer screening recommendations. JAMA Intern Med. 2017;177(6):763–4.
14. Berg W, Mendelson EB, Merritt CB. ACRIN 6666: screening breast ultrasound in high risk women. https://www.acrin.org/portals/0/protocols/6666/a6666partial_summary.pdf.
15. Kennedy DA, Lee T, Seely D. A comparative review of thermography as a breast cancer screening technique. Integr Cancer Ther. 2009;8(1):9–16.
16. Gautherie M. Thermobiological assessment of benign and malignant breast diseases. Am J Obstet Gynecol. 1983;147(8):861–9.
17. Alcantara D, Leal MP, Garcia-Bocanegra I, Garcia-Martin ML. Molecular imaging of breast cancer: present and future directions. Front Chem. 2014;2:112.
18. O'Connor MK. Molecular breast imaging: an emerging modality for breast cancer screening. Breast Cancer Manag. 2015;4(1):33–40.

Breast Cancer Screening Modalities

28

Kerry-Ann McDonald and Jessica Young

28.1 Introduction

Breast cancer is the most common malignancy in women and a leading cause of morbidity and mortality in them. Breast cancer survival varies by stage at diagnosis. According to the 2017 Surveillance, Epidemiology, and End Results (SEER) data, the overall 5-year relative survival rate is 99% for localized disease, 85% for regional disease, and 27% for distant-stage disease [1]. Breast cancer screening is used to identify women with asymptomatic cancer so that cases are picked up and treated early leading to better outcomes. Presently, breast cancer detection relies on mammography as the main screening modality, but mammography has high false-positive rates and limited sensitivity for detection of lesions in dense breast tissues. Biomarkers that can predict early disease are a welcome addition to the imaging methods used for breast cancer screening. Imaging techniques for screening have been discussed in detail in Chap. 27, and the role of clinical examination and biomarkers will be dealt with in this chapter.

K.-A. McDonald · J. Young (✉)
Breast Surgery Division, Department of Surgical Oncology, Roswell Park Comprehensive Cancer Center, Buffalo, NY, USA
e-mail: jessica.young@roswellpark.org

28.2 Breast Self-Examination

Breast self-examination (BSE) has been promoted earlier as a screening method to diagnose breast cancer at an earlier age. It may help in the detection of lager lesions but is associated with increased false positives and more frequent physician referrals and biopsies.

A large randomized trial of breast self-examination in 266,064 women was carried out by Gao et al. in Shanghai, China, in 2005. The women were randomly assigned to a BSE instruction group or a control group. Breast cancer was detected in 864 women, and 133 breast cancer deaths were observed in the BSE group versus 896 cancers and 130 deaths in the control group. This was not found to be statistically significant, and so they concluded that intensive BSE cannot reduce mortality rate of breast cancer but will detect a higher number of smaller and benign breast lumps [2]. Baxter N in collaboration with the Canadian Task Force on Preventive Health Care evaluated the role of breast self-examination in screening for breast cancer. BSE failed to show a benefit in picking up significant cases of breast cancer but significantly increased the number of physician visits for evaluation of benign breast lesions and number of breast biopsies [3].

Following this, the Canadian Task Force on Preventive Health Care gave the following recommendations:

S. Mehta, A. Singla (eds.), *Preventive Oncology for the Gynecologist*,
https://doi.org/10.1007/978-981-13-3438-2_28

Women between 40 and 70 years: No need to routinely teach BSE during the periodic health examination in this age group.

Women <40 years: Due to the lack of sufficient data in this age group and low incidence of breast cancer in them, the risk of net harm from BSE and BSE instruction is high.

Women >70 years: In spite of high incidence of breast cancer in women of this age group, evidence is insufficient to make a recommendation regarding BSE.

A 2003 cochrane review based its recommendations on data from two large population-based studies (388,535 women) from Russia and Shanghai comparing BSE with no intervention. They did not find any statistically significant difference in breast cancer mortality in both groups, RR (95% CI 0.9–1.24), but women who were randomized to breast self-examination were almost twice as likely to undergo a biopsy of the breast. There were 3406 biopsies performed in the screening group as compared to 1856 biopsies in the control group. They recommended that BSE should not be used for breast cancer screening; but women should seek medical help if they find any changes in their breasts [4].

28.2.1 Breast Self-Awareness

Public education is an important component of early detection, and increasing breast awareness among women is an important aspect of it. The terms breast self-examination and breast awareness are often used loosely [5]. No expert group now recommends SBE, but they all do recommend that women should be familiar with the appearance and feel of their breasts. Any changes detected by the woman should be promptly reported to the physician. The changes to be looked for include:

- Any palpable lump
- Discharge from nipples, especially bloody discharge
- Change in shape or size of the breast
- Skin changes such as erythema, scaling, or dimpling
- Swollen lymph nodes in axilla

Breast health awareness is the key element of interventions done for early detection of breast cancer.

28.3 Clinical Breast Examination

Clinical breast exams (CBE) are manual examinations performed by a clinician, usually a primary care provider or OB/GYN specialist. CBE also offers an opportunity to educate women about the importance of early detection, the risks of breast cancer, and breast awareness.

There are different palpation techniques for CBE. But the key to successful examination is careful observation and systemic palpation. The time required for conducting CBE is 2–5 min.

Steps for CBE include [6]:

- With the woman sitting up with arms at her side, an observation of shape, color, and skin characteristic of the breast should be done. Any skin retraction, ulceration, erythema, crusting, inversion, or eversion of nipples should be noted.
- Now the woman is asked to raise her arms over the head. A note of movement of breast tissue (can also be done by asking to arch her back with hands on hips) and any tethering of breast tissue to the chest is done.
- With the woman sitting up, palpation should be done with the flat of the finger pads, not the tips. To increase the sensitivity should remain cognizant of the nipples. The main purpose is to evaluate all tissue between skin and chest wall.
- The movement of fingers can follow any of the three patterns. (a) In "radial spoke" technique, wedges of the tissues are examined beginning at the periphery toward the nipple in a radial manner. (b) Palpation can be done in overlapping "vertical strips" across the chest wall from medial portion of the chest wall below the clavicle and progress down and then up. (c) The breast can be examined

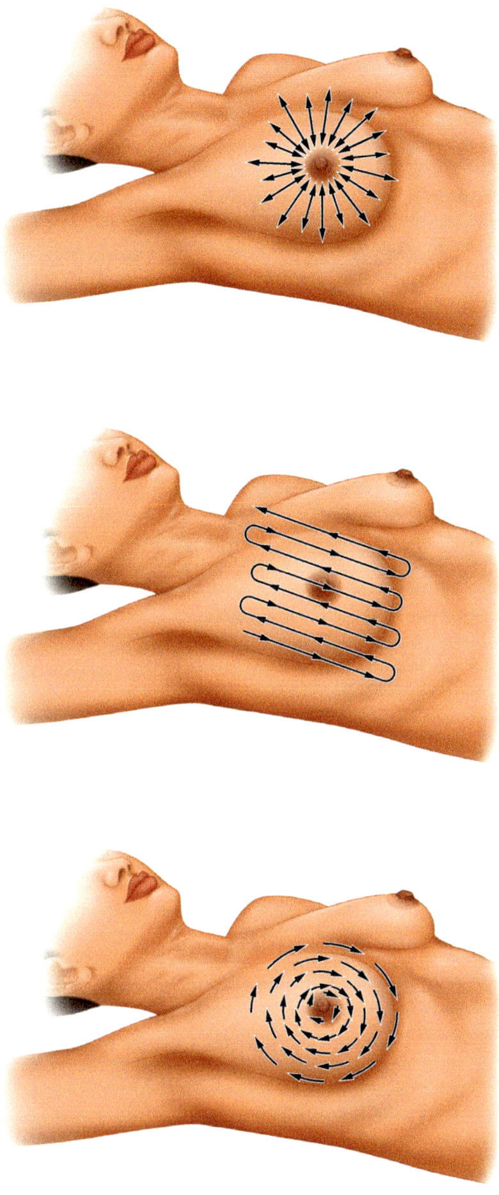

Fig. 28.1 Patterns of hand movement during CBE

in "concentric circles" method, starting from the nipple and areola (Fig. 28.1).

- It is possible to repeat the palpation pattern using different degrees of pressure (to assess different depths of tissue), but more efficient approach is to spiral in each position from superficial to deep; thus, tissue at each level is evaluated.
- The opposite breast is examined in the same manner.
- Now, the woman is asked to lie flat with arm of the examining breast behind the woman's head which causes the breast tissue to stretch against the chest wall, which particularly helps in examining the lower quadrants. The breast can be examined by using any palpatory method described above.
- Evaluation of supraclavicular and axillary node is always performed to complete the CBE. Examination of the axilla is best done in sitting position with raised arms. The examiner inserts her hand in the axilla, just behind the pectoralis major muscle and parallel to the plane of the muscle. The woman lowers her arms with examiner's hand in place. The examiner then rotates her palm perpendicular to the plane and sweeps downward, palpating for nodes. Nodes that are hard, fixed to underlying structures, or greater than 1 cm may be pathological and need evaluation.
- Supraclavicular nodes are best palpated in sitting upright position.
- Please note that nodal basins should be compared bilaterally for symmetry.

If any abnormality is identified, it should be noted. The lesion is described with respect to nipple and relative depth from the skin. It can be documented more objectively using a diagram, or by describing the location of the lesion as a time on a clockface (i.e. 1 cm mass @ 2:00, 2 cm from the nipple).

It is estimated that between 5% and 10% of breast cancers may be detected by CBE. The sensitivity of CBE alone is only 21%, and it is not comparable to the sensitivity of mammography, but the two combined tend to improve the sensitivity of breast cancer detection to 82%. In the Cairo breast screening trial, 4116 women between 35 and 64 years underwent CBE at a primary health center. Eight of 1000 women were detected with breast cancer at the time of examination, and two among those were rescreened. The initial high prevalence of advanced cancer showed that women in the community did not seek medical help until their disease is advanced. This study highlights the importance of educating women and increasing their awareness about breast health [7].

Dinshaw et al. undertook a community-based, controlled cohort study on breast and cervical cancer screening in 150,000 women aged 35–64 years. The average compliance to getting investigations done was 73% among women with breast cancer, and compliance to treatment was 95%. This study showed that screening programs with CBE were feasible and acceptable in Indian population [8]. However, routine CBE is not recommended in screening-based programs due to the lack of evidence [9–13].

28.4 Imaging Tools for Breast Cancer Screening

Mammography is the gold standard for detecting early breast cancer in screening programs. Other imaging diagnostic techniques include ultrasonography and MRI of the breast. These have been discussed in detail in Chap. 27, and only a brief mention is made here.

28.4.1 Mammography

Mammography is the gold standard for breast cancer screening. It has an overall sensitivity of 85% and specificity of 92–97% [14, 15]. For average-risk women older than 40 years of age, mammography is the only recommended imaging modality to screen for breast cancer.

During the procedure the breast tissue is compressed between two clear plates which are attached to an X-ray machine. This results in pictures being taken from two directions. Standard mammographic projections include craniocaudal (CC), mediolateral oblique (MLO), and mediolateral (ML). Mass lesions, calcifications, and asymmetric densities can be seen on mammographic images. Conventional methods of mammography include film mammography, and advances in technology have paved the way for digital (2D) and 3D (tomosynthesis) mammography.

Film Mammography—In film-screen mammography, X-rays from a stationary X-ray tube are absorbed by a phosphor screen, which emits light and exposes it to the film to create the mammographic image [16]. This labor-intensive technique exposes patients to an average radiation dose of 2.377 mGy per view [17]. As a result of image processing errors, digital mammography has quickly replaced film.

Digital Mammography—It was approved in 2000 by the US Food and Drug Administration (FDA) and is a similar technique to film mammography with the exception that the X-rays used in digital mammography are converted to an electrical signal by the digital detector [16]. This allows for improved image quality and more efficient electronic-based image management [16]. This technique also exposes the patient to less radiation, with two-view digital mammography having an average radiation dose of 1.86 mGy per view [17]. The main shortcoming of digital mammography is the overlap of normal breast tissue which can obscure small cancers [18]. It is important to remind women that palpable lesions need to be evaluated even if they recently had a negative mammogram. The newest form of mammography, tomosynthesis, has overcome this problem of overlapping breast tissue.

Tomosynthesis digital breast tomosynthesis (DBT) represents a newer modality in mammographic imaging which was approved by the FDA in 2011. It is generally used in combination with full-field digital mammography [19]. The X-ray tube rotates over an arc and thus is able to get low-dose images from multiple angles. These are then reconstructed into a series of high-resolution "slices" and displayed in a dynamic three-dimensional ciné mode [19]. It increases the cancer detection rate by 29% and decreases the recall rate of the patient by 15% [19, 20].

The STORM trial confirmed that DBT detected more cancers compared to standard mammography. This trial prospectively compared the effect of integrated 2D and 3D mammography in a population-based breast cancer screening of 7292 women [18, 21]. The cancer detection rates were higher for the integrated screening, 8.1 cancers per 1000 screens [18, 21]. DBT was also better at localizing lesions for biopsy, accurately characterizing the size of lesions, and requires less compression than conventional mammography [16].

The main disadvantages of DBT include increased radiation exposure to patients; limited evaluation of calcifications, with overall calcification detection sensitivity of 75% versus 84% for digital mammography; longer procedure time; and increased cost compared to standard mammography [22].

28.4.2 Mammography as a Screening Modality

False-Positive Results—The false-positive results of mammography vary from 61% for women aged 40 to 50 years to 49.7% for women in the age group 66 to 74 years [23]. False-positive results can lead to a tremendous amount of anxiety for the patient, increased healthcare costs, and overdiagnosis.

Pain and Discomfort—Mammography is associated with pain and discomfort for a majority of women, with up to 35% of women reporting pain with the procedure [24]. This pain often stems from compression, which makes the breast density more uniform, but can deter some women from having screening mammograms. One study found that pain is often associated with patient's anticipation of pain rather than the actual compression itself [25]. Multiple interventions are available to relieve the pain, such as providing women with verbal information before the procedure, pain relief medication taken before the procedure, use of a breast cushion, patient-controlled compression of the breast, and reduced compression. The breast cushion was found to interfere with image quality, and all maneuvers were associated with decreased pain except for the technologist's reduction of compression [24]. With the advent of 3D mammography, less compression can be used, thus alleviating some of the pain.

28.4.3 Breast Ultrasound

Breast ultrasound is a useful adjunctive tool for women with dense breasts and in characterizing abnormalities seen on mammography [15, 18]. It is also used for evaluating focal breast symptoms in women younger than 40 years, due to their breast density [26]. Unlike mammography, breast ultrasound defines cystic versus solid lesions and their characteristics, such as simple or complex with smooth or irregular margins [15, 18]. Its other advantages include low cost and no requirement of dye or ionizing radiation. The shortcomings are the technical differences between exams and the time and skill necessary to detect small, non-palpable tumors [15]. In 2014, the SomoInsight study showed that screening breast ultrasound can detect more cancers in conjunction with mammography as opposed to mammography alone [18, 27]. Specifically, 82 cancers were detected with screening mammography and an additional 30 cancers with ultrasound out of 112 women. Addition of ultrasound to screening mammography yielded an additional 1.9 detected cancers per 1000 women screened supporting the role of breast ultrasound as a good adjunctive tool [27].

28.4.4 Breast MRI

Breast MRI is a highly sensitive screening modality. Studies suggest that MRI offers a significantly higher sensitivity of 91% compared to mammography in higher-risk patients, with equivalent specificity of 97.2% [28]. Despite this benefit, to our knowledge no studies have definitively demonstrated decreased breast cancer-specific mortality in high-risk patients [14]. In addition to increased sensitivity, MRI does not use radiation. However, MRI does require the administration of IV gadolinium contrast load to delineate areas of enhancement and washout kinetics, which can give clues about the suspiciousness of a lesion within the breast. It is also one of the most expensive screening modalities and costs approximately ten times more than standard mammography [18, 29]. Therefore, some institutions are investigating the usefulness of abbreviated MRIs to reduce cost and scan times. The use of breast MRI for screening is limited primarily to women with a greater than or equal to 20% lifetime risk of breast cancer [18, 30] or for the diagnosis of palpable breast cancer not seen on mammography.

28.5 Biomarkers

Mammography is associated with overdiagnosis and high false-positive and false-negative rates. To overcome this, biomarkers have been developed which can help in generating cost-effective assays feasible for routine screening. As they are still in early stages of development, none of them are sensitive enough for the early detection of breast cancer.

Promising candidate biomarkers include proteins, autoantibodies, miRNAs [31], nucleic acid methylation, metabolites, exosomes [32], glycans [33], plasma proneurotensin [34], CA15-3, RANTES, IGFBP3, OPN, PAI-1, SLPI, HSP90A, PAPPA and APOC1 [35], and phospholipids [36].

Established biomarkers already in use for diagnosis and prognosis of breast cancer are:

- Estrogen receptor (ER): ER (α) expression is a surrogate marker for sensitivity to endocrine treatment and response to neoadjuvant chemotherapy. Tumors which are positive for estrogen receptors have a lower rate of complete response (pCR) to neoadjuvant chemotherapy than ER-negative tumors [37]. However, ER positive tumors generally have a better prognosis than ER negative.
- Progesterone receptor (PgR): PgR expression in the breast cancer tissue is directly related to better outcomes [38].
- HER2: HER2-positive malignancy has a poorer outcome compared to HER2-negative cancer. Trastuzumab, which is a monoclonal antibody targeted to HER2, has helped in developing HER2 as a predictive biomarker as well as greatly decreasing the mortality of HER2-positive patients. Other HER2-targeted therapies, including pertuzumab, are also routinely given to HER2-positive patients [39].

Emerging biomarkers for diagnosis and prognosis of breast cancer are:

- Ki67: This biomarker predicts whether chemotherapy will be helpful in early or locally advanced cancer. Measurement of Ki67 after neoadjuvant chemotherapy predicts recurrences and overall survival [40].
- Cyclin D1: Amplification of cyclin D1 predicts early relapse and poor prognosis [41, 42].
- Cyclin E: Two types of cyclin E have been studied—low-molecular-weight and total cyclin E. Their levels help to discriminate overall and disease-free survival. They have proved to be better than even the clinical and pathological biomarkers [43].
- ERβ: Though ERβ protein levels are generally predictive of good prognosis, prolonged disease-free survival, and response to Tamoxifen [44, 45], more studies are needed for confirmation.

Multigene parameters: Several genomic tests like MammaPrint, Oncotype DX, Genomic Grade Index, and Rotterdam signature based on genomic profiling are developed with the expectation that this might better predict for clinical outcome than the standard pathological and clinical markers [46]. Oncotype DY and MammaPrint tests are routinely used for ER/PR-positive HER2-negative patients to help determine the need for adjuvant chemotherapy.

28.5.1 Circulating Tumor Cells and Tumor-Specific DNA

Increased serum levels of cell-free DNA (cfDNA) were shown in breast cancer patients by Leon et al. [47]. As an apoptotic biomarker, cfDNA gives valuable information regarding diagnosis and therapy response prediction [48].

Potential biomarkers under research for the diagnosis and prognosis of breast cancer are the urokinase-dependent plasminogen activator system (uPA), the plasminogen activator inhibitor (PAI), mammaglobin, osteopontin, fibroblast growth factor receptor 2 (FGFR2), sirtuins (SIRT), snail, twist, and Zeb-1 [49].

28.6 Average-Risk Screening Recommendations in the United States

Average-risk women include those who are asymptomatic without any history of high-risk or malignant lesion of the breast, are not at high risk for a known underlying genetic mutation (such as a BRCA1 or BRCA2 gene mutation or other familial breast cancer syndromes), do not have multiple family members with breast cancer and also have no history of chest radiation at a young age [50, 51]. Recommendations may vary for each national society/task force.

28.6.1 United States Preventive Service Task Force (USPSTF)

The USPSTF recommends biennial screening mammography for women aged 50 to 74 years, using the rationale that most of the benefit of mammography is derived at this time. They state that the decision to start screening at an earlier age needs to be individualized, as screening mammography in women aged 40 to 49 may result in unnecessary biopsies and also the number of deaths averted is smaller than that in older women [50].

28.6.2 American Cancer Society (ACS)

The American Cancer Society [51] breast cancer screening recommendations (2015) are as follows:

Screening mammography should start at 45 years in average-risk women, using the rationale that mammographic screening reduces mortality and increases life expectancy.

Women who are ages 45 to 54 years should be screened annually, as they report that annual screening yielded a larger reduction in breast cancer mortality than biennial screening.

Biennial screening or annual screening should be done in women who are 55 years and older.

Opportunity to begin annual screening between the ages of 40 and 44 years should be given to women, as long as they understand the risks and benefits.

The ACS also states that women should continue screening mammography as long as their overall health is good with a life expectancy of 10 years or more. Finally, the ACS does not recommend CBE for breast cancer screening among average-risk women at any age, as there is no evidence that points toward improved outcomes.

28.6.3 American College of Obstetricians and Gynecologists (ACOG)

The updated 2017 breast cancer screening recommendations from ACOG are as follows:

Screening mammography should start at 40 years in women at average risk of breast cancer.

Women at average risk of breast cancer should have screening mammography every 1 or 2 years and should continue screening mammography until at least 75 years of age.

Screening mammography may be discontinued after 75 years of age depending on the patient's health status and life expectancy [52].

28.6.4 American College of Physicians (ACP)

For women at average risk of breast cancer between the ages of 50 and 74 years, physicians should encourage mammography screening every 2 years in average-risk women. It is further stated that for women at average risk of breast cancer between the ages of 40 and 49 years, mammography screening should be done every 2 years if the woman requests it. They do not recommend screening beyond 74 years of age [53].

28.6.5 American Academy of Family Physicians (AAFP)

The AAFP recommends that women aged 50 to 74 years should have biennial screening mammography and if earlier screening is required, then it should be an individualized decision.

28.6.6 National Comprehensive Cancer Network (NCCN)

The NCCN recommends annual screening mammogram for asymptomatic average-risk women aged 40 years and older, with reduction in breast cancer-related mortality being the major benefit of screening mammography.

For women less than 40 years of age, at minimum a medical and family history should be obtained, and clinical referral should include risk assessment, counseling for risk reduction, as well as a clinical breast examination every 1 to 3 years. They have not decided on the upper age limit for screening.

In summary, most of the US groups advocate for screening starting at age 40–50 years and discontinuing screening after 74 years of age.

28.7 International Breast Cancer Screening Guidelines (Other than United States)

28.7.1 The Canadian Task Force on Preventive Health

They do not recommend routine screening mammography for women 40–49 years of age. They calculated that the number needed to screen to prevent one death from breast cancer for women aged 40–49 years is 2108, as compared with 721 for women aged 50–69 years. Therefore, women in the age group of 50–74 years should have mammography every 2 to 3 years. They also recommend against MRI screening and CBEs, as there is no evidence that it reduces mortality [54].

28.7.2 European Commission Initiative on Breast Cancer (ECIBC)

ECIBC is a patient-centered initiative aiming to improve breast cancer care in Europe. For women at average risk of breast cancer between the ages of 45 and 74 years, physicians should encourage mammography screening. They recommend not implementing screening for asymptomatic women aged 40–44 years with an average risk of breast cancer due to concerns about false-positive rates and overdiagnosis.

28.7.3 Breast Cancer Screening in India

Indian practitioners stress the importance of patient recognition and early detection of breast cancer. Awareness and education start at the age of 30 years as the peak incidence of breast cancer in India is in younger women. Since resources are limited, screening mammography for the entire population is not an affordable approach. Therefore, CBEs combined with diagnostic ultrasound are deemed fundamental instruments for breast assessment and are used as a routine method for breast cancer diagnosis, especially in women younger than 50 years. When mammography is available, its primary use is diagnostic [55].

28.8 Screening Guidelines in Low- and Middle-Income Countries

Formulation and implementation of breast cancer screening guidelines in LMICs were finalized in the third Global Summit of Breast Health Global Initiative (BHGI) in 2007 [56].

The programs must be culturally sensitive and should be in the language understood by the people of region. In LMICs most of the women do not have access or the finances for mammography screening. So the goal in such *places with basic resources* should be to downstage the disease by teaching women the importance of seeking timely help when breast symptoms occur. These women can then undergo CBE by a health worker who can refer her for further diagnostic tests if required. Education should emphasize that survival is better when cancer is treated at an early stage (Table 28.1).

When the resources are limited, education programs stressing the importance of breast awareness can be implemented at the district level with the help of local midwives. The training of healthcare provider in CBE is the key to successful implementation of the screening program. If the CBE is positive, a diagnostic ultrasound or mammography can

Table 28.1 BGHI guidelines for LMICs (2007)

Resources	Awareness	Detection methods	Evaluation goal
Basic	Development of culturally sensitive appropriate local education programs for target populations to teach value of early detection, breast cancer risk factors, and breast health awareness	Clinical history and CBE	Breast health awareness regarding value of early detection in improving breast cancer outcome
Limited	Culturally appropriate targeted outreach/ education encouraging CBE for age groups at higher risk administered at district/ provincial level using healthcare providers in the field	Diagnostic breast USG and/ or diagnostic mammography in women with positive CBE Mammographic screening of target group	Downsizing of symptomatic disease
Enhanced	Regional awareness programs regarding breast health linked to general health and women's health programs	Mammographic screening every 2 years in women aged 50–69 Consider mammographic screening every 12–18 months in women aged 40–49	Downsizing and/or downstaging of asymptomatic disease in women in highest yield target groups
Maximal	National awareness campaigns regarding breast health using media	Consider annual mammographic screening in women ages 40 and older Other imaging technologies as appropriate for high-risk groups	Downsizing and/or downstaging of asymptomatic disease in women in all risk groups

be done. At least it will help in picking up early-stage tumors which have a better prognosis. Though wherever finances permit, mammography should be offered to women.

28.9 Screening in Special Populations

In the United States, despite some controversies, the most common recommendation for screening is still annually starting at age 40, without a specific age to stop. The following scenarios are special populations for which other recommendations might be made. These do not include women at higher risk of breast cancer from gene mutations or family history, which will be addressed elsewhere.

28.9.1 Younger Women (<40 Years)

Women <40 years at average risk should not have routine screening, given the low rate of cancer, increased breast density leading to less accurate screening, and false-positive/false-negative results. The National Comprehensive Cancer Network (NCCN) guidelines recommend that women of average risk between the ages of 25 and 40 have a clinical exam every 1–3 years and that they be familiar with their breasts and report any changes to their healthcare provider [13]. For women with specific complaints of pain or a mass, the best imaging modality under the age of 40 years would be ultrasound, followed by mammogram if needed. However, mammograms are of lesser utility in this age group due to breast density.

28.9.2 Elderly

While there are some differences, most large national groups advocate breast cancer screening with mammography starting between ages 40 and 50 for women of average risk. However, there is no consensus as to when a woman should stop screening for breast cancer. As the population ages, this is becoming a more and more important question.

Most randomized control trials did not include elderly women, especially over the age of 80. More importantly, the health and longevity of a woman are just as important as her actual age. Observational studies and computer models show a mortality benefit to screening up to age 80–84 [12, 57]. The mortality benefit of screening is often delayed about 5–7 years in RCTs that emphasize the importance of life expectancy and overall health when considering the age at which to stop screening [58].

Therefore, screening is generally recommended for women with at least a 5–10 life expectancy, as studies show that it takes approximately 10 years before a screening-detected breast cancer is shown to impact an older woman's survival. Screening beyond age 70 is estimated to help 2 out of 1000 women avoid breast cancer death.

There are considerable disadvantages to continued screening in older women, including anxiety about abnormal findings that may be false positive and the trauma of unnecessary benign biopsies. Discussing the risks and benefits of routine screening in older women, in the context of their overall health and quality of life, can help them make an informed decision in line with their preferences and values. For example, if a woman would decide not to have treatment, even if she was found to have breast cancer, it would be more prudent to stop screening. In the discussion with these women, it should be emphasized that there is insufficient evidence to show that routine screening at this age increases survival. However, more RCTs are needed to make an informed decision.

If the patient has severe comorbid conditions which would limit her life expectancy to less than 10 years and any intervention based on the screening findings would not be beneficial, then the recommendations are to stop screening her, regardless of her age [58, 59]. It can certainly be a difficult discussion to have with patients, as the idea of letting a potential cancer go untreated can be uncomfortable for most people. However, a thorough discussion of the risks and benefits should help with their concerns.

28.9.3 Thoracic Radiation

Younger women who receive thoracic mantle radiation are more prone to develop breast cancer. Women who undergo chest irradiation before 30 years of age have the highest risk of developing breast cancer. This is usually seen in women with Hodgkin's lymphoma who receive mantle radiation. Their CBE is recommended annually if they received the radiation between ages of 10 and 25 years, and the current age of the patient is <25 years. If the patient is over the age of 25, there should be a clinical breast exam every 6–12 months, starting 8–10 years after the radiation was given. Mammograms and MRI of the breasts should also be initiated if the patient is >25 years and at least 8 years after radiation was given.

Thoracic irradiation given when a patient is in their 20s–30s substantially increases the risk of developing breast cancer by age 40 [60–65]. There is some concern for cumulative radiation exposure in these young women, but the additional radiation is negligible compared to the overall lifetime radiation exposure. The use of MRI can also alleviate these concerns.

28.9.4 Dense Breasts

In the United States, many states have passed legislation which requires them to inform women if they have dense breasts. This was first passed in Connecticut in 2009, with more than 30 states joining to date. The notification was put into place, as there is evidence that women who have dense breast tissue are at an increased risk of breast cancer (up to 3–5 times greater lifetime risk) compared to women with entirely fatty breasts [66–68]. However, currently there is little evidence that additional screening would have any mortality benefit.

28.10 Conclusion

Breast cancer is the most common malignancy in women and a leading cause of morbidity and mortality in them. Screening for breast cancer relies mainly on education programs stressing the importance of breast awareness and clinical breast examination by health workers. Healthcare guidelines for early detection, diagnosis, and treatment should be implemented in all countries depending on the resources they have, but all the programs must be culturally sensitive and should be in the language of the region. Screening mammography is currently the gold standard for early detection of breast cancer though other imaging modalities can also be used. Newer noninvasive strategies for breast cancer screening which include blood-based biomarkers are not sensitive enough for early detection of breast cancer, but some promising biomarkers such as proteins, miRNAs, exosomes, glycans, etc. have shown great potential in detection of breast cancer at the preinvasive stages of the disease.

Key Points

- Breast cancer screening is used to identify women with asymptomatic cancer.
- Presently, breast cancer detection relies on mammography as the main screening modality.
- Public education is an important component of early detection and increasing breast awareness among women.
- Clinical breast examination also offers an opportunity to educate women about the importance of early detection, the risks of breast cancer, and breast awareness.
- Breast ultrasound is a useful adjunctive tool for women with dense breasts and in characterizing abnormalities seen on mammography.
- There is a need to identify reliable biomarkers from an easily accessible source that could generate cost-effective assays feasible for routine screening.

References

1. American Cancer Society. Breast Cancer Facts & Figures 2017–2018. Atlanta: American Cancer Society, Inc.; 2017.
2. Gao DL, Thomas DB, Ray RM, Wang WW, Allison CJ, Chen FL, Porter P, Hu YW, Zhao GL, Pan LD, Li WJ, Wu CY, Coriaty Z, Evans I, Lin MG, Stalsberg H, Self SG. Randomized trial of breast self-examination in 266,064 women in Shanghai. Zhonghua Zhong Liu Za Zhi. 2005;27:350–4.
3. Baxter N, Canadian Task force on Preventive Health Care. Preventive health care, 2001 update: should women be routinely taught breast self-examination to screen for breast cancer? CMAJ. 2001;164(13):1837–46.
4. Kosters JP, Gotzsche PC. Regular self-examination or clinical examination for early detection of breast cancer. Cochrane Database Syst Rev. 2003;(2):CD003373. https://doi.org/10.1002/14651858.CD003373.
5. Thornton H, Pillarisetti R. Breast awareness and breast self examination are not the same. What do these terms mean? Why are they confused? What can we do? Eur J Cancer. 2008;44(15):2118–21.
6. Grethelin SJ. Breast examination technique. Updated on 21 Jan 2016. https://emedicine.medscape.com/article/1909276-technique.
7. Boulos S, Gadallah M, Neguib S, et al. Breast screening in the emerging world: high prevalence of breast cancer in Cairo. Breast. 2005;14:340–6.
8. Dinshaw K, Mishra G, Shastri S, et al. Determinants of compliance in a cluster randomised controlled trial on screening of breast and cervix cancer in Mumbai, India. 2. Compliance to referral and treatment. Oncology. 2007;73:154–61.
9. Nelson HD, Tyne K, Naik A, Bougatsos C, Chan BK, Humphrey L, On Behalf of the U.S. Preventive Services Task Force. Screening for breast cancer: an update for the U.S. Preventive Services Task Force. Ann Intern Med. 2009;151:727–37, W237–42. https://doi.org/10.7326/0003-4819-151-10-200911170-00009.
10. Tonelli M, Connor Gorber S, Joffres M, et al. On Behalf of the Canadian Task Force on Preventive Health Care Recommendations on screening for breast cancer in average-risk women aged 40–74 years. CMAJ. 2011;183:1991–2001. https://doi.org/10.1503/cmaj.110334.
11. U.S. Preventive Services Task Force. Screening for breast cancer: U.S. Preventive Services Task Force recommendation statement. Ann Intern Med. 2009;151:716–26, W236. https://doi.org/10.7326/0003-4819-151-10-200911170-00008.
12. Oeffinger KC, Fontham ET, Etzioni R, et al. Breast cancer screening for women at average risk: 2015 guideline update from the American Cancer Society. JAMA. 2015;314:1599–614. https://doi.org/10.1001/jama.2015.12783.
13. National Comprehensive Cancer Network (NCCN). NCCN clinical practice guidelines in oncology: breast cancer screening and diagnosis ver 1.2014. Fort Washington, PA: NCCN; 2014. Current version available online at: https://www.nccn.org/professionals/physician_gls/pdf/breast-screening.pdf (free registration required). Cited 3 June 2016.
14. Gillman J, Toth HK, Moy L. The role of dynamic contrast-enhanced screening breast MRI in populations at increased risk for breast cancer. Womens Health (Lond). 2014;10(6):609–22.

15. Chetlen A, Mack J, Chan T. Breast cancer screening controversies: who, when, why, and how? Clin Imaging. 2016;40(2):279–82.
16. Moseley TW. Digital mammography and digital breast tomosynthesis. Clin Obstet Gynecol. 2016;59(2):362–79.
17. Hendrick RE, Pisano ED, Averbukh A, Moran C, Berns EA, Yaffe MJ, et al. Comparison of acquisition parameters and breast dose in digital mammography and screen-film mammography in the American College of Radiology Imaging Network digital mammographic imaging screening trial. AJR Am J Roentgenol. 2010;194(2):362–9.
18. Fiorica JV. Breast cancer screening, mammography, and other modalities. Clin Obstet Gynecol. 2016;59(4):688–709.
19. Morris E, Feig SA, Drexler M, Lehman C. Implications of overdiagnosis: impact on screening mammography practices. Popul Health Manag. 2015;18(Suppl 1):S3–11.
20. Friedewald SM, Rafferty EA, Rose SL, Durand MA, Plecha DM, Greenberg JS, et al. Breast cancer screening using tomosynthesis in combination with digital mammography. JAMA. 2014;311(24):2499–507.
21. Ciatto S, Houssami N, Bernardi D, Caumo F, Pellegrini M, Brunelli S, et al. Integration of 3D digital mammography with tomosynthesis for population breast-cancer screening (STORM): a prospective comparison study. Lancet Oncol. 2013;14(7):583–9.
22. Spangler ML, Zuley ML, Sumkin JH, Abrams G, Ganott MA, Hakim C, et al. Detection and classification of calcifications on digital breast tomosynthesis and 2D digital mammography: a comparison. AJR Am J Roentgenol. 2011;196(2):320–4.
23. Pace LE, Keating NL. A systematic assessment of benefits and risks to guide breast cancer screening decisions. JAMA. 2014;311(13):1327–35.
24. Miller D, Livingstone V, Herbison P. Interventions for relieving the pain and discomfort of screening mammography. Cochrane Database Syst Rev. 2008;(1):CD002942.
25. Armstrong K, Moye E, Williams S, Berlin JA, Reynolds EE. Screening mammography in women 40 to 49 years of age: a systematic review for the American College of Physicians. Ann Intern Med. 2007;146(7):516–26.
26. Loving VA, DeMartini WB, Eby PR, Gutierrez RL, Peacock S, Lehman CD. Targeted ultrasound in women younger than 30 years with focal breast signs or symptoms: outcomes analyses and management implications. AJR Am J Roentgenol. 2010;195(6):1472–7.
27. Brem RF, Tabar L, Duffy SW, Inciardi MF, Guingrich JA, Hashimoto BE, et al. Assessing improvement in detection of breast cancer with three-dimensional automated breast US in women with dense breast tissue: the SomoInsight Study. Radiology. 2015;274(3):663–73.
28. Kuhl CK, Schrading S, Leutner CC, Morakkabati-Spitz N, Wardelmann E, Fimmers R, et al. Mammography, breast ultrasound, and magnetic resonance imaging for surveillance of women at high familial risk for breast cancer. J Clin Oncol. 2005;23(33):8469–76.
29. Moore SG, Shenoy PJ, Fanucchi L, Tumeh JW, Flowers CR. Cost-effectiveness of MRI compared to mammography for breast cancer screening in a high risk population. BMC Health Serv Res. 2009;9:9. https://doi.org/10.1186/1472-6963-9-9.
30. Saslow D, Boetes C, Burke W, Harms S, Leach MO, Lehman CD, et al. American Cancer Society guidelines for breast screening with MRI as an adjunct to mammography. CA Cancer J Clin. 2007;57(2):75–89.
31. Fu SW, Chen L, Man Y. miRNA biomarkers in breast cancer detection and management. J Cancer. 2011;2:116–22. https://doi.org/10.7150/jca.2.116.
32. Muralidharan-Chari V, Clancy JW, Sedgwick A, D'souza-schorey C. Microvesicles: mediators of extracellular communication during cancer progression. J Cell Sci. 2010;123:1603–11.
33. van't Veer LJ, Dai H, van de Vijver MJ, He YD, Hart AAM, Mao M, et al. Gene expression profiling predicts clinical outcome of breast cancer. Nature. 2002;415(6871):530–6.
34. Melander O, Belting M, Manjer J, Maisel AS, Hedblad B, Engström G, Nilsson P, Struck J, Hartmann O, Bergmann A, Orho-Melander M. Validation of plasma proneurotensin as a novel biomarker for the prediction of incident breast cancer. Cancer Epidemiol Biomarkers Prev. 2014;23(8):1672–6. https://doi.org/10.1158/1055-9965.EPI-13-1200.
35. Kazarian A, Blyuss O, Metodieva G, et al. Testing breast cancer serum biomarkers for early detection and prognosis in pre-diagnosis samples. Br J Cancer. 2017;116(4):501–8. https://doi.org/10.1038/bjc.2016.433.
36. Menendez J, Lupu R, Colomer R. Targeting fatty acid synthase: potential for therapeutic intervention in Her-2/neu-overexpressing breast cancer. Drug News Perspect. 2005;18:375.
37. Colleoni M, Viale G, Zahrieh D, Pruneri G, Gentilini O, Veronesi P, Gelber RD, Curigliano G, Torrisi R, Luini A, Intra M, Galimberti V, Renne G, Nolè F, Peruzzotti G, Goldhirsch A. Chemotherapy is more effective in patients with breast cancer not expressing steroid hormone receptors: a study of preoperative treatment. Clin Cancer Res. 2004;10(19):6622–8.
38. Dowsett M, Houghton J, Iden C, et al. Benefit from adjuvant tamoxifen therapy in primary breast cancer patients according estrogen receptor, progesterone receptor, EGF receptor and HER2 status. Ann Oncol. 2006;17:818–26.
39. Slamon DJ, Leyland-Jones B, Shak S, et al. Use of chemotherapy plus a monoclonal antibody against HER2 for metastatic breast cancer that overexpresses HER2. N Engl J Med. 2001;344:783–92.
40. Chang J, Ormerod M, Powles TJ, Allred DC, Ashley SE, Dowsett M. Apoptosis and proliferation as predic-

tors of chemotherapy response in patients with breast carcinoma. Cancer. 2000;89:2145–52. https://doi.org/10.1002/1097-0142(20001201)89:11<2145::AID-CNCR1>3.0.CO;2-S.
41. Gillett C, Smith P, Gregory W, Richards M, Millis R, Peters G, Barnes D. Cyclin D1 and prognosis in human breast cancer. Int J Cancer. 1996;69:92–9. https://doi.org/10.1002/(SICI)1097-0215(19960422)69:2<92::AID-IJC4>3.0.CO;2-Q.
42. Seshadri R, Lee CS, Hui R, McCaul K, Horsfall DJ, Sutherland RL. Cyclin DI amplification is not associated with reduced overall survival in primary breast cancer but may predict early relapse in patients with features of good prognosis. Clin Cancer Res. 1996;2:1177–84.
43. Keyomarsi K, Tucker SL, Buchholz TA, Callister M, Ding Y, Hortobagyi GN, Bedrosian I, Knickerbocker C, Toyofuku W, Lowe M, et al. Cyclin E and survival in patients with breast cancer. New Engl J Med. 2002;347:1566–75. https://doi.org/10.1056/NEJMoa021153.
44. Skliris GP, Munot K, Bell SM, Carder PJ, Lane S, Horgan K, Lansdown MR, Parkes AT, Hanby AM, Markham AF, et al. Reduced expression of oestrogen receptor beta in invasive breast cancer and its re-expression using DNA methyl transferase inhibitors in a cell line model. J Pathol. 2003;201:213–20. https://doi.org/10.1002/path.1436.
45. Hopp TA, Weiss HL, Parra IS, Cui Y, Osborne CK, Fuqua SA. Low levels of estrogen receptor beta protein predict resistance to tamoxifen therapy in breast cancer. Clin Cancer Res. 2004;10:7490–9. https://doi.org/10.1158/1078-0432.CCR-04-1114.
46. Weigel MT, Dowsett M. Current and emerging biomarkers in breast cancer: prognosis and prediction. Endocr Relat Cancer. 2010;17(4):R245–62.
47. Leon SA, Shapiro B, Sklaroff DM, Yaros MJ. Free DNA in the serum of cancer patients and the effect of therapy. Cancer Res. 1977;37:646–50.
48. Stoetzer OJ, Fersching DM, Salat C, Steinkohl O, Gabka CJ, Hamann U, et al. Prediction of response to neoadjuvant chemotherapy in breast cancer patients by circulating apoptotic biomarkers nucleosomes, DNAse, cytokeratin-18 fragments and survivin. Cancer Lett. 2013;336:140–8.
49. Dos Anjos Pultz B, da Luz FA, de Faria PR, Oliveira AP, de Araújo RA, Silva MJ. Far beyond the usual biomarkers in breast cancer: a review. J Cancer. 2014;5(7):559–71.
50. Siu AL, U.S. Preventive Services Task Force. Screening for breast cancer: U.S. preventive services task force recommendation statement. Ann Intern Med. 2016;164(4):279–96.
51. Oeffinger KC, Fontham ET, Etzioni R, Herzig A, Michaelson JS, Shih YC, et al. Breast cancer screening for women at average risk: 2015 guideline update from the American Cancer Society. JAMA. 2015;314(15):1599–614.
52. Committee on Practice Bulletins-Gynecology. Practice bulletin number 179: breast cancer risk assessment and screening in average-risk women. Obstet Gynecol. 2017;130(1):e1–16.
53. Wilt TJ, Harris RP, Qaseem A, High Value Care Task Force of the American College of Physicians. Screening for cancer: advice for high-value care from the American College of Physicians. Ann Intern Med. 2015;162(10):718–25.
54. Canadian Task Force on Preventive Health Care, Tonelli M, Connor Gorber S, Joffres M, Dickinson J, Singh H, et al. Recommendations on screening for breast cancer in average-risk women aged 40-74 years. CMAJ. 2011;183(17):1991–2001.
55. Rajaraman P, Anderson BO, Basu P, Belinson JL, Cruz AD, Dhillon PK, et al. Recommendations for screening and early detection of common cancers in India. Lancet Oncol. 2015;16(7):e352–61.
56. Yip CH, Smith RA, Anderson BO, Miller AB, et al. Guideline implementation for breast healthcare in low and middle income countries. Cancer. 2008;113:2244–56.
57. Mandelblatt JS, Cronin KA, Bailey S, Berry DA, de Koning HJ, Draisma G, et al. Effects of mammography screening under different screening schedules: model estimates of potential benefits and harms. Ann Intern Med. 2009;151(10):738–47.
58. Walter LC, Covinsky KE. Cancer screening in elderly patients: a framework for individualized decision making. JAMA. 2001;285(21):2750–6.
59. Smith RA, Saslow D, Sawyer KA, Burke W, Costanza ME, Evans WP 3rd, et al. American cancer society guidelines for breast cancer screening: update 2003. CA Cancer J Clin. 2003;53(3):141–69.
60. Bhatia S, Robison LL, Oberlin O, Greenberg M, Bunin G, Fossati-Bellani F, et al. Breast cancer and other second neoplasms after childhood Hodgkin's disease. N Engl J Med. 1996;334(12):745–51.
61. Bhatia S, Yasui Y, Robison LL, Birch JM, Bogue MK, Diller L, et al. High risk of subsequent neoplasms continues with extended follow-up of childhood Hodgkin's disease: report from the Late Effects Study Group. J Clin Oncol. 2003;21(23):4386–94.
62. Hancock SL, Tucker MA, Hoppe RT. Breast cancer after treatment of Hodgkin's disease. J Natl Cancer Inst. 1993;85(1):25–31.
63. Metayer C, Lynch CF, Clarke EA, Glimelius B, Storm H, Pukkala E, et al. Second cancers among long-term survivors of Hodgkin's disease diagnosed in childhood and adolescence. J Clin Oncol. 2000;18(12):2435–43.
64. van Leeuwen FE, Klokman WJ, Stovall M, Dahler EC, van't Veer MB, Noordijk EM, et al. Roles of radiation dose, chemotherapy, and hormonal factors in breast cancer following Hodgkin's disease. J Natl Cancer Inst. 2003;95(13):971–80.
65. Yahalom J, Petrek JA, Biddinger PW, Kessler S, Dershaw DD, McCormick B, et al. Breast cancer in patients irradiated for Hodgkin's disease: a clinical

and pathologic analysis of 45 events in 37 patients. J Clin Oncol. 1992;10(11):1674–81.
66. McCormack VA, dos Santos Silva I. Breast density and parenchymal patterns as markers of breast cancer risk: a meta-analysis. Cancer Epidemiol Biomarkers Prev. 2006;15(6):1159–69.
67. Byrne C, Schairer C, Wolfe J, Parekh N, Salane M, Brinton LA, et al. Mammographic features and breast cancer risk: effects with time, age, and menopause status. J Natl Cancer Inst. 1995;87(21):1622–9.
68. Boyd NF, Guo H, Martin LJ, Sun L, Stone J, Fishell E, et al. Mammographic density and the risk and detection of breast cancer. N Engl J Med. 2007;356(3):227–36.

Breast Cancer Risk Assessment and Genetic Testing

29

Nidhi Arora and Sumita Mehta

29.1 Introduction

Breast cancer is a heterogeneous disorder and is the most common cancer in women all over the world [1], and its incidence has increased in the last few decades. According to the 2012 statistics [2], almost 1.7 million new breast cancer cases were diagnosed which account for approximately 12% of all new cancer cases. Thirty percent of all new cancer cases in women have been reported due to breast cancer [3]. Of all the causes of death from cancer, this is the fifth most common cause of death. The reasons contributing to its increased incidence are timely detection due to the rapid improvement in the screening strategies all over the world. The factor increasing the prevalence of this cancer is the advancement in the treatment protocols all over the world that have helped in improving the survival rate after the diagnosis. The 5-year survival rate has improved to 90% as compared to 75% in 1975 [4].

N. Arora
Department of Fetal Medicine, Rainbow Hospital, New Delhi, India

S. Mehta (✉)
Department of Obstetrics and Gynecology, Babu Jagjivan Ram Memorial Hospital, New Delhi, India

29.2 Risk Factors

The most important risk factors for breast cancer are increasing age and female sex. Other risk factors are mentioned in Table 29.1.

29.2.1 Gender/Sex

Breast cancer is primarily seen in women with 99% of cases diagnosed in women and approximately 1% of breast malignancy in men. The risk factor for breast cancer in men includes obesity, Klinefelter syndrome, heavy alcohol use, family

Table 29.1 Risk factors for breast cancer

Female sex
Advancing age
Pathogenic germline mutations
Family history: breast, ovary, pancreas or prostate cancer (features of HBOC)
Ethnic origins: Ashkenazi Jewish population
Reproductive factors: nulliparity, early age at menarche, delayed menopause
Hormonal factors
Modifiable risk factors: obesity, alcohol, smoking, inadequate physical activity
Previous biopsy results: atypical hyperplasia, LCIS
Radiation exposure between 10 and 30 years

S. Mehta, A. Singla (eds.), *Preventive Oncology for the Gynecologist*,
https://doi.org/10.1007/978-981-13-3438-2_29

history, previous estrogenic hormonal therapy, and previous radiation exposure to chest.

29.2.2 Age

This is the strongest factor known to affect the breast cancer risk. The risk increases with increasing age. It is seen most commonly in the postmenopausal age group when the risk doubles with every decade till 80 years of life [5]. After that, there is a decrease in the incidence of breast cancer which could be because of inadequate screening. In men, the risk of breast cancer also increases with increasing age.

29.2.3 Race and Socioeconomic Status

Risk of breast cancer is highest in Caucasian women, followed by Hispanics and African-American population. It is seen lowest in Asian women [5]. It is seen more commonly in women in the higher socioeconomic status which could be due to the change in lifestyle and reproductive factors [6].

29.2.4 Radiation Exposure

Therapeutic chest radiation increases the risk of breast cancer. This risk correlates with the doses received, the age at which there has been exposure to the radiation, and the time elapsed since the exposure [7]. Effect of ionizing radiation is most pronounced at the time of puberty, even at low doses [8].

29.2.5 Family History

Breast cancer has a familial predilection. If there is a family history of breast cancer, especially in the first-degree relative, the risk of developing cancer almost becomes twice the population-based risk [9].

29.2.6 Hereditary Breast Cancers

There is an earlier onset of breast cancer in women (and men) in syndrome-associated familial breast cancers. About 2–5% of all breast cancers are inherited [10]. Approximately, 4–5% of breast cancer is thought to be inherited with autosomal dominant predisposing gene mutation [11]. The most common genes searched after gene linkage analysis are BRCA1 and BRCA2. They are associated with hereditary breast and ovarian cancer (HBOC). In a study by Lalloo et al., almost 20% of breast cancer patients less than or equal to 30 years were caused by well-known genes, BRCA1, BRCA2, and TP53 [12]. The types of pathogenic variants of BRCA gene are described along with their cancer risk in Table 29.2.

BRCA 1 and BRCA 2: BRCA1 (on chromosome 17) and BRCA2 (on chromosome 13) are tumor suppressor genes with multitudinous cell functions, such as transcription, regulation of cell cycle, genomic stability, and DNA repair [24]. Its prevalence in the general population (excluding Ashkenazi Jewish population) is approximately 1:400 to 1:500 [25, 26].

The modes of inheritance for these genes are autosomal dominant. The various other genes associated with inherited breast cancer are enumerated along with their breast cancer risk in Table 29.3.

Table 29.2 Risk of various types of malignancies in individuals of BRCA1/BRCA2 pathogenic variants [13–23]

Cancer	Population risk	BRCA1	BRCA2
Breast	12%	46–87%	38–84%
Second primary breast	2% in 5 years	21.1% in 10 years	10.8% in 10 years
Ovarian	1–2%	39–63%	16.5–27%
Male breast cancer	0.1%	1.2%	8.9%
Prostate	6% by 69 years	8.6% by 65 years	15% by 65 years, 29% by lifetime
Pancreatic	0.5%	1–3%	2–7%
Melanoma	1.6%		Increased risk

Table 29.3 Various cancer-specific syndromes and their breast cancer risk

Cancer-specific syndrome	Gene	Inheritance	Breast cancer risk	Associated tumors
Li–Fraumeni syndrome [27]	TP53	AD	≤79% (premenopausal)	Soft tissue sarcoma, osteosarcoma, brain tumors, adrenocortical cancer, leukemias •Occur in childhood or young adulthood
Cowden syndrome [28]	PTEN	AD	25–50%	Thyroid cancer Renal cell carcinoma Endometrial carcinoma Colorectal cancer Hamartomas Trichilemmomas Papillomatous papules •Present some features by 20 years
Hereditary diffuse gastric cancer [29]	CDH1	AD	39–52%	Diffuse gastric cancer •Present before 40 years
CHEK2 [30]	CHEK	AD	25–39%	Prostate cancer Stomach cancer Sarcoma Kidney cancer
ATM heterozygotes [31]	*ATM*	AD	17–52%	
PALB2 [32]	PALB2	AD	≤58%	Male breast cancer Pancreatic cancer
Peutz–Jeghers syndrome [27]	SKT11	AD	32–54%	Gastrointestinal malignancies Ovary, cervix, uterus, pancreas Sertoli cell testicular and lung cancer Gastrointestinal polyposis
Bloom syndrome	BLM	AR	Increased risk	Epithelial carcinoma Lymphoma, leukemia Severe pre- and postnatal growth deficiency, sparse subcutaneous fat tissue, short stature, sun-sensitive, erythematous skin lesion of the face
Werner syndrome [33]	WRN	AR	Increased risk	Sarcomas Melanoma Thyroid cancer Hematologic malignancies

29.2.7 Reproductive Factors

These are early menarche, late menopause, nulliparity, longer interval between menarche and first pregnancy, and decreased breastfeeding. All these reflect the risks arising from the hormonal changes in estrogen and progesterone in the life of a woman. These factors mainly carry risks for hormone receptor-positive cancer.

29.2.7.1 Early Menarche and Late Menopause

The risk of developing breast cancer decreases by almost 5% with increase in every 1 year of decreased age of menarche [34]. The increased age at the menopause, on the other hand, increases the breast cancer risk.

29.2.7.2 Parity and Breastfeeding

In comparison to nulliparous females, the parous females have almost 17–41% lower risk of developing breast cancer [34]. The risk with each added pregnancy is reduced by approximately 7% [35], and with each year of breastfeeding, the relative risk of developing breast cancer decreases by 4.3%. With the hormonal milieu during pregnancy and breastfeeding, the breast epithelial cells become time and again well differentiated saving them from the damage that is bound to happen because of DNA damage during the reproductive period [36].

29.2.7.3 Age at the First Birth

Apart from the number of pregnancies, the age at the first pregnancy becomes an important determining factor of breast cancer. This could be attributed to the advantage provided by the early onset of the final terminal duct maturation of the breast [37]. If a woman has the first pregnancy at or after 35 years of age, her risk of having breast cancer is 60% more as compared to women with the first pregnancy at 18 years of age [34].

29.2.8 Hormonal Therapy

29.2.8.1 Oral Contraceptive Pills (OCPs)

The association between the use of OCP and breast cancer is well established with an overall 20% increased risk among women currently using OCP as compared to women who have never used [38]. Mørch et al. [39], in a recently published large prospective study in women younger than 50 years, observed a 20% higher risk of breast cancer among women who were currently using or had recently used hormonal contraceptives, and the risk increased with the duration of contraceptive used. This relative risk increased from 1.09 with less than 1 year of use to 1.38 with more than 10 years of use. Every different formulation of birth control pill as well as the intrauterine device (IUD) that releases the hormone levonorgestrel (a progestin) was associated with a higher risk of breast cancer.

Increased risk with the use of hormonal contraceptive in women at higher risk for developing breast cancer due to strong family history or due to the presence of *BRCA1* or *BRCA2* mutation is controversial till date. A meta-analysis looking at the increased risk of breast cancer in such population suggested that associations between ever use of OCPs and breast cancer among women who are *BRCA1* or *BRCA2* mutation carriers are similar to those reported for the general population [40].

29.2.8.2 Postmenopausal Hormone Therapy

Long-term estrogen replacement (more than 5 years) post menopause has been shown to increase the risk of breast cancer; however, it has not been seen when used for short term to treat menopausal symptoms. On the contrary, combined short-term estrogen-progestin use has shown increased risk [41]. Estrogen antagonists (selective estrogen receptor modulators) on the contrary have shown a protective effect on breast cancer incidence [42].

29.2.9 Benign Breast Disorders

Women with histological diagnosis of atypical ductal/lobular hyperplasia and lobular carcinoma in situ on biopsy specimens from suspected benign breast lesions have a four times higher risk of developing breast cancer [43]. The various histological types of benign breast disorder that are seen associated with breast cancer risks [44] are tabulated with their relative risks in Table 29.4.

The relative risks differ with the menopausal status [45]. It is 5.9 (95% CI, 2.9–13.2) in premenopausal group with atypical hyperplasia, whereas in the postmenopausal age group, it is less 2.3 (95% CI, 0.9–5.9). The type of histology also affects the breast cancer risk, with lobular hyperplasia having a fivefold increase in cancer risk as compared to ductal hyperplasia (2.4-fold increase). Both have a higher risk when compared to women with nonproliferative breast lesions [46].

Table 29.4 The pathological types of benign breast diseases and their breast cancer risks [42]

Breast disease	Breast cancer risk	OR (95% CI)
Benign disease without hyperplasia	1.5-fold	1.5 (1.3–1.9)
Hyperplasia with atypia	2.6-fold	2.6 (1.6–4.1)
Hyperplasia without atypia	1.8-fold	1.8 (1.1–2.5)
Fibroadenoma	1.7-fold	1.7 (1.1–2.5)

29.2.9.1 Density of the Breast

Women with higher breast density have a higher risk of development of breast cancer [47]. Also, there is difficulty in detecting cancer in dense breasts. Among women with more than 75% breast density, the risk of breast cancer is more than four times that of women with much less dense breasts [48]. The density of the breast is measured by the amount of radiodense areas. This represents the epithelial tissue and the stroma [49]. It correlates with epithelial proliferation and stromal fibrosis.

29.3 Modifiable Risk Factors

29.3.1 Obesity and Physical Activity

Increasing body mass index (BMI) especially at adult onset has been associated with an increased risk for breast cancer in postmenopausal women, while this association is not seen in premenopausal women [50]. However, an increased BMI becomes a protective factor for young adolescent girls. This could be explained by the early age for menarche with obesity in these girls. Physical activity decreases the breast cancer risk in postmenopausal women; however, it has not been proven for premenopausal women [51].

29.3.2 Alcohol

Intake of alcohol at any age is considered a risk factor for breast cancer. The risk with alcohol is usually dose-dependent, and it increases to around 7.1% for every 10 g of alcohol consumed each day [52]. This alcohol-related risk can be attributed to the effects of alcohol on folate metabolism which is required for the action of the hormones [53].

29.3.3 Smoking

There have been multiple studies on association of smoking with breast cancer; however, the results have been inconclusive. A meta-analysis by Gaudet et al. that included 15 prospective cohort studies till 2013 on association of smoking with breast cancer showed that smoking any time in life whether current or former increases the breast cancer risk [54]. In a recent study by Catsburg et al., it was concluded that women with history of smoking for more than 40 cigarettes in a day for over 40 years are at the highest risk of breast cancer [55].

The relative risk for breast cancer associated with various risk factors is shown in Table 29.5.

Table 29.5 Relative risk of known breast cancer risk factors

Relative risk <2	Relative risk 2–4	Relative risk >4
Early menarche	One first-degree relative with breast cancer	Mutation *BRCA1* or *BRCA2*
Late menopause		LCIS
Nulliparity	*CHEK2* mutation	Atypical hyperplasia
Hormone replacement therapy	Age >35 years for the first birth	Radiation exposure before 30
Alcohol use	Proliferative breast disease	
Postmenopausal obesity		

29.4 Breast Cancer Risk Assessment

As detailed, the breast cancer risk is based on the combination of the above risk factors (see Table 29.2). In the initial history taking, it is important to include the reproductive factors, hormone use, BMI, radiation exposure, and any specific family history of breast and other cancers, i.e., ovarian, pancreatic, colon, prostate, and other types of germline cancers in first-, second-, and third-degree relative. The biopsy reports should also be reviewed for the type of lesions diagnosed earlier.

With respect to family history, it is also important to take into consideration the age of the affected family member at the time of diagnosis. The incidence of bilateral breast cancer in the affected relative is important. It can be counted as

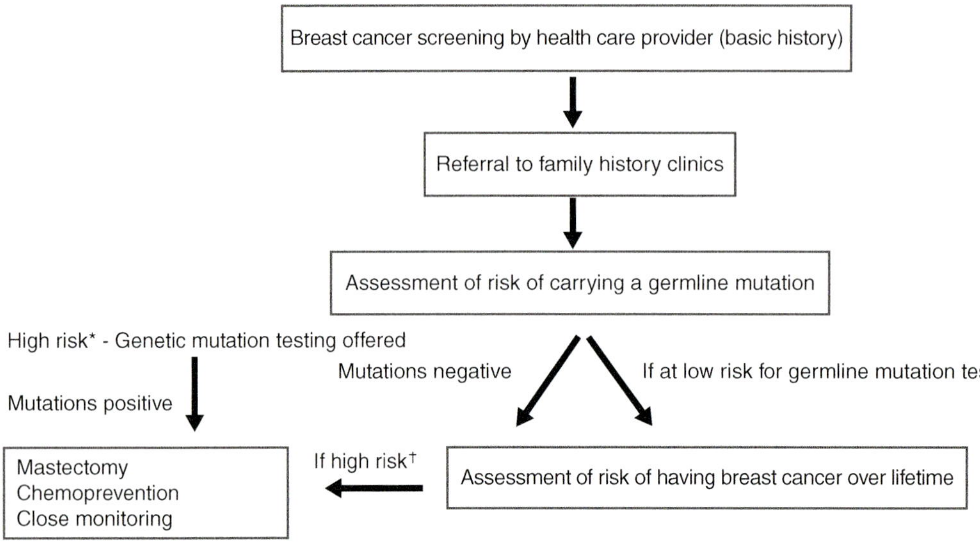

*High risk is labelled as with greater than 10% risk of carrying the pathological mutation and low risk as 10% or less. †High risk usually defined as a 5-year risk of developing breast cancer more than 1.67%, and low risk usually defined as a 5-year risk of developing breast cancer 1.67% or lower. Reproduced from Amir et al. [57]. By permission of Oxford University Press

Fig. 29.1 Breast cancer screening and mutation testing.

two affected relatives for the calculation of the overall risk. The number of members affected particularly on one side is another aspect of risk calculation. The frequency of unaffected members should also be taken into account as with big families and few affected individuals, the chances of a germline predisposing gene would be less.

The family history of breast cancer is very important to look for the predisposing gene in the family since, apart from BRCA1/BRCA2 dominantly inherited genes, hereditary factors are also important in association with sporadic cancers but at present are difficult to be evaluated, and more genome-wide studies are required in the future [56].

The factors like early age at the diagnosis of cancers and more than one cancer in a single individual in the pedigree give a clue toward the possibility of germline mutations in the family. The risk calculated varies with the age of onset in a family member in relation to the degree of relationship. For instance, if we compare with respect to the age group, the risk is three times if a first-degree relative has been affected at less than 40 years of age in comparison to the age group of greater than 65 years. Again, this becomes two times, if the age group is between 40 and 50 years and is one and half times if the age group is 50–65 years. All these are the risks calculated for the first-degree family members affected [9].

Women who become positive with any of these risk factors should be further assessed by any of the web tools for breast cancer risk assessment like Gail, BRCAPRO, Breast and Ovarian Analysis of Disease Incidence and Carrier Estimation Algorithm, International Breast Cancer Intervention Studies, or Claus model. Figure 29.1 describes the breast cancer screening and mutation testing algorithm in low- and high-risk women [57].

Types of risk assessment—two groups [57]:

1. The risk of carrying a mutation in a known high-risk gene such as BRCA1 or BRCA2
2. Chances of developing breast cancer over a given life span in the presence or absence of such mutation

Different online tools take into consideration either one of or both these aspects. However, it is very important to assess all known risk contributors to evaluate the breast cancer risks over a time period.

There are two types of risk assessment models [57]:

1. Empirical model
2. Genetic risk prediction model

The first type (empirical) calculates the probability of detecting BRCA mutations without any explicit assumption of the underlying genetic risks like the type of inheritance, the frequency of mutations, or the penetrance, whereas the genetic risk prediction models make these assumptions regarding the number of susceptible genes involved and the frequency of alleles in the population along with their cancer risks.

29.4.1 Empirical Models

These are Shattuck–Eidens model (Myriad 1) and Couch model (UPenn or Penn). These were the earliest models developed even before the genetic testing evolved. Nowadays, these have been modified further with incorporation of risk factors including individual and family history. The Penn II model [58] now includes more comprehensive personal and family cancer histories. Furthermore, the scoring systems were developed, and cutoffs were defined to estimate the risk of carrying the germline mutation. These were used in the family history assessment tool [59] and the Manchester model [60]. Other examples are the Myriad II, National Cancer Institute, and the Australian LAMBDA models.

29.4.2 Genetic Risk Prediction Models

These can calculate the cancer risks and mutation carrier probability irrespective of family structure and the disease type. These specifically involve the use of family pedigree to extract the exact family relationships, and the cancer risks are computed. But, their calculations are merely based on the estimated assumptions. Also, since the cancer susceptibility genes are still under evaluation, these models can give only approximate risks. The various models under this subgroup are BRCAPRO model, Yale University model, International Breast Cancer Intervention Study (IBIS) model, and the Breast and Ovarian Analysis of Disease Incidence and Carrier Estimation Algorithm (BOADICEA).

29.4.3 Limitations of Various Models

The different models consume varying time intervals for the risk assessment depending upon the scoring systems and the computerized calculations.

The most important risk factor is family history apart from the age. Detailed family history is difficult to be reproduced as it is a retrospective data. Also, emotional and ethical issues with respect to adoption come into play. With the nuclear family concept [61], the knowledge about distant family is scarce. Patients are also reluctant to discuss the illness of their family sometimes due to social issues. It is a mistaken assumption to consider only maternal family history in cases of breast and ovarian cancer [62], and it has been reported in the literature [63, 64] that parental medical illness is not precisely reproduced and discussed by the offspring.

An important limitation is the incorporation of history of cancers of the breast and ovary only with respect to first- and second-degree relatives in different models. This can further underestimate the risks calculated. So despite continuous improvement in various types of models, the data collection is limited especially with respect to family history. In some models the family history of other BRCA-associated cancers like pancreatic and prostate is not evaluated [65]. In order to improve these algorithms, these models should consider including the population-specific risks, the prevalence of various genetic mutations, and/or the cancer-specific characteristics. The latest literature has improved the accuracy of risk calculation by addition of pathological features of the various types of breast and ovarian cancer [66, 67].

The most commonly used models are discussed below.

29.4.3.1 Gail Model

It is the most frequently used method [68] and was developed by Dr. Mitchell Gail in 1989. A screening study (1973–1980) of 300,000 women aged between 35 and 74 years, as a part of the Breast Cancer Detection and Demonstration Project, was conducted to draft this online tool. Subsequently, it has been validated in the Nurses' Health Study [69], and modification was done in 1999 [70].

The modified model (NCI Gail model) differs from the original draft in three aspects. The original model considers both invasive and in situ cancers, whereas the modified version only incorporates the invasive cancers. The age-specific incidence rates have been gathered by the Surveillance, Epidemiology, and End Results database rather than from the Breast Cancer Detection and Demonstration Project in the modified tool. And lastly, the composite incidence rates for African-American patients have been incorporated in the modification.

It comprises of seven key factors: age; age at menarche; age at the first pregnancy; family history of breast cancer in mother, daughter, or sister; previous breast biopsy and their number; biopsy with atypical hyperplasia; and race/ethnicity. A 5-year risk of greater than or equal to 1.67% is defined as "high risk" and is an indication to start with risk-lowering drugs.

It is not appropriate to be used in women less than 35 years of age, women with family history of breast cancer on paternal side, and in second-degree relative, and it also doesn't take into account the history of other cancers related with germline mutations. Another important limitation of this model is that the biopsy results not with atypical hyperplasia are not included while calculating the risk. In such situations the other online models can be of appropriate use. Of the current available evidence, this is the only tool that has been validated in large population-based databases [69, 70]; however, it has limited discriminatory accuracy [71]. It can therefore not be used in higher-risk groups, for example, in the family history clinics [72].

29.4.3.2 Claus Model [11]

This has been developed using data from Cancer and Steroid Hormone Study, conducted from 1980 to 1982 in which the patients enrolled from eight Surveillance, Epidemiology, and End Results regions. It uses just the family history to estimate risk as compared to the abovementioned Gail model where many other factors are also considered. But the advantage over the Gail model is that the family history is taken extensively, and both first- and second-degree relatives are taken into account. Also, their age at the onset of breast cancer is included. Paternal family history is also incorporated in the pedigree. The family history of only breast cancer was initially asked, but recent modification also questions about the ovarian cancer history. The tables were further drafted giving the lifetime risks of first- and second-degree relatives [73].

Limitations of Claus Model

The first drawback is that only the hereditary factors are incorporated, so the individual hormonal and reproductive associated individual risks are not evaluated. The risks calculated are still based on the data collected from North American women in the 1980s. However, the current studies show that the incidence of breast cancer in the same population as well as in some European groups is higher as compared to the incidence rates collected for the model. Another very important limitation is the difference between the published tables and the computerized versions [74]. The computerized risks are considerably lower than those calculated from the tables. This could be explained by the advantage of computerized adjustments due to the included unaffected family members. A large unaffected population definitely reduces the inherent risk of inheriting a germline mutation. It could also be due to noninclusion of population-based risks in the computerized model or because of the level at which the adjustments are done for the unaffected family members.

An important thing to consider is the huge differences in the risk calculation by the Claus and the NCI Gail model. This was largely seen in women with nulliparity, with multiple benign breast biopsies, or with paternal or first-degree family history [75, 76].

29.4.3.3 BRCAPRO Model

This online model was developed by Parmigiani et al. [77] at the Institute of Statistics and Decision Sciences, Duke University, USA. It is used to predict the probability of mutation in BRCA1 and BRCA2 genes in the individual. This model calculates the risk of breast cancer on the basis of Bayes rules of determining probability of a mutation, once the family history is provided. The mutation frequencies in the general population and in the Ashkenazi Jews give an estimate of the probability of the mutation in the studied subject, before checking the family history [78–80]. It includes the history of first- and second-degree relatives.

The main feature of this model is that family history of both affected and unaffected relatives is used for the risk calculation. It was initially validated only for female population but at present is used for both men and women.

Limitations: Just like the Claus model, only hereditary factors are taken into consideration without incorporating other individual risk factors.

29.4.3.4 Jonker Model [81]

This is a combination of features from the Claus and the BRCAPRO models. Family history of both breast and ovarian cancers is included. It is based upon the hypothesis that hereditary breast cancer can be due to three types of genes—BRCA1, BRCA2, and an unknown gene named as BRCAu. This can explain all non-BRCA germline mutation cancers. This also doesn't include non-hereditary risk factors and thereby can underestimate the overall risks.

29.4.3.5 IBIS Model

This is also known as the Tyrer–Cuzick model [82]. The main advantage of this model is that it includes the family history, reproductive risk factors, and also the history of benign breast disease. Data has been collected from the International Breast Intervention Study. This model includes the presence of multiple genes of differing penetrance.

29.4.3.6 BOADICEA Model

The concept of segregation analysis has been used here, which explains the mutation in BRCA genes along with polygenic inheritance, which defines the combined effect of multiple small genes [83]. Initial design calculated only the risk of carrying a germline mutation [83], but the latest validation also gives the risk of developing breast cancer over lifetime [66].

Even after extensive studies by various probability models, there is no clearly defined risk threshold that can be used in determining the appropriate use of genetic testing (American Society of Clinical Oncology 2003) [84]. However, the use of these models has somehow helped to discriminate which individuals are likely to have pathological variants of BRCA gene.

A comparison of various probability models is shown in Table 29.6.

Table 29.6 Comparison of risk assessment models

Method	Empirical model (myriad prevalence tables) [58–60]	NCI Gail model [70]	BRCAPRO [77]	BOADICEA [83]	IBIS model [82]
Description	Calculates the probability of detecting BRCA mutations without any explicit assumption of the underlying genetic risks Uses only history (both self and family) documented in the forms	Statistical model, absolute risk is calculated for the next 5 years and over lifetime	Statistical model, assumption based on autosomal dominant inheritance of BRCA1/2	Statistical model, assumption based on polygenic risk	Statistical model, assumption based on autosomal dominant inheritance of BRCA1/2
	Tested individual (proband) may be affected or unaffected by breast or ovarian cancer	Tested individual is unaffected by breast cancer	Tested individual may be affected or unaffected by breast or ovarian cancer	Tested individual may be affected or unaffected by breast or ovarian cancer	Tested individual should be unaffected by breast or ovarian cancer
	Age at time of onset of breast cancer is taken as greater or less than 50 years		Exact age at the time of onset of breast cancer is incorporated	Exact age at the time of onset of breast cancer is incorporated	
	Family history significant only if ≥1 relative with breast cancer at age ≥50 years	Only first-degree relatives with breast cancer are considered	Includes all first- and second-degree family members with or without cancer	Includes all first- and second-degree family members with or without cancer	
		Age, reproductive history, and previous history of breast disease also considered			Reproductive history, BMI, and history of benign breast disease also considered
	Includes Ashkenazi Jewish ancestry		Includes Ashkenazi Jewish ancestry	Includes Ashkenazi Jewish ancestry	
Limitations	Simplified and easy to use		Requires computer software and time-consuming data entry	Requires computer software and time-consuming data entry	Requires computer software and time-consuming data entry
	Early age of breast cancer onset	Limited discriminatory accuracy, cannot be used in higher-risk groups	Risk factors other than the family history are not evaluated	Risk factors other than the family history are not evaluated	

29.5 Genetic Mutation Analysis

The various genes associated with breast cancer risk have been tabulated in Table 29.3 along with their mode of inheritance.

According to US Preventive Services Task Force [85] and NICE guidelines [86], women who have the following risk factors are further offered BRCA testing.

- More than one first-degree relative affected with breast cancer and one of them affected ≤50 years of age
- Greater than three first-degree relatives affected irrespective of their age of presentation
- Combination of both ovarian cancer and breast cancer in first- and second-degree relative
- Cancer affecting both breasts in any first-degree relative
- Greater than two first- or second-degree relatives with ovarian cancer irrespective of the age at presentation
- Breast cancer and ovarian cancer at any age in a first- or second-degree relative
- Any male relative affected with breast cancer
- Women with Ashkenazi Jewish heritage with first-degree relative (or two second-degree relatives) with breast/ovarian cancer

It is important to know that even after mutation analysis for BRCA genes in women with significant family history of breast cancer, results can come as negative. These are termed as a "wild type." Of these wild-type cases, around 12% can still have a large genomic deletion or duplication in one of these genes, and approximately 5% are likely to have a mutation in the rest of the breast cancer-predisposing genes [87].

According to the National Comprehensive Cancer Network (NCCN) Clinical Practice Guidelines in Oncology [88], there are some added scenarios in which genetic testing for Hereditary Breast and Ovarian Cancer can be offered.

- Triple-negative breast cancer, especially when diagnosed before age 60 years
- Individuals with pancreatic cancer and/or prostate cancer (Gleason score ≥7) along with breast cancer and/or ovarian cancer (any of these combinations)

29.5.1 Diagnosis

Molecular genetic testing is used to identify heterozygous germline pathogenic variants in BRCA1 or BRCA2 [89].

1. *Targeted analysis*. It is used for founder germline pathogenic variants—BRCA1 c.68_69delAG (BIC: 185delAG), BRCA1 c.5266dupC (BIC: 5382insC), and BRCA2 c.5946delT (BIC: 6174delT).
2. *BRCA1 and BRCA2 gene panel*. Both sequence analyses along with deletion/duplication analysis of BRCA1 and BRCA2 are done.
3. *Multigene panel*. This includes testing for other genes of interest along with BRCA1 and BRCA2. It is very important to understand what kind of testing should be preferred in different individuals.

For example, in individuals with Ashkenazi Jewish descent, the targeted analysis can be performed as there is a high population frequency of the three founder pathogenic variants. Also, coexistence of more than one of these three variants has been reported in few families. On the other hand, if there is a knowledge of BRCA1 or BRCA2 pathogenic variant on one side of the family along with the typical features of HBOC on the other side, sequence and deletion/duplication analysis of *BRCA1* and *BRCA2* can be performed.

The clinicians should also be aware of the various genes available in the multigene panel along with their sensitivities as this may vary from lab to lab and over time. All these options should be weighed according to the affording cost of the individual.

29.5.2 Interpretation of Results

Once an individual has been identified as positive for germline pathogenic variant in *BRCA1* or

BRCA2, proper counselling of available options of surveillance and prevention should be discussed.

The prevention strategies are prophylactic bilateral mastectomy, prophylactic bilateral oophorectomy, and chemoprevention.

29.5.3 Surveillance [88, 89]

In women:

- Self-examination of the breast every month.
- Annual or 6-monthly clinical breast examination starting at 25 years of age.
- Breast MRI yearly to be initiated at 25 years. It can be advised early if the onset of cancer in the family is at age less than 30 years.
- Yearly mammography starting at 30 years of age.
- Transvaginal sonography and serum CA 125 evaluation yearly ≥35 years.

This is important if a woman has not opted for prophylactic mastectomy/oophorectomy.

In men:

- Self-breast examination of the breast every month after training starting at 35 years of age
- Yearly clinical breast examination at age 35.
- Annual screening for prostate cancer starting at age 45.

The prevention and treatment strategies are beyond the scope of this chapter.

29.6 Genetic Counselling for Breast Cancer Risk Assessment [90]

Genetic counselling is the process in which the individuals and families are provided information relevant to the nature, inheritance, and implications of genetic disorders in order to help them take medical and personal decisions.

As described in the beginning, the inheritance of most of the breast cancer predisposing genes is autosomal dominant. This implies that offspring of an individual identified as having a pathogenic gene variant have a 50% chance of inheriting the same and the risk that the sibling of an index case will inherit the same variant is 50%.

Though most of the individuals with pathogenic variants in BRCA1 or BRCA2 have got it from either of the parents, but due to incomplete penetrance, gender of the parent, varying age of onset of cancer, prophylactic surgeries, and early death, all individuals with such pathological variants may not have a parent with the diagnosis of cancer.

Once an individual is tested positive for BRCA1/BRCA2 pathogenic variants, both parents should be offered molecular testing so as to identify the side of the family is at risk. In most of the cases, the pedigree analysis representing the cancers in the family of the proband gives us the information as to which parent is tested first.

Rarely, when neither of the parents come as positive for any of these variants, it can be of a de novo origin; it has been reported as less than 5% only [91–93]. Also, before attributing the negative testing of both parents to de novo origin, alternate paternity or maternity and adoption should be ruled out. Due to the rapid advancement in prenatal and preconception counselling, many young couples may come up to clinicians for genetic counselling regarding breast cancer issues. The best time to offer such counselling is before planning of pregnancy.

It is definitely important to discuss potential risks to the offspring and provide the available reproductive options to the affected couples or who are found to be at risk as part of the same pedigree. The position of the particular individual in that pedigree will help the geneticist to identify the risks and offer further counselling.

Prenatal testing can be discussed, but ethical and legal issues vary with the country of origin as it would lead to the termination of pregnancy rather than the need for early testing of the offspring. Still, these issues should be discussed specially in the current scenario.

29.6.1 Genetic Evaluation of Younger Age Group

According to the available recommendations by the American College of Medical Genetics and the American Society of Human Genetics, it is not advisable to offer genetic testing at less than 18 years of age. Genetic testing for HBOC is not recommended for at-risk individuals younger than age 18 years. However, it can be done if required for medical management in certain cases. Since the management of such inherited cancers begins at 25 years of age, one should ideally wait for an individual to be capable of making independent decisions.

29.6.2 Pros and Cons of Genetic Testing for Inherited Breast Cancers

1. The proband once identified as a carrier for the pathogenic germline variant gets an advantage of early detection by screening at a younger age and can opt for the preventive strategies for cancer reduction.
2. Those that have been identified as negative for these mutations along with their offspring have the benefit of cost reduction over various expensive screening strategies. This also decreases the level of anxiety and stress for the development of breast cancer.
3. The decision of genetic testing by one member in the family and the final results can have implications to the rest of the family [94].

Genetic testing is also performed once diagnosis of cancer is made in the patient for the surveillance post therapy and to calculate the probability of other organs being affected in the lifetime. And here, it is a very mixed psychological feeling when one receives inconclusive results despite significant family history. This could imply that even if they are negative for the known mutant genes, they have no assurance that they are not at any risk for hereditary cancers in self or the offspring. In such cases, further testing the patient and the family becomes important, and there is a possibility of genes other than the known BRCA1 and BRCA2 variants to be involved.

Key Points

- Breast cancer contributes to 30% of all new cancers identified in women.
- Risk assessment is based on the interplay of multiple risk factors.
- Clinicians and health workers should evaluate the risk factors and distinguish between the average-risk and high-risk population by the available and most appropriate models for risk assessment.
- Family history must be taken in detail, and referral can be made to family history clinics.
- If there is high risk based on the family history, genetic mutation testing should be offered.
- An appropriate gene panel should be offered for the genetic testing keeping in mind the affordability.
- Once declared as positive on mutation testing, adequate counselling by the genetic counsellor should be offered.

References

1. Torre LA, Bray F, Siegel RL, Ferlay J, Lortet-Tieulent J, Jemal A. Global cancer statistics, 2012. CA Cancer J Clin. 2015;65(2):87–108.
2. Ferlay J, Soerjomataram I, Ervik M, Dikshit R, Eser S, Mathers C, et al. GLOBOCAN 2012 v1.1, Cancer Incidence and Mortality Worldwide: IARC Cancer Base No. 11.
3. Siegel RL, Miller KD, Jemal A. Cancer statistics, 2017. CA Cancer J Clin. 2017;67:7–30.
4. Howlader N, Noone AM, Krapcho M, Miller D, Bishop K, Altekruse SF, et al., editors. SEER cancer statistics review, 1975–2013 (Level II–3). Bethesda, MD: National Cancer Institute.
5. Ries LAG, Melbert D, Krapcho M, et al. SEER cancer statistics review, 1975–2004. Bethesda, MD: National Cancer Institute. http://seer.cancer.gov/csr/1975_2004/, based on November 2006 SEER data submission, posted to the SEER web site, 2007.
6. Krieger N. Social class and the black/white crossover in the age-specific incidence of breast cancer: a study linking census-derived data to population-based registry records. Am J Epidemiol. 1990;131(5):804–14.

7. Boice JD Jr. Radiation and breast carcinogenesis. Med Pediatr Oncol. 2001;36(5):508–13.
8. Modan B, Chetrit A, Alfandary E, Katz L. Increased risk of breast cancer after low-dose irradiation. Lancet. 1989;1(8639):629–31.
9. Collaborative Group on Hormonal Factors in Breast Cancer. Familial breast cancer: collaborative reanalysis of individual data from 52 epidemiological studies including 58,209 women with breast cancer and 101,986 women without the disease. Lancet. 2001;358(9291):1389–99.
10. Hennekens CH, Buring JE, Manson JE, Stampfer M, Rosner B, Cook NR, et al. Lack of effect of long-term supplementation with beta carotene on the incidence of malignant neoplasms and cardiovascular disease. N Engl J Med. 1996;334:1145–9.
11. Claus EB, Risch N, Thompson WD. Genetic analysis of breast cancer in the cancer and steroid hormone study. Am J Hum Genet. 1991;48(2):232–42.
12. Lalloo F, Varley J, Ellis D, Moran A, O'Dair L, Pharoah P, et al. Prediction of pathogenic mutations in patients with early-onset breast cancer by family history. Lancet. 2003;361(9363):1101–2.
13. Ford D, Easton DF, Bishop DT, Narod SA, Goldgar DE. Risks of cancer in BRCA1-mutation carriers. Breast Cancer Linkage Consortium. Lancet. 1994;343:692–5.
14. Easton DF, Ford D, Bishop DT. Breast and ovarian cancer incidence in BRCA1-mutation carriers. Breast Cancer Linkage Consortium. Am J Hum Genet. 1995;56:265–71.
15. Robson M, Gilewski T, Haas B, Levin D, Borgen P, Rajan P, et al. BRCA-associated breast cancer in young women. J Clin Oncol. 1998;16:1642–9.
16. Breast Cancer Linkage Consortium. Cancer risks in BRCA2 mutation carriers. J Natl Cancer Inst. 1999;91:1310–6.
17. Van den Broek AJ, Schmidt MK, van't Veer LJ, Tollenaar RA, van Leeuwen FE. Worse breast cancer prognosis of BRCA1/BRCA2 mutation carriers: what's the evidence? A systematic review with meta-analysis. PLoS One. 2015;10:e0120189.
18. Mavaddat N, Peock S, Frost D, Ellis S, Platte R, Fineberg E, et al. Cancer risks for BRCA1 and BRCA2 mutation carriers: results from prospective analysis of EMBRACE. J Natl Cancer Inst. 2013;105:812–22.
19. Kote-Jarai Z, Leongamornlert D, Saunders E, Tymrakiewicz M, Castro E, Mahmud N, et al. BRCA2 is a moderate penetrance gene contributing to young-onset prostate cancer: implications for genetic testing in prostate cancer patients. Br J Cancer. 2011;105:1230–4.
20. Iqbal J, Ragone A, Lubinski J, Lynch HT, Moller P, Ghadirian P, et al. The incidence of pancreatic cancer in BRCA1 and BRCA2 mutation carriers. Br J Cancer. 2012;107:2005–9.
21. Leongamornlert D, Mahmud N, Tymrakiewicz M, Saunders E, Dadaev T, Castro E, et al. BRCA1 mutations increase prostate cancer risk. Br J Cancer. 2012;106:1697–701.
22. Graeser MK, Engel C, Rhiem K, Gadzicki D, Bick U, Kast K, et al. Contralateral breast cancer risk in BRCA1 and BRCA2 mutation carriers. J Clin Oncol. 2009;27:5887–92.
23. Van Asperen CJ, Brohet RM, Meijers-Heijboer EJ, Hoogerbrugge N, Verhoef S, Vasen HF, et al. Cancer risks in BRCA2 families: estimates for sites other than breast and ovary. J Med Genet. 2005;42:711–9.
24. Abbott DW, Thompson ME, Robinson-Benion C, Tomlinson G, Jensen RA, Holt JT. BRCA1 expression restores radiation resistance in BRCA1-defective cancer cells through enhancement of transcription-coupled DNA repair. J Biol Chem. 1999;274(26):18808–12.
25. Anglian Breast Cancer Study Group. Prevalence and penetrance of BRCA1 and BRCA2 mutations in a population-based series of breast cancer cases. Br J Cancer. 2000;83:1301–8.
26. Whittemore AS, Gong G, John EM, McGuire V, Li FP, Ostrow KL, et al. Prevalence of BRCA1 mutation carriers among U.S. non-Hispanic Whites. Cancer Epidemiol Biomark Prev. 2004b;13:2078–83.
27. Ruijs MW, Verhoef S, Rookus MA, Pruntel R, van der Hout AH, Hogervorst FB, et al. TP53 germline mutation testing in 180 families suspected of Li-Fraumeni syndrome: mutation detection rate and relative frequency of cancers in different familial phenotypes. J Med Genet. 2010;47:421–8.
28. Hobert JA, Eng C. PTEN hamartoma tumor syndrome: an overview. Genet Med. 2009;11:687–94.
29. Brooks-Wilson AR, Kaurah P, Suriano G, Leach S, Senz J, Grehan N, et al. Germline E-cadherin mutations in hereditary diffuse gastric cancer: assessment of 42 new families and review of genetic screening criteria. J Med Genet. 2004;41:508–17.
30. Weischer M, Bojesen SE, Tybjaerg-Hansen A, Axelsson CK, Nordestgaard BG. Increased risk of breast cancer associated with CHEK2*1100delC. J Clin Oncol. 2007;25:57–63.
31. Renwick A, Thompson D, Seal S, Kelly P, Chagtai T, Ahmed M, et al. ATM mutations that cause ataxia-telangiectasia are breast cancer susceptibility alleles. Nat Genet. 2006;38:873–5.
32. Antoniou AC, Casadei S, Heikkinen T, Barrowdale D, Pylkäs K, Roberts J, et al. Breast-cancer risk in families with mutations in PALB2. N Engl J Med. 2014;371:497–506.
33. Lauper JM, Krause A, Vaughan TL, Monnat RJ Jr. Spectrum and risk of neoplasia in Werner syndrome: a systematic review. PLoS One. 2013;8:e59709.
34. Kelsey JL, Gammon MD, John EM. Reproductive factors and breast cancer. Epidemiol Rev. 1993;15(1):36–47.
35. Collaborative Group. Breast cancer and breastfeeding: collaborative reanalysis of individual data from 47 epidemiological studies in 30 countries, including 50302 women with breast cancer and 96973 women without the disease. Lancet. 2002;360(9328):187–95.
36. Trichopoulos D, Hsieh CC, MacMahon B, Lin TM, Lowe CR, Mirra AP, et al. Age at any birth and breast cancer risk. Int J Cancer. 1983;31(6):701–4.

37. Russo J, Russo IH. Toward a physiological approach to breast cancer prevention. Cancer Epidemiol Biomark Prev. 1994;3(4):353–64.
38. Collaborative Group on Hormonal Factors in Breast Cancer. Breast cancer and hormonal contraceptives: further results. Contraception. 1996;54(3 Suppl):1S–106S.
39. Mørch LS, Skovlund CW, Hannaford PC, Iversen L, Fielding S, Lidegaard Ø. Contemporary hormonal contraception and the risk of breast cancer. N Engl J Med. 2017;377:2228–39.
40. Moorman PG, Havrilesky LJ, Gierisch JM, Coeytaux RR, Lowery WJ, Peragallo Urrutia R, et al. Oral contraceptives and risk of ovarian cancer and breast cancer among high-risk women: a systematic review and meta-analysis. J Clin Oncol. 2013;31(33):4188–98.
41. Chlebowski RT, Hendrix SL, Langer RD, Stefanick ML, Gass M, Lane D, et al. Influence of estrogen plus progestin on breast cancer and mammography in healthy postmenopausal women: the Women's Health Initiative Randomized Trial. JAMA. 2003;289:3243–53.
42. Smith CL, Santen RJ, Komm B, Mirkin S. Breast-related effects of selective estrogen receptor modulators and tissue-selective estrogen complexes. Breast Cancer Res. 2014;16(3):212. https://doi.org/10.1186/bcr3677.
43. Dyrstad SW, Yan Y, Fowler AM, Colditz GA. Breast cancer risk associated with benign breast disease: systematic review and meta-analysis. Breast Cancer Res Treat. 2015;149:569–75.
44. McDivitt RW, Stevens JA, Lee NC, Wingo PA, Rubin GL, Gersell D. Histologic types of benign breast disease and the risk for breast cancer. The Cancer and Steroid Hormone Study Group. Cancer. 1992;69(6):1408–14.
45. London SJ, Connolly JL, Schnitt SJ, Colditz GA. A prospective study of benign breast disease and the risk of breast cancer. JAMA. 1992;267(7):941–4.
46. Marshall LM, Hunter DJ, Connolly JL, et al. Risk of breast cancer associated with atypical hyperplasia of lobular and ductal types. Cancer Epidemiol Biomark Prev. 1997;6(5):297–301.
47. Boyd NF. Mammography density and risk of breast cancer. Am Soc Clin Oncol Educ Book. 2013. https://doi.org/10.1200/EdBook_AM.2013.33.e57.
48. Boyd NF, Rommens JM, Vogt K, Lee V, Hopper JL, Yaffe MJ, et al. Mammographic breast density as an intermediate phenotype for breast cancer. Lancet Oncol. 2005;6(10):798–808.
49. Ursin G, Ma H, Wu AH, Bernstein L, Salane M, Parisky YR, et al. Mammographic density and breast cancer in three ethnic groups. Cancer Epidemiol Biomark Prev. 2003;12(4):332–8.
50. Van den Brandt PA. Pooled analysis of prospective cohort studies on height, weight, and breast cancer risk. Am J Epidemiol. 2000;152(6):514–27.
51. Friedenreich CM, Orenstein MR. Physical activity and cancer prevention: etiologic evidence and biological mechanisms. J Nutr. 2002;132(11 Suppl):3456S–64S.
52. Collaborative Group. Alcohol, tobacco and breast cancer–collaborative reanalysis of individual data from 53 epidemiological studies, including 58,515 women with breast cancer and 95,067 women without the disease. Br J Cancer. 2002;87(11):1234–45.
53. Boffetta P, Hashibe M. Alcohol and cancer. Lancet Oncol. 2006;7:149–56.
54. Gaudet MM, Gapstur SM, Sun J, Diver WR, Hannan LM, Thun MJ. Active smoking and breast cancer risk: original cohort data and meta-analysis. J Natl Cancer Inst. 2013;105:515–25.
55. Catsburg C, Miller AB, Rohan TE. Active cigarette smoking and risk of breast cancer. Int J Cancer. 2015;136:2204–9. https://doi.org/10.1002/ijc.29266.
56. Easton DF, Pooley KA, Dunning AM, Pharoah PD, Thompson D, Ballinger DG, et al. Genome-wide association study identifies novel breast cancer susceptibility loci. Nature. 2007;447(7148):1087–93.
57. Amir E, Freedman OC, Seruga B, Evans DG. Assessing women at high risk of breast cancer: a review of risk assessment models. J Natl Cancer Inst. 2010;102(10):680–69.
58. University of Pennsylvania Abramson Cancer Center. The Penn II BRCA1 and BRCA2 mutation risk evaluation model. Philadelphia, PA. https://www.afcri.upenn.edu:8022/itacc/penn2/index.asp. Accessed 29 May 2009.
59. Gilpin CA, Carson N, Hunter AG. A preliminary validation of a family history assessment form to select women at risk for breast or ovarian cancer for referral to a genetics center. Clin Genet. 2000;58(4):299–308.
60. Evans DGR, Eccles DM, Rahman N, Young K, Bulman M, Amir E, et al. A new scoring system for the chances of identifying a BRCA1/2 mutation, outperforms existing models including BRCAPRO. J Med Genet. 2004;41(6):474–80.
61. Weitzel JN, Lagos VI, Cullinane CA, Gambol PJ, Culver JO, Blazer KR, et al. Limited family structure and BRCA gene mutation status in single cases of breast cancer. JAMA. 2007;297(23):2587–95.
62. Quillin JM, Ramakrishnan V, Borzelleca J, Bodurtha J, Bowen D, Baer Wilson D. Paternal relatives and family history of breast cancer. Am J Prev Med. 2006;31(3):265–8.
63. Murabito JM, Nam BH, D'Agostino RB Sr, Lloyd-Jones DM, O'Donnell CJ, Wilson PW. Accuracy of offspring reports of parental cardiovascular disease history: the Framingham Offspring Study. Ann Intern Med. 2004;140(6):434–40.
64. Douglas FS, O'Dair LCO, Robinson M, Evans DGR, Lynch SA. The accuracy of diagnosis as reported by the proband in families with cancer: a retrospective study. J Med Genet. 1999;36(4):309–12.
65. Liede A, Karlan BY, Narod SA. Cancer risks for male carriers of germline mutations in BRCA1 or BRCA2: a review of the literature. J Clin Oncol. 2004;22(4):735–42.
66. Antoniou AC, Cunningham AP, Peto J, Evans DG, Lalloo F, Narod SA, et al. The BOADICEA model of genetic susceptibility to breast and ovarian

cancers: updates and extensions. Br J Cancer. 2008;98(8):1457–66.
67. Evans DG, Lalloo F, Cramer A, Jones EA, Knox F, Amir E, et al. Addition of breast cancer pathological correlates significantly improves the performance of the Manchester scoring system for BRCA1 and BRCA2 testing. J Med Genet. 2009;46(12):811–7.
68. Gail MH, Brinton LA, Byar DP, Corle DK, Green SB, Schairer C, et al. Projecting individualized probabilities of developing breast cancer for white females who are being examined annually. J Natl Cancer Inst. 1989;81(24):1879–86.
69. Spiegelman D, Colditz GA, Hunter D, Hertzmark E. Validation of the Gail et al. model for predicting individual breast cancer risk. J Natl Cancer Inst. 1994;86(8):600–7.
70. Costantino JP, Gail MH, Pee D, Anderson S, Redmond CK, Benichou J, et al. Validation studies for models projecting the risk of invasive and total breast cancer incidence. J Natl Cancer Inst. 1999;91(18): 1541–8.
71. Cummings SR, Tice JA, Bauer S, Browner WS, Cuzick J, Ziv E, et al. Prevention of breast cancer in postmenopausal women: approaches to estimating and reducing risk. J Natl Cancer Inst. 2009;101(6):384–98.
72. Pankratz VS, Hartmann LC, Degnim AC, Vierkant RA, Ghosh K, Vachon CM, et al. Assessment of the accuracy of the Gail model in women with atypical hyperplasia. J Clin Oncol. 2008;26(33):5374–9.
73. Claus EB, Risch N, Thompson WD. Autosomal dominant inheritance of early onset breast cancer: implications for risk prediction. Cancer. 1994;73(3):643–51.
74. Tischkowitz M, Wheeler D, France E, Chapman C, Lucassen A, Sampson J, et al. A comparison of methods currently used in clinical practice to estimate familial breast cancer risks. Ann Oncol. 2000;11(4):451–4.
75. McGuigan KA, Ganz PA, Breant C. Agreement between breast cancer risk estimation methods. J Natl Cancer Inst. 1996;88(18):1315–7.
76. McTiernan A, Kuniyuki A, Yasui Y, Bowen D, Burke W, Culver JB, et al. Comparisons of two breast cancer risk estimates in women with a family history of breast cancer. Cancer Epidemiol Biomark Prev. 2001;10(4):333–8.
77. Parmigiani G, Berry DA, Aguilar O. Determining carrier probabilities for breast cancer-susceptibility genes BRCA1 and BRCA2. Am J Hum Genet. 1998;62:145–58.
78. Claus EB, Schildkraut JM, Thompson WD, Risch NJ. The genetic attributable risk of breast and ovarian cancer. Cancer. 1996;77:2318–24.
79. Ford D, Easton DF, Stratton M, Narod S, Goldgar D, Devilee P, et al. Genetic heterogeneity and penetrance analysis of the BRCA1 and BRCA2 genes in breast cancer families. Am J Hum Genet. 1998;62:676–89.
80. Struewing JP, Hartge P, Wacholder S, Baker SM, Berlin M, McAdams M, et al. The risk of cancer associated with specific mutations of BRCA1 and BRCA2 among Askenazi Jews. N Engl J Med. 1997;336:1401–8.
81. Jonker MA, Jacobi CE, Hoogendoorn WE, Nagelkerke NJ, de Bock GH, van Houwelingen JC. Modeling familial clustered breast cancer using published data. Cancer Epidemiol Biomark Prev. 2003;12(12):1479–85.
82. Tyrer J, Duffy SW, Cuzick J. A breast cancer prediction model incorporating familial and personal risk factors. Stat Med. 2004;23(7):1111–30.
83. Antoniou AC, Pharoah PP, Smith P, Easton DF. The BOADICEA model of genetic susceptibility to breast and ovarian cancer. Br J Cancer. 2004;91(8): 1580–90.
84. American Society of Clinical Oncology. Policy statement update: genetic testing for cancer susceptibility. J Clin Oncol. 2003;21:2397–406.
85. U.S. Preventive Services Task Force. Risk assessment, genetic counseling, and genetic testing for *BRCA*-related cancer in women: recommendation statement. Am Fam Physician. 2015;91(2):online.
86. National Collaborating Centre for Cancer (UK). National Institute for Health and Care Excellence. Familial breast cancer: classification, care and managing breast cancer and related risks in people with a family history of breast cancer. Cardiff: National Collaborating Centre for Cancer; 2013.
87. Walsh T, Casadei S, Coats KH, Swisher E, Stray SM, Higgins J, et al. Spectrum of mutations in BRCA1, BRCA2, CHEK2, and TP53 in families at high risk of breast cancer. JAMA. 2006;295(12):1379–88.
88. NCCN clinical practice guidelines in oncology: genetic/familial-high-risk assessment: breast and ovarian. Version 2.2016. NCCN.org.
89. Petrucelli N, Daly MB, Pal T. *BRCA1*- and *BRCA2*-associated hereditary breast and ovarian cancer. In: GeneReviews. Seattle, WA: University of Washington; 2016.
90. PDQ® Cancer Genetics Editorial Board. PDQ cancer genetics risk assessment and counseling. Bethesda, MD: National Cancer Institute. Updated 30 Nov 2017.
91. Kwong A, Ng EK, Tang EY, Wong CL, Law FB, Leung CP, et al. A novel de novo BRCA1 mutation in a Chinese woman with early onset breast cancer. Familial Cancer. 2011;10:233–7.
92. Zhang L, Fleischut MH, Kohut K, Spencer S, Wong K, Stadler ZK, et al. Assessment of the prevalence of de novo mutations in the BRCA1 and BRCA2 genes. Clin Genet. 2011;80:97–8.
93. De Leeneer K, Coene I, Crombez B, Simkens J, van den Broecke R, Bols A, Stragier B, Vanhoutte I, De Paepe A, Poppe B, Claes K. Prevalence of BRCA1/2 mutations in sporadic breast/ovarian cancer patients and identification of a novel de novo BRCA1 mutation in a patient diagnosed with late onset breast and ovarian cancer: implications for genetic testing. Breast Cancer Res Treat. 2012;132:87–95.
94. Gaff C, Collins V, Symes T, Halliday J. Facilitating family communication about predictive testing: probands' perspectives. J Genet Couns. 2005;14:133–40.

30 Preinvasive Breast Lesions: Detection and Management

Sumit Goyal and Niti Raizada

30.1 Introduction and Epidemiology

Breast cancer is the commonest and the lead cause of cancer deaths worldwide, which accounts for 23% of total cancer load and 14% of cancer-related mortalities [1] with a lifetime risk of breast cancer in women ebbing as high as 1 in 8. Women 65 and above account for 40% of cases with a fatality rate of almost 60%. The estimated risk <49 years is 1 in 43 at 50–59, 1 in 23 at 60–69, and 1 in 15 at the age >70 years [2].

The age-adjusted incidence rate among Indian female is 25.8 per lac with a mortality rate of 12.7 per lac, becoming the number one cancer. Since 1982 till 2014, a statistically significant increase in age-adjusted rates of breast cancer incidence was noted from all major cities. Delhi ranked the highest with 41 per lac followed by Chennai with 37.9, Bangalore with 34.4, and Thiruvananthapuram district with 33.7 when age-adjusted incidence rates were compared [3].

S. Goyal (✉)
Department of Medical oncology, Rajiv Gandhi Cancer Institute and Research Centre, New Delhi, India

N. Raizada
Department of Medical Oncology and Hemato-Oncology, Health Care Global Enterprises, Bangalore, Karnataka, India

30.2 Preinvasive Stages of Breast Cancer

Preinvasive epithelial lesions of the breast are defined as neoplastic proliferation of epithelial cells confined to the ductal lobular network without invasion of the basement membrane and surrounding stroma. According to SEER (Surveillance, Epidemiology, and End Results Program) statistics, in situ breast cancer ranks fourth after invasive breast, lung, and colorectal cancer with an estimated 63,410 new cases being diagnosed only in 2017 [4].

30.2.1 Histopathological Review

The architecture of the breast is formed of progressively branching ducts originating at the nipple and ending in the terminal ductal lobular units (TDLUs). A TDLU, the smallest functioning unit of the breast, has a specialized stroma with single terminal duct and multiple end acini. Both the systems are two cell layered. The inner epithelial layer with a terminal ductile was being lined with columnar and acini by cuboidal cell. The outer myoepithelial layer abuts the basement membrane [5].

Wellings and Jensen and Wellings et al. challenged the concept that the different histological verities arose from distinct microanatomical structures within the breast tissue. They

S. Mehta, A. Singla (eds.), *Preventive Oncology for the Gynecologist*,
https://doi.org/10.1007/978-981-13-3438-2_30

Table 30.1 Histology of preinvasive lesions of the breast

Type	Differentiation
FEA	Minimal proliferation of TDLU, one to several layers of cuboidal or columnar epithelial cells, low-grade cytological atypia
ADH	Differ from FEA in pseudostratified manner with secondary architectural atypia in the form of micropapillae
Low-grade DCIS	Small, cohesive, polarized, uniform cells of low proliferative capacity
Intermediate-grade DCIS	Small- to medium-sized, polarized cells with moderate nuclear pleomorphism and low proliferative capacity with or without necrosis
High-grade DCIS	Large, pleomorphic cells of high proliferative capacity with necrosis

demonstrated that in situ lesions as well as invasive counterparts despite differing histology originate from the TDLU [6, 7].

The terms ductal or lobular cancer are based on their discrete architectural patterns, cytological features, and immunohistochemical features.

The preinvasive lesions of the lobular type include [8]:

- Atypical lobular hyperplasia (ALH).
- Lobular carcinoma in situ (LCIS).

The extent of proliferation and distension of the acini within the TDLU differentiate ALH and LCIS.

LCIS is subdivided into pleomorphic and the classical type. The pleomorphic variety has loosely cohesive cell variable in size and shape, whereas the cells in the classical type are small, uniform, and non-polarized.

The preinvasive stages of the ductal type are [8]:

- Flat epithelial atypia (FEA).
- Atypical ductal hyperplasia (ADH).
- Ductal carcinoma in situ (DCIS) (Table 30.1).

30.2.2 Natural History

In the prescreening era, DCIS presented mainly as a palpable mass with mastectomy being the mainstay of treatment; thus, by default the natural history is poorly understood. In a 30-year follow-up study by Sanders et al., of the 28 women treated for low-grade DCIS with biopsy, 11 developed IVC in the same breast and quadrant (7 within 10 years, 1 after 12 years, and 3 over a period of 23–42 years). Five of these 11 developed distant metastasis [9].

Similar results were reported by Page and colleagues who reviewed 11,760 biopsies and identified 28 women of DCIS. They reported that 28% women treated with biopsy alone will develop invasive cancer in approximately 15 years of follow-up [10].

King et al. reviewed the risk factors associated with LCIS over a period of 29 years in 1060 women. The median age was 50 years (27–83 years) with an annual incidence of 2% for breast cancer with no dominant histological subtype in women of LCIS cohort. Age and family history were not associated with an increased risk. Chemoprevention was the only factor associated with a significant decrease (7% vs. 21%, $p < 0.001$) (Figs. 30.1 and 30.2).

30.2.2.1 Molecular Classification

In an effort to identify diagnostic, prognostic, and predictive classifications, in an aid to decision-making, a plethora of research on genome-wide expression profiling studies have been done. A molecular classification scheme by which breast cancers can be categorized into different varieties was given by Perou et al. [11]. Four distinct intrinsic categories were identified that include (a) two subtypes of estrogen receptor (ER)-negative tumors, the basal-like and the ERBB2, and (b) two ER-positive tumors, the luminal A and the luminal B subtypes. A lack of expression of ER, progesterone receptor (PR), and human epidermal growth factor receptor 2 (HER2) and expression of cytokeratins 5/6 (basal cytokeratins) and epidermal growth factor receptor (EGFR) is seen in basal-like, whereas the ERBB2 tumors are characterized by the expression of HER2 but not ER and PR. Luminal A tumors show ER and PR expression with no HER2 overexpression, but luminal B tumors express ER and overexpress HER2 with or without PR expression. These four specific molecular subtypes have been found to have distinct clinical outcomes [12, 13].

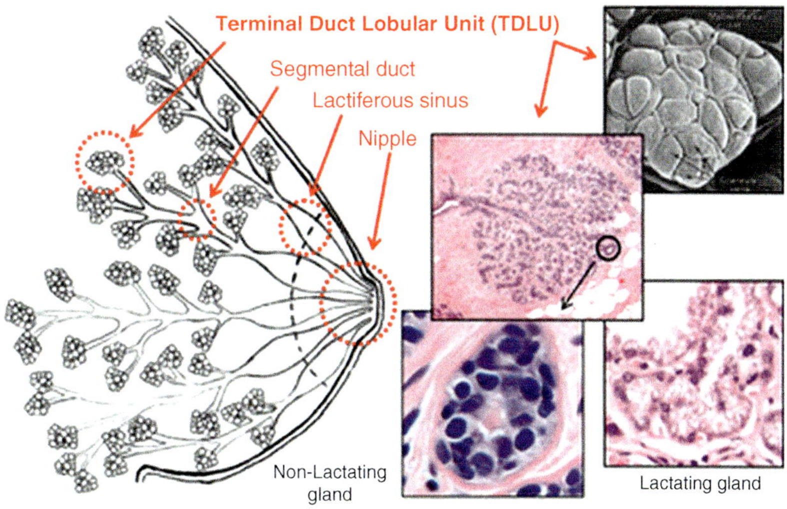

Fig. 30.1 Anatomy of female breast

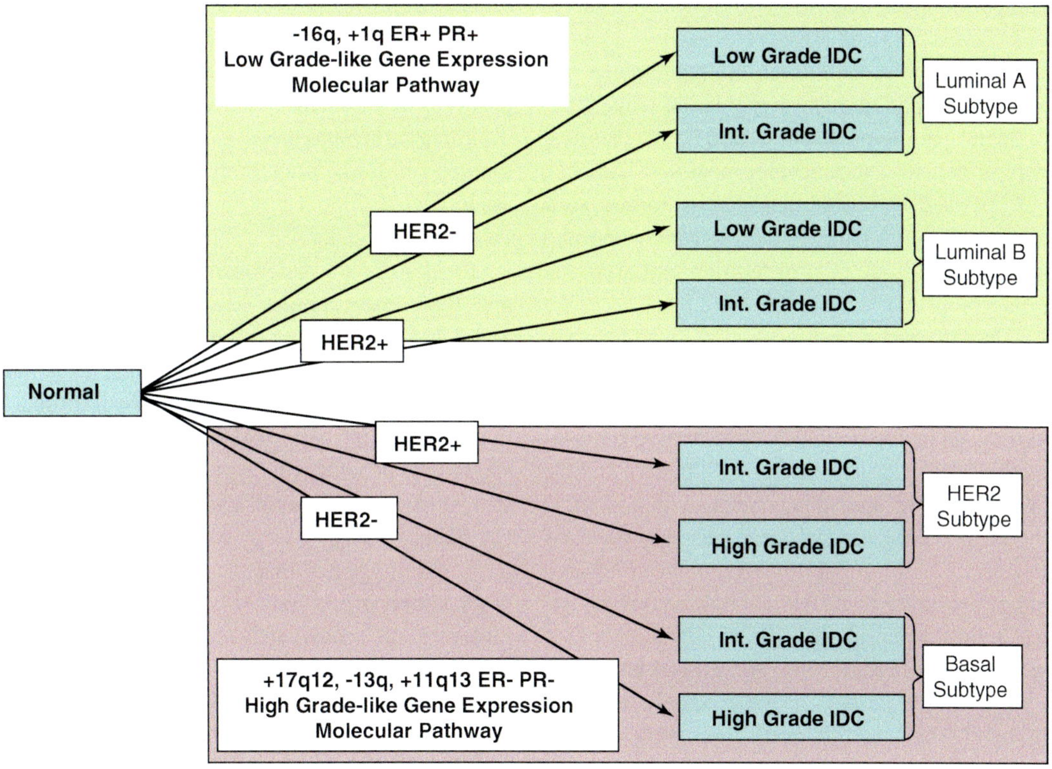

Fig. 30.2 Molecular classification of breast cancers

Fan et al. in their study used five gene expression-based models to look for concordance in their outcome predictors for individual samples. They found that four of the tested five models showed significant concordance that was probably due to the common biological phenotype. All the four signatures were equally useful in distributing patients to either the low- or the high-risk groups. Cell proliferation was the common biological principal and is the main force which drives the prognostic power of these biomarkers [14].

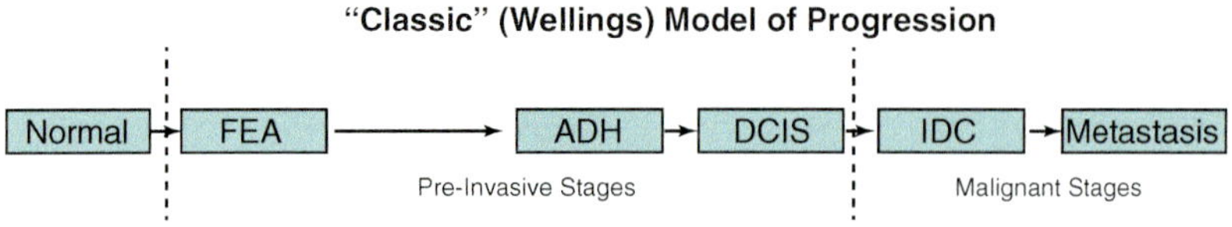

Fig. 30.3 Concepts for progression from pre-invasive to invasive cancer

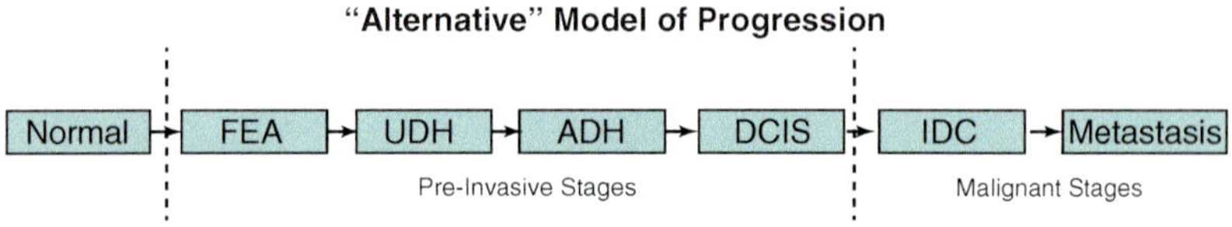

Fig. 30.4 Concepts for progression from pre-invasive to invasive cancer

30.2.3 Models of Progression

Two well-recognized linear models of breast cancer progression have been the result of enormous epidemiological and histopathological observations (Figs. 30.3 and 30.4).

Transition from normal epithelial cells via hyperplasia and atypical hyperplasia (Fig. 30.3) to ductal carcinoma in situ (DCIS) is the classical way of breast cancer development and has been corroborated by mouse mammary tumor models and by epidemiological studies, which revealed that increased rate of proliferation and atypia in breast biopsies.

The intraductal proliferation that can be associated with invasive breast cancer is CIS. CIS can be further divided into LCIS and DCIS, and DCIS in turn can be further subclassified based on cytonuclear characteristics and growth pattern and the absence or presence of necrosis. A hypothetical model of cancer progression was described by Page et al. In this model, UDH replaced FEA as a direct precursor to ADH. Though epidemiological studies supported the role of UDH, as women whose benign breast biopsies showed UDH had a slight increased risk of malignancy to the tune of 1.5–2.0 times the general population. But the recent evidence suggests that the alternate model is invalid and UDH is precursor to ADH [15–18].

30.2.4 Gene Expression Profiles of Breast Cancer Progression

Linear model of breast cancer progression was though to provide an earlier insight into the diagnosis and treatment of breast cancer. But DCIS and IDC are heterogeneous with respect to mitotic activity and cellular differentiation both intra- and intertumor. Thus, several tumor-grading systems were evolved which are used clinically to subtype DCIS and IDC into three tumor grades I, II, and III corresponding to well, moderately, and poorly differentiated breast tumors, respectively. Tumor grading has been a valuable prognostic marker for fairly poor clinical outcome that is associated with poorly differentiated, high-grade DCIS or IDC lesions.

To identify the heterogeneity between DCIS and IDC, laser capture microdissection (LCM) and DNA microarray technologies to perform cellular-based gene expression profile analyses were used. LCM was highly accurate in procuring the specific cells which form the different stages of progression avoiding contamination with surrounding stromal and inflammatory cells [19] (Fig. 30.5).

It was suggested that the transcriptional program which drives cancer cells to an advanced tumor grade may also confer invasiveness. Ribonucleotide Reductase Regulatory subunit (RRM2) is a gene which has been identified and correlates well with both advanced tumor grade and stage. RRM2 is the rate-limiting step in DNA synthesis which facilitates conversion of ribonucleotides to deoxyribonucleotides; thus, increased expression may support the rapid cell division characteristic of high-grade tumors. RRM2 acts as ion conjunction with a wide variety of oncogenes like H-Ras, Rac-1, v-fms, v-Src, A-raf, v-fes, and c-Myc, thus promoting metastatic potential [19].

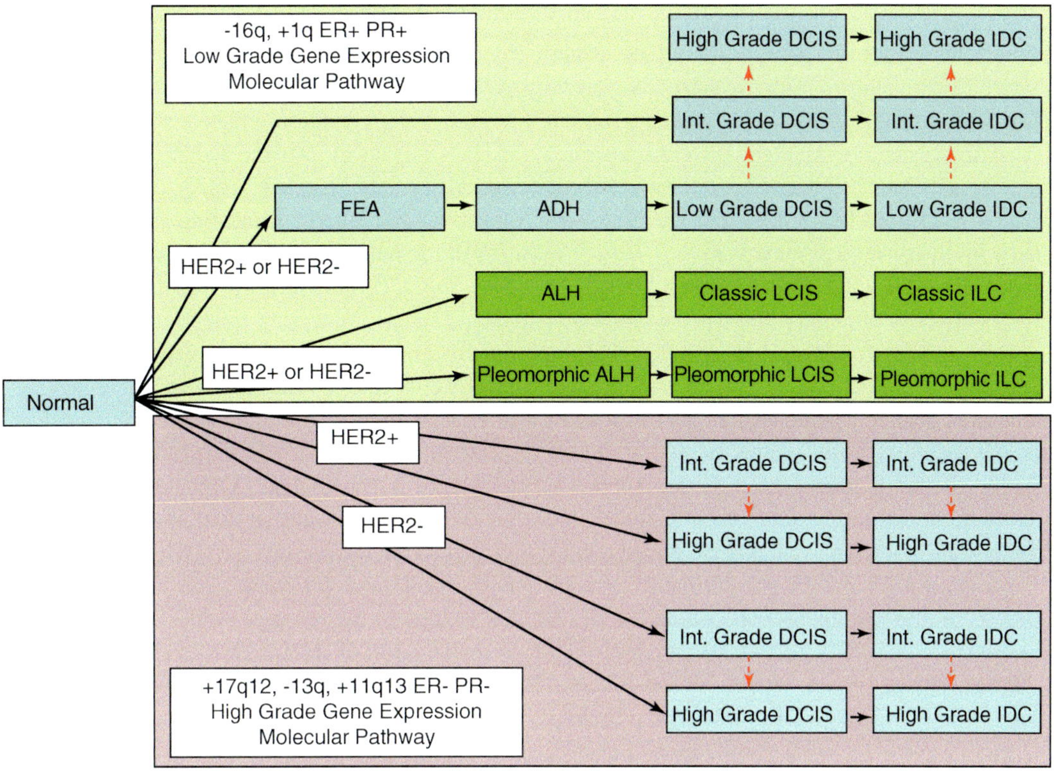

Fig. 30.5 Molecular gene expression profiles of pre-invasive and invasive breast cancers

30.2.4.1 Genomic Analysis of Preinvasive Stages of Ductal Breast Cancer

Buerger et al. on a comparative genomic hybridization (CGH)-based analysis of DCIS and invasive carcinoma showed that losses of 16q were limited to low- and intermediate-grade DCIS, whereas 1q main and 11q loss were majorly associated with intermediate-grade DCIS. High-grade DCIS was associated with complex genomic alterations like loss of 8p, 11q, 13q, and 14q; gain of 1q, 5p, 8q, and 17q; and high-level amplifications of 17q12 and 11q13 [20].

O'Connell and colleagues analyzed the loss of heterozygosity (LOH) in 399 preinvasive breast lesions. 42% and 44% of ADH lesions were found to have LOH in at least 1 of 15 loci studied. 16q was identified as an LOH hot spot in ADH and was found to be more associated with low-grade DCIS than high-grade DCIS [21].

30.2.4.2 Genetic Alterations in Preinvasive Lesions

Ductal carcinoma in situ: A number of methods to characterize preinvasive breast lesions have been used like immunohistochemistry, fluorescent in situ hybridization (FISH), analysis of loss of heterozygosity (LOH), comparative genomic hybridization (CGH), and, more recently, cDNA microarrays and proteomic analysis.

Alterations detected on CGH analysis of DCIS are gain in 1q, 5p, 6q, 8q, 17q, 19q, 20p, 20q, and Xq and loss of 2q, 5q, 6q, 8p, 9p, 11q, 13q, 14q, 16q, 17p, and 22q which are similar to in invasive carcinoma, thus confirming that DCIS is a precursor lesion.

Alterations at 16q occur majorly in low-grade DCIS than in high-grade DCIS where alterations in 13q, 17q, and 20q are more frequent, thus supporting the idea that low-grade and high-grade lesions develop through distinct pathways rather than by dedifferentiation [19].

O'Connell and colleagues reported that 50% of the proliferative and 80% of the DCIS lesions shared LOH patterns with invasive carcinoma [21]. Stratton and colleagues [13] using a limited set of microsatellite markers on chromosomes 7q, 16q, 17p, and 17q found a similarity of LOH in subsets of pure DCIS only and DCIS associated with invasive carcinoma [22].

c-erbB2 (Her-2/neu) protein is identified in as high as 60–80% of DCIS though is uncommon in the low-grade forms. Allred et al. noted that the expression of this oncogene is higher in invasive carcinoma associated with DCIS than those without. Though very rarely overexpressed in classic lobular carcinoma in situ (LCIS), overexpression has been occasionally seen with pleomorphic lobular carcinoma in situ variety. No evidence of overexpression in benign proliferative breast diseases or atypical ductal hyperplasia (ADH) is seen [23].

Lobular carcinoma in situ: LCIS is an uncommon lesion with a distinctive appearance formed of discohesive cells with small, monomorphic, hyperchromatic nuclei, though a pleomorphic variant is also known. However, studies have shown that the biological behavior and clinical implications of LCIS are very different from those of DCIS.

Usually diagnosed aged between 40 and 50 years, approximately one-fifth of the cases often progress to invasive cancer over a period of 20 to 25 year. Although invasive ductal carcinomas, especially of tubular type, do occur after LCIS, majority cases associated with LCIS are infiltrating lobular carcinoma, though tubular type cancers can also occur after LCIS. The risk is equal for the two breasts, but literature suggests that the risk is more for ipsilateral breast. Despite these thorny dilemmas, LCIS is considered a "marker of increased risk" than a true precursor.

CGH analysis done on LCIS and ALH demonstrated chromosomal imbalance with loss of 16p, 16q, 17p, and 22q and gain at 6q at similarly between LCIS and ALH. Losses at 1q, 16q, and 17p are seen in invasive lobular carcinomas. LOH data in LCIS are limited but show a similarity between LCIS and ILC [24].

E-cadherin is a tumor suppressor protein coded by a gene on 16q22.1 through the β-catenin/Wnt pathway which helps in cell-to-cell adhesion and in cell cycle regulation. Positive staining on IHC is shown by most invasive ductal cancers though majority of the invasive lobular carcinomas are negative. E-cadherin truncating mutations with loss of the wild-type allele (LOH at 16q) are seen both in LCIS and invasive lobular carcinomas [25], though truncating mutations in invasive ductal carcinomas of NST or medullary carcinomas in congruence with Roylance and colleagues [19] have not been seen.

Atypical ductal hyperplasia: Lakhani et al. [26] demonstrated that LOH identified at loci on 16q and 17p in invasive carcinoma and DCIS is also similarly present in ADH in congruence with Amari and colleague [27]. O'Connell and colleagues in 51 cases of ADH at 15 polymorphic loci noted LOH in 42% of the cases, demonstrating that morphological overlaps are reflected at the molecular level and raise questions about the validity of separating ADH from DCIS. CGH analysis of nine cases of ADH showed chromosomal abnormalities in five. Due to the similar morphology between low-grade DCIS and ADH, the loss of 16q and 17p is the most frequent change found in ADH [16, 17].

30.3 Diagnostic Techniques of Preinvasive Breast Cancer

Diagnostic modalities of choice for any suspicious breast mass are a combination of clinical examination, imaging, and biopsy. Clinical examination to assess palpable abnormalities should include axillary and lymph node assessment.

30.3.1 Imaging

30.3.1.1 Mammography

The initial years of screening mammography saw a whooping 75% rise in the incidence of DCIS. Presently, DCIS are diagnosed by the presence of microcalcifications on mammogram with a sensitivity of 86% [28].

Microcalcifications seen in DCIS are due to cellular necrosis. With limited accuracy some of the calcification patterns can suggest architectural type of DCIS. Fine, linear, and branching calcifications also referred to as casting calcification could suggest calcification of comedocarcinoma. However, mammography can underestimate the size of DCIS lesions because of its inability to detect non-calcified lesions.

Choi and his group retrospectively analyzed imaging findings of nine cases pathologically diagnosed as pure LCIS according to the BI-RADS lexicon. The most common ultrasound findings suggestive of LCIS were irregular shape in five, ill-defined margins in eight, hypoechogenicity in seven, and microcalcifications in two. All cases had elongated or round shape parallel to the skin. The BI-RADS was category 3 in one, category 4A in two, and category 4B in six cases [28].

30.3.1.2 Ultrasonography

Ultrasound detects almost 85% of pure DCIS with 15% seen on ultrasound being not localized on a mammogram. DCIS without calcifications are architecturally distorted, isoechoic to hypoechoic heterogenous multilobulated with a ductal extension. In contrast DCIS with microcalcifications on mammography usually appear as non-mass hypoechoic abnormalities [29].

30.3.1.3 MRI

Morphologic patterns of malignancy on MRI are irregular, spiculated, or microlobulated borders, early rim enhancement, and peripheral washout. A more variable pattern on MRI is seen for pure DCIS in comparison to invasive carcinoma. The commonest presentation on MRI is a non-mass enhancement and may or may not have a clumped or linear pattern that follows a ductal distribution [30].

A recent meta-analysis on the diagnostic accuracy of MRI reported a sensitivity of 90% and a specificity of 72% for diagnosis of malignant breast lesions [31].

In LCIS, NCCN guidelines recommend considering breast MRI screening [32]. A study of enhanced screening with MRI in patients with LCIS showed that 4% of patients had cancer on MRI with a negative mammogram.

30.3.2 Biopsy

Core needle biopsy and fine needle aspiration (FNA) have outdone the need for open biopsy/frozen section to diagnose breast cancer, though not without diagnostic dilemmas to the pathologist.

30.3.2.1 Fine Needle Aspiration (FNA)

FNA was initially introduced to replace incisional biopsy for the diagnosis of breast lesions and presently is a part of the triple regimen to diagnose breast cancer. The superficial nature of breast lesions makes FNA highly sensitive and specific for diagnosis but still has a number of limitations. Unquestionable advantages are the simple technique, low cost and risk of complications, minimally invasive, and a ready availability in most setups [33].

In cystic lesions of the breast, FNA can be both diagnostic and therapeutic with an incidence of cancer being 2% in these. The problems associated with cystic lesions are collapse of the cyst, stripping of the epithelium, and acellular fluid. A variety of cells seen are foam cells, inflammatory cells, benign epithelium, and apocrine cells. If cytological atypia is detected, it should raise a suspicion. FNA for solid lesion can be important for prompt diagnosis.

FNA has technical, intrinsic limitations and limitation with the type of lesion. False negative may be due to improper technique, contamination with blood, thick and nonuniform smear, improper training, small mobile fibrous lesions, and dense fibrotic stroma.

Role of cytology in the evaluation of prognostic markers. Aspirate can be used to evaluate the expression of receptors like ER and PR, E-cadherin, and p53. Cytocentrifuged material is better for the same [34]. The expression of HER-2 by FISH and immunocytochemistry using aspiration material has been reported [35].

30.3.2.2 Core Needle Biopsy

The role of core needle biopsy has been widely accepted with the advent of smaller gauge needles used under stereotactic guidance; complications of trauma, pain, the use of anesthetic agents, and tumor implantation in the biopsy tract have decreased. Accurate subcategorization of the pathology, study of hormone receptors, and other prognostic markers has become possible. The false-positive rate is very low (0.2–0.3%) and is minimally higher for nonpalpable lesions [36].

Fibroadenoma and phyllodes tumor pose a difficulty on core biopsy. Stromal cellularity, vesicular nuclei of stromal cells, mitotic figures, and epithelial hyperplasia should raise a suspicion of phyllodes tumor. Thus, excisional biopsy is recommended for difficult cases [37].

Loose papillary fragments can cause difficulty and distortion of papillary architecture and in turn cause stromal invasion. Irfan and coworkers [38] demonstrated that 14.3% of the papillary lesions on stereo core biopsy showed cancer on further excision. Thus, papillary lesions should undergo complete excision regardless of cytological and architectural atypia.

Due to the limited amount of material obtained on core biopsy, the distinction between low-grade DCIS and ADH is usually difficult. Bonnett et al. reported that severe atypical hyperplasia on core biopsy is associated with a high probability of DCIS on further follow-up excision; thus, complete excision should be done [39].

30.3.2.3 Ductal Lavage

The recently developed less invasive techniques like ductal lavage, ductoscopy, and nipple discharge on examination are more attractive for patients and physicians. Ductal lavage, with or without ductoscopy, is less invasive and technically not complicated. With cost being comparable to FNA and results are obtained more quickly. Domchek et al. [40] showed that a large yield of breast epithelial cells can be collected by ductal lavage, though the reliability is limited. The main factors responsible are varied and degenerated cellularity of the sample, thus limiting the specificity as these cells can be mistakenly diagnosed as malignant. Lower sensitivity may be due to lower cell output, but still lavage is potentially a more sensitive method than nipple aspiration in detecting cellular atypia.

30.3.3 Immunohistochemistry of Ductal or Lobular Carcinomas

Hematoxylin-eosin stain can distinguish between invasive and in situ ductal and lobular carcinomas, though categorization may require IHC and E-cadherin with E-cadherin being expressed in ductal and not lobular carcinomas.

High molecular weight CK (clone 34βE12) is usually expressed by lobular carcinomas, and usually low or absent levels are seen in most cases of DCIS. Also, CK8 staining in peripheral cytoplasm is seen in ductal carcinoma, while perinuclear staining is a characteristic of lobular carcinoma [41].

30.4 Recent Trends in Treatment

30.4.1 Mastectomy

In DCIS, survival rates with mastectomy are excellent. But these excellent survival rates lead to more conservative approach. Still mastectomy holds a place in the management of DCIS when either lesion is too extensive, high grade, patient is not eligible for radiation therapy, pregnant women or with previous history of radiation on chest.

In LCIS generally mastectomy is not required unless pleomorphic LCIS is found on biopsy.

30.4.2 Breast-Conserving Therapy (BCT)

BCT is the main treatment modality by which 75% of DCIS lesions are treated. DCIS lesions detected by mammography should be localized with wire or radioactive seed prior to excision under imaging guidance. Wire localization involves two wires which crosses the sire of lesion under stereotactic guidance or ultrasound. Radioactive seed localization involves a percutaneous placement of a radioactive seed at the site of the lesion under stereotactic or ultrasound guidance with the benefit of flexibility in scheduling the surgery as seed placement can be done several days to weeks in advance.

Bruno et al. retrospectively analyzed 200 cases of pure LCIS in seven centers from 1990 to 2008. Median age was 52 years. Of 200 women, 176 had breast-conserving surgery (BCS) and 24 mastectomy. Of the BCS group, 17 received whole breast irradiation (WBRT) and 20 hormonal treatments. During the 144-month follow-up, no local recurrences (LR) were noted among 24 mastectomized women. But, three late recurrences occurred in women treated by BCS and WBRT. Among 159 women treated with BCS alone, 13% developed LR with only a 72-month FU. No specific LR risk factors were identified [42].

Surgical margins: The width of margin for breast-conserving surgery is debatable. There is a general agreement that less than 1 mm is not ideal. However, the ideal margin width is less clear. Most surgeons prefer to achieve a 2 mm radial margin. It is notable that the margin width is considered more with DCIS than with invasive breast cancer. This is related to the growth pattern in a linear and branching pattern compared to an expanding invasive cancer mass.

In general, with resection margins greater than 10 mm, there is a low recurrence rate, but the absolute benefit of radiation is low. However, considerations of other factors such as young age, high tumor grade, and large tumors give more impetus for radiation despite wide margins. Cases with margins under 1 mm derive the greatest benefit from radiation.

A recent analysis suggests that patients with Van Nuys scores of 4–6 or 7 with a margin width above 3 mm can be treated with excision alone and achieve local recurrence rates of below 6%. The addition of radiation achieves acceptable rates of local control (<20% local recurrence at 12 years) for those with score 7 and have margins under 3 mm, for patients who score 8 and have margins equal to 3 mm, and for patients who score 9 and have margins equal to 5 mm [43].

A meta-analysis of 4660 patients treated with lumpectomy and radiation showed that negative margins were associated with substantially lower risk of local recurrences compared to positive margins. A margin of 2 mm was superior for local control compared to less than 2 mm, with a relative reduction of local recurrence of 47%. There was no additional advantage for margins greater than 5 mm [44].

30.4.3 Sentinel Lymph Node Biopsy (SLNB)

A sentinel lymph node (SLN) is the first lymph node to which cancer cells drain. A SLNB is a procedure in which the SLN is identified, removed, and examined to determine whether cancer cells are present or not. A positive SLNB indicates that cancer is present in the sentinel lymph node and the decision whether to do regional lymphadenectomy has to be taken.

In women with invasive breast carcinoma, SLNB can help avoid the potential morbidity of an axillary dissection. DCIS being considered as preinvasive axillary staging is unnecessary, except for women undergoing mastectomy and those with lesions in the upper outer quadrant of the breast command axillary dissection. In both scenarios, the extent of primary procedure compromises SLNB if invasive disease is discovered on the final pathology. Whether SLNB at the time of DCIS treatment be considered in other clinical scenarios is debatable. Some argue that SLNB should not be considered given the low rate of node positivity with DCIS and the little influence this has on subsequent therapy.

Van and colleagues tried to validate whether SLNB is justified in patients with DCIS on core biopsy in current understanding. Clinically node-negative DCIS patients diagnosed between 2004 and 2013 on core biopsy were enrolled. A total of 910 patients were recruited and SLNB was done in 471. Women undergoing mastectomy had 7% SLN metastases versus 3.5% for breast-conserving surgery (BCS). The two factors which correlated with SLN metastases were smaller core needle size and invasive cancer. Histopathologically diagnosed invasive cancer was found in 16.7% with 15.6% SLN metastases but only 2% in pure DCIS. They concluded that SLNB is not required for DCIS on core biopsy undergoing BCS. If definitive histopathology showed invasive cancer, SLNB can be considered later [45].

30.5 Adjuvant Therapy

30.5.1 Role of Radiation

In 1993 National Surgical Adjuvant Breast and Bowel Project (NSABP) trial was done to evaluate radiation therapy after lumpectomy and concluded that the combination was better than lumpectomy alone for localized DCIS. They included 818 women with localized DCIS who were randomly assigned to either group (lumpectomy or lumpectomy plus radiation), and they followed up patients for 90 months. The result of the trial demonstrated that the benefit of lumpectomy plus radiation was seen between 5 and 8 years of follow-up and was due to a decrease in invasive and noninvasive ipsilateral breast tumors (IBTs). Locoregional and distant metastasis were similar. Regardless of clinical or mammographic tumor characteristics, radiation benefits were seen for all [46].

A randomized controlled trial from Australia and New Zealand recruited 1701 DCIS women for 8 years. Ipsilateral invasive disease was not reduced by tamoxifen, but recurrence of overall DCIS was decreased. Radiotherapy reduced the incidence of ipsilateral invasive disease and ipsilateral ductal carcinoma in situ but did not affect the occurrence of contralateral disease. Thus, post the complete local excision of DCIS, radiotherapy can be given, but tamoxifen has a little role to play if any [47].

30.5.2 Hormonal Therapy

Estrogen receptor (ER) is not only a powerful predictive and prognostic marker but also a target for the treatment of hormone-dependent breast cancer.

National Surgical Adjuvant Breast and Bowel Project B-24 was a randomized controlled trial done to evaluate the efficacy of tamoxifen in DCIS. One thousand and eight hundred four women with DCIS even with involved margins were randomly allocated equally to lumpectomy, radiation therapy, and placebo or lumpectomy, radiation therapy, and tamoxifen. After 5 years of follow-up, women in the tamoxifen group had fewer reported breast cancer events than placebo. In the tamoxifen group, the cumulative incidence of all invasive breast cancer events were 4.1% at 5 years: 2.1% in the ipsilateral breast, 1.8% in the contralateral breast, and 0.2% at regional or distant sites [48].

In 2002 the American Society of Clinical Oncology provided guidelines for pharmacological intervention in breast cancer [49].

30.6 Prognosis

Approximately 15–30% of women with pure DCIS develop a subsequent breast tumor event within the first decade after lumpectomy; though a majority (70%) with pure DCIS are treated with lumpectomy, radiation, and anti-hormonal treatment, it is opt to say that many are being over treated. Thus, identification of a prognostic biomarker to predict the clinical behavior of DCIS is the need of the hour so that the line of treatment between lumpectomy alone and lumpectomy with adjuvant therapy can be reliably decided upon.

Narod et al. in their observational study reported that among the 108,196 women with DCIS, the mean age at diagnosis of DCIS was 53.8 (15–69) years and the mean duration of follow-up was 7.5 (0–23.9) years. At 20 years, the overall breast cancer-specific mortality was 3.3% and was higher for women diagnosed before 35 years and for black ethnicity [50].

Five hundred seventeen women died of breast cancer following a DCIS diagnosis with a mean follow-up of 7.5 years without being diagnosed with invasive breast cancer. Among patients who underwent lumpectomy, radiotherapy reduced the risk of ipsilateral invasive recurrence at

10 years but not of breast cancer-specific mortality at 10 years. Understanding the prognostic factors that influence recurrence after treatment of DCIS is important, as roughly 50% of recurrences are invasive cancers and thus an increased mortality risk [50].

Chuba et al. investigated the incidence rates of invasive breast cancer (IBC) in 4853 women having a diagnosis of primary LCIS from 1973 to 1998. The incidence of IBC increased over time from the diagnosis of LCIS, with 7.1 ± 0.5% incidence of IBC at 10 years. IBCs detected after partial mastectomy occurred in either breast (46% ipsilateral and 54% contralateral); however, after mastectomy, most IBCs were contralateral (94.7%). IBCs occurring after LCIS were mainly of lobular histology (23.1%) compared with the primary IBCs (6.5%) [51].

30.7 Conclusion

Preinvasive lesions of breast carcinoma are the fourth most common cancer diagnosed in women after invasive breast, lung, and colorectal cancer. These are mainly grouped into the lobular and ductal in situ carcinomas. There are two models suggested for progression of preinvasive lesions to invasive cancer, and genetic aberrations in both groups can be studied via IHC, FISH, LOH, CGH, or proteomics. The diagnosis of preinvasive lesions requires a careful clinical examination followed by imaging and biopsy of the lump. Imaging can be done by mammography, ultrasonography, or MRI. FNA and core biopsy have virtually eliminated the need for open biopsy or frozen section in diagnosis of breast cancer. Breast-conserving therapy in the form of localized excision followed by adjuvant radiation or pharmacological intervention is the cornerstone of treatment.

Key Points

- Breast cancer is the leading cause of cancer deaths in women worldwide, accounting for 23% of total cancer cases and 14% of all cancer-related mortalities.
- The preinvasive lesions of lobular type include atypical lobular hyperplasia, and ductal precancer includes flat epithelial hyperplasia, ADH, and DCIS.
- The gold standard for the diagnosis of any concerning breast lesion involves a triple assessment, including clinical examination, imaging, and biopsy.
- Seventy-five percent of DCIS cases present as microcalcifications on mammography, while the MRI picture is of a non-mass enhancement with a clumped or linear pattern.
- Fine needle aspiration (FNA) and core biopsy are now universally accepted as methods that virtually eliminate the need for open biopsy or frozen sections in diagnosis of breast cancer.
- Immunohistochemistry can be used to differentiate ductal and lobular in situ and invasive carcinomas. The majority of ductal carcinomas express cytoplasmic E-cadherin and lack high molecular weight CK, whereas most lobular carcinomas lack expression of E-cadherin but express CK.
- Today, almost 75% of newly diagnosed patients with DCIS are treated with BCT, while mastectomy is not needed for LCIS. The ideal margin width is not clear, and most surgeons prefer to achieve a 2 mm radial margin.
- Adjuvant therapy in the form of radiation or chemotherapy improves prognosis in women treated for preinvasive in situ lesions of the breast.

References

1. Jemal A, Bray F, Center MM, Ferlay J, Ward E, Forman D. Global cancer statistics. CA Cancer J Clin. 2011;61(2):69–90.
2. McGuire A, Brown JA, Malone C, McLaughlin R, Kerin MJ. Effects of age on the detection and management of breast cancer. Cancers (Basel). 2015;7(2):908–29.
3. Malvia S, Bagadi SA, Dubey US, Saxena S. Epidemiology of breast cancer in Indian women. Asia Pac J Clin Oncol. 2017;13(4):289–95.
4. Sgroi DC. Preinvasive breast cancer. Annu Rev Pathol. 2010;5:193–221.

5. American Cancer Society. Breast cancer facts & figures. https://www.cancer.org/research/cancer-facts-statistics/breast-cancer-facts-figures.html. Accessed 10 Sept 2018.
6. Wellings SR, Jensen HM. On the origin and progression of ductal carcinoma in the human breast. J Natl Cancer Inst. 1973;50:1111–8.
7. Wellings SR, Jensen HM, Marcum RG. An atlas of subgross pathology of the human breast with special reference to possible precancerous lesions. J Natl Cancer Inst. 1975;55:231–73.
8. Hanby AM, Hughes TA. In situ and invasive lobular neoplasia of the breast. Histopathology. 2008;52:58–66.
9. Sanders ME, Schuyler PA, Dupont WD, Page DL. The natural history of low-grade ductal carcinoma in situ of the breast in women treated by biopsy only revealed over 30 years of long-term follow-up. Cancer. 2005;103(12):2481–4.
10. Page DL, Dupont WD, Rogers LW, Landenberger M. Intraductal carcinoma of the breast: follow-up after biopsy only. Cancer. 1982;49(4):751–8.
11. Perou CM, Sorlie T, Eisen MB, van de Rijn M, Jeffrey SS, Rees CA, Pollack JR, et al. Molecular portraits of human breast tumours. Nature. 2000;406:747–52.
12. Sorlie T, Tibshirani R, Parker J, Hastie T, Marron JS, Nobel A, et al. Repeated observation of breast tumor subtypes in independent gene-expression data sets. Proc Natl Acad Sci U S A. 2003;100:8418–23.
13. Sorlie T, Perou CM, Tibshirani R, Aas T, Geisler S, Johnsen H, et al. Gene-expression patterns of breast carcinomas distinguish tumor subclasses with clinical implications. Proc Natl Acad Sci U S A. 2001;98:10869–74.
14. Bergers E, Baak JP, van Diest PJ, van Gorp LH, Kwee WS, Los J, et al. Prognostic implications of different cell cycle analysis models of flow cytometric DNA histograms of 1,301 breast cancer patients: results from the Multicenter Morphometric Mammary Carcinoma Project (MMMCP). Int J Cancer. 1997;74:260–9.
15. Page DL, Dupont WD, Rogers LW, Rados MS. Atypical hyperplastic lesions of the female breast. A long-term follow-up study. Cancer. 1985;55:2698–708.
16. Dupont WD, Page DL. Risk factors for breast cancer in women with proliferative breast disease. N Engl J Med. 1985;312:146–51.
17. Van de Vijver MJ, Peterse H. The diagnosis and management of pre-invasive breast disease: pathological diagnosis—problems with existing classifications. Breast Cancer Res. 2003;5(5):269.
18. Page DL, Rogers LW. Combined histologic and cytologic criteria for the diagnosis of mammary atypical ductal hyperplasia. Hum Pathol. 1992;23(10):1095–7.
19. Roylance R, Gorman P, Hanby A, Tomlinson I. Allelic imbalance analysis of chromosome 16q shows that grade I and grade III invasive ductal breast cancers follow different genetic pathways. J Pathol. 2002;196(1):32–6.
20. Buerger H, Otterbach F, Simon R, Poremba C, Diallo R, Decker T, et al. Comparative genomic hybridization of ductal carcinoma in situ of the breast-evidence of multiple genetic pathways. J Pathol. 1999;187:396–402.
21. O'Connell P, Pekkel V, Fuqua SA, Osborne CK, Clark GM, Allred DC. Analysis of loss of heterozygosity in 399 premalignant breast lesions at 15 genetic loci. J Natl Cancer Inst. 1998;90:697–703.
22. Stratton MR, Collins N, Lakhani SR, Sloane JP. Loss of heterozygosity in ductal carcinoma in situ of the breast. J Pathol. 1995;175(2):195–201.
23. Gusterson BA, Machin LG, Gullick WJ, Gibbs NM, Powles TJ, Elliott C, et al. c-erbB-2 expression in benign and malignant breast disease. Br J Cancer. 1988;58(4):453–7.
24. Lu YJ, Osin P, Lakhani SR, Di Palma S, Gusterson BA, Shipley JM. Comparative genomic hybridization analysis of lobular carcinoma in situ and atypical lobular hyperplasia and potential roles for gains and losses of genetic material in breast neoplasia. Cancer Res. 1998;58:4721–7.
25. Berx G, Van Roy F. The E-cadherin/catenin complex: an important gatekeeper in breast cancer tumorigenesis and malignant progression. Breast Cancer Res. 2001;3(5):289–93.
26. Lakhani SR, Collins N, Stratton MR, Sloane JP. Atypical ductal hyperplasia of the breast: clonal proliferation with loss of heterozygosity on chromosomes 16q and 17p. J Clin Pathol. 1995;48(7):611–5.
27. Amari M, Suzuki A, Moriya T, Yoshinaga K, Amano G, Sasano H, et al. LOH analyses of premalignant and malignant lesions of human breast: frequent LOH in 8p, 16q, and 17q in atypical ductal hyperplasia. Oncol Rep. 1999;6(6):1277–80.
28. Choi BB, Kim SH, Park CS, Cha ES, Lee AW. Radiologic findings of lobular carcinoma in situ: mammography and ultrasonography. J Clin Ultrasound. 2011;39(2):59–63.
29. Lee MH, Ko EY, Han BK, Shin JH, Ko ES, Hahn SY. Sonographic findings of pure ductal carcinoma in situ. J Clin Ultrasound. 2013;41(8):465–71.
30. Macura KJ, Ouwerkerk R, Jacobs MA, Bluemke DA. Patterns of enhancement on breast MR images: interpretation and imaging pitfalls. Radiographics. 2006;26(6):1719–34.
31. Zhang Y, Ren H. Meta-analysis of diagnostic accuracy of magnetic resonance imaging and mammography for breast cancer. J Cancer Res Ther. 2017;13(5):862–8.
32. Gradishar WJ, Anderson BO, Balassanian R, Blair SL, Burstein HJ, Cyr A, et al. NCCN guidelines insights: breast cancer, version 1.2017. J Natl Compr Canc Netw. 2017;15(4):433–51.
33. Łukasiewicz E, Ziemiecka A, Jakubowski W, Vojinovic J, Bogucevska M, Dobruch-Sobczak K. Fine-needle versus core-needle biopsy - which one to choose in preoperative assessment of focal lesions in the breasts? Literature review. J Ultrason. 2017;17(71):267–74.

34. Kuenen-Boumeester V, Timmermans AM, De Bruijn EM, Henzen-Logmans SC. Immunocytochemical detection of prognostic markers in breast cancer; technical considerations. Cytopathology. 1999;10(5):308–16.
35. Solomides CC, Zimmerman R, Bibbo M. Semiquantitative assessment of c-erbB-2 (HER-2) status in cytology specimens and tissue sections from breast carcinoma. Anal Quant Cytol Histol. 1999;21(2):121–5.
36. Denley H, Pinder SE, Elston CW, Lee AH, Ellis IO. Preoperative assessment of prognostic factors in breast cancer. J Clin Pathol. 2001;54(1):20–4.
37. Hoda SA, Rosen PP. Practical considerations in the pathologic diagnosis of needle core biopsies of breast. Am J Clin Pathol. 2002;118(1):101–8.
38. Irfan K, Brem RF. Surgical and mammographic follow-up of papillary lesions and atypical lobular hyperplasia diagnosed with stereotactic vacuum-assisted biopsy. Breast J. 2002;8(4):230–3.
39. Bonnett M, Wallis T, Rossmann M, Pernick NL, Bouwman D, Carolin KA, et al. Histopathologic analysis of atypical lesions in image-guided core breast biopsies. Mod Pathol. 2003;16(2):154–60.
40. Domchek SM. The utility of ductal lavage in breast cancer detection and risk assessment. Breast Cancer Res. 2002;4(2):51–3.
41. Zaha DC. Significance of immunohistochemistry in breast cancer. World J Clin Oncol. 2014;5(3):382–92.
42. Cutuli B, De Lafontan B, Kirova Y, Auvray H, Tallet A, Avigdor S, et al. Lobular carcinoma in situ (LCIS) of the breast: is long-term outcome similar to ductal carcinoma in situ (DCIS)? Analysis of 200 cases. Radiat Oncol. 2015;10:110.
43. Gilleard O, Goodman A, Cooper M, Davies M, Dunn J. The significance of the Van Nuys prognostic index in the management of ductal carcinoma in situ. World J Surg Oncol. 2008;6:61.
44. Dunne C, Burke JP, Morrow M, Kell MR. Effect of margin status on local recurrence after breast conservation and radiation therapy for ductal carcinoma in situ. J Clin Oncol. 2009;27(10):1615–20.
45. van Roozendaal LM, Goorts B, Klinkert M, Keymeulen KBMI, De Vries B, Strobbe LJA, et al. Sentinel lymph node biopsy can be omitted in DCIS patients treated with breast conserving therapy. Breast Cancer Res Treat. 2016;156(3):517–25.
46. Fisher B, Dignam J, Wolmark N, Mamounas E, Costantino J, Poller W, et al. Lumpectomy and radiation therapy for the treatment of intraductal breast cancer: findings from National Surgical Adjuvant Breast and Bowel Project B-17. J Clin Oncol. 1998;16(2):441–52.
47. Cuzick J, Sestak I, Pinder SE, Ellis IO, Forsyth S, Bundred NJ, et al. Effect of tamoxifen and radiotherapy in women with locally excised ductal carcinoma in situ: long-term results from the UK/ANZ DCIS trial. Lancet Oncol. 2011;12(1):21–9.
48. Fisher B, Dignam J, Wolmark N, Wickerham DL, Fisher ER, Mamounas E, et al. Tamoxifen in treatment of intraductal breast cancer: National Surgical Adjuvant Breast and Bowel Project B-24 randomised controlled trial. Lancet. 1999;353(9169):1993–2000.
49. Chlebowski RT, Col N, Winer EP, Collyar DE, Cummings SR, Vogel VG 3rd, American Society of Clinical Oncology Breast Cancer Technology Assessment Working Group, et al. American Society of Clinical Oncology technology assessment of pharmacologic interventions for breast cancer risk reduction including tamoxifen, raloxifene, and aromatase inhibition. J Clin Oncol. 2002;20(15):3328–4.
50. Narod SA, Iqbal J, Giannakeas V, Sopik V, Sun P. Breast cancer mortality after a diagnosis of ductal carcinoma in situ. JAMA Oncol. 2015;1(7):888–96.
51. Chuba PJ, Hamre MR, Yap J, Severson RK, Lucas D, Shamsa F, et al. Bilateral risk for subsequent breast cancer after lobular carcinoma-in-situ: analysis of surveillance, epidemiology, and end results data. J Clin Oncol. 2005;23(24):5534–41.

Part VI

Newer Concepts

31 Contribution of the Gut and Vaginal Microbiomes to Gynecological Cancers

R. S. Jayshree and Rekha V. Kumar

31.1 Introduction

The saying "No man is an island.....every man is a piece of the continent, a part of the main" is very apt in the context of microbiomes in health and disease. Just as man is affected by the surrounding environment, likewise the cells of the body too are in tune with their microenvironment. The term "microbiota" refers to complex ecological communities of microbes in aggregate that are in a reciprocal relationship with the host at a specific site, while "microbiome" or metagenome of microbiota, by definition, is the collective genetic map of the entire microbiota residing in a specific niche [1] (Fig. 31.1). The term "microbiome," however, has often been used as a substitute for "microbiota." Within the human body, there are an estimated 100 trillion microbes, tenfold more in number than human cells [2, 3], that interact with the cells of the host constantly at numerous sites including the skin and mucosal surfaces such as the gastrointestinal (GI) tract. The GI tract houses the major share of the total human microbiome and exerts both local and far-reaching effects [4]. These microbes are capable of expressing many more distinctive genes than their host cells, providing remarkable enzymatic potential and imparting an essential role in many aspects of host physiology [5]. Thus, the gut microbes that have coevolved with their hosts for millions of years are no longer considered passive travelers but are intricately associated with a vast range of host activities like development and maturation of immune system [6], digestion and nutrition [6, 7], and detoxification and body defense [8]. The term microbiota encompasses various types of microorganisms like bacteria, viruses, fungi, parasites, etc. [9]. The normal microbial flora of any site is commonly referred to as commensals; however, technically they could be classified as *truly commensals*, *symbionts*, *parasites*, or *pathogens* depending on the resultant action at specific sites in the host. This relationship however is entirely context driven, depending on the diet/nutritional status, hormones, genetic makeup of the host, age, race, underlying diseases, and other coinfecting pathogens [10]. At each specific site of the body, these members need to be maintained in a "eubiotic" state—a state of equilibrium for sustaining the health of that site [4]. It is when there is disequilibrium, e.g., during inflammatory processes, that the microbial community changes, resulting in dysbiosis [4]. Dysbiosis, therefore, is an imbalance in the microbial ecology, i.e., variation in the proportions and/or strains of commensals, symbionts, and pathogens at a particular niche

R. S. Jayshree (✉)
Center for Molecular Oncology, Kidwai Cancer Institute, Bangalore, Karnataka, India

R. V. Kumar
Department of Oncopathology, Kidwai Cancer Institute, Bangalore, Karnataka, India

S. Mehta, A. Singla (eds.), *Preventive Oncology for the Gynecologist*,
https://doi.org/10.1007/978-981-13-3438-2_31

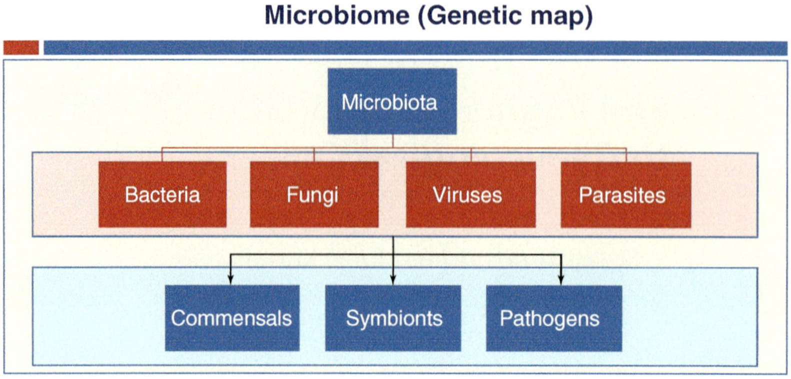

Fig. 31.1 Composition of the microbiome. Microbiome is the genetic content in toto of the microbiota present at a specific site [1]. The term microbiota is inclusive of all types of microorganisms like bacteria, fungi, viruses, and parasites which are in a constant relationship with the host cells. The host-microbe relationship can be classified under three broad types, viz., commensalism wherein the microorganism (commensal) neither harms or benefits the host; symbiosis where both the host and the microbe (symbiont) derive benefit from each other; and parasitism where the microbe (pathogen) harms the host

[4]. A persistent state of dysbiosis could further aid pathogen establishment, inflammation, production of genotoxins, and other carcinogenic microbial metabolites, all of which need not be mutually exclusive [4]. We are now tempted to agree with the old Ayurvedic adage that "gut health is critical to overall health" [11, 12], and varied types of diseases including depression, obesity, diabetes, chronic fatigue syndrome, rheumatoid arthritis, and cancer are associated with an unhealthy gut [13, 14]. In this chapter, we explain in detail the role of the gut and vaginal microbiota in gynecological malignancies.

31.2 The Role of the Gut Microbiome in Health and Gynecologic Cancers

The science of microbiomes has progressed exponentially in the last decade – thanks to the advances in sequencing technologies and bioinformatics. The resultant discoveries have revolutionized our perception about the composition, capability, and activity of the human intestinal microbiome. Microbes in the GI tract control several features of gut physiology, like digestion of complex foods, intestinal permeability, prevention of pathogen colonization, synthesis of vitamins, and metabolism. These have far-reaching effects well beyond the local GI compartment [13, 15]. Microbiota influence oncogenesis in various ways: (1) by the direct oncogenic action of specific pathogens or their products, e.g., *Helicobacter pylori* and gastric cancer and with reference to gynecologic malignancies, human papillomavirus (HPV) and cervical cancer (this aspect has been covered separately; please see Chap. 9); (2) by inducing pro-inflammatory and/or immunosuppressive activity, thereby subverting anticancer immunosurveillance [16, 17]; and (3) aids in the trafficking of numerous metabolites including hormones which favor tumor growth [18, 19].

31.2.1 Gut Microbiome Modulates the Systemic Immune and Inflammatory Responses

A healthy gut microbiome primarily comprises four phyla: *Bacteroidetes*, *Firmicutes*, *Actinobacteria*, and *Proteobacteria*. In order to maintain a healthy epithelial barrier, intestinal immunity, and homeostasis, the combined abundance of the former two phyla should be >90% of species, with a lower *Firmicutes*/*Bacteroidetes* (F/B) ratio [20]. The interaction between unique gut microbiota ("keystone species") and the gut epithelium drives the development and function of the immune system: Segmented filamentous bacteria (SFB) promote the differentiation of pro-inflammatory Th17 cells in the intestinal lamina propria, which has a substantial impact on the pathogenesis of autoimmune disorders [21, 22], whereas *Bacteroides fragilis* [23] and some species of *Clostridia* [24] direct the development and function of IL10-secreting regulatory T cells (Tregs) in the gut to actively induce gut mucosal tolerance and hence prevention of inflammatory bowel disease [25]. Likewise, nutrients and their metabolites influence the composition and functions of gut microbiota and their interaction with the immune system, e.g., tryptophan metabolites in the GI tract comprise those derived both from the GI host cells (endogenous catabolism: kynurenines, serotonin, and melatonin) and GI microbiota (indole, indolic acid, skatole, and tryptamine). The gut flora in turn influences absorption and metabolism of tryptophan by the host's cells and thus regulates host immunological responses [26]. The crucial role of normal gut flora in the development of the immune system is affirmed by a defective immune system in germ-free mice [27, 28]. Alteration in the types and/or abundance of the normal flora can even regulate immunity and inflammation in organs distal from the intestine [29]: gut microbiota-driven TLR5 signaling upregulated circulatory levels of tumor-promoting IL6, with subsequent mobilization of myeloid-derived suppressor cells (MDSCs) into ovarian cancer resulting in inflammatory and immunosuppressive microenvironment leading to malignant progression [30]. This is relevant considering that gene polymorphisms for pathogen recognition receptors (PRRs) [31] including TLR5 are common in the population [32].

31.2.2 Gut Microbiota Regulate Circulatory Hormone Levels

Peyer's patches in the gut-associated lymphoid tissue (GALT) have recently been recognized as sites for estradiol (E2) synthesis in mice, where the total quantity of the hormone exceeds that of the gonads [33]. Briefly, E2 acts canonically/genomically by binding to estrogen receptors (ERs), causing downstream gene activation and epigenetic modifications and eventually sets off signaling cascades within the cells. The net outcome of these series of events is physiological alterations across various estrogen-responsive tissues [14]. E2 regulates proliferation and homeostasis of lymphocytes locally in the gut and ultimately alters the diversity of the microbiome of the gut lumen [34]. The hormone in addition is also a potent immunosuppressor and acts by boosting suppressor cells like Tregs [35–38], M2 subtype of tumor-associated macrophages [39], and MDSCs [40]. Estradiol also upregulates expression of granzyme B inhibitor, proteinase inhibitor-9, which thereby protects cancer cells against apoptosis induced by immune effectors like natural killer and cytotoxic T cells [41]. In postmenopausal women, the gut microbiota plays a primary physiological role in the regulation of circulating estrogen levels [42]. Thus, dysbiosis in the gut could influence the risk of developing estrogen-related diseases including cancers [42]. Estradiol possesses pro-tumorigenic potential acting via both genomic and non-genomic pathways and has been incriminated in a variety of malignancies, predominantly breast, endometrial [43–45], and ovarian cancers [46], and, as described later in the chapter, in the etiopathogenesis of cervix cancer as well [38, 47].

31.2.2.1 Estrogen Metabolism in the Gut and Liver

Estrogens (C18) are derived from cholesterol (C27) through a series of reduction steps. There are three main forms of endogenous estrogens in the human female body: (1) Estradiol (E2) is the predominant premenopausal estrogen in non-pregnant women. It is majorly synthesized by the ovaries, Peyer's patches in mice (yet to be demonstrated in human Peyer's patches), and, to a small extent, adrenal glands and adipose tissue, through aromatization of testosterone [33, 34]. Androstenedione is aromatized to (2) estrone (E1), which in turn gets converted to E2 by 17β-hydroxysteroid dehydrogenases. Estrone predominates after menopause. (3) Estriol (E3) is

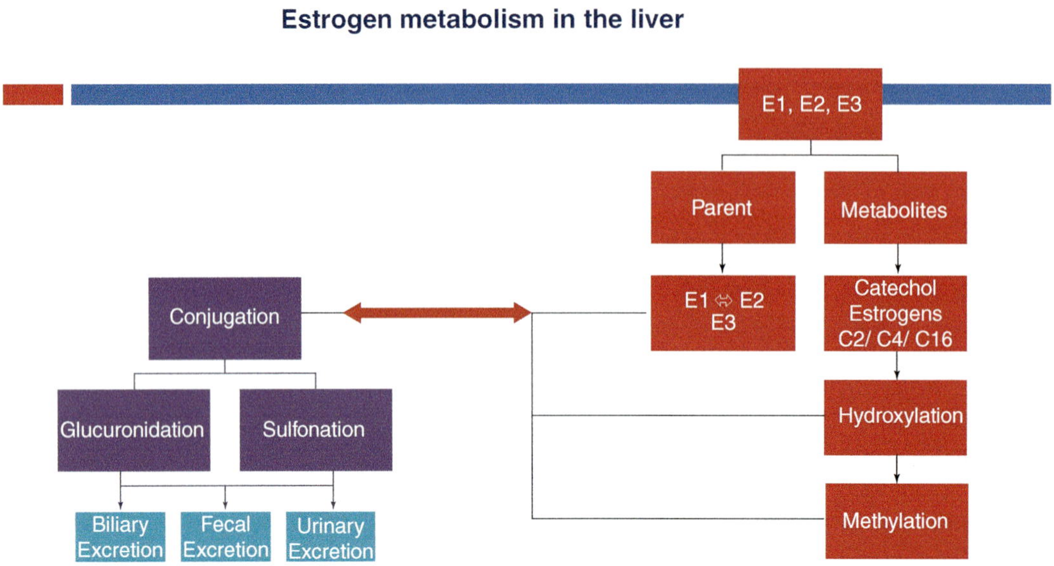

Fig. 31.2 Estrogen metabolism in the liver. Parent estrogens: *E1* estrone, *E2* estradiol, *E3* estriol. The steroid ring in the parent hormone undergoes irreversible hydroxylation and subsequent methylation at the C-2, C-4, or C-16 positions resulting in different types and concentration of estrogen metabolites. Both the parent molecules and the metabolites get conjugated via glucuronidation and sulfonation, and the resultant end products get excreted via the bile, feces, and urine [49–56]

highest during pregnancy [48]. Estrogens are largely transported in the plasma either in the free form, which is biologically active, or bound to proteins.

Phase I metabolism of estrogens (Fig. 31.2): Parent estrogens (E2, E1) undergo phase I metabolism in the liver; the steroid ring in the hormone undergoes irreversible hydroxylation at the C-2, C-4, or C-16 positions resulting in estrogen metabolites with varied hormone potency and half-life [49].

Phase II metabolism of estrogens: Further, both the parent hormone molecules and their metabolites (including cathechol estrogens derived via hydroxylation and subsequent methylation [50] get conjugated through glucuronidation or also through sulfonation, which then get readily excreted in the bile [51, 52], urine, and feces [50, 53]. Approximately 65%, 48%, and 23% of circulating forms of E2, E1, and E3, respectively, are recovered in bile [54], and accordingly about 10–15% of circulating E2, E1, and E3 are found in the conjugated form in the feces [55, 56]. An important aspect of estrogen metabolism is that β-glucuronidase- and β-glucosidase-expressing gut microbes deconjugate these estrogen glucuronides [57–61], resulting in reabsorption of a biologically significant proportion of estrogens into the circulation [42]. Analysis of fecal estrogen metabolites in humans after exposure to antibiotics [56, 62–64] and experiments with germ-free animals offer further support for the crucial role of gut microbiota in estrogen metabolism [65, 66]. The term "estrobolome" refers to the collective gut microbial genes whose expression is capable of metabolizing estrogens [18] (Fig. 31.3), which essentially modulates enterohepatic circulation of estrogens. In healthy men and postmenopausal women, fecal β-glucuronidases inversely correlated with total fecal estrogens and directly correlated with increased ratios of parent estrogen concentrations vs. estrogen metabolites in the serum, putting such women at an increased risk of breast cancer [67–70]. The right proportions of gut microbes contribute to the estrobolome, which regulates estrogen homeostasis at intestinal and distal mucosal sites [14, 71]. However, when gut

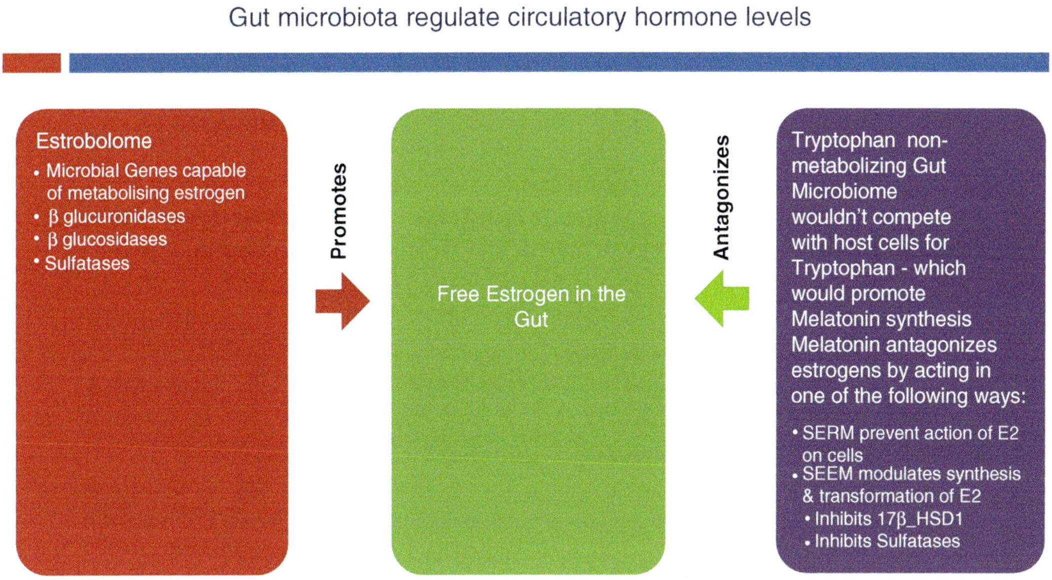

Fig. 31.3 Estrogen metabolism by the gut microbiome. At one end of the spectrum is the "estrobolome"—the overall gut microbial genes which can metabolize estrogens: e.g., β-glucuronidases and sulfatases. These enzymes deconjugate estrogens (both parent and metabolites) and release free estrogens in the gut lumen which can get absorbed into the circulation. At the other end is tryptophan non-metabolizing microbiome (e.g., *Klebsiella* spp.)—which doesn't compete with the host cells for tryptophan and thereby promotes the synthesis of melatonin in the gut. Melatonin antagonizes estrogens by acting as a selective estrogen receptor modulator (SERM) and a selective estrogen enzyme modulator (SEEM) by inhibiting enzymes which synthesize estradiol (E2), viz., 17β-hydroxysteroid dehydrogenase 1 (17β-HSD1), sulfatases, and aromatase [14, 18, 19, 26, 55, 77–80]

dysbiosis occurs, ratios of deconjugated-conjugated estrogens get altered resulting in either hyper- or hypoestrogenism, thus promoting the development of estrogen-related pathologies [18]. Thus, host-mediated glucuronidation of estrogens, which was once considered to primarily serve a classical excretory role, is challenged by microbial β-glucuronidases resulting in recycling of estrogens [55]. Microbial β-glucuronidases could thus be considered a boon for normal estrogen physiology but a bane for malignancies.

31.2.2.2 Melatonin, Estrogen, and the Gut Microbiome

While microbiota producing β-glucuronidases are at one end of the spectrum, at the other end are tryptophan-metabolizing and tryptophan-non-metabolizing gut microbes like *Escherichia coli* (*E. coli*) and *Klebsiella* spp., respectively (see Fig. 31.3). Melatonin, an indole hormone which is a by-product of tryptophan metabolism, is produced by the pineal gland and in addition is also synthesized by the cells of the GI tract, retina, leucocytes, and the skin [72]. The quantity of melatonin released in the GI tract is up to 400 times the concentration produced by the pineal gland [73]. The synthesis of melatonin in the gut partly depends on the dominant microbiome: for instance, microbes like *Klebsiella* spp. do not compete with the host cells for tryptophan and hence would promote melatonin synthesis, whereas tryptophan-utilizing microbes like *E. coli* eventually end up regulating serotonin and downstream melatonin synthesis in the gut [19, 26]. In addition to regulation of the circadian rhythm, melatonin also has other properties, such as regulation of gut permeability and immunomodulatory, anti-inflammatory, antioxidant, oncostatic, and antiproliferative properties [74]. The latter two effects of melatonin have been well established in estrogen-dependent breast cancer and endometrial cancer as well [75, 76]. Melatonin (1) interferes with the activation of ER and is thus akin to a selective estrogen receptor modulator (SERM) [77, 78]; (2) inhibits enzymes involved in the synthesis of estrogen, leading to lower plasma levels [79]; and (3) promotes metabolism of E2 into its inactive estrogen sulfate (E1S) form. The latter two properties are termed selective estrogen enzyme modulator (SEEM) [80]. Diet influences both the microbiome and in turn the estrobolome. A vegetarian diet has been proven to discourage the growth of β-glucuronidase-expressing microbes and accordingly vegetarians have higher concentrations of conjugated estrogens in the feces and lower serum levels of estrogens [51]. Hence, having the right species and/or proportions of gut bacteria would help them bind to fiber and excrete both excess human estrogen and chemical estrogens from the body [51].

31.2.2.3 Estrobolomes and Gynecological Malignancies

The metabolic functioning of the estrobolome is considered to be partly responsible for the lifetime burden of exposure to estrogen in a woman [18]. An estrobolome enriched in gene products promoting estrogen metabolite deconjugation reactions including but not limited to fecal β-glucuronidase levels may end up in greater reabsorption of free estrogens, thus influencing development of estrogen-driven neoplasia [18] (see Fig. 31.3). A phylogenetic diverse gut microbiome favors metabolism of conjugated estrogens. While the field of estrobolomes in gynecological malignancies remains to be explored, it may be very pertinent considering that excess circulatory and/or tissue estrogen may be a risk factor for the development of these cancers [38, 43, 81, 82].

31.2.2.4 Cervical Cancer

Several lines of evidence support a role of E2 in human cervical cancer (CxCa): firstly, long-term estrogen exposure by way of use of oral contraceptives/multiparity has been proven to increase the risk of cancer cervix [83, 84]. Secondly, in transgenic mouse models of cervical carcinogenesis, E2 has been proven to be a necessity for induction of oncogenesis [47, 85, 86]. Thirdly, in human disease, high intratumoral concentrations of the hormone were localized within both the tumor and stromal cells, in the absence of raised plasma levels [38]. However, since E1 is the predominant form of estrogen in postmenopausal women [48], it may be worth correlating plasma E1 levels with estrobolomes in this malignancy.

31.2.2.5 Endometrial Hyperplasia and Endometrial Cancer

High levels of estrogen unopposed by progesterone are thought to be a primary driver in both endometrial hyperplasia (EH) and endometrial carcinoma (EC) (OR 2.1–4.1) [87–90]. Hyperestrinism in the form of nulliparity, early menarche, and late menopause are known risk factors [91], and progestins, which are antiestrogens, are used in the therapy of atypical hyperplasia and EC [92]. High plasma levels of E1 in postmenopausal women is thought to originate by aromatization of adipose tissue [90, 93], which is relevant considering that majority of EC patients in developed countries are obese. Bariatric surgery, which modifies both the metabolic profile and the microbiome composition – and perhaps the estrobolome—thus reduces the risk of developing EH in obese women [94, 95]. The scenario regarding obesity and risk of cancer in the Asian-Indian population was not a concern until recently when 23% of females in India were reported to be either obese or overweight [96]. Furthermore, an increasing concern is that in the Indian population, the ill effects of obesity might be evident even at a lower BMI (<25 kg/m^2) [97]. Hence, characterizing the estrobolome vis-a-vis tryptophan metabolizing microbial genes which influence melatonin production is indeed required to understand whether gut microbes contribute to raised plasma levels of the hormone in EC.

31.2.2.6 Ovarian Cancer

The role of hormones in the etiology of ovarian cancer is controversial. There is only one prospective study which demonstrated that women with high circulatory E2 had three times the risk of developing ovarian cancer (OR 3.0) compared to women with the lowest E2 levels [98]. Estrogen may possibly be involved in the early steps of malignant transformation of ovarian tumors: ~60 to 100% of ovarian tumors express both types of estrogen receptors (ERα and ERβ) [99]; ERβ, which inhibits cell proliferation, gets downregulated with disease progression [100–102]. Additionally, through the non-genomic pathway involving NFκB, E2 promotes proliferation of ovarian granulosa cells which also downregulates ERβ [103]. Further, E2-ERα signaling may be playing an indirect role by potentiating the suppressive function of MDSCs in the tumor microenvironment [40].

31.3 Vaginal Microbiome in Gynecological Malignancies

Alteration in the flora of any site could play a role in the pathogenesis of various diseases including cancer broadly by promoting the establishment of pathogens/by modulating the local immune responses/metabolism [104]. In this section, we will review altered local microbial flora and its relevance to pathogen colonization and invasion in gynecological cancers.

31.3.1 The Normal Microbiota of the Vagina in Healthy Women

Both by forming communities and through elaboration of various metabolites like lactic acid, hydrogen peroxide, etc., the normal vaginal flora act as a crucial crusader against pathogen establishment including sexually transmitted infections (STIs) [105–110]. The flora is influenced by the microenvironment and by factors like age, sexual activity, antibiotic usage, use of oral contraceptives/hormone replacement therapy, and pregnancy [111, 112]. Long before the bacterial culture era, lactobacilli representing the normal vaginal flora were recognized as "gatekeepers" of the vaginal ecosystem. However, since more than 80% of vaginal microbiota is not culturable [113, 114], the actual composition of the normal vaginal flora was not known until recently. The dawn of the genomic era, and advances in sequencing technologies, has truly been a blessing to establish a "normogram" of the vagina through "The Human Microbiome Project," which the National Institutes of Health, USA, embarked upon from 2007 [9]. Various methods are used to characterize the microbiome at any site: viz., 16S rDNA amplification by polymerase chain reaction and pyrosequencing or whole genome sequencing. The microbiome profiles are classified by clustering them into community state types (CST), based on the predominant taxa present in the specimens. Such a method of classification is useful for studying the dynamics of microbiome, especially where large inter-subject heterogeneity and/or intra-subject temporal variability is found, which may be difficult to quantify but is nevertheless critically important, e.g., in bacterial vaginosis (BV) [115]. Overall, bacteria comprising a healthy vagina are classifiable into six major phyla—*Bacteroidetes*, *Fusobacteria*, *Actinobacteria*, *Tenericutes*, *Proteobacteria*, and *Firmicutes* [116]—and are typically dominated by members of the latter phyla, viz., *Lactobacillus crispatus* (*L. crispatus*), *L. gasseri*, *L. iners*, and *L. jensenii* [117]. The predominant species of lactobacilli, however, varies based on geography [118]. A reduction in the overall abundance of lactobacilli and variability in the predominant species has been observed in the vaginal microbiome from pre-, peri- to postmenopausal women: *L. crispatus* and *L. iners* dominated in premenopausal women; in perimenopausal women *L. gasseri* was predominant, whereas postmenopausal women had microbial species from diverse genera including *Proteobacteria*, *Porphyromonas*, *Streptococcus*, *Sphingomonas*, *Campylobacter*, and *Peptoniphilus* [116, 119, 120]. This fluctuation in vaginal microbiota observed during the lifetime of women is probably influenced by epithelial thickness and intraepithelial glycogen synthesis which is under the control of estrogen [116, 121].

31.3.2 Bacterial Vaginosis

In women of the reproductive age, bacterial vaginosis (BV) is one of the most common causes of abnormal vaginal discharge [122]. It is a condition that is marked by vaginal dysbiosis, wherein the normal vaginal flora comprising majorly of lactobacilli is replaced by varied combinations of anaerobic and facultatively anaerobic bacteria. Although there is inter-individual variation in the microbiota reported in BV, the most frequent ones observed are *Gardnerella*, *Prevotella*, *Atopobium*, *Sneathia*, *Mycoplasma*, *Megasphaera*, *Dialister*, *Bifidobacterium*, *Leptotrichia*, and *Clostridium* species [123–125]. Bacterial vaginosis can promote colonization and establishment of pathogens including STIs like HIV [126], *Chlamydia trachomatis* (*C. trachomatis*), *Neisseria gonorrhoeae* [127, 128], and HPV [129]. The diagnosis of BV is presently based on "Nugent" criteria—an objective microscopic reporting system of Gram-stained smears of vaginal discharge that evaluates bacteria on morphotypes [130]. Nugent score is the ratio of "beneficial" lactobacilli to other flora, which in BV is reversed sometimes to the extent of 100–1000 times compared to a healthy vagina. However, the diagnosis of BV is not free from problems: (1) there are difficulties in differentiating between normal flora and BV-predominant bacteria based on morphology; (2) inability to detect biofilm formation, which is an important pathogenetic mechanism in BV; (3) the dynamic nature of vaginal flora, which is swayed by various factors; (4) absence of lactobacilli in healthy women from certain geographic regions (African and Hispanics) where some other lactic acid-producing bacteria predominate; and/or (5) variable concentrations of facultative or anaerobic bacteria—microbiota that have been traditionally associated with BV [131].

31.3.3 The Vaginal Microbiome in HPV Infection, Precancer, and Invasive Cervical Cancer

Persistent infection with one of the high-risk genotypes of HPV has been proven to be necessary but not sufficient for initiation or progression of CxCa [132]. It is a well-established fact that 70% of HPV infections resolve within a year of infection [133] and <1% of these will progress to cancer [134]. Microbes sharing the same niche could be additional cofactors that either reduce the host's ability to clear HPV, increase the risk of acquisition, enhance HPV replication, and/or accelerate cancer progression [135]. Bacterial vaginosis [118, 136] or coinfections with other STIs are implicated in the acquisition, persistence, and progression of HPV infection to CxCa [132], aided by cytokines in the microenvironment [137]. Of the various STIs associated with genital HPV infection, two prominent ones relevant for monitoring progression of an HPV-infected lesion will be reviewed here, viz., *C. trachomatis* and human immunodeficiency virus (HIV) infections [138].

31.3.4 Bacterial Vaginosis in Cervical Carcinogenesis

There has been a great deal of interest in characterizing the vaginal microbiota in HPV-infected women, basically with an intent to identify other possible cofactors. No consistent pattern of microbes has been found in the composition of the cervicovaginal microbiomes across various stages of progression of HPV infection to invasive cancer [139]; however, a vast diversity of vaginal microbiomes was a common feature observed [116, 118, 140]. Briefly, vaginal dysbiosis was characterized by a decrease in lactobacilli and a concomitant increase in the diversity and number of anaerobic bacteria including species of *Gardnerella* [118, 141], *Fusobacteria* including *Sneathia* spp. [116, 139], *Atopobium* [141–143], *Prevotella* [116], and *Clostridia* [116]. Such a changed microenvironment is known to increase susceptibility to genital infections [144]. Cervical microbiome has been well characterized across all stages of cervical carcinogenesis only in one landmark study [139]: wherein samples were clustered into CSTs based on the histopathological findings (Table 31.1). Though the study was limited in numbers, it laid the foundation for further studies on microbiota in CxCa. A recent reanalysis of published microbiome data assessed the functional relevance of CSTs over time and observed *Gardnerella vaginalis*

Table 31.1 Clustering of cervical microbiome-based histopathological criteria [139]

No.	Cluster	Histopathology of cervical lesions	Predominant microbe
1.	CST I	Non-cervical lesion (HPV negative)	*L. crispatus* (21%)
2.	CST II	Non-cervical lesion (HPV positive)	*L. iners* (17%)
3.	CST III	Non-cervical lesion (HPV positive)	*Pseudomonas oleovorans* (10%)
4.	CST IV	SIL (HPV positive)	*Sneathia* (17%)
5.	CST V	Cervical lesion regardless of HPV status	*G. vaginalis* (7%)
6.	CST VI	Not done	*S. agalactiae* (7%)
7.	CST VII	Predominantly CxCa	*F. necrophorum* (7%)
8.	CST VIII	Only CxCa	*Fusobacteria* spp. (14%)

(*G. vaginalis*) to be a strong predictor of an upcoming CST change [145]. An inverse correlation has been reported between decreased relative abundance of *Lactobacillus* spp. with a concomitant increase in the abundance of *L. iners* in the vaginal flora and increasing severity of SIL disease [146]. This paradox of higher *L. iners* with higher grades of SIL may be due to the inability of *L. iners* to produce antimicrobials, lactic acid and hydrogen peroxide [144, 146], and hence may be aiding acquisition and/or persistence of the viral infection [116, 117, 139, 147, 148]. A predominance of *A. vaginae*, *G. vaginalis*, and *L. iners* with a concomitant paucity of *L. crispatus* in the cervical microbiota was associated with higher risk of SIL disease progression, suggesting that bacterial dysbiosis and its combination with oncogenic HPV types may be risk factors for cervical neoplasia [149].

31.3.5 HPV and Other Coinfections

31.3.5.1 *Chlamydia Trachomatis*

C. trachomatis is one of the most common STIs producing chronic inflammation [150, 151] and pelvic inflammatory disease (PID) and increases the risk of cervical neoplasia [152–155]. It is an intracellular Gram-negative bacterium, which infects the epithelium of the genital tract. The association of *C. trachomatis* infection was higher in HPV-positive women when compared to HPV-negative ones [156–158]. Both the microbes—HPV and *C. trachomatis*—reciprocally aid each other's acquisition [156–159]. *C. trachomatis* facilitates access of HPV to the basal cells of the cervical epithelium and may accelerate cell proliferation, inhibit apoptosis of infected cells, and even promote host DNA damage [160–162], which is a necessary condition for cell transformation [162]. *C. trachomatis* prevalence in CxCa is known to vary based on geography, detection method employed, and number of specimens sampled, and some studies have reported specific serotypes to be associated with the disease [162]. Large seroepidemiological studies across Europe have confirmed *C. trachomatis* to be a significant risk factor for high-grade SIL, carcinoma in situ, and invasive cancer cervix (ICC) [152, 163, 164] (OR 4.03 for the latter) [165]. This observation is of direct prognostic value, and it is therefore important to test women for *C. trachomatis*, particularly those who have tested positive for HPV. The advantage of such an approach could be twofold: it could protect against PID and may also prevent invasive cancer [165].

31.3.5.2 Human Immunodeficiency Virus

The second co-pathogen of relevance is the human immunodeficiency virus (HIV). HIV-mediated immunodeficiency adversely impacts the natural history of HPV infection, being associated with increased acquisition [166], and persistence [167] of the viral infection, and also with increased risk of progression to high-grade SIL [168, 169] and ICC [169–171] as compared to the general population. Both the viruses share common behavioral characteristics, use the cervix as the site of entry, and mutually complement each other in pathogenesis [172]. Mechanistically, inflammatory cytokines produced by the infected cells in response to HIV glycoproteins disrupt tight junctions and epithelial barrier function [173], which could then facilitate access and entry of HPV to basal epithelial cells [172, 174]. The rate of clearance of HPV infections is inversely proportional to the degree of immunosuppression represented by peripheral CD4 T-cell count in the HIV infected [175]. After the advent of highly active antiretroviral therapy (HAART), a reduction in the persistence of HPV and regression of low-grade SIL, signifying HPV clearance, has been observed in coinfected women [176, 177]. Decreasing HIV viral load however is not effective for reducing the prevalence of ICC in HIV-infected women [178]. Thus, HIV infection confers lifelong risk for the development of HPV-associated cervix carcinoma. Conversely, it has been observed worldwide that the risk for acquiring HIV infections in HPV-infected women is doubled [179–181]. Hence, besides protecting against HPV-associated cancers, prophylactic vaccination programs against HPV will have an added advantage of reducing the risk for HIV infection as well.

31.3.6 Modulation of Local Immune Responses by the Vaginal Microbiome

Chronic inflammation has a role to play in carcinogenesis of most solid tumors [182]. Some members of the cervicovaginal microbiota can translocate the epithelium, leading to low-grade inflammation which contributes to carcinogenesis [4]. Conversely, the inflammatory response to the tumors may cause dysbiosis, resulting in a positive feedback loop further promoting disease [4]. Accordingly, high expression of immunosuppressive cytokines IL4 and TGF-β1 have been observed within the lesions of cervical precancer and cancer in the CST dominated by *Fusobacterium* spp. indicating thereby that these microorganisms could be setting the stage by creating an immunosuppressive microenvironment, thus aiding HPV in cervical carcinogenesis [139].

31.3.7 Vaginal Microbiome and Endometrial Cancers

Although estrogen excess and metabolism are strong etiological factors in the pathogenesis of endometrial cancer, vaginal dysbiosis, as seen in BV resulting in PID, is considered a strong and independent risk factor for endometrial cancer (OR 1.79) [183–185]. Pelvic inflammatory disease results when pathogenic bacteria ascend through the cervix into the upper genital tract and cause inflammation of the uterus, fallopian tubes, and/or ovaries [185]. This is understandable with the growing consensus that the endometrial cavity is not sterile [186]. A large multicentric prospective study on vaginal microbiome (VMB) revealed that in patients with BV, a marked decrease in the abundance of lactobacilli and a relative abundance of anaerobic organisms including *G. vaginalis*, *Mycoplasma hominis*, *Ureaplasma urealyticum*, *Prevotella*, *Atopobium*, and *Mobiluncus* and anaerobic Gram-negative bacilli were significantly more likely to develop PID [184]. Hence, altered VMB is a risk factor for PID. A similar abundance of *Atopobium vaginae* and a *Porphyromonas* species was observed in the uterine microbiome from patients with EC [187].

31.3.8 Vaginal Microbiome and Ovarian Cancer

The upper female reproductive tract was once considered "sterile." A recent study, however, has refuted this fact: unique microbiomes have been demonstrated in the ovaries and fallopian tubes suggesting that the composition of upper genital tract microbiomes may be different in patients with epithelial ovarian cancer when compared to cancer-free controls [188]. Hence, chronic inflammation may play a role in the etiology of ovarian cancer [189]. One school of thought believes that following BV, the dysbiotic vaginal microflora ascend to the upper reproductive tract (uterus and fallopian tubes) [186, 190–193], especially to the latter site [194] leading to inflammation.

31.3.9 Prevention of Gynecological Malignancies

31.3.9.1 Diagnosis and Treatment of Vaginal Infections

Prompt diagnosis of the etiology and treatment of abnormal vaginal discharge may help prevent establishment of pathogens including STIs [131].

Also, in HIV-positive patients, it may be useful to screen for HPV infections for the long-term management of cervical precancer [195]. Likewise, in HPV-infected patients, it would help to know the presence of coinfections like *C. trachomatis* [196] since treatment of these infections may check the persistence of the viral infection [167] and help prevent progression to cervical precancer [176, 177].

31.3.9.2 Metabolic Products of Microbes

Besides their antioxidant, anti-inflammatory, and pro-apoptotic characteristics, the anticancer properties of phytochemicals can be ascribed to phytoestrogens, which are polyphenols structurally similar to estrogens but are of plant origin. There are three main types of phytoestrogens—isoflavones, ellagitannins, and lignans, which are metabolized by the gut microbiota into equol, urolithins, and enterolignans, respectively [197]. The estrogenic/antiestrogenic characteristics and the bioavailability of these metabolites are higher than the parent compound [198, 199]. Also, this dual activity of eliciting estrogenic/antiestrogenic properties gives phytoestrogens the therapeutic advantage in both hyper- and hypoestrogenism including cancers of the reproductive and nonreproductive tissue [198, 199]. However, inter-individual variation in the composition of host indigenous gut microbiota causes inconsistency in the ability to produce the final metabolites, and accordingly a variation is observed in the health benefits attributed to their consumption [200]. Antibiotics [201] and hormonal contraceptives [202] alter the gut microbiota, which may in turn reflect on the estrobolome. Since the gut microbiome plays an important role in regulating the metabolism of phenolic compounds [203], supplementation with probiotics might help counter the disease-promoting effects of these drugs.

Key Points

- Specific types and proportions of microbes comprise the normal eubiotic state at specific sites in the body; and dysbiosis is a deviation from this state.
- Eubiotic microbial flora in the gut is essential for the development and function of the normal immune system. Gut dysbiosis can induce systemic inflammation which could promote malignancies in distal organs.
- Gut microbiota or their by-products influence metabolism of hormones like estrogen and melatonin and thereby could either promote or inhibit oncogenesis, respectively, in various distant organs.
- Dysbiosis of the cervicovaginal microbiota aids gynecological malignancies either by promoting pathogen colonization/invasion or by suppressing the local immune response to favor oncogenesis.
- Dysbiotic vaginal flora in CxCa is characterized by a decrease in the overall abundance of lactobacilli and dominated by microbial species from diverse genera: Characteristically *Sneathia* in SIL and *Fusobacteria* in invasive cancer. These flora create an immunosuppressive microenvironment thus preparing the ground for establishment of other pathogens. Sexually transmitted infections like HIV, *C. trachomatis*, and *G. vaginalis* aid in HPV acquisition and/or persistence and/or progression to CxCa.
- Ascending dysbiotic vaginal microbiome causing PID has also been recognized to be a risk factor for both endometrial and ovarian cancers.
- Diet containing phytoestrogens counteracts the ill effects of estrogen metabolizing gut microbiota and hence is preventive against oncogenesis including gynecological malignancies.
- Treating PID and STIs would also form a first line of action for prevention of gynecological malignancies.

Acknowledgments We wish to acknowledge the help of Mr. G. R. Chandran, Project Management Consultant in making the figures; Prof. Rita Christopher, Department of Neurochemistry, National Institute of Mental Health and Neurosciences; and Dr. Sandhya Ravi, Consultant Surgeon and Managing Director, Prameya Health Pvt. Ltd., Bangalore, for reviewing the chapter and for offering useful suggestions.

References

1. Ursell LK, Metcalf JL, Parfrey LW, Knight R. Defining the human microbiome. Nutr Rev. 2012;70:S38–44.
2. Savage DC. Microbial ecology of the gastrointestinal tract. Annu Rev Microbiol. 1977;31:107–33.
3. Gill SR, Pop M, Deboy RT, Eckburg PB, Turnbaugh PJ, Samuel BS, et al. Metagenomic analysis of the human distal gut microbiome. Science. 2006;312:1355–9.
4. Schwabe RF, Jobin C. The microbiome and cancer. Nat Rev Cancer. 2013;13:800–12.
5. Ley RE, Peterson DA, Gordon JI. Ecological and evolutionary forces shaping microbial diversity in the human intestine. Cell. 2006;124:837–48.
6. Turnbaugh PJ, Gordon JI. The core gut microbiome, energy balance and obesity. J Physiol. 2009;587:4153–8.
7. Hehemann JH, Correc G, Barbeyron T, Helbert W, Czjzek M, Michel G. Transfer of carbohydrate-active enzymes from marine bacteria to Japanese gut microbiota. Nature. 2010;464:908–12.
8. Relman DA. The human microbiome: ecosystem resilience and health. Nutr Rev. 2012;70:S2–9.
9. Turnbaugh PJ, Ley RE, Hamady M, Fraser-Liggett CM, Knight R, Gordon JI. The human microbiome project. Nature. 2007;449:804–10.
10. Liang D, Leung RK, Guan W, Au WW. Involvement of gut microbiome in human health and disease: brief overview, knowledge gaps and research opportunities. Gut Pathog. 2018;10:3.
11. Peterson CT, Denniston K, Chopra D. Therapeutic uses of Triphala in Ayurvedic medicine. J Altern Complement Med. 2017;23:607–14.
12. Eswaran HT, Kavita MB, Tripaty TB, Shivakumar. Formation and validation of questionnaire to assess Jātharāgni. Anc Sci Life. 2015;34:203–9.
13. Belkaid Y, Hand TW. Role of the microbiota in immunity and inflammation. Cell. 2014;157:121–41.
14. Baker JM, Al-Nakkash L, Herbst-Kralovetz MM. Estrogen-gut microbiome axis: physiological and clinical implications. Maturitas. 2017;103:45–53.
15. Trompette A, Gollwitzer ES, Yadava K, Sichelstiel AK, Sprenger N, Ngom-Bru C, et al. Gut microbiota metabolism of dietary fiber influences allergic airway disease and hematopoiesis. Nat Med. 2014;20:159–66.
16. Guo Y, Qi Y, Yang X, Zhao L, Wen S, Liu Y, et al. Association between polycystic ovary syndrome and gut microbiota. PLoS One. 2016;11:e0153196.
17. Markle JG, Frank DN, Mortin-Toth S, Robertson CE, Feazel LM, Rolle-Kampczyk U, et al. Sex differences in the gut microbiome drive hormone-dependent regulation of autoimmunity. Science. 2013;339:1084–8.
18. Plottel CS, Blaser MJ. Microbiome and malignancy. Cell Host Microbe. 2011;10:324–35.
19. Wikoff WR, Anfora AT, Liu J, Schultz PG, Lesley SA, Peters EC, et al. Metabolomics analysis reveals large effects of gut microflora on mammalian blood metabolites. Proc Natl Acad Sci U S A. 2009;106:3698–703.
20. Turnbaugh PJ, Ley RE, Mahowald MA, Magrini V, Mardis ER, Gordon JI. An obesity-associated gut microbiome with increased capacity for energy harvest. Nature. 2006;444:1027–31.
21. Ivanov II, Atarashi K, Manel N, Brodie EL, Shima T, Karaoz U, et al. Induction of intestinal Th17 cells by segmented filamentous bacteria. Cell. 2009;139:485–98.
22. Wu HJ, Ivanov II, Darce J, Hattori K, Shima T, Umesaki Y, et al. Gut-residing segmented filamentous bacteria drive autoimmune arthritis via T helper 17 cells. Immunity. 2010;32:815–27.
23. Mazmanian SK, Round JL, Kasper DL. A microbial symbiosis factor prevents intestinal inflammatory disease. Nature. 2008;453:620–5.
24. Atarashi K, Tanoue T, Oshima K, Suda W, Nagano Y, Nishikawa H, et al. Treg induction by a rationally selected mixture of Clostridia strains from the human microbiota. Nature. 2013;500:232–6.
25. Round JL, Mazmanian SK. Inducible Foxp3+ regulatory T-cell development by a commensal bacterium of the intestinal microbiota. Proc Natl Acad Sci U S A. 2010;107:12204–9.
26. Gao J, Xu K, Liu H, Liu G, Bai M, Peng C, et al. Impact of the gut microbiota on intestinal immunity mediated by tryptophan metabolism. Front Cell Infect Microbiol. 2018;8:13.
27. Huang T, Wei B, Velazquez P, Borneman J, Braun J. Commensal microbiota alter the abundance and TCR responsiveness of splenic naive CD4+ T lymphocytes. Clin Immunol. 2005;117:221–30.
28. Ostman S, Rask C, Wold AE, Hultkrantz S, Telemo E. Impaired regulatory T cell function in germ-free mice. Eur J Immunol. 2006;36:2336–46.
29. Belkaid Y, Naik S. Compartmentalized and systemic control of tissue immunity by commensals. Nat Immunol. 2013;14:646–53.
30. Rutkowski MR, Stephen TL, Svoronos N, Allegrezza MJ, Tesone AJ, Perales-Puchalt A, et al. Microbially driven TLR5-dependent signaling governs distal malignant progression through tumor-promoting inflammation. Cancer Cell. 2015;27:27–40.
31. Casanova JL, Abel L, Quintana-Murci L. Human TLRs and IL-1Rs in host defense: natural insights from evolutionary, epidemiological, and clinical genetics. Annu Rev Immunol. 2011;29:447–91.
32. Hawn TR, Verbon A, Lettinga KD, Zhao LP, Li SS, Laws RJ, et al. A common dominant TLR5 stop codon polymorphism abolishes flagellin signaling and is associated with susceptibility to legionnaires' disease. J Exp Med. 2003;198:1563–72.
33. Oakley OR, Kim KJ, Lin PC, Barakat R, Cacioppo JA, Li Z, et al. Estradiol synthesis in gut-associated lymphoid tissue: leukocyte regulation by a

sexually monomorphic system. Endocrinology. 2016;157:4579–87.
34. Barakat R, Oakley O, Kim H, Jin J, Ko CJ. Extra-gonadal sites of estrogen biosynthesis and function. BMB Rep. 2016;49:488–96.
35. Tai P, Wang J, Jin H, Song X, Yan J, Kang Y, et al. Induction of regulatory t cells by physiological level estrogen. J Cell Physiol. 2008;214:456–64.
36. Polanczyk MJ, Carson BD, Subramanian S, Afentoulis M, Vandenbark AA, Ziegler SF, et al. Cutting edge: estrogen drives expansion of the cd4+cd25+ regulatory t cell compartment. J Immunol. 2004;173:2227–30.
37. Polanczyk MJ, Hopke C, Vandenbark AA, Offner H. Treg suppressive activity involves estrogen dependent expression of programmed death-1 (PD-1). Int Immunol. 2007;19:337–43.
38. Adurthi S, Kumar MM, Vinodkumar HS, Mukherjee G, Krishnamurthy H, Acharya KK, et al. Oestrogen Receptor-α binds the FOXP3 promoter and modulates regulatory T-cell function in human cervical cancer. Sci Rep. 2017;7:17289–304.
39. Svensson S, Abrahamsson A, Rodriguez GV, Olsson AK, Jensen L, Cao Y, et al. CCL2 and CCL5 are novel therapeutic targets for estrogen-dependent breast cancer. Clin Cancer Res. 2015;21:3794–805.
40. Svoronos N, Perales-Puchalt A, Allegrezza MJ, Rutkowski MR, Payne KK, Tesone AJ, et al. Tumor cell-independent estrogen signaling drives disease progression through mobilization of myeloid-derived suppressor cells. Cancer Discov. 2017;7:72–85.
41. Jiang X, Orr BA, Kranz DM, Shapiro DJ. Estrogen induction of the granzyme B inhibitor, proteinase inhibitor 9, protects cells against apoptosis mediated by cytotoxic T lymphocytes and natural killer cells. Endocrinology. 2006;147:1419–26.
42. Chen KL, Madak-Erdogan Z. Estrogen and microbiota crosstalk: should we pay attention? Trends Endocrinol Metab. 2016;27:752–5.
43. Grady D, Gebretsadik T, Kerlikowske K, Ernster V, Petitti D. Hormone replacement therapy and endometrial cancer risk: a meta-analysis. Obstet Gynecol. 1995;85:304–13.
44. Guo RX, Wei LH, Tu Z, Sun PM, Wang JL, Zhao D, et al. 17 beta-estradiol activates PI3K/Akt signaling pathway by estrogen receptor (ER)-dependent and ER-independent mechanisms in endometrial cancer cells. J Steroid Biochem Mol Biol. 2006;99:9–18.
45. Zhang Y, Zhao D, Gong C, Zhang F, He J, Zhang W, et al. Prognostic role of hormone receptors in endometrial cancer: a systematic review and meta-analysis. World J Surg Oncol. 2015;13:208.
46. Lacey JV, Mink PJ, Lubin JH, Sherman ME, Troisi R, Hartge P, et al. Menopausal hormone replacement therapy and risk of ovarian cancer. J Am Med Assoc. 2002;288:334–41.
47. Brake T, Lambert PF. Estrogen contributes to the onset, persistence, and malignant progression of cervical cancer in a human papillomavirus-transgenic mouse model. Proc Natl Acad Sci U S A. 2005;102:2490–5.
48. Gruber CJ, Tschugguel W, Schneeberger C, Huber JC. Production and actions of estrogens. N Engl J Med. 2002;346:340–52.
49. Zhu BT, Han GZ, Shim JY, Wen Y, Jiang XR. Quantitative structure-activity relationship of various endogenous estrogen metabolites for human estrogen receptor alpha and beta subtypes: insights into the structural determinants favoring a differential subtype binding. Endocrinology. 2006;147:4132–50.
50. Raftogianis R, Creveling C, Weinshilboum R, Weisz J. Estrogen metabolism by conjugation. J Natl Cancer Inst Monogr. 2000;27:113–24.
51. Kwa M, Plottel CS, Blaser JM, Adams S. The intestinal microbiome and estrogen receptor–positive female breast cancer. J Natl Cancer Inst. 2016;108:djw029.
52. Ebner T, Remmel RP, Burchell B. Human bilirubin UDP-glucuronosyl- transferase catalyzes the glucuronidation of ethinylestradiol. Mol Pharmacol. 1993;43:649–54.
53. Bongiovanni AM, Cohn RM. Clinical aspects of steroid conjugation. In: Bernstein S, Solomon S, editors. Chemical and biological aspects of steroid conjugation, chap. 9. New York: Springer; 1970.
54. Sandberg AA, Slaunwhite WR Jr. Studies on phenolic steroids in human subjects. II. The metabolic fate and hepato-biliary-enteric circulation of C14-estrone and C14-estradiol in women. J Clin Invest. 1957;36:1266–78.
55. Adlercreutz H, Martin F. Biliary excretion and intestinal metabolism of progesterone and estrogens in man. J Steroid Biochem. 1980;13:231–44.
56. Adlercreutz H, Jarvenpaa P. Assay of estrogens in human feces. J Steroid Biochem. 1982;17:639–45.
57. Cole CB, Fuller R, Mallet AK, Rowland IR. The influence of the host on expression of intestinal microbial enzyme activities involved in metabolism of foreign compounds. J Appl Bacteriol. 1985;59:549–53.
58. Dabek M, McCrae SI, Stevens VJ, Duncan SH, Louis P. Distribution of beta-glucosidase and beta-glucuronidase activity and of beta-glucuronidase gene gus in human colonic bacteria. FEMS Microbiol Ecol. 2008;66:487–95.
59. Gadelle D, Raibaud P, Sacquet E. beta-Glucuronidase activities of intestinal bacteria determined both in vitro and in vivo in gnotobiotic rats. Appl Environ Microbiol. 1985;49:682–5.
60. Gloux K, Berteau O, El Oumami H, Beguet F, Leclerc M, Dore J. A metagenomic beta-glucuronidase uncovers a core adaptive function of the human intestinal microbiome. Proc Natl Acad Sci U S A. 2011;108:4539–46.
61. McBain AJ, Macfarlane GT. Ecological and physiological studies on large intestinal bacteria in relation to production of hydrolytic and reductive enzymes

involved in formation of genotoxic metabolites. J Med Microbiol. 1998;47:407–16.
62. Martin F, Peltonen J, Laatikainen T, Pulkkinen M, Adlercreutz H. Excretion of progesterone metabolites and estriol in faeces from pregnant women during ampicillin administration. J Steroid Biochem. 1975;6:1339–46.
63. Adlercreutz H, Martin F, Lindström B. Gas chromatographic and mass spectrometric studies on oestrogens in bile—2. Men and non-pregnant women. J Steroid Biochem. 1978;9:1197–205.
64. Adlercreutz H, Martin F, Järvenpää P, Fotsis T. Steroid absorption and enterohepatic recycling. Contraception. 1979;20:201–23.
65. Eriksson H, Gustafsson JA, Sjovall J. Steroids in germfree and conventional rats. Free steroids in faeces from conventional rats. Eur J Biochem. 1969;9:286–90.
66. Shimizu K, Muranaka Y, Fujimura R, Ishida H, Tazume S, Shimamura T. Normalization of reproductive function in germfree mice following bacterial contamination. Exp Anim. 1998;47:151–8.
67. Falk RT, Brinton LA, Dorgan JF, Fuhrman BJ, Veenstra TD, Xu X, et al. Relationship of serum estrogens and estrogen metabolites to postmenopausal breast cancer risk: a nested case-control study. Breast Cancer Res. 2013;15:R34.
68. Flores R, Shi J, Fuhrman B, Xu X, Veenstra TD, Gail MH, et al. Fecal microbial determinants of fecal and systemic estrogens and estrogen metabolites: a cross-sectional study. J Transl Med. 2012;10:253.
69. Sampson JN, Falk RT, Schairer C, Moore SC, Fuhrman BJ, Dallal CM, et al. Association of estrogen metabolism with breast cancer risk in different cohorts of postmenopausal women. Cancer Res. 2017;77:918–25.
70. Fuhrman BJ, Schairer C, Gail MH, Boyd-Morin J, Xu X, Sue LY, et al. Estrogen metabolism and risk of breast cancer in postmenopausal women. J Natl Cancer Inst. 2012;104:326–39.
71. Sommer F, Backhed F. The gut microbiota – masters of host development and physiology. Nat Rev Microbiol. 2013;11:227–38.
72. Radogna F, Diederich M, Ghibelli L. Melatonin: a pleiotropic molecule regulating inflammation. Biochem Pharmacol. 2010;80:1844–52.
73. Bubenik GA, Brown GM, Grota LJ. Immunohistological localization of melatonin in the rat digestive system. Experientia. 1977;33:662–3.
74. Talib WH. Melatonin and cancer hallmarks. Molecules. 2018;23:E518.
75. Viswanathan A, Hankinson SE, Schernhammer ES. Night shift work and the risk of endometrial cancer. Cancer Res. 2007;67:10618–22.
76. Viswanathan AN, Schernhammer ES. Circulating melatonin and the risk of breast and endometrial cancer in women. Cancer Lett. 2009;281:1–7.
77. Blask DE, Hill SM. Effects of melatonin on cancer: studies on MCF-7 human breast cancer cells in culture. J Neural Transm. 1986;21:433–49.
78. Hill SM, Blask DE. Effects of the pineal hormone melatonin on the proliferation and morphological characteristics of human breast cancer cells (MCF-7) in culture. Cancer Res. 1988;48:6121–6.
79. Martínez-Campa C, González A, Mediavilla MD, Alonso-González C, Alvarez-García V, Sánchez-Barceló EJ, et al. Melatonin inhibits aromatase promoter expression by regulating cyclooxygenases expression and activity in breast cancer cells. Br J Cancer. 2009;101:1613–9.
80. Gonzalez A, Cos S, Martinez-Campa C, Alonso-Gonzalez C, Sanchez-Mateos S, Mediavilla MD, et al. Selective estrogen enzyme modulator actions of melatonin in human breast cancer cells. J Pineal Res. 2008;45:86–92.
81. Xu D, Lin TH, Yeh CR, Cheng MA, Chen LM, Chang C, et al. The wedelolactone derivative inhibits estrogen receptor-mediated breast, endometrial, and ovarian cancer cells growth. Biomed Res Int. 2014;2014:713263.
82. Antunes CM, Strolley PD, Rosenshein NB, Davies JL, Tonascia JA, Brown C, et al. Endometrial cancer and estrogen use. Report of a large case-control study. N Engl J Med. 1979;300:9–13.
83. Moreno V, Bosch FX, Muñoz N, Meijer CJ, Shah KV, Walboomers JM, et al. Effect of oral contraceptives on risk of cervical cancer in women with human papillomavirus infection: the IARC multicentric case-control study. Lancet. 2002;359:1085–92.
84. Muñoz N, Franceschi S, Bosetti C, Moreno V, Herrero R, Smith JS, et al. Role of parity and human papillomavirus in cervical cancer: the IARC multicentric case-control study. Lancet. 2002;359:1093–101.
85. Arbeit JM, Howley PM, Hanahan D. Chronic estrogen-induced cervical and vaginal squamous carcinogenesis in human papillomavirus type 16 transgenic mice. Proc Natl Acad Sci U S A. 1996;93:2930–5.
86. Park JS, Rhyu JW, Kim CJ, Kim HS, Lee SY, Kwon YI, et al. Neoplastic change of squamo-columnar junction in uterine cervix and vaginal epithelium by exogenous estrogen in hpv-18 URR E6/E7 transgenic mice. Gynecol Oncol. 2003;89:360–8.
87. Lukanova A, Kaaks R. Endogenous hormones and ovarian cancer: epidemiology and current hypotheses. Cancer Epidemiol Biomark Prev. 2005;14:98–107.
88. Allen NE, Key TJ, Dossus L, Rinaldi S, Cust A, Lukanova A, et al. Endogenous sex hormones and endometrial cancer risk in women in the European Prospective Investigation into Cancer and Nutrition (EPIC). Endocr Relat Cancer. 2008;15:485–97.
89. Gunter MJ, Hoover DR, Yu H, Wassertheil-Smoller S, Manson JE, Li J, et al. A prospective evaluation of insulin and insulin-like growth factor I as risk factors for endometrial cancer. Cancer Epidemiol Biomark Prev. 2008;17:921–9.
90. Charalampakis V, Tahrani AA, Helmy A, Gupta JK, Singhal R. Polycystic ovary syndrome and endometrial hyperplasia: an overview of the role of bariatric surgery in female fertility. Eur J Obstet Gynecol Reprod Biol. 2016;207:220–6.

91. Purdie DM, Green AC. Epidemiology of endometrial cancer. Best Pract Res Clin Obstet Gynaecol. 2001;15:341–54.
92. Carlson MJ, Thiel KW, Leslie KK. Past, present, and future of hormonal therapy in recurrent endometrial cancer. Int J Womens Health. 2014;6:429–35.
93. Siiteri PK. Adipose-tissue as a source of hormones. Am J Clin Nutr. 1987;45:277–82.
94. Upala S, Sanguankeo A. Bariatric surgery and risk of postoperative endometrial cancer: a systematic review and meta-analysis. Surg Obes Relat Dis. 2015;11:949–55.
95. Kaska L, Sledzinski T, Chomiczewska A, Dettlaff-Pokora A, Swierczynski J. Improved glucose metabolism following bariatric surgery is associated with increased circulating bile acid concentrations and remodeling of the gut microbiome. World J Gastroenterol. 2016;22:8698–719.
96. Gouda J, Prusty RK. Overweight and obesity among women by economic stratum in urban India. J Health Popul Nutr. 2014;32:79–88.
97. Yajnik CS. Confessions of a thin-fat Indian. Eur J Clin Nutr. 2018;72:469–73.
98. Helzlsouer KJ, Alberg AJ, Gordon GB, Longcope C, Bush TL, Hoffman SC, et al. Serum gonadotropins and steroid hormones and the development of ovarian cancer. JAMA. 1995;274:1926–30.
99. Lindgren PR, Cajander S, Backstrom T, Gustafsson JA, Makela S, Olofsson JI. Estrogen and progesterone receptors in ovarian epithelial tumors. Mol Cell Endocrinol. 2004;221:97–104.
100. Lau KM, Mok SC, Ho SM. Expression of human estrogen receptor-a and -b, progesterone receptor, and androgen receptor mRNA in normal and malignant ovarian epithelial cells. Proc Natl Acad Sci U S A. 1999;96:5722–7.
101. Bardin A, Boulle N, Lazennec G, Vignon F, Pujol P. Loss of ERb expression as a common step in estrogen-dependent tumor progression. Endocr Relat Cancer. 2004;11:537–51.
102. Lazennec G. Estrogen receptor b, a possible tumor suppressor involved in ovarian carcinogenesis. Cancer Lett. 2006;23:151–7.
103. Chu S, Nishi Y, Yanase T, Nawata H, Fuller PJ. Transrepression of estrogen receptor b signaling by nuclear factor-kb in ovarian granulosa cells. Mol Endocrinol. 2004;18:1919–28.
104. Avilés-Jiménez F, Guoqin Y, Torres-Poveda K, Madrid-Marina V, Torres J. On the search to elucidate the role of microbiota in the genesis of cancer: the cases of gastrointestinal and cervical cancer. Arch Med Res. 2017;48:754–65.
105. Boskey ER, Cone RA, Whaley KJ, Moench TR. Origins of vaginal acidity: high D/L lactate ratio is consistent with bacteria being the primary source. Hum Reprod. 2001;16:1809–13.
106. Aroutcheva A, Gariti D, Simon M, Shott S, Faro J, Simoes JA, et al. Defense factors of vaginal lactobacilli. Am J Obstet Gynecol. 2001;185:375–9.
107. Ocana VS, Pesce De Ruiz Holgado AA, Nader-Macias ME. Characterization of a bacteriocin-like substance produced by a vaginal Lactobacillus salivarius strain. Appl Environ Microbiol. 1999;65:5631–5.
108. Reid G, Heinemann C, Velraeds M, van der Mei HC, Busscher HJ. Biosurfactants produced by Lactobacillus. Methods Enzymol. 1999;310:426–33.
109. Boris S, Barbés C. Role played by lactobacilli in controlling the population of vaginal pathogens. Microbes Infect. 2000;2:543–6.
110. McMillan A, Dell M, Zellar MP, Cribby S, Martz S, Hong E, et al. Disruption of urogenital biofilms by lactobacilli. Colloids Surf B Biointerfaces. 2011;86:58–64.
111. Evans JM, Morris LS, Marchesi JR. The gut microbiome: the role of a virtual organ in the endocrinology of the host. J Endocrinol. 2013;218:R37–47.
112. Freestone PP, Sandrini SM, Haigh RD, Lyte M. Microbial endocrinology: how stress influences susceptibility to infection. Trends Microbiol. 2008;16:55–64.
113. Amann RI, Ludwig W, Schleifer KH. Phylogenetic identification and in situ detection of individual microbial cells without cultivation. Microbiol Rev. 1995;59:143–69.
114. Eckburg PB, Bik EM, Bernstein CN, Purdom E, Dethlefsen L, Sargent M, et al. Diversity of the human intestinal microbial flora. Science. 2005;308:1635–8.
115. Ma ZS, Li L. Quantifying the human vaginal community state types (CSTs) with the species specificity index. PeerJ. 2017;5:e3366.
116. Lee JE, Lee S, Lee H, Song YM, Lee K, Han MJ, et al. Association of the vaginal microbiota with human papillomavirus infection in a Korean twin cohort. PLoS One. 2013;8:e63514.
117. Ravel J, Gajer P, Abdo Z, Schneider GM, Koenig SS, McCulle SL, et al. Vaginal microbiome of reproductive-age women. Proc Natl Acad Sci U S A. 2011;108(Suppl 1):4680–7.
118. Gao W, Weng J, Gao Y, Chen X. Comparison of the vaginal microbiota diversity of women with and without human papillomavirus infection: a cross-sectional study. BMC Infect Dis. 2013;13:271.
119. Brotman RM, Shardell MD, Gajer P, Fadrosh D, Chang K, Silver MI, et al. Association between the vaginal microbiota, menopause status, and signs of vulvovaginal atrophy. Menopause. 2014;21:450–8.
120. Pabich WL, Fihn SD, Stamm WE, Scholes D, Boyko EJ, Gupta K. Prevalence and determinants of vaginal flora alterations in postmenopausal women. J Infect Dis. 2003;188:1054–8.
121. Hillier SL, Lau RJ. Vaginal microflora in postmenopausal women who have not received estrogen replacement therapy. Clin Infect Dis. 1997;25:S123.
122. Kenyon C, Colebunders R, Crucitti T. The global epidemiology of bacterial vaginosis: a systematic review. Am J Obstet Gynecol. 2013;209:505–23.

123. Srinivasan S, Hoffman NG, Morgan MT, Matsen FA, Fiedler TL, Hall RW, et al. Bacterial communities in women with bacterial vaginosis: high resolution phylogenetic analyses reveal relationships of microbiota to clinical criteria. PLoS One. 2012;7:e37818.
124. Ling Z, Kong J, Liu F, Zhu H, Chen X, Wang Y, et al. Molecular analysis of the diversity of vaginal microbiota associated with bacterial vaginosis. BMC Genomics. 2010;11:488.
125. Cox C, Watt AP, McKenna JP, Coyle PV. Mycoplasma hominis and Gardnerella vaginalis display a significant synergistic relationship in bacterial vaginosis. Eur J Clin Microbiol Infect Dis. 2016;35:481–7.
126. Atashili J, Poole C, Ndumbe PM, Adimora AA, Smith JS. Bacterial vaginosis and HIV acquisition: a meta-analysis of published studies. AIDS. 2008;22:1493–501.
127. Gallo MF, Macaluso M, Warner L, Fleenor ME, Hook EW, Brill I, et al. Bacterial vaginosis, gonorrhea, and chlamydial infection among women attending a sexually transmitted disease clinic: a longitudinal analysis of possible causal links. Ann Epidemiol. 2012;22:213–20.
128. Aghaizu A, Reid F, Kerry S, Hay PE, Mallinson H, Jensen JS, et al. Frequency and risk factors for incident and redetected Chlamydia trachomatis infection in sexually active, young, multi-ethnic women: a community based cohort study. Sex Transm Infect. 2014;90:524–8.
129. Gillet E, Meys JF, Verstraelen H, Bosire C, De Sutter P, Temmerman M, et al. Bacterial vaginosis is associated with uterine cervical human papillomavirus infection: a meta-analysis. BMC Infect Dis. 2011;11:10.
130. Nugent RP, Krohn MA, Hillier SL. Reliability of diagnosing bacterial vaginosis is improved by a standardized method of gram stain interpretation. J Clin Microbiol. 1991;29:297–301.
131. Nasioudis D, Linhares IM, Ledger WJ, Witkin SS. Bacterial vaginosis: a critical analysis of current knowledge. BJOG. 2017;124:61–9.
132. Castellsague X, Munoz N. Chapter 3: Cofactors in human papillomavirus carcinogenesis—role of parity, oral contraceptives, and tobacco smoking. J Natl Cancer Inst Monogr. 2003;(31):20–8.
133. Winer RL, Hughes JP, Feng Q, Xi LF, Cherne S, O'Reilly S, et al. Early natural history of incident, type-specific human papillomavirus infections in newly sexually active young women. Cancer Epidemiol Biomark Prev. 2011;20:699–707.
134. Castellsague X, Bosch FX, Munoz N. Environmental co-factors in HPV carcinogenesis. Virus Res. 2002;89:191–9.
135. Guidry JT, Scott RS. The interaction between human papillomavirus and other viruses. Virus Res. 2017;231:139–47.
136. Guo YL, You K, Qiao J, Zhao YM, Geng L. Bacterial vaginosis is conducive to the persistence of HPV infection. Int J STD AIDS. 2012;23:581–4.
137. Behbakht K, Friedman J, Heimler I, Aroutcheva A, Simoes J, Faro S. Role of the vaginal microbiological ecosystem and cytokine profile in the promotion of cervical dysplasia: a case-control study. Infect Dis Obstet Gynecol. 2002;10:181–6.
138. Grce M, Husnjak K, Matovina M, Milutin N, Magdic L, Husnjak O, et al. Human papillomavirus, cytomegalovirus, and adeno-associated virus infections in pregnant and nonpregnant women with cervical intraepithelial neoplasia. J Clin Microbiol. 2004;42:1341–4.
139. Audirac-Chalifour A, Torres-Poveda K, Bahena-Román M, Téllez-Sosa J, Martínez-Barnetche J, Cortina-Ceballos B, et al. Cervical microbiome and cytokine profile at various stages of cervical cancer: a pilot study. PLoS One. 2016;11:e0153274.
140. Di Pietro M, Filardo S, Porpora MG, Recine N, Latino MA, Sessa R. HPV/Chlamydia trachomatis co-infection: metagenomic analysis of cervical microbiota in asymptomatic women. New Microbiol. 2018;41:34–41.
141. Oh HY, Kim BS, Seo SS, Kong JS, Lee JK, Park SY, et al. The association of uterine cervical microbiota with an increased risk for cervical intraepithelial neoplasia in Korea. Clin Microbiol Infect. 2015;21:674.e1–9.
142. Brotman RM, Shardell MD, Gajer P, Tracy JK, Zenilman JM, Ravel J, et al. Interplay between the temporal dynamics of the vaginal microbiota and human papillomavirus detection. J Infect Dis. 2014;210:1723–33.
143. Seo SS, Oh HY, Lee JK, Kong JS, Lee DO, Kim MK. Combined effect of diet and cervical microbiome on the risk of cervical intraepithelial neoplasia. Clin Nutr. 2016;35:1434–41.
144. Lewis FM, Bernstein KT, Aral SO. Vaginal microbiome and its relationship to behavior, sexual health, and sexually transmitted diseases. Obstet Gynecol. 2017;129:643–54.
145. Brooks JP, Buck GA, Chen G, Diao L, Edwards DJ, Fettweis JM, et al. Changes in vaginal community state types reflect major shifts in the microbiome. Microb Ecol Health Dis. 2017;28:1303265.
146. Mitra A, MacIntyre DA, Lee YS, Smith A, Marchesi JR, Lehne B, et al. Cervical intraepithelial neoplasia disease progression is associated with increased vaginal microbiome diversity. Sci Rep. 2015;5:16865.
147. Smith SB, Ravel J. The vaginal microbiota, host defence and reproductive physiology. J Physiol. 2017;595:451–63.
148. Chase D, Goulder A, Zenhausern F, Monk B, Herbst-Kralovetz M. The vaginal and gastrointestinal microbiomes in gynecologic cancers: a review of applications in etiology, symptoms and treatment. Gynecol Oncol. 2015;138:190–200.
149. Zhang C, Liu Y, Gao W, Pan Y, Gao Y, Shen J, et al. The direct and indirect association of cervical microbiota with the risk of cervical intraepithelial neoplasia. Cancer Med. 2018;7:2172. https://doi.org/10.1002/cam4.1471.
150. Fernández-Benítez C, Mejuto-López P, Otero-Guerra L, Margolles-Martins MJ, Suárez-Leiva P, Vazquez F, Chlamydial Primary Care Group. Prevalence of genital Chlamydia trachomatis infection among

young men and women in Spain. BMC Infect Dis. 2013;13:388.
151. Lewis D, Newton DC, Guy RJ, Ali H, Chen MY, Fairley CK, et al. The prevalence of Chlamydia trachomatis infection in Australia: a systematic review and meta-analysis. BMC Infect Dis. 2012;12:113.
152. Castellsague X, Pawlita M, Roura E, Margall N, Waterboer T, Bosch FX, et al. Prospective seroepidemiologic study on the role of human papillomavirus and other infections in cervical carcinogenesis: evidence from the EPIC cohort. Int J Cancer. 2014;135:440–52.
153. Arnheim Dahlstrom L, Andersson K, Luostarinen T, Thoresen S, Ögmundsdottír H, Tryggvadottír L, et al. Prospective seroepidemiologic study of human papillomavirus and other risk factors in cervical cancer. Cancer Epidemiol Biomark Prev. 2011;20:2541–50.
154. Bebear C, de Barbeyrac B. Genital Chlamydia trachomatis infections. Clin Microbiol Infect. 2009;15:4–10.
155. Ohman H, Tiitinen A, Halttunen M, Lehtinen M, Paavonen J, Surcel HM, et al. Cytokine polymorphisms and severity of tubal damage in women with Chlamydia-associated infertility. J Infect Dis. 2009;199:1353–9.
156. Muñoz N, Kato I, Bosch FX, Eluf-Neto J, De Sanjosé S, Ascunce N, et al. Risk factors for HPV DNA detection in middle-aged women. Sex Transm Dis. 1996;23:504–10.
157. Seraceni S, De Seta F, Colli C, Del Savio R, Pesel G, Zanin V, et al. High prevalence of HPV multiple genotypes in women with persistent chlamydia trachomatis infection. Infect Agent Cancer. 2014;9:30.
158. Silva J, Cerqueira F, Ribeiro J, Sousa H, Osório T, Medeiros R. Is Chlamydia trachomatis related to human papillomavirus infection in young women of southern European population? A self-sampling study. Arch Gynecol Obstet. 2013;288:627–33.
159. Castle PE, Escoffery C, Schachter J, Rattray C, Schiffman M, Moncada J, et al. Chlamydia trachomatis, herpes simplex virus 2, and human T-cell lymphotrophic virus type 1 are not associated with grade of cervical neoplasia in Jamaican colposcopy patients. Sex Transm Dis. 2003;30:575–80.
160. Samoff E, Koumans EH, Markowitz LE, Sternberg M, Sawyer MK, Swan D, et al. Association of Chlamydia trachomatis with persistence of high-risk types of human papillomavirus in a cohort of female adolescents. Am J Epidemiol. 2005;162:668–75.
161. Vriend HJ, Bogaards JA, van Bergen JEAM, Brink AATP, van den Broek IVF, Hoebe CJPA, et al. Incidence and persistence of carcinogenic genital human papillomavirus infections in young women with or without Chlamydia trachomatis co-infection. Cancer Med. 2015;4:1589–98.
162. Karim S, Souho T, Benlemlih M, Bennani B. Cervical cancer induction enhancement potential of Chlamydia trachomatis: a systematic review. Curr Microbiol. 2018;75:1667. https://doi.org/10.1007/s00284-018-1439-7.
163. Koskela P, Anttila T, Bjørge T, Brunsvig A, Dillner J, Hakama M, et al. Chlamydia trachomatis infection as a risk factor for invasive cervical cancer. Int J Cancer. 2000;85:35–9.
164. Smith JS, Bosetti C, Muñoz N, Herrero R, Bosch FX, Eluf-Neto J. Chlamydia trachomatis and invasive cervical cancer: a pooled analysis of the IARC multicentric case-control study. Int J Cancer. 2004;111:431–9.
165. Zhu H, Shen Z, Luo H, Zhang W, Zhu X. Chlamydia trachomatis infection-associated risk of cervical cancer: a meta-analysis. Medicine (Baltimore). 2016;95:e3077.
166. Massad LS, Xie X, Burk R, Keller MJ, Minkoff H, D'Souza G, et al. Long-term cumulative detection of human papillomavirus among HIV seropositive women. AIDS. 2014;28:2601–8.
167. Rowhani-Rahbar A, Hawes SE, Sow PS, Toure P, Feng Q, Dem A, et al. The impact of HIV status and type on the clearance of human papillomavirus infection among Senegalese women. J Infect Dis. 2007;196:887–94.
168. Massad LS, Xie X, D'Souza G, Darragh TM, Minkoff H, Wright R, et al. Incidence of cervical precancers among HIV seropositive women. Am J Obstet Gynecol. 2015;212:606.e1–8.
169. Clifford GM, Franceschi S, Keiser O, Schöni-Affolter F, Lise M, Dehler S, et al. Immunodeficiency and the risk of cervical intraepithelial neoplasia 2/3 and cervical cancer: a nested case-control study in the Swiss HIV cohort study. Int J Cancer. 2016;138:1732–40.
170. Abraham AG, Strickler HD, D'Souza G. Invasive cervical cancer risk among HIV infected women is a function of CD4 count and screening. J Acquir Immune Defic Syndr. 2013;63:e163.
171. Grulich AE, van Leeuwen MT, Falster MO, Vajdic CM. Incidence of cancers in people with HIV/AIDS compared with immunosuppressed transplant recipients: a meta-analysis. Lancet. 2007;370:59–67.
172. Reusser NM, Downing C, Guidry J, Tyring SK. HPV carcinomas in immunocompromised patients. J Clin Med. 2015;4:260–81.
173. Nazli A, Chan O, Dobson-Belaire WN, Ouellet M, Tremblay MJ, Gray-Owen SD, et al. Exposure to HIV-1 directly impairs mucosal epithelial barrier integrity allowing microbial translocation. PLoS Pathog. 2010;6:e1000852.
174. Tugizov SM, Herrera R, Chin-Hong P, Veluppillai P, Greenspan D, Michael Berry J, et al. HIV-associated disruption of mucosal epithelium facilitates paracellular penetration by human papillomavirus. Virology. 2013;446:378–88.
175. Palefsky J. Human papillomavirus-related disease in people with HIV. Curr Opin HIV AIDS. 2009;4:52–6.
176. Blitz S, Baxter J, Raboud J, Walmsley S, Rachlis A, Smaill F, et al. Evaluation of HIV and highly active antiretroviral therapy on the natural history of human papillomavirus infection and cervical cytopathologic findings in HIV-positive and high-risk HIV-negative women. J Infect Dis. 2013;208:454–62.

177. Konopnicki D, Manigart Y, Gilles C, Barlow P, de Marchin J, Feoli F, et al. Sustained viral suppression and higher CD4+ T-cell count reduces the risk of persistent cervical high-risk human papillomavirus infection in HIV-positive women. J Infect Dis. 2013;207:1723–9.
178. Frisch M, Biggar RJ, Goedert JJ. Human papillomavirus-associated cancers in patients with human immunodeficiency virus infection and acquired immunodeficiency syndrome. J Natl Cancer Inst. 2000;92:1500–10.
179. Houlihan CF, Larke NL, Watson-Jones D, Smith-McCune KK, Shiboski S, Gravitt PE, et al. Human papillomavirus infection and increased risk of HIV acquisition. A systematic review and meta-analysis. AIDS. 2012;26:2211–22.
180. Averbach SH, Gravitt PE, Nowak RG, Celentano DD, Dunbar MS, Morrison CS, et al. The association between cervical human papillomavirus infection and HIV acquisition among women in Zimbabwe. AIDS. 2010;24:1035–42.
181. Smith-McCune KK, Shiboski S, Chirenje MZ, Magure T, Tuveson J, Ma Y, et al. Type-specific cervico-vaginal human papillomavirus infection increases risk of HIV acquisition independent of other sexually transmitted infections. PLoS One. 2010;5:e10094.
182. Liu M, Kalbasi A, Beatty GL. Functio laesa: cancer inflammation and therapeutic resistance. J Oncol Pract. 2017;13:173–80.
183. Yang TK, Chung CJ, Chung SD, Muo CH, Chang CH, Huang CY. Risk of endometrial cancer in women with pelvic inflammatory disease: a nationwide population-based retrospective cohort study. Medicine (Baltimore). 2015;94:e1278.
184. Ness RB, Kip KE, Hillier SL, Soper DE, Stamm CA, Sweet RL, et al. A cluster analysis of bacterial vaginosis–associated microflora and pelvic inflammatory disease. Am J Epidemiol. 2005;162:585–90.
185. Sharma H, Tal R, Clark NA, Segars JH. Microbiota and pelvic inflammatory disease. Semin Reprod Med. 2014;32:43–9.
186. Mitchell CM, Haick A, Nkwopara E, Garcia R, Rendi M, Agnew K, et al. Colonization of the upper genital tract by vaginal bacterial species in nonpregnant women. Am J Obstet Gynecol. 2015;212:611.e1–9.
187. Walther-Antonio MR, Chen J, Multinu F, Hokenstad A, Distad TJ, Cheek EH, et al. Potential contribution of the uterine microbiome in the development of endometrial cancer. Genome Med. 2016;8:122.
188. Brewster WR, Ko EM, Keku TO. An evaluation of the microbiota of the upper genital tract of women with benign changes and epithelial ovarian cancer. J Clin Oncol. 2016;34(15_suppl):5568.
189. Poole EM, Lee IM, Ridker PM, Buring JE, Hankinson SE, Tworoger SS. A prospective study of circulating C-reactive protein, interleukin-6, and tumor necrosis factor alpha receptor 2 levels and risk of ovarian cancer. Am J Epidemiol. 2013;178:1256–64.
190. Krohn MA, Hillier SL, Nugent RP, Cotch MF, Carey JC, Gibbs RS, et al. The genital flora of women with intraamniotic infection. Vaginal Infection and Prematurity Study Group. J Infect Dis. 1995;171:1475–80.
191. Silver HM, Sperling RS, St Clair PJ, Gibbs RS. Evidence relating bacterial vaginosis to intraamniotic infection. Am J Obstet Gynecol. 1989;161:808–12.
192. Hillier SL, Krohn MA, Cassen E, Easterling TR, Rabe LK, Eschenbach DA. The role of bacterial vaginosis and vaginal bacteria in amniotic fluid infection in women in preterm labor with intact fetal membranes. Clin Infect Dis. 1995;20:S276–8.
193. Hillier SL, Kiviat NB, Hawes SE, Hasselquist MB, Hanssen PW, Eschenbach DA, et al. Role of bacterial vaginosis-associated microorganisms in endometritis. Am J Obstet Gynecol. 1996;175:435–41.
194. Tone AA, Salvador S, Finlayson SJ, Tinker AV, Kwon JS, Lee CH, et al. The role of the fallopian tube in ovarian cancer. Clin Adv Hematol Oncol. 2012;10:296–306.
195. Massad LS, Ahdieh L, Benning L, Minkoff H, Greenblatt RM, Watts H, et al. Evolution of cervical abnormalities among women with HIV-1: evidence from surveillance cytology in the women's interagency HIV study. J Acquir Immune Defic Syndr. 2001;27:432–42.
196. Silva J, Cerqueira F, Medeiros R. Chlamydia trachomatis infection: implications for HPV status and cervical cancer. Arch Gynecol Obstet. 2014;289:715–23.
197. Gaya P, Medina M, Sánchez-Jiménez A, Landete JM. Phytoestrogen metabolism by adult human gut microbiota. Molecules. 2016;21:E1034.
198. Rietjens IMCM, Louisse J, Beekmann K. The potential health effects of dietary phytoestrogens. Br J Pharmacol. 2017;174:1263–80.
199. Landete JM, Arqués JL, Medina M, Gaya P, de las Rivas B, Muñoz R. Bioactivation of phytoestrogens: intestinal bacteria and health. Crit Rev Food Sci Nutr. 2016;56:1826–43.
200. Selma MV, Beltrán D, Luna MC, Romo-Vaquero M, García-Villalba R, Mira A, et al. Isolation of human intestinal bacteria capable of producing the bioactive metabolite isourolithin A from ellagic acid. Front Microbiol. 2017;8:1521.
201. Velicer CM, Heckbert SR, Lampe JW, Potter JD, Robertson CA, Taplin SH. Antibiotic use in relation to the risk of breast cancer. JAMA. 2004;291:827–35.
202. Javurek AB, Spollen WG, Johnson SA, Bivens NJ, Bromert KH, Givan SA, et al. Effects of exposure to bisphenol A and ethinyl estradiol on the gut microbiota of parents and their offspring in a rodent model. Gut Microbes. 2016;7:471–85.
203. Clavel T, Mapesa JO. Phenolics in human nutrition: importance of the intestinal microbiome for isoflavone and lignan bioavailability. In: Ramawat K, Mérillon JM, editors. Natural products. Berlin: Springer; 2013.

32 HPV Infection and Gynecological Cancers

Vani Bharani, Rajesh Kumar, and Bharti Bharani

32.1 Introduction

In the 1970s, Harald zur Hausen (Fig. 32.1), a German virologist, discovered the human papillomavirus (HPV) in warts and cervical cancer. His interests in these viruses led him to isolate them and clone various strains of HPV. His discovery concluded that infection with HPV strain 16 and HPV 18 have a high risk of causing cancers. His profound work was recognized when he was awarded the Nobel Prize in Physiology or Medicine in 2008 [1]. Now, it is identified that HPV is an etiology for nearly 5% of all cancers worldwide [2]. The cervical cancers are almost always related to HPV infection; however, HPV is associated with anogenital cancers (vulval, vaginal, penile, and anal) and significant cases of oropharyngeal cancers [3]. Most of the individuals are asymptomatic, and HPV infection is taken care by host immune response. However, a small proportion of these infections persist and progress to precancerous and cancerous lesions.

In the current chapter, we review the HPV biology, epidemiology of HPV infection, life cycle of HPV infection, and factors that influence the progression of infection. We also discuss briefly regarding the gynecological cancers and their association with HPV infection.

V. Bharani · R. Kumar · B. Bharani (✉)
Dysplasia Clinic, Indore, Madhya Pradesh, India

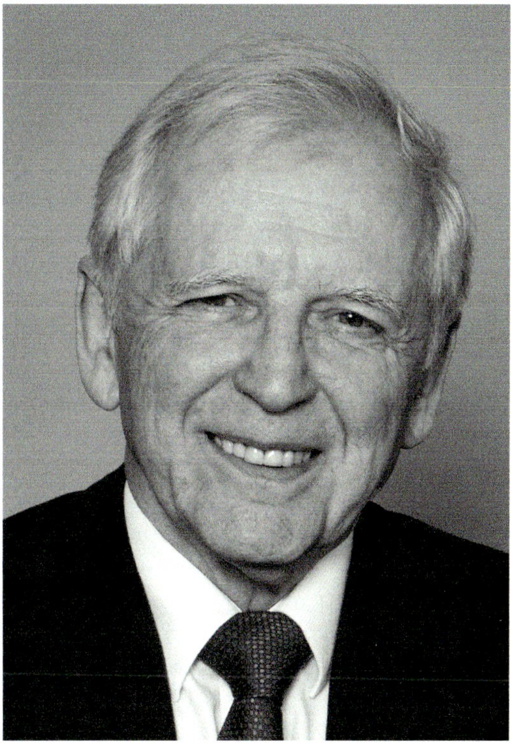

Fig. 32.1 Harald zur Hausen discovered HPV causes cervical cancer [1]. ©The Nobel Foundation Photo: Ulla Montan

32.2 HPV Structure

Papillomaviruses (PVs) are oncogenic DNA viruses which are small sized and infect a wide range of vertebrate hosts including human,

S. Mehta, A. Singla (eds.), *Preventive Oncology for the Gynecologist*,
https://doi.org/10.1007/978-981-13-3438-2_32

Table 32.1 Classification of alpha human papillomavirus (HPV) based on carcinogenic risk [6]

Oncogenicity	IARC category	Types[a]
High risk	1	**16, 18**, 31, 33, 35, 39, 45, 51, 52, 56, 58, 59
Possibly carcinogenic	2A	68
Probably carcinogenic	2B[b]	26, 30, 53, 66, 67, 69, 70, 73, 82, 85
Low risk	3	2, **6**, 7, **11**,13, 27, 28, 29,32, 40, 44, 57, 61, 62, 72, 74, 77, 81, 83, 84, 86, 87, 89, 90, 91, 106

[a]Common types highlighted
[b]Limited epidemiologic data. Phylogenetically related to carcinogenic types

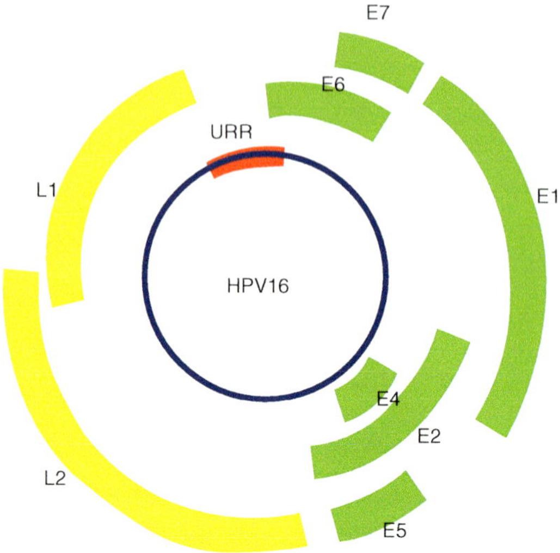

Fig. 32.2 Diagrammatic representation of HPV 16 genome. Early genes (green), late genes (yellow), and upstream regulatory region (red)

nonhuman mammals, reptiles, birds, and fishes. These are non-enveloped viruses, measuring approximately 55 nm in diameter, and have an 8-kb double-stranded circular DNA genome. Over 350 PV types have been identified and classified into 45 genera. *Papillomaviridae* family includes about 200 HPV types that belong to five genera, namely, alpha, beta, gamma, mu, and nu. HPV can be classified based on their tissue tropism and oncogenic potential. The alpha HPVs display a mucosal tropism, while the other genera infect mostly the skin [4, 5].

The International Agency for Research on Cancer (IARC) lists 12 high-risk oncogenic HPV (HR-HPV) types (HPV 16, 18, 31, 33, 35, 39, 45, 51, 52, 56, 58, and 59). These HR-HPVs are from alpha genus. Low-risk HPV (LR-HPV) types like HPV 6 and HPV 11 cause benign cutaneous and mucosal lesions like warts. The oncogenicity of certain types remains unclear; these have been classified as probably or possibly carcinogenic [6] (Table 32.1).

32.3 HPV Genome [4, 5, 7]

The genome structure and organization are similar across the papillomavirus family. The genome has three main regions, which encode eight open reading frames (ORFs) or genes (Fig. 32.2):

1. Early region (E1, E2, E4, E5, E6, E7): These ORFs are required for viral replication, virion protein synthesis, and release. These play a key role in cell transformation.
2. Late region (L1, L2): This region encodes capsid proteins.
3. Upstream regulatory region/long control region: This is the noncoding region that controls viral gene transcription.

Among all papillomaviruses, the ORFs L1, L2, E1, and E2 are well conserved, while E4–E7 show greater diversity. The taxonomic classification of papillomavirus into types, subtypes, and variants is based on the degree of difference in the sequence of their L1 genes.

E1 gene encodes a helicase that is virus-specific and necessary for viral replication. E2 binds to sites in viral and host genome and is involved in viral transcription, followed by replication and genome partitioning. Probably as a result of an error in genome sequencing gene, E3 does not exist. E4 protein facilitates in viral assembly and release; E5 is involved in immune evasion.

E6 and E7 genes are primary oncoproteins which inhibit tumor suppressor pathways. E6 degrades tumor suppressor gene p53 by the ubiquitination mediated pathway, while E7 does so by

Table 32.2 HPV genes/open reading frames and functions of their proteins [6]

Region	Genes	Functions
Early	E1	Essential for viral DNA replication, attaches to viral origin of DNA replication as a hexameric complex. Has adenosine triphosphatase (ATPase) and DNA helicase activity
	E2	Main regulator of viral transcription, involved in replication and genome partitioning
	E4	Facilitates in virus assembly and release
	E5	Involved in evasion of host immune response, inhibits transfer of major histocompatibility complexes to the cell surface
	E6	Utilizes the ubiquitination mediated pathway for degrading p53, induces telomerase, and prevents cell differentiation
	E7	Induces unscheduled cell proliferation, inhibits the retinoblastoma protein, and activates the oncogenic transcription pathways
Late	L1	Major viral structural protein, assembles in capsomeres and capsids, interacts with L2, interacts with cell receptors, and encodes neutralizing epitopes
	L2	Minor viral structural protein, contributes to infectivity, and involved in viral trafficking, encapsulation of viral DNA, and virion release
URR	NCR	Regulate DNA replication by controlling the viral gene transcription

URR upstream regulatory region, *NCR* noncoding region

inhibiting the retinoblastoma gene. Both E6 and E7 deregulate pathways involved in cellular proliferation, apoptosis, telomerase maintenance, and cell cycle regulation. They help create a favorable condition for epithelial cell transformation.

L1 and L2 are part of the viral capsid: L1 is part of external viral capsid, while L2 lies in the inner surface. The details of HPV ORFs and their functions are shown in Table 32.2.

32.4 Modes of Transmission

Genital HPV is the most common sexually transmitted infection [6]. Other possible modes of transmission include vertical transmission, transmission through fomites, and skin-to-skin contact; nonsexual modes of transmission are however rare [8, 9].

32.4.1 Horizontal Transmission

Sexual contact is the major route of transmission of HPV with an infected partner through cervical, vulvovaginal, anal, or penile epithelia. The infection is presumably spread through the microscopic abrasions in mucosa or skin. Several observations support this, including transmission of genital warts and concordance of HPV types in sex partners, low rates of genital HPV in virgins, and increase risk of infection with new sex partners [6].

Self-inoculation from one anogenital site to another has been demonstrated [10]. Also, hand carriage of genital HPV, possibly leading to digital-genital transmission, has been identified [11].

Though HPV is easily transmitted, the degree of transmissibility varies with the type and across populations [12–14].

32.4.2 Vertical Transmission

Vertical transmission of HPV was first seen with a case of juvenile laryngeal papillomatosis. The rate of transmission from mother to child remains unclear. HPV type concordance has been shown in mother-infant pair [15], wherein same HPV types were demonstrated in both. The possible modes of direct transmission include during vaginal delivery or at cesarean section occurring with rupture of membranes or in the form of ascending infection from the maternal genital tract [16]. Few cases of transplacental spread have also been demonstrated [16–18].

32.5 Life Cycle of HPV Infection

HPVs display a high degree of epitheliotropism and establish productive infections in skin and mucosal surfaces lined by stratified squamous epithelium. Following mucosal microtrauma,

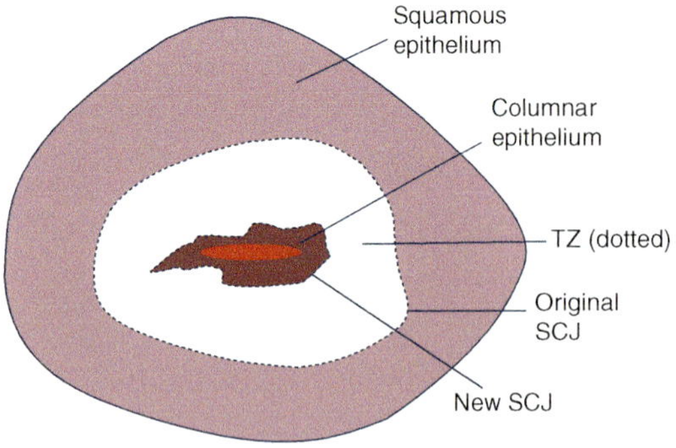

Fig. 32.3 Transformation zone (TZ, dotted). Region of the cervix lined by metaplastic squamous epithelium. Area is bound by original squamocolumnar junction (SCJ) distally and new SCJ proximally. Area is susceptible to persistent HPV infections and carcinogenesis due to active proliferation of basal/reserve cells

HPV infects the basal layer of epithelial cells. The transformation zone (TZ) (Fig. 32.3) is susceptible to preneoplastic and neoplastic disease, especially at the onset of puberty and later on with sexual activity [19], due to basal/reserve cell proliferation. The infection of the basal stem cells is key to formation of persistent lesions [20, 21].

The cellular entry of HPV 16 is mediated via interaction of L1 protein with proteoglycans. After cellular internalization, L1 is uncoated and L2 associated with HPV DNA migrates through the Golgi system and endoplasmic reticulum. The viral DNA finally reaches the nucleus and remains in extrachromosomal episomal form, where replication can occur [22].

The initial infection of HPV occurs in basal cells of squamous epithelium. There is a phase of genome amplification and viral episome maintenance at low copy number [23–25]. In the normal viral life cycle, copy numbers of HPV genome are about 50–100/basal cell. Within the basal layer, the early HPV genes including E1 and E2 are expressed at low levels [26, 27]. E1 and E2 genes are required for the initial amplification phase [28]. E2 is involved in genome partitioning and regulating viral transcription.

During the process of normal epithelial maturation when basal cells divide, the daughter cells withdraw from the cell cycle, migrate to the suprabasal compartment, and initiate the process of terminal differentiation. But, in HPV-infected suprabasal cells, the E6 and E7 viral genes induce reentry of these cells into S-phase of cell cycle [29]. Thus, there is reactivation of the host replication machinery, which supports viral genome amplification [30]. The viral capsid proteins L1 and L2 are expressed in superficial layers. Viral assembly and release of new virions occur from the surface epithelium. Thus, the life cycle of HPV and time duration for basal layer cells to mature, migrate to superficial layers, undergo senescence, and die are same, around 2–3 weeks [31]. Hence, in such productive infections, the viral oncogenes are expressed in compartment that is destined to be shed from the cervical epithelium.

32.6 HPV and Carcinogenesis

HPV-induced carcinogenesis has been studied in context of cervical carcinoma; the mechanisms at other sites appear to be similar. The present discussion is in reference to cervical carcinomas. The viral life cycle associated with cervical carcinogenesis shows two significant alterations: first, the loss of terminal differentiation of keratinocytes in the epithelium and, second, integration of the viral genome into the host DNA. The ordered viral gene expression is lost in HPV-induced neoplasia. The dysregulation of viral gene expression is due to alterations in cell signaling induced by changes in the hormonal milieu [32] or by epigenetic modifications like viral DNA methylation [33]. There is an increased level of expression of E6 and E7 proteins, which facilitates viral integration in the host chromosome. Though the likely site for integration is the common fragile site hotspot in the host genome, integration is always a chance event. Integration leads to disruption of E2, which normally regulates the E6 and E7 abundance. This leads to high-level unregulated E6 and E7 gene expression [34, 35] which leads to unforced accumulation of genetic errors and finally to precancerous lesions and cancer [36].

Integrated HPV 16 sequences are seen in 70% of cervical cancers, while all HPV 18 associated cancers show integration in host genome [37]. In both conditions, long-term overexpression of E6 and E7 along with accumulation of genetic errors is responsible for progression from precancerous lesions to cervical cancer.

32.7 Differences in HR-HPV and LR-HPV

The differences in the E6 and E7 oncoprotein functions of LR-HPV and HR-HPV lead to differences in the pathogenesis in the two types. The E6/E7 proteins of HR-HPV promote proliferation of the basal and parabasal cells and an increase in lesion size. The E6 proteins in both LR-HPV and HR-HPV inactivate p53, but its ubiquitination and proteosome-dependent degradation occur in HR-HPV infections only [38–40]. The HR-HPV E6 can upregulate the telomerase activity. This leads to a maintained telomere length during multiple cell divisions [41–43]. The LR-HPV and HR-HPV E7 proteins show difference in their abilities to bind to retinoblastoma protein family. The HR-HPV E7 binds and degrades p105, p107, and p103. These proteins are involved in the cell cycle entry in the basal cell layer (p105 and p107) and upper layers (p103) [44, 45]. The LR-HPV E7 has low affinity for p105 and p107; however, it can bind and degrade p103 [46, 47].

32.8 Host Immune Response

Over 90% of HPV infections are cleared within a few years, and nearly half of these are cleared in the first 6 months [48, 49]. These are often referred to as acute, transient, nonpersistent, or cleared infections [50]. These infections establish within the host successfully, replicate, and are cleared by the host immune response.

Certain infections appear to have cleared, and the viral genome is not detected due to low levels. These are the latent infections. Reactivation of such an infection may be triggered later, due to immunosuppression [51] or without any obvious reason.

Infections where the viral activity is maintained and the infection is not cleared are called as chronic infections or persistent infections. Persistence of infection is defined as detection of same HPV type (or the same intratypic variant) over a certain period of time. The duration after which an infection should be termed as persistent is not well defined; however, a duration of minimum 6 months to 1 year is usually chosen [52, 53]. These infections can potentially develop into precancerous and cancerous lesions.

HPV evades the host immune response, which leads to persistence and subsequent progression of infection. The infection is maintained with a low level of gene expression. The infection is intraepithelial and does not lead to cell lysis; thus, there is no associated pro-inflammatory signal generation [54]. There is minimal or absent cytokine release or Langerhans cell recruitment for antigen presentation [55]. Several other mechanisms of immune evasion are seen in the alpha type HR-HPV. E6 protein of HPV16 interferes with tyrosine kinase 2 function and affects STAT signaling [56, 57]. Induction of interferon response factor 1 is affected by E7. Both E6 and E7 proteins can reduce the surface expression of E cadherin. This reduction in E cadherin levels results in a reduced number of Langerhans cells around the lesion [58–61]. E5 protein of the HR-HPV can compromise the MHC-associated display of viral particles on epithelial cells [62]. Thus, the immune evasion and low-level genome expression promote immunological tolerance rather than clearance of infection.

Despite these mechanisms, majority of HPV infections are successfully resolved. Cell-mediated immune response is implicated in clearance of infection. The infection leads to sensitization of dendritic cells followed by a T-cell-mediated response which stops the viral gene expression.

Antibodies to L1 protein can be demonstrated 6 months after infection [63]. These may be detected even after the clearance of HPV infection [64], and the presence of L1 antibody may indicate a past or persistent infection. Almost half of individuals never seroconvert [65], and whether naturally induced L1 antibodies have protective response against new infections is unclear.

32.9 HPV Prevalence

32.9.1 Women Without Cytological Abnormalities

The lifetime risk of acquiring HPV infection by sexual transmission is 50% [66], and most women will acquire a HPV infection at some time. A global meta-analysis including publications from 1999 to 2005 provides the HPV prevalence in 157,897 women without any cytological abnormalities [67, 68]. Women with any cytological abnormality (atypical squamous cells of undetermined significance ASCUS, low-grade squamous intraepithelial lesion LSIL, or higher) were specifically excluded from the study. The study constituted women visiting referral clinics and general population as well. HPV DNA prevalence in the cervix was found to be 10.4% (95% confidence interval (CI): 10.2–10.7) worldwide. HPV prevalence was higher in the less developed regions of the world (13.4%; 95% CI: 13.1–13.7) as compared to the more developed regions (8.4%; 95% CI: 8.3–8.6). The highest HPV prevalence was seen in African women (22.1%; 95% CI: 20.9–23.4). The Eastern African region had the highest rates in Africa (31.6%; 95% CI: 29.5–33.8). The lowest rates of HPV prevalence are seen in Southeastern Asia (6.2%; 95% CI: 5.5–7.0). Another large-scale population-based survey showed an overall point prevalence of HPV DNA as 10.5% (95% CI: 9.9–11.0). The survey included 15,613 women, between the ages 15 and 74 years [69].

HPV 16 was found to be the commonest HPV type across all continents, and the prevalence was 2.6% (95% CI: 2.5–2.8). The prevalence is higher in Northern America (3.5%; 95% CI: 2.8–4.3) than in Europe (2.3%; 95% CI: 2.0–2.5). In Central America, South America, and Europe, HPV 18 was the second commonest type. In Africa, the common types are HPV 16 and HPV 52, followed by HPV 18. While in Asia and Northern America, HPV 18 was the fourth commonest type. In Asia, the commonest types were HPV 16, HPV 52, and HPV 58 and in Northern America, these are HPV 16, HPV 53, and HPV 52. All HPV types other than HPV 16 had a prevalence of <1% in Europe, Asia, and Northern America. However, in other parts of the world, several other HPV types had a prevalence of 1% or more [67].

A high prevalence of HPV (up to 30%) is observed in young women, which falls in the middle age group. A second peak is seen in the fourth to fifth decade of life. This rise in HPV prevalence can be attributed to acquisition of new HPV infections as a result of change in sexual activity or reactivation of latent infections [67, 68].

32.9.2 High-Grade Cervical Lesions

In a large meta-analysis from 38 nations, HPV DNA was identified in 85% high-grade squamous intraepithelial lesions (HSILs), ranging from 78% in Asia to 95.8% in Oceania. The variation in estimate of HPV prevalence is explained by the difference in quality of the specimens and sensitivity of the assays used for HPV detection. The detection of various HPV types is however less affected by sensitivity of tests utilized. No significant differences have been found across various laboratories and assays for HPV 16, 18, 33, and 45 detections. However, detection of HPV 31, 35, 52, and 6 is affected by sensitivity and specificity of the assay used [70].

HPV 16 was the commonest type detected in HSIL prevalence of 45.4% worldwide. The highest prevalence was noted in Europe (51.8%; 95% CI: 50.1–53.5), while the lowest was 33.3% (95% CI: 20.4–48.4) in Oceania. Geographic variation in the other common types of HPV was noted. The second and third common HPV types were worldwide, Africa, and Europe (HPV 31 and HPV 33), Northern America (HPV 6 and HPV 18), Latin America and Caribbean (HPV 58 and HPV 18), Oceania (HPV 31 and HPV 18), and Asia (HPV 58 and HPV 52) [67, 68].

32.9.3 Invasive Cervical Cancer

Data from large meta-analysis and pooled studies show that HPV 16 and HPV 18 account for nearly 70% of all invasive cervical carcinomas. The other common types besides these were HPV 33, 45, 31, 58, 52, and 35. In all continents, the third to fifth commonest HPV types were HPV 33, 45, and 31, while in Asia they were HPV 58, 33, and 52 [67, 68].

HPV 16 is the commonest type detected not only in normal cytology samples but also in HSIL and invasive cervical carcinomas including squamous cell carcinomas and adenocarcinomas. HPV 18 is the second type, and it dominates in the adenocarcinoma group [71]. HPV 45 has a prevalence of 2.3% in HSIL and 4.6–5% in invasive cervical cancer. It is interesting to note that HPV 45 is uncommon in women without cytological abnormalities. HPV58 is common in normal cytology samples and HSILs, while it has a lower frequency in invasive cervical cancers.

Adenocarcinomas represent around 16% of all cervical cancers [72]. HPV 16 and HPV 18 are the commonest types detected. HPV 18 is more common in adenocarcinomas as compared to squamous cell carcinomas (36.3% in adenocarcinoma vs. 12.8% squamous cell carcinoma). Increasing rates and relative frequencies are being reported from developed nations, possibly due to lower frequency of detection of precursor lesion in cytology-based tests and increased HPV exposure [67].

32.10 Infection with Multiple HPV Types

The frequency of multiple type HPV infections is variable across different geographic regions and certain special population groups. These infections are found in both sexes. In women without any cytological abnormalities, single type infection is more common than multiple type infection [69]. The prevalence rates of infection with two types of HPV range from 0.2 to 5% in various parts of the world, with an overall prevalence of 1.7%. The infection with three or more types of HPV is seen in 0.9% women without cytological abnormalities. The highest prevalence of three or more HPV infections is seen in Nigeria (3.3%).

The number of HPV types detected increase in SILs as compared to women with normal cytology. Infection with two or more HPV types was detected in nearly 60% of LSILs evaluated in the ASCUS/LSIL Triage Study (ALTS) [73]. Ho et al. reported infection with two or more HPV types in 45% CIN 1 and CIN 2 lesions and 34% in CIN 3 lesions [74].

Multiple HPV type infection confers a greater risk for untoward outcomes, which is a sum of the various types and does not show synergistic effects. An increased risk of persistence of infection is seen in women infected with multiple HPV types [75].

A single HPV type is demonstrated in invasive cancers; this is in conjunction with the known monoclonal development of HPV-induced cancers. The presence of multiple HPV types in about 4% invasive cancers may be a result of a concomitant CIN lesion along with the invasive cancer [76].

32.11 HPV Infections in India

A meta-analysis of nine studies from India estimated a 12% prevalence of any HPV type in women without cytological abnormalities. The prevalence in LSIL, HSIL, and invasive carcinoma was 65.4%, 86.5%, and 94.6%, respectively [77].

HPV 16 is the commonest type seen in 70–90% of Indian women with cervical cancer, while HPV 18 has been observed in 3–20% [78]. HPV 16 has been identified in several regions of India and appears to be most ubiquitous. HPV 18 is shown to be more oncopotent as compared to HPV 16, with development of cancerous lesions from precancerous lesions in a shorter time [79].

A higher incidence of HPV 56 and HPV 42 has been reported in IARC surveys from Southern Tamil Nadu [80]. HPV 42 is a low-risk type, while HPV 56 is high-risk type. A higher prevalence of HPV 16 and HPV 18 has been shown in Hindus (9.6%) as compared to Muslims (7.5%)

in rural regions of West Bengal [81]. Male circumcision appears to play a protective role in the Muslim population.

A study from Odisha, Eastern India [82], showed an HPV prevalence of 60.33% in 595 women. HPV prevalence was highest in invasive cancer (93.80%) and was 19.11% in women with normal cytology. Similar to other studies, the commonest HPV type was HPV 16 (87.28%). Next, the most prevalent types were HPV18 (24.56%) and HPV 51 (3.46%). A single HPV type infection was seen in 76.58% cases. In cases with more than one type of HPV infection, the commonest combination was HPV 16 with HPV 18 (9.4%) followed by HPV 16 with HPV 66 and HPV 68 (2.7%). The latter combination was commonly observed with inflammatory cytology.

The common HPV types reported in women from various parts of India are HPV 16 followed by HPV 18. However, data from Manipur [83] showed a higher prevalence of HPV 18. The study found an overall prevalence of HPV infection in women without cytological abnormalities to be 6.70% in Manipur, 11.14% in Sikkim, and 11.60% in West Bengal. In Manipur, the prevalence of HPV 16 was 1.2%, while that of HPV 18 was higher at 2.1%. In the other two regions, the prevalence of HPV 16 was higher than HPV 18. A possible explanation is the geographically contiguity of Manipur to Southeast Asia, from where HPV 18 may have been introduced. Southeast Asian nations like Thailand and the Philippines show a higher frequency of HPV 18 despite lower HPV prevalence rates [84–86].

A study conducted by Sharma et al. [87] in tribal districts of Madhya Pradesh, Jharkhand, and Chhattisgarh showed a high prevalence of HPV infection at 12.9%. Majority of these infections (65%) were with HR-HPV types. HPV 16 was the commonest type detected (54%). The prevalence in different age groups was 6.6% (9–12 years), 11.4% (13–17 years), and 19.2% (18–25 years). Similar studies with urine sampling technique have reported a significantly lower HPV prevalence rate. A 0.85% HPV infection was reported in 8–13 years and 2.3% in 13–17 years [88]. A study from New Delhi reported a prevalence of 6% in the 17–25-year age group [89], while the prevalence in college goers in Tamil Nadu was found to be 9.2% [90].

32.12 Cofactors in HPV Carcinogenesis

It is well established that the HPV infection is necessary but not sufficient for progression to cervical cancer. Several endogenous and exogenous cofactors have been identified in various epidemiological studies which act together with HPV and affect the risk of progression to an invasive malignancy. The important ones are described in the following sections.

32.12.1 Noninfectious Cofactors

32.12.1.1 Oral Contraceptive Use

The use of combined hormonal oral contraceptive (OC) formulations influences the development of preinvasive lesions and cancer in the cervix [91]. However, not all epidemiologic studies have found an association between OC use and cervical cancer. Lacey et al. [92] found an odds ratio (OR) of 17.1 for current vs never OC users in cases of adenocarcinoma in situ. A study from Costa Rica by Hildesheim et al. [93] showed a 3.1-fold increase in risk of carcinoma in OC users of ≥5 years as compared to never users. This association was noted in women with ≤2 pregnancies, and the study population was small. Moreno et al. [94] showed that ever use of OCs was associated with cancer risk with an OR of 1.4. There was no significant increase in the risk for up to 4 years of OC use, but there was a strong dose-response relationship after 5 years of OC use (OR 3.4; 95% CI: 2.1–5.5).

Data elucidating the mechanism of hormonal influences on the progression of cervical cancer are limited. Steroid hormones are thought to increase the expression of E6 and E7 oncoproteins and may contribute to carcinogenesis [95].

32.12.1.2 Parity

High parity increases the risk of in situ and invasive cervical cancer. IARC-pooled analysis shows a fourfold higher risk of cervical cancer in women with ≥7 full-term pregnancies than the nulliparous group [94]. Also, a linear increase in the risk with an increasing number of pregnancies has been demonstrated [96]. A significant increase in the risk for adenocarcinoma in women with ≤2 full-term pregnancies was also seen. This did not show a linear relation with parity [94]. An increase in the risk of HSIL/cervical cancer was seen with an increased number of live births [93].

Repeated pregnancies maintain the TZ on the ectocervix for prolonged duration [97]. The presence of TZ on ectocervix facilitates exposure to HPV and other cofactors. Hormonal changes like elevated estrogen and progesterone levels seen in pregnancy may influence the persistence and clearance of HPV infection [96, 98].

32.12.1.3 Tobacco Smoking

Smoking shows a significant association with cervical cancer. The ORs for HPV-positive smokers range from 2 to 5. Kjaer et al. reported a twofold increase in the risk of SIL or ASCUS in current and former smokers as compared to never smokers [99]. Olsen et al. showed a 4.6-fold increased risk of CIN 2/3 among smokers [100]. A study from Sweden demonstrated an approximately twofold increase in the risk for carcinoma in situ in both former and current smokers as compared to never smokers. Both groups were matched by HPV status [101]. Pooled data analyzed from eight case-control studies showed twofold higher risk for cervical cancer in reformed and current smokers [102]. Increasing exposure to tobacco, estimated with intensity, duration, and pack years, increases the risk of invasive cancer.

Prospective studies have demonstrated that smoking alters the natural history of HPV infections. Giuliano et al. showed a lower probability of clearance and longer duration of HR-HPV infections in smokers [103]. Higher incidence of persistent HPV infections has been shown in current smokers [104].

The chemical carcinogens from tobacco may have a mitogenic effect leading to DNA damage. Cervical mucus of smokers shows nicotine and other tobacco-related carcinogens [105]. Tobacco can affect the local host immune response against viral infections [106]. A reduction in number of Langerhans cells has been seen in smokers.

32.12.1.4 Other Cofactors

Other cofactors in cervical carcinogenesis include micronutrient deficiencies, genetic susceptibility, and human leukocyte antigen (HLA) polymorphisms. Deficiencies of vitamins and micronutrients have been evaluated as cofactors. Familial studies show familial clustering and moderately increased risk of in situ and invasive cervical carcinoma among women who had a first- or a second-degree relative with cervical cancer. These reports cannot separate the effect of genetic susceptibility from the effects of common environmental and behavioral traits in the family members. Several allele groups in HLA class II have been identified that confer the risk of cervical cancer including DRB1*11, DRB1*15, and DQB1*06, while some can protect against the development of cervical cancer, like DRB1*13 and the DRB1*13–DQB1*06 haplotype [6].

32.12.1.5 Infectious Cofactors

Coinfection with other sexually transmitted infections like *Chlamydia trachomatis* has been inconsistently linked with the risk of progression to cancer. Safaeian et al. did not find any association between chlamydia infection in HPV-positive women and the risk of preneoplastic lesions [107], while Zhu et al. [108] report a significant increase of cervical cancer risk associated to *C. trachomatis*.

HIV can induce progression of HPV infection to cancer; this is mediated by the immunosuppression seen in active HIV infection. Women on anti-retroviral therapy have a lower risk of acquisition of HR-HPV types and lower incidence of intraepithelial lesions and their progression [109].

32.13 HPV Infection and Gynecological Cancers

32.13.1 Cervical Cancer

Cervical cancer is the fourth most common cancer of women in the world and second most common cancer in the 15–44-year age group. In the year 2012, 528,000 new cervical cancer cases and 266,000 cervical cancer-related deaths were reported [110]. Most cases (85%) and associated cancer deaths (87%) occur in the less developed nations [110].

India contributed to 25% of global cervical cancer burden in 2000. Cervical cancer ranks second among all malignancies affecting Indian women. India harbors a large at-risk population above the age of 15 years [111].

The development of cervical cancer begins with a HR-HPV infection, followed by persistence of the infection at the transformation zone, development of precancerous lesions, and progression to invasive cancer. The precancerous lesions have been categorized by a three-tier system into cervical intraepithelial neoplasia (CIN) 1, 2, and 3 depending on the severity of the lesion. They can also be categorized into low-grade and high-grade squamous intraepithelial lesions (SILs). The two-tier system is now recommended, as it is consistent with our understanding of HPV biology and is more reproducible [112].

The LSIL/CIN 1 (Fig. 32.4a) lesions typically regress and do not have the risk of progression to cancer. LSILs show proliferation of squamous cells with increased nuclear to cytoplasmic ratio

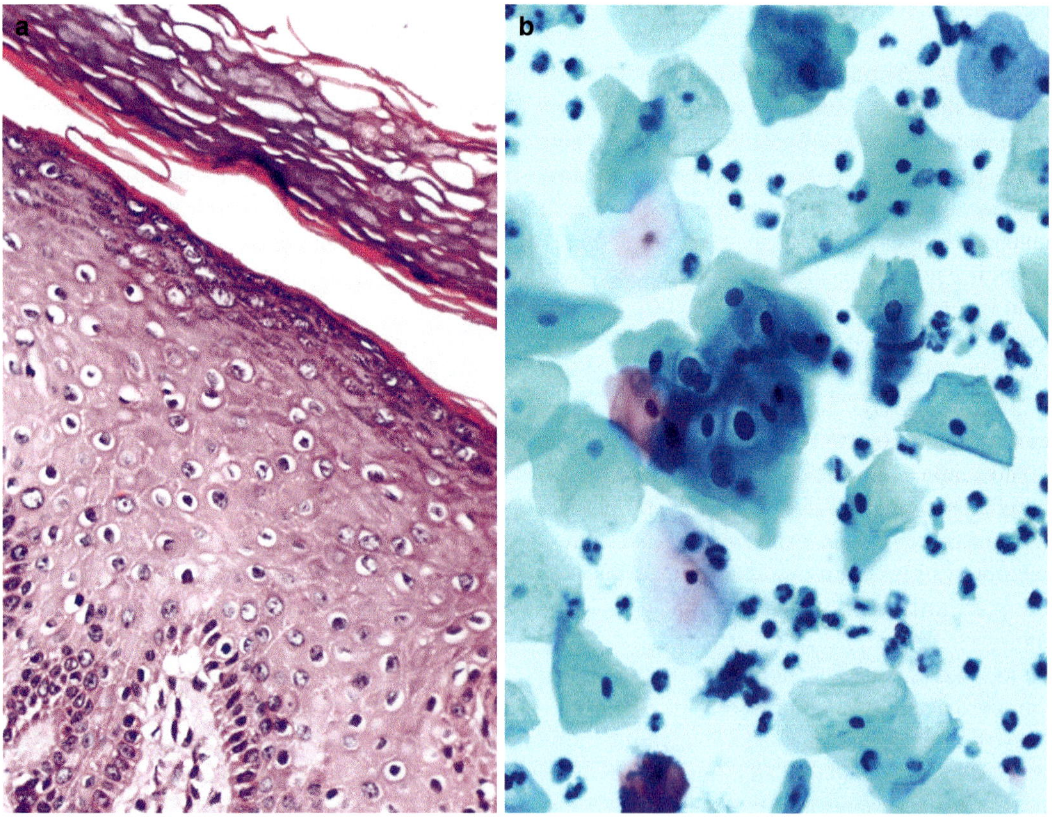

Fig. 32.4 LSIL/CIN 1. (**a**) The lower third of the epithelium showing nuclear enlargement, nuclear membrane irregularity, and increased nucleocytoplasmic ratio (H&E stain ×200). (**b**) Typical koilocytic change with nuclear hyperchromasia, nuclear membrane irregularity, and a well-defined perinuclear halo (BD Sure Path, ×400)

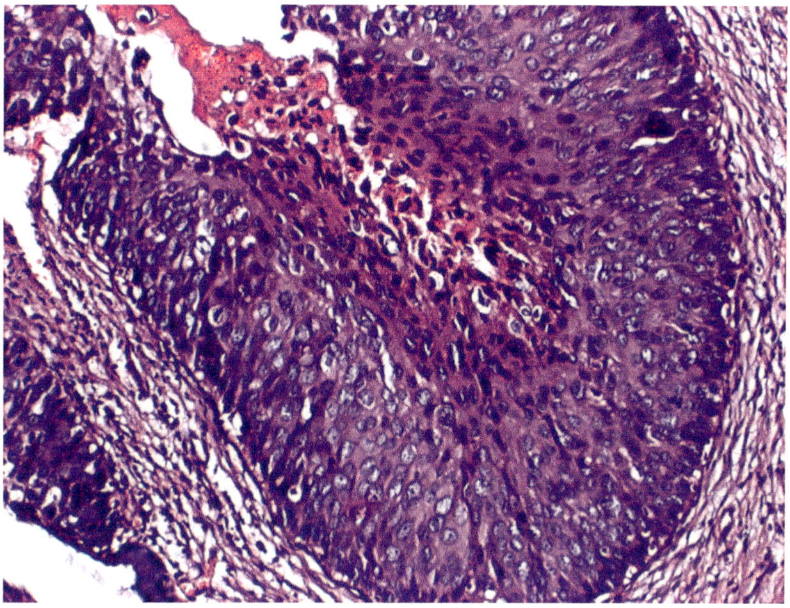

Fig. 32.5 HSIL/CIN 2/3. The entire thickness of the epithelium showing nuclear hyperchromasia, nuclear enlargement, and increased nuclear cytoplasmic ratio (H&E stain ×200)

(n:c ratio), increased nuclear size, and irregular nuclear membrane. This proliferation is limited to basal−/parabasal-like cells and lower one-third of the epithelium. Cytoplasmic maturation is seen in upper layers. Mitotic figures can be seen in the lower one-third of the squamous epithelium. The characteristic viral cytopathic change of nuclear hyperchromasia, nuclear membrane irregularity, and a well-defined perinuclear halo is seen. This is known as kilocytosis, koilocytic atypia, or HPV cytopathic effect (Fig. 32.4b).

HSIL or CIN 2/3 (Fig. 32.5) have a significant risk of progression to invasive carcinoma if not treated. Proliferation of squamous or metaplastic squamous cells which show high n:c ratio, increase in nuclear size and nuclear membrane irregularity is seen. Mitotic figures are seen in all layers of squamous epithelium, and atypical mitosis is not uncommon. These lesions show similar HPV profile as invasive carcinomas.

The further progression of HSIL to invasive carcinoma is a slow process and may take decades. The carcinogenic events occur at transformation zone near the squamocolumnar junction (Fig. 32.6) and can be readily detected by cytological examination.

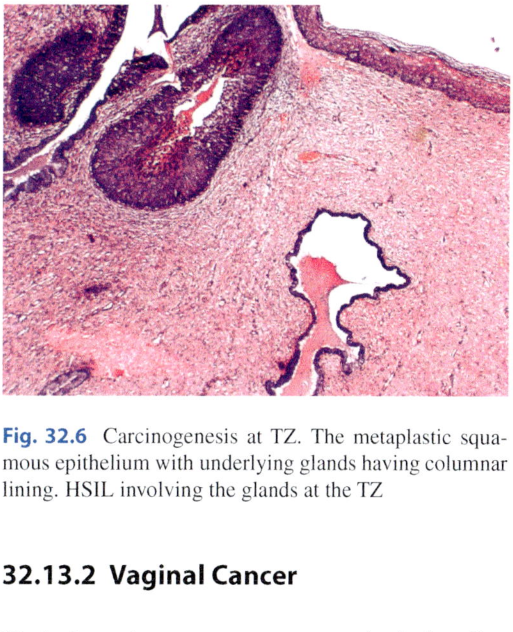

Fig. 32.6 Carcinogenesis at TZ. The metaplastic squamous epithelium with underlying glands having columnar lining. HSIL involving the glands at the TZ

32.13.2 Vaginal Cancer

Vaginal carcinomas are rare gynecological malignancies and account for 2% of all gynecologic cancers [2]. Majority of these occur in the less developed countries. Squamous cell carcinoma is the most common invasive cancer in the vagina. The median age of diagnosis is 68 years, with 70% cases diagnosed over 50 years of age. Majority of vaginal SCC (70%) are associated with HR-HPV, similar to the cervix. HR-HPV DNA is detected in

91% high-grade precursor lesions (vaginal intraepithelial neoplasia (VaIN) 2/3). HPV16 is the commonest type detected in both high-grade precancerous lesions and invasive carcinomas [2].

32.13.3 Vulvar Cancer

Vulvar carcinomas are rare tumors and constitute 4% of all gynecological malignancies worldwide. Nearly 27,000 new cases were diagnosed in the year 2008 [2]. Squamous cell carcinoma is the most common vulvar cancer, and it has two distinct histological patterns: (1) basaloid/warty types and (2) keratinizing types. Both of these show a different risk factor profile. The former is common in young women and often associated with HR-HPV (75–100%). Their risk profile is similar to cervical cancer. These are often found adjacent to vulval intraepithelial neoplasia (VIN). High-grade VIN (VIN 2/3) shows HPV DNA in 85.3% cases. HPV 16 and HPV 33 are the commonest types detected. Keratinizing vulvar carcinomas are more common (>60% cases) and occur in older women. These are rarely related to HPV (only 6% cases). These lesions develop in the setting of chronic vulvar dermatoses like lichen sclerosus and lichen planus; the precursor lesion is a non-HPV-related, differentiated type VIN.

32.14 HPV Detection

The cytopathic effect of HPV infection can be seen on cytological/histological examination, which can be further confirmed by serology and molecular tests. The molecular techniques have an advantage of being more accurate and are helpful in subtyping the infection [113]. The material for molecular techniques can be retrieved from the cell block or samples sent for sure path or thin prep. There are three molecular methods to detect HPV, which can be classified on the basis of primary technique used:

1. Nucleic acid hybridization technique
2. Signal amplification technique
3. Nucleic acid amplification technique [114]

The hybridization techniques include Southern blot, in situ hybridization, and dot blot hybridization. Their advantages are low cost and ease of availability. The disadvantage is low sensitivity and requiring high DNA load. It is a time-consuming procedure and other methods preferred [113].

The Food and Drug Administration (FDA) have approved two different techniques [115] for HPV detection by signal amplification 1: Hybrid Capture® 2 and Cervista®. In Hybrid Capture 2, the signal amplification is done through hybridization of target HPV DNA to RNA-labeled probes [116]. It can detect 13 HR-HPV subtypes and 5 LR types [115]. Cervista also follows the similar principle and can detect HR-HPV types. It is more sensitive and specific for detecting HPV 16/18 [117, 118].

There are various nucleic acid amplification techniques which utilize heat-stable DNA polymerases to amplify the known sequences of interests. These techniques are more reliable and have high sensitivity and specificity [119]. The advantage is it can amplify partially degenerated DNA fragment's which are not useful in other techniques. The NA amplification techniques are more helpful in detecting multiple infections, can estimate viral load on real time, and are more reproducible [120]. Various techniques for HPV detection are shown in Table 32.3 [121].

Table 32.3 Molecular techniques to detect HPV

NA hybridization technique	Signal amplification technique[a]	NA amplification techniques[a]
Southern blot	Hybrid Capture 2	Real-time PCR-based: Cobas 4800 HPV test and Abbott RealTime
Dot blot	Cervista	mRNA-based transcription-mediated amplification tests: APTIMA HPV test and APTIMA HPV 16, 18/45 test
In situ hybridization		

[a]Approved by the FDA

32.15 HPV Vaccination

According to WHO, the primary prevention of cancers can be done by restricting the HPV virus during the early period of a woman's life [122]. The secondary preventions can be done by screening methods and treating the precancerous lesions. Palliative treatment and cancer treatment are required for women with higher stage of disease.

FDA has approved bivalent and quadrivalent vaccines for HPV prevention, and both of these are available commercially [123]. Bivalent vaccine (Cervarix) protects against HPV 16/18, and quadrivalent vaccine (Gardasil) protects against HPV 16/18/6/11. These vaccines are recommended for girls in the age group 11–12 years and for women in the age groups 13–26 years if they have not been vaccinated previously [124]. Quadrivalent vaccine is also recommended for men in 22–26-year age group if they are immunocompromised or are gay, bisexual, and transgender who were not vaccinated previously. Persons allergic to latex and yeast are contraindicated for bivalent and quadrivalent vaccinations, respectively. The protection provided by these vaccines is effective for 10 years [124].

Two doses (0, 6–12 months) of these vaccinations have been recommended for females <15 years. The second dose is given between 6 and 12 months after the first dose. For females older than 15 years, three dose schedules are recommended (0, 1–2, 6 months), i.e., the second dose is given 1–2 months after the first dose and the third dose is given at 6 months [123] of the first dose. The idea is keeping a minimum gap of 5 months between the first and last doses in bivalent vaccination. Similarly, a gap of 4–5 months is recommended between the second and third doses where the second dose can be given after 3–4 weeks of the first dose [123].

Protection against additional five HPV viruses can be done through nano-valent vaccine (Gardasil 9) approved by the FDA recently [125]. The recommendation for dosing and age groups are similar to quadrivalent vaccines.

32.16 Conclusion

Human papilloma viruses (HPVs) are sexually transmitted, double-stranded oncogenic DNA viruses, and HPV infections account for approximately 5% of all malignancies worldwide. They are responsible for causing almost all cervical carcinomas and a significant proportion of other anogenital carcinomas (vulvovaginal, anal, penile carcinomas) and oropharyngeal carcinomas. Most HPV infections are cleared within 6–12 months by the cell-mediated host immune response. A small proportion of infections that persist can develop into preinvasive lesions and finally can progress to malignancy. The cofactors for persistence and progression of infection are smoking, parity, hormonal influences, and other sexually transmitted infections like HIV. There are now many tests commercially available for detection of HPV. Primary prevention of HPV infection through vaccination of young girls and screening and treatment of preinvasive lesions can help to bring down the burden of disease.

Key Points

- HPV infections account for approximately 5% of all malignancies worldwide.
- Majority of HPV infections are successfully resolved through cell-mediated immune response of the host. The infection leads to sensitization of dendritic cells followed by a T-cell-mediated response that stops the viral gene expression.
- The lifetime risk of acquiring HPV infection by sexual transmission is 50% [66], and most women will acquire a HPV infection at some time.
- The cofactors for persistence and progression of HPV infection are smoking, parity, hormonal influences, and other sexually transmitted infections like HIV.
- The important methods to detect HPV are nucleic acid hybridization, signal amplification, and nucleic acid amplification technique.
- FDA has approved bivalent, quadrivalent, and nonavalent vaccines for HPV prevention, and all of these are available commercially.

References

1. Nobel Media. Harald zur Hausen – Biographica [internet]. Available from: <http://www.nobelprize.org/nobel_prizes/medicine/laureates/2008/hausen-bio.html>.
2. de Martel C, Ferlay J, Franceschi S, Vignat J, Bray F, Forman D, et al. Global burden of cancers attributable to infections in 2008: a review and synthetic analysis. Lancet Oncol. 2012;13:607–15.
3. Bosch FX, Broker TR, Forman D, Moscicki AB, Gillison ML, Doorbar J, et al. Comprehensive control of human papillomavirus infections and related diseases. Vaccine. 2013;31(Suppl 8):I1–31.
4. Bernard HU, Burk RD, Chen Z, van Doorslaer K, zur Hausen H, de Villiers EM. Classification of papillomaviruses (PVs) based on 189 PV types and proposal of taxonomic amendments. Virology. 2010;401:70–9.
5. de Villiers EM. Cross-roads in the classification of papillomaviruses. Virology. 2013;445:2–10.
6. IARC Working Group on the Evaluation of Carcinogenic Risks to Humans. Human papillomaviruses. IARC Monogr Eval Carcinog Risks Hum. 2007;90:1–636.
7. Doorbar J, Egawa N, Griffin H, Kranjec C, Murakami I. Human papillomavirus molecular biology and disease association. Rev Med Virol. 2015;25(Suppl 1):2–23.
8. Mindel A, Tideman R. HPV transmission — still feeling the way. Lancet. 1999;354:2097–8.
9. Frega A, Cenci M, Stentella P, Cipriano L, De Ioris A, Alderisio M, et al. Human papillomavirus in virgins and behaviour at risk. Cancer Lett. 2003;194:21–4.
10. Winer RL, Lee SK, Hughes JP, Adam DE, Kiviat NB, Koutsky LA. Genital human papillomavirus infection: incidence and risk factors in a cohort of female university students. Am J Epidemiol. 2003;157:218–26.
11. Sonnex C, Strauss S, Gray JJ. Detection of human papillomavirus DNA on the fingers of patients with genital warts. Sex Transm Infect. 1999;75:317–9.
12. Franco EL, Villa LL, Ruiz A, Costa MC. Transmission of cervical human papillomavirus infection by sexual activity: differences between low and high oncogenic risk types. J Infect Dis. 1995;172:756–63.
13. Kjaer SK, van den Brule AJC, Bock JE, Poll PA, Engholm G, Sherman ME, et al. Determinants for genital human papillomavirus (HPV) infection in 1000 randomly chosen young Danish women with normal Pap smear: are there different risk profiles for oncogenic and nononcogenic HPV types? Cancer Epidemiol Biomark Prev. 1997;6:799–805.
14. Rousseau MC, Franco EL, Villa LL, Sobrinho JP, Termini L, Prado JM, et al. A cumulative case–control study of risk factor profiles for oncogenic and nononcogenic cervical human papillomavirus infections. Cancer Epidemiol Biomark Prev. 2000;9:469–76.
15. Tenti P, Zappatore R, Migliora P, Spinillo A, Belloni C, Carnevali L. Perinatal transmission of human papillomavirus from gravidas with latent infections. Obstet Gynecol. 1999;93:475–9.
16. Syrjänen S, Puranen M. Human papillomavirus infections in children: the potential role of maternal transmission. Crit Rev Oral Biol Med. 2000;11:259–74.
17. Sedlacek TV, Lindheim S, Eder C, Hasty L, Woodland M, Ludomirsky A, et al. Mechanism for human papillomavirus transmission at birth. Am J Obstet Gynecol. 1989;161:55–9.
18. Armbruster-Moraes E, Ioshimoto LM, Leao E, Zugaib M. Detection of human papillomavirus deoxyribonucleic acid sequences in amniotic fluid during different periods of pregnancy. Am J Obstet Gynecol. 1993;169:1074.
19. Grayson W, Rhemtula HA, Taylor LF, Allard U, Tiltman AJ. Detection of human papillomavirus in large cell neuroendocrine carcinoma of the uterine cervix: a study of 12 cases. J Clin Pathol. 2002;55:108–14.
20. Egawa K. Do human papillomaviruses target epidermal stem cells? Dermatology. 2003;207:251–4.
21. Schmitt A, Rochat A, Zeltner R, Borenstein L, Barrandon Y, Wettstein FO, et al. The primary target cells of the high-risk cottontail rabbit papillomavirus colocalize with hair follicle stem cells. J Virol. 1996;70:1912–22.
22. Aksoy P, Gottschalk EY, Meneses PI. HPV entry into cells. Mutat Res Rev Mutat Res. 2017;772:13–22.
23. Pyeon D, Pearce SM, Lank SM, Ahlquist P, Lambert PF. Establishment of human papillomavirus infection requires cell cycle progression. PLoS Pathog. 2009;5:e1000318.
24. Parish JL, Bean AM, Park RB, Androphy EJ. ChlR1 is required for loading papillomavirus E2 onto mitotic chromosomes and viral genome maintenance. Mol Cell. 2006;24:867–76.
25. McBride AA. Replication and partitioning of papillomavirus genomes. Adv Virus Res. 2008;72:155–205.
26. Hubert WG, Laimins LA. Human papillomavirus type 31 replication modes during the early phases of the viral life cycle depend on transcriptional and posttranscriptional regulation of E1 and E2 expression. J Virol. 2002;76:2263–73.
27. Stubenrauch F, Colbert AM, Laimins LA. Transactivation by the E2 protein of oncogenic human papillomavirus type 31 is not essential for early and late viral functions. J Virol. 1998;72:8115–23.
28. Egawa N, Nakahara T, Ohno S, Narisawa-Saito M, Yugawa T, Fujita M, et al. The E1 protein of human papillomavirus type 16 is dispensable for maintenance replication of the viral genome. J Virol. 2012;86:3276–83.

29. Cheng S, Schmidt-Grimminger DC, Murant T, Broker TR, Chow LT. Differentiation-dependent up-regulation of the human papillomavirus E7 gene reactivates cellular DNA replication in suprabasal differentiated keratinocytes. Genes Dev. 1995;9:2335–49.
30. Peh WL, Middleton K, Christensen N, Nicholls P, Egawa K, Sotlar K, et al. Life cycle heterogeneity in animal models of human papillomavirus-associated disease. J Virol. 2002;76:10401–16.
31. Stanley M. Pathology and epidemiology of HPV infection in females. Gynecol Oncol. 2010;117:S5–S10.
32. Gariglio P, Gutiérrez J, Cortés E, Vázquez J. The role of retinoid deficiency and estrogens as cofactors in cervical cancer. Arch Med Res. 2009;40:449–65.
33. Ding DC, Chiang MH, Lai HC, Hsiung CA, Hsieh CY, Chu TY. Methylation of the long control region of HPV16 is related to the severity of cervical neoplasia. Eur J Obstet Gynecol Reprod Biol. 2009;147:215–20.
34. Jeon S, Allen-Hoffmann BL, Lambert PF. Integration of human papillomavirus type 16 into the human genome correlates with a selective growth advantage of cells. J Virol. 1995;69:2989–97.
35. Jeon S, Lambert PF. Integration of human papillomavirus type 16 DNA into the human genome leads to increased stability of E6 and E7 mRNAs: implications for cervical carcinogenesis. Proc Natl Acad Sci U S A. 1995;92:1654–8.
36. Pett MR, Alazawi WO, Roberts I, Dowen S, Smith DI, Stanley MA, et al. Acquisition of high-level chromosomal instability is associated with integration of human papillomavirus type 16 in cervical keratinocytes. Cancer Res. 2004;64:1359–68.
37. Badaracco G, Venuti A, Sedati A, Marcante ML. HPV16 and HPV18 in genital tumors: significantly different levels of viral integration and correlation to tumor invasiveness. J Med Virol. 2002;67:574–82.
38. Fu L, Van Doorslaer K, Chen Z, Ristriani T, Masson M, Travé G, et al. Degradation of p53 by human Alphapapillomavirus E6 proteins shows a stronger correlation with phylogeny than oncogenicity. PLoS One. 2010;5(9):e12816.
39. Zanier K, ould M'hamed ould Sidi A, Boulade-Ladame C, Rybin V, Chappelle A, Atkinson A, et al. Solution structure analysis of the HPV16 E6 oncoprotein reveals a self-association mechanism required for E6-mediated degradation of p53. Structure. 2012;20:604–17.
40. Pim D, Banks L. Interaction of viral oncoproteins with cellular target molecules: infection with high-risk vs low-risk human papillomaviruses. APMIS. 2010;118:471–93.
41. Galloway DA, Gewin LC, Myers H, Luo W, Grandori C, Katzenellenbogen RA, et al. Regulation of telomerase by human papillomaviruses. Cold Spring Harb Symp Quant Biol. 2005;70:209–15.
42. Gewin L, Galloway DA. E box-dependent activation of telomerase by human papillomavirus type 16 E6 does not require induction of c-myc. J Virol. 2001;75:7198–201.
43. Klingelhutz AJ, Foster SA, McDougall JK. Telomerase activation by the E6 gene product of human papillomavirus type 16. Nature. 1996;380:79–82.
44. Barrow-Laing L, Chen W, Roman A. Low- and high-risk human papillomavirus E7 proteins regulate p130 differently. Virology. 2010;400:233–9.
45. Roman A. The human papillomavirus E7 protein shines a spotlight on the pRB family member, p130. Cell Cycle. 2006;5:567–8.
46. Klingelhutz AJ, Roman A. Cellular transformation by human papillomaviruses: lessons learned by comparing high- and low-risk viruses. Virology. 2012;424:77–98.
47. Felsani A, Mileo AM, Paggi MG. Retinoblastoma family proteins as key targets of the small DNA virus oncoproteins. Oncogene. 2006;25:5277–85.
48. Rodríguez AC, Schiffman M, Herrero R, Hildesheim A, Bratti C, Sherman ME, et al. Longitudinal study of human papillomavirus persistence and cervical intraepithelial neoplasia grade 2/3: critical role of duration of infection. J Natl Cancer Inst. 2010;102:315–24.
49. Winer RL, Hughes JP, Feng Q, Xi LF, Cherne S, O'Reilly S, et al. Early natural history of incident, type-specific human papillomavirus infections in newly sexually active young women. Cancer Epidemiol Biomark Prev. 2011;20:699–707.
50. Alizon S, Murall CL, Bravo IG. Why human papillomavirus acute infections matter. Viruses. 2017;9(10):e293.
51. Maglennon GA, McIntosh PB, Doorbar J. Immunosuppression facilitates the reactivation of latent papillomavirus infections. J Virol. 2014;88:710–6.
52. Muñoz N, Hernandez-Suarez G, Méndez F, Molano M, Posso H, Moreno V, et al. Persistence of HPV infection and risk of high-grade cervical intraepithelial neoplasia in a cohort of Colombian women. Br J Cancer. 2009;100:1184–90.
53. Marks MA, Castle PE, Schiffman M, Gravitt PE. Evaluation of any or type-specific persistence of high-risk human papillomavirus for detecting cervical precancer. J Clin Microbiol. 2012;50:300–6.
54. Stanley MA. Epithelial cell responses to infection with human papillomavirus. Clin Microbiol Rev. 2012;25:215–22.
55. Kanodia S, Fahey LM, Kast WM. Mechanisms used by human papillomaviruses to escape the host immune response. Curr Cancer Drug Targets. 2007;7:79–89.
56. Li S, Labrecque S, Gauzzi MC, Cuddihy AR, Wong AH, Pellegrini S, et al. The human papilloma virus (HPV)-18 E6 oncoprotein physically associates with Tyk2 and impairs Jak-STAT activation by interferon-alpha. Oncogene. 1999;18:5727–37.

57. Nees M, Geoghegan JM, Hyman T, Frank S, Miller L, Woodworth CD. Papillomavirus type 16 oncogenes downregulate expression of interferon-responsive genes and upregulate proliferation-associated and NF-kappaB-responsive genes in cervical keratinocytes. J Virol. 2001;75:4283–96.
58. Perea SE, Massimi P, Banks L. Human papillomavirus type 16 E7 impairs the activation of the interferon regulatory factor-1. Int J Mol Med. 2000;5:661–6.
59. Um SJ, Rhyu JW, Kim EJ, Jeon KC, Hwang ES, Park JS. Abrogation of IRF-1 response by high-risk HPV E7 protein in vivo. Cancer Lett. 2002;179:205–12.
60. Caberg JH, Hubert PM, Begon DY, Herfs MF, Roncarati PJ, Boniver JJ, et al. Silencing of E7 oncogene restores functional E-cadherin expression in human papillomavirus 16-transformed keratinocytes. Carcinogenesis. 2008;29:1441–7.
61. Matthews K, Leong CM, Baxter L, Inglis E, Yun K, Bäckström BT, et al. Depletion of Langerhans cells in human papillomavirus type 16-infected skin is associated with E6-mediated down regulation of E-cadherin. J Virol. 2003;77:8378–85.
62. Ashrafi GH, Haghshenas M, Marchetti B, Campo MS. E5 protein of human papillomavirus 16 downregulates HLA class I and interacts with the heavy chain via its first hydrophobic domain. Int J Cancer. 2006;119:2105–12.
63. Carter JJ, Koutsky LA, Hughes JP, Lee SK, Kuyper J, Kiviat N, et al. Comparison of human papillomavirus types 16, 18, and 6 capsid antibody responses following incident infection. J Infect Dis. 2000;181:1911–9.
64. Wang SS, Schiffman M, Herrero R, Carreon J, Hildesheim A, Rodriguez AC, et al. Determinants of human papillomavirus 16 serological conversion and persistence in a population-based cohort of 10 000 women in Costa Rica. Br J Cancer. 2004;91:1269–74.
65. Carter JJ, Madeleine MM, Shera K, Schwartz SM, Cushing-Haugen KL, Wipf GC, et al. Human papillomavirus 16 and 18 L1 serology compared across anogenital cancer sites. Cancer Res. 2001;61:1934–40.
66. Handler MZ, Handler NS, Majewski S, Schwartz RA. Human papillomavirus vaccine trials and tribulations: clinical perspectives. J Am Acad Dermatol. 2015;73:743–56.
67. de Sanjose S, Diaz M, Castellsague X, Clifford G, Bruni L, Munoz N, et al. Worldwide prevalence and genotype distribution of cervical human papillomavirus DNA in women with normal cytology: a meta-analysis. Lancet Infect Dis. 2007;7:453–9.
68. Castellsague X, de Sanjose S, Aguado T, Louie KS, Bruni L, Munoz J, et al., editors. HPV and cervical cancer in the world. 2007 report. WHO/ICO Information Centre on HPV and Cervical Cancer (HPV Information Centre). Vaccine. 2007;25(Suppl 3):C1–224.
69. Clifford GM, Gallus S, Herrero R, Munoz N, Snijders PJ, Vaccarella S, et al. Worldwide distribution of human papillomavirus types in cytologically normal women in the International Agency for Research on Cancer HPV prevalence surveys: a pooled analysis. Lancet. 2005;366:991–8.
70. Quint WG, Pagliusi SR, Lelie N, de Villiers EM, Wheeler CM. Results of the first World Health Organization international collaborative study of detection of human papillomavirus DNA. J Clin Microbiol. 2006;44:571–9.
71. Castellsague X, Diaz M, de Sanjose S, Munoz N, Herrero R, Franceschi S, et al. Worldwide human papillomavirus etiology of cervical adenocarcinoma and its cofactors: implications for screening and prevention. J Natl Cancer Inst. 2006;98:303–15.
72. Parkin DM, Whelan SLFJ, Teppo L, Thomas DB. Cancer incidence in five continents, volume VIII. IARC scientific publications no. 155. Lyon: IARC Press; 2003.
73. Human papillomavirus testing for triage of women with cytologic evidence of low-grade squamous intraepithelial lesions: baseline data from a randomized trial. The Atypical Squamous Cells of Undetermined Significance/Low-Grade Squamous Intraepithelial Lesions Triage Study (ALTS) Group. J Natl Cancer Inst. 2000;92:397–402.
74. Ho GY, Kadish AS, Burk RD, Basu J, Palan PR, Mikhail M, et al. HPV 16 and cigarette smoking as risk factors for high-grade cervical intra-epithelial neoplasia. Int J Cancer. 1998;78:281–5.
75. Ho GY, Bierman R, Beardsley L, Chang CJ, Burk RD. Natural history of cervicovaginal papillomavirus infection in young women. N Engl J Med. 1998;338:423–8.
76. Clifford GM, Smith JS, Plummer M, Munoz N, Franceschi S. Human papillomavirus types in invasive cervical cancer worldwide: a meta-analysis. Br J Cancer. 2003;88:63–73.
77. Bhatla N, Lal N, Bao YP, Ng T, Qiao YL. A meta-analysis of human papillomavirus type-distribution in women from South Asia: implications for vaccination. Vaccine. 2008;26(23):2811–7.
78. World Health Organization. Human papilloma virus and related cancers summary report update. 3rd ed. Geneva: WHO; 2010.
79. Berlin Grace VM. HPV type 18 is more oncopotent than HPV16 in uterine cervical carcinogenesis although HPV16 is the prevalent type in Chennai, India. Indian J Cancer. 2009;46:203e7.
80. Franceschi S, Rajkumar R, Snijders PJ, Arslan A, Mahé C, Plummer M, et al. Papillomavirus infection in rural women in southern India. Br J Cancer. 2005;92:601e6.
81. Duttagupta C, Sengupta S, Roy M, Sengupta D, Bhattacharya P, Laikangbam P, et al. Are Muslim women less susceptible to oncogenic human papilloma virus infection? A study from the rural eastern India. Int J Gynecol Cancer. 2004;14:293–e303.
82. Senapati R, Nayak B, Kar SK, Dwibedi B. HPV genotypes distribution in Indian women with and without cervical carcinoma: implication for HPV

vaccination program in Odisha, Eastern India. BMC Infect Dis. 2017;17:30.
83. Laikangbam P, Sengupta S, Bhattacharya P, Duttagupta C, Dhabali Singh T, Verma Y, et al. A comparative profile of the prevalence and age distribution of human papillomavirus type 16/18 infections among three states of India with focus on Northeast India. Int J Gynecol Cancer. 2007;17:107–17.
84. Schellekens MC, Dijkman A, Aziz MF, Siregar B, Cornain S, Kolkman-Uljee S, et al. Single and multiple HPV types in cervical carcinomas in Jakarta, Indonesia. Gynecol Oncol. 2004;93:49–53.
85. Ngelangel C, Munoz N, Bosch FX, Limson GM, Festin MR, Deacon J, et al. Causes of cervical cancer in the Philippines: a case-control study. J Natl Cancer Inst. 1998;90:43–9.
86. Chicharen S, Herrero R, Munoz N, Bosch FX, Jacobs MV, Deacon J, et al. Risk factors for cervical cancer in Thailand: a case-control study. J Natl Cancer Inst. 1998;90:50–7.
87. Sharma K, Kathait A, Jain A, Kujur K, Raghuwanshi S, Bharti AC, et al. Higher prevalence of human papillomavirus infection in adolescent and young adult girls belonging to different Indian tribes with varied socio-sexual lifestyle. PLoS One. 2015;10:e0125693.
88. Hussain S, Bharadwaj M, Nasare V, Kumari M, Sharma S, Hedau S, et al. Human papillomavirus infection among young adolescents in India: impact of vaccination. J Med Virol. 2012;84:298–305.
89. Prusty BK, Kumar A, Arora R, Batra S, Das BC. Human papillomavirus (HPV) DNA detection in self-collected urine. Int J Gynaecol Obstet. 2005;90:223–7.
90. Thilagavathi A, Shanmughapriya S, Vinodhini K, Das BC, Natarajaseenivasan K. Prevalence of human papillomavirus (HPV) among college going girls using self collected urine samples from Tiruchirappalli, Tamilnadu. Arch Gynecol Obstet. 2012;286:1483–6.
91. Castellsagué X, Muñoz N. Chapter 3: cofactors in human papillomavirus carcinogenesis — role of parity, oral contraceptives, and tobacco smoking. J Natl Cancer Inst Monogr. 2003;31:20–8.
92. Lacey JV Jr, Brinton LA, Abbas FM, Barnes WA, Gravitt PE, Greenberg MD, et al. Oral contraceptives as risk factors for cervical adenocarcinomas and squamous cell carcinomas. Cancer Epidemiol Biomark Prev. 1999;8:1079–85.
93. Hildesheim A, Herrero R, Castle PE, Wacholder S, Bratti MC, Sherman ME, et al. HPV co-factors related to the development of cervical cancer: results from a population-based study in Costa Rica. Br J Cancer. 2001;84:1219–26.
94. Moreno V, Bosch FX, Munoz N, Meijer CJ, Shah KV, Walboomers JM, et al. Effect of oral contraceptives on risk of cervical cancer in women with human papillomavirus infection: the IARC multicentric case–control study. Lancet. 2002;359:1085–92.
95. Moodley M, Moodley J, Chetty R, Herrington CS. The role of steroid contraceptive hormones in the pathogenesis of invasive cervical cancer: a review. Int J Gynecol Cancer. 2003;13:103–10.
96. Munoz N, Franceschi S, Bosetti C, Moreno V, Herrero R, Smith JS, et al. Role of parity and human papillomavirus in cervical cancer: the IARC multicentric case–control study. Lancet. 2002;359:1093–101.
97. Autier P, Coibion M, Huet F, Grivegnee AR. Transformation zone location and intraepithelial neoplasia of the cervix uteri. Br J Cancer. 1996;74:488–90.
98. Sethi S, Muller M, Schneider A, Blettner M, Smith E, Turek L, et al. Serologic response to the E4, E6, and E7 proteins of human papillomavirus type 16 in pregnant women. Am J Obstet Gynecol. 1998;178:360–4.
99. Kjaer SK, van den Brule AJC, Bock JE, Poll PA, Engholm G, Sherman ME, et al. Human papillomavirus — the most significant risk determinant of cervical intraepithelial neoplasia. Int J Cancer. 1996;65:601–6.
100. Olsen AO, Dillner J, Skrondal A, Magnus P. Combined effect of smoking and human papillomavirus type 16 infection in cervical carcinogenesis. Epidemiology. 1998;9:346–9.
101. Ylitalo N, Sørensen P, Josefsson A, Frisch M, Sparén P, Pontén J, et al. Smoking and oral contraceptives as risk factors for cervical carcinoma in situ. Int J Cancer. 1999;81:357–65.
102. Plummer M, Herrero R, Franceschi S, Meijer CJLM, Snijders P, Bosch FX, et al. Smoking and cervical cancer: pooled analysis of the IARC multicentric case–control study. Cancer Causes Control. 2003;14:805–14.
103. Giuliano AR, Harris R, Sedjo RL, Baldwin S, Roe D, Papenfuss MR, et al. Incidence, prevalence, and clearance of type-specific human papillomavirus infections: the young women's health study. J Infect Dis. 2002;186:462–9.
104. Minkoff H, Feldman JG, Strickler HD, Watts DH, Bacon MC, Levine A, et al. Relationship between smoking and human papillomavirus infections in HIV-infected and -uninfected women. J Infect Dis. 2004;189:1821–8.
105. Prokopczyk B, Cox JE, Hoffmann D, Waggoner SE. Identification of tobacco-specific carcinogen in the cervical mucus of smokers and non-smokers. J Natl Cancer Inst. 1997;89:868–73.
106. Poppe WA, Ide PS, Drijkoningen MP, Lauweryns JM, Van Assche FA. Tobacco smoking impairs the local immunosurveillance in the uterine cervix. An immunohistochemical study. Gynecol Obstet Investig. 1995;39:34–8.
107. Safaeian M, Quint K, Schiffman M, Rodriguez AC, Wacholder S, Herrero R, et al. Chlamydia trachomatis and risk of prevalent and incident cervical premalignancy in a population-based cohort. J Natl Cancer Inst. 2010;102:1794–804.

108. Zhu H, Shen Z, Luo H, Zhang W, Zhu X. Chlamydia trachomatis infection-associated risk of cervical Cancer: a Meta-analysis. Medicine (Baltimore). 2016;95:e3077.
109. Kelly H, Weiss HA, Benavente Y, de Sanjose S, Mayaud P, ART and HPV Review Group. Association of antiretroviral therapy with high-risk human papillomavirus, cervical intraepithelial neoplasia, and invasive cervical cancer in women living with HIV: a systematic review and meta-analysis. Lancet HIV. 2018;5:e45–58.
110. Bruni L, Barrionuevo-Rosas L, Albero G, Serrano B, Mena M, Gómez D, et al. ICO/IARC Information Centre on HPV and Cancer (HPVInformation Centre). Human papillomavirus and related diseases in the world. Summary report 27 July 2017. [Assessed on 18 March 2018].
111. Bruni L, Barrionuevo-Rosas L, Albero G, Serrano B, Mena M, Gómez D, et al. ICO/IARC Information Centre on HPV and Cancer (HPV Information Centre). Human papillomavirus and related diseases in India. Summary report 27 July 2017. [Assessed on 18 March 2018].
112. Darragh TM, Colgan TJ, Cox JT, Heller DS, Henry MR, Luff RD, et al. The lower anogenital squamous terminology standardization project for HPV-associated lesions: background and consensus recommendations from the College of American Pathologists and the American Society for Colposcopy and Cervical Pathology. Arch Pathol Lab Med. 2012;136:1266–97.
113. Villa LL, Denny L. Methods for detection of HPV infection and its clinical utility. Int J Gyn Obst. 2006;94:71–80.
114. Shen-Gunther J, Yu X. HPV molecular assays: defining analytical and clinical performance characteristics for cervical cytology specimens. Gynecol Oncol. 2011;123:263–71.
115. Hwang SJ, Shroyer KR. Biomarkers of cervical dysplasia and carcinoma. J Oncol. 2012;2012:507286.
116. Bozzetti M, Nonnenmacher B, Mielzinska II, Villa L, Lorincz A, Breitenbach VV, et al. Comparison between hybrid capture II and polymerase chain reaction results among women at low risk for cervical cancer. Ann Epidemiol. 2000;10:466.
117. Einstein MH, Martens MG, Garcia FA, Ferris DG, Mitchell AL, Day SP, et al. Clinical validation of the Cervista HPV HR and 16/18 genotyping tests for use in women with ASC-US cytology. Gynecol Oncol. 2010;118:116–22.
118. Bartholomew DA, Luff RD, Quigley NB, Curtis M, Olson MC. Analytical performance of Cervista HPV 16/18 genotyping test for cervical cytology samples. J Clin Virol. 2011;51:38–43.
119. Kocjan BJ, Seme K, Poljak M. Comparison of the Abbott real time high risk HPV test and INNO-LiPA HPV genotyping extra test for the detection of human papillomaviruses in formalin-fixed, paraffinembedded cervical cancer specimens. J Virol Methods. 2011;175:117–9.
120. Roberts I, Ng G, Foster N, Stanley M, Herdman MT, Pett MR, et al. Critical evaluation of HPV16 gene copy number quantification by SYBR green PCR. BMC Biotechnol. 2008;8:57.
121. Choi YJ, Park JS. Clinical significance of human papillomavirus genotyping. J Gynecol Oncol. 2016;27:e21.
122. WHO, UN Population Fund. Preparing for the introduction of HPV vaccine: policy and programme guideance for countries. Geneva: WHO; 2006.
123. Meites E, Kempe A, Markowitz LE. Use of a 2-dose schedule for human papillomavirus vaccination—updated recommendations of the advisory committee on immunization practices. MMWR Morb Mortal Wkly Rep. 2016;65:1405–8.
124. Markowitz LE, Dunne EF, Saraiya M, Chesson HW, Curtis CR, Gee J, et al. Human papillomavirus vaccination: recommendations of the advisory committee on immunization practices (ACIP). MMWR Recomm Rep. 2014;63:1–30.
125. Petrosky E, Bocchini JA Jr, Hariri S, Chesson H, Curtis CR, Saraiya M, et al. Use of 9-valent human papillomavirus (HPV) vaccine: updated HPV vaccination recommendations of the advisory committee on immunization practices. MMWR Morb Mortal Wkly Rep. 2015;64:300–4.

Advances in Colposcopy

33

Bindiya Gupta

The science of today is the technology of tomorrow

33.1 Introduction

Colposcopy helps in identification of abnormalities of the lower genital tract (cervix, vulva, and vagina) by using principles of magnification (3–15 times) and illumination. Various stains like acetic acid, Lugol's iodine, toluidine blue, etc. are used to identify the abnormalities. It helps to identify the color of the epithelium, the surface contour, and vasculature both before and after application of the various stains. It can be a binocular colposcope mounted on a tripod with a light source and mirror or a modern-day video colposcope which has a zoom capacity and photographic, video, and analytic facilities [1].

Colposcopy is not a screening tool, rather it's a diagnostic tool to confirm the presence of precancerous or cancerous lesions once a screening test is positive. It can also be done in situations when the cervix is looking abnormal or there is a history of postcoital bleeding.

The accuracy of diagnosis in colposcopy has interobserver and intraobserver variability and depends on operator skill and experience. Among experienced colposcopists, the level of agreement is higher with high-grade lesions compared to diagnosing low-grade disease. In meta-analysis by Mitchell et al. in 1998, the sensitivity and specificity of colposcopy for CIN2+ disease were 96% and 48%, respectively [2]. For the threshold normal cervix compared with all abnormalities, the area under the curve (AUC) was 0.80, while for the threshold normal cervix and low-grade SIL compared with high-grade SIL and cancer, the AUC was 0.82.

Another systematic review by Hopman EH et al. showed a positive predictive value of a colposcopy for CIN3 as 78% [3]. Baseline colposcopy could only identify 54% CIN3+ in women with ASCUS or 56% of CIN3+ cases diagnosed in women with low-grade squamous intraepithelial lesions in the ALTS trial [4]. In a systematic review of colposcopy-directed punch biopsy, the pooled sensitivity for a punch biopsy to diagnose CIN2+ disease was 91.3% (95% CI 85.3–94.9%), and the specificity was 24.6% (95% CI 16.0–35.9%) [5].

Various new technologies have been introduced to improve the diagnostic accuracy of colposcopy, and they will be discussed in this chapter. Not only the adjunct use of technology but portable user-friendly devices have been developed which have increased the provision of colposcopy in remote areas.

B. Gupta (✉)
Department of Obstetrics and Gynaecology,
UCMS & GTB Hospital, New Delhi, India

S. Mehta, A. Singla (eds.), *Preventive Oncology for the Gynecologist*,
https://doi.org/10.1007/978-981-13-3438-2_33

33.2 Spectroscopy

33.2.1 Dynamic Spectral Imaging System (DySIS)

DySIS (DySIS Medical Ltd., Livingston) is a digital video colposcope that uses dynamic spectral imaging to measure the rate, extent, and duration of acetowhitening of cervical epithelium. This serves as a guide to identify the area to be biopsied [6]. It measures the effect of application of acetic acid on every image pixel of the cervix by kinetic mapping of the cervix. A colored grading of the acetowhite change (or DySISmap) is superimposed on a live color image of the cervix which helps to determine the presence and grade of a neoplastic lesion and thereby select the site for biopsy [7].

The patient has to remain still at the time of DySIS colposcopy and examination, and the time taken for this takes slightly longer than that of a standard colposcopy. According to a study, almost one third of women felt less discomfort during Pap smear than DySIS, and 6.5% of women felt that DySIS colposcopy was more time consuming [8]. It is used in NHS, United Kingdom, and it is recommended that colposcopists should perform 20 examinations to become familiar with the use of DySIS and interpretation of its findings. Various studies on efficacy of DySIS taking CIN2+ as cutoff are summarized in Table 33.1. In a systematic review, it was seen that DySIS treatment options are more cost-effective than colposcopy alone [14].

33.2.2 LuViva Advanced Cervical Scan (Guided Therapeutics, Norcross)

It uses multimodal hyperspectroscopy (MHS) and analyzes fluorescence and reflectance spectra from the cervix. The emitted and reflected light is measured which is determined by the characteristics of the epithelium such as nuclear density, thickness, and neovascularization. The metabolic alterations that occur in dysplastic tissue are also analyzed [15]. The results are available in about a minute. The learning curve for the procedure is small, and it takes only about 2–3 weeks of training to use the machine. It is currently under US Food and Drug Administration premarket approval review. Besides an adjunct to colposcopy, it has a potential to be used as a screening

Table 33.1 Evidence for accuracy of DySIS

Studies	Sensitivity	Specificity	Others
Soutter et al. [9]; (DySIS vs colposcopy)	79% (95% CI; 68–88) for DySIS and 49% (95% CI; 37–61) for colposcopy		PPV for DySIS was 50% versus conventional colposcopy was 58%. DySIS detected 62.9% more high-grade cases than colposcopy ($p = 0.0001$)
Louwers et al. [10]; (DySIS vs conventional colposcopy)	DySIS colposcopy was 79% (95% CI 70–88); 55% (95% CI 44–65) for colposcopy alone	DySIS colposcopy was 77% (95% CI 69–86); 85% (95% CI 77–92) for colposcopy	The PPVs for DySIS and conventional colposcopy 76%
Roensbo et al. [11]; (DySIS colposcopy with histology as gold standard)	32.4%	83%	
Coronado and Fasero [12]; (DySIS map with histology as reference standard)	84%	89%	
Zaal et al. [13]; (DySIS colposcopy with histology and HPV testing)	CIN2+/HPV 16 +ve: 97%; CIN2+/high-risk HPV +ve (nonHPV 16) 74%		

Table 33.2 Studies on LuViva TM

Studies	Sensitivity	Specificity	Others
Ferris et al. [16]	95%	83%	Sensitivity was increased from 72% with conventional cytology at the time of colposcopy to 97% for LuViva for a matched specificity of 70%
DeSantis et al. [17]	95% (95% CI; 92–99)	55% (95% CI; 69–81)	
Winter and Sternfield (2012; unpublished) (LuViva), used in combination with an HPV test	LuViva combined with HPV testing produced both a sensitivity and negative predictive value of 99%	83%	Could safely reduce the number of unnecessary colposcopies by 33%
Twiggs LB [18] (LuViva), used without an HPV test	91%	39%	
Flowers et al. (2012; unpublished) [19]	60%	88%	This compared favorably with the performance of cytology, which had a surprisingly poor sensitivity (20–35%) but higher specificity (90–95%)

device since results for guiding management are immediately available. The accuracy of the device for the detection of CIN2 or greater is summarized in Table 33.2.

33.2.3 LUMA Cervical Imaging System

It is a non-contact optical imaging device that has been approved by FDA in 2006 for supplementing colposcopy as a diagnostic modality. It uses a combination of fluorescence spectroscopy, white-light diffuse reflectance spectroscopy, and video imaging for scanning the tissue which is completed in 12 s. Optical sources used are a 337 nm UV nitrogen laser to induce fluorescence and two xenon flash lamps [20, 21]. In a prospective, randomized controlled trial, using LUMA imaging with colposcopy increased the rate of true positives by 25% for women with atypical squamous cell or low-grade squamous intraepithelial lesions on Pap smear [22].

33.2.4 Trimodal Spectroscopy

As it uses a combination of intrinsic fluorescence, diffuse reflectance, and light scattering, it is a superior tool for the detection of precancer and cancer. However, the complexity and the cost of this multifunctional equipment are high. In a study by Georgakoudi et al., the sensitivity for high-grade and low-grade CIN compared with histopathologically proven normal cervices was 92%, with a specificity of 71% [23].

33.2.5 Electrical Impedance Spectroscopy, Zedscan™ (Zilico Ltd., Manchester)

It maps the impedance profile of cervical epithelium and thus helps in directing the site of biopsy. The Zedscan is held against the squamocolumnar junction after acetic acid application at 10 points which are pre-designated. A small amount of current is then passed through the 5.5 mm diameter tip. The device measures the resistance of the tissue which depends on the capacitance of cell membranes and extra- and intracellular spaces. Zedscan is done prior to colposcopy and helps in guiding the site for biopsy which is taken from the area with abnormal signals.

In a study by Tidy et al., including 474 women, PPV increased with Zedscan from 54% (95% CI 45–62) to 67% for predicting high-grade CIN ($p = 0.0006$) [24]. In their study using the presence of disease as reference standard (colposcopy+ biopsy) for CIN2/CIN3, sensitivity and specificity were 92% and 51.6%, respectively. Various other studies to identify CIN2+ lesions using first- and second-generation prototypes have reported sensitivity ranging from 73 to 75% and specificity of 43 to 63% [25–27].

33.2.6 TruScreen® (Polartechnics Ltd., Sydney)

It is a hybrid optoelectronic device that measures the response to optical and electrical stimulation of the cervix and returns a screening result in real time. It is a portable device, which is placed in contact with different predetermined points on the cervix. Electrical decay curves combine information from reflected light from four discrete visible and infrared wavelengths. This real-time device can be used as an adjunct to cervical cytology and colposcopy [28].

In a study by Singer et al., sensitivity for CIN1+ detection increased in comparison to cytology (67% vs. 45%), but there was loss of specificity. The sensitivities for histologically confirmed CIN2 and CIN3 lesions by TruScreen, Pap, and TruScreen and Pap combined were 70% (95% CI 67–74), 69% (CI 65–72), and 93% (CI 91–95), respectively [29].

33.2.7 Niris (Imalux Corporation, Cleveland)

The technique used is called optical coherence tomography which utilizes near-infrared light to detect small changes in refraction between intracellular structures in about 2 min. Niris visualizes tissue microstructure to a depth of 1.6 mm which is similar to the precision of histopathology and helps in determining the site of biopsy. The procedure can be learnt within a couple of hours.

There is insufficient evidence to use Niris as a colposcopic adjunct as two studies on Niris have shown increased specificity for CIN2+ disease but with a significant loss of sensitivity which is similar to visual inspection with acetic acid [30, 31].

33.3 Digital Imaging

Digital imaging colposcopy has been developed to characterize colposcopic features that predict histological grade. The specific areas can be enlarged, enhanced, or measured using image processing techniques [32]. Images can be stored and retrieved for comparison at future visits or for consultation with expert colposcopists. The main advantage of these systems allows an element of operator independence and that less experienced people can perform colposcopy. The images stored can even be sent across other experienced colposcopists, i.e., telecolposcopy.

33.4 Potential for Future Diagnostic Techniques

33.4.1 Mueller Polarimetric Colposcope (MPC)

Polarimetric imaging enables the detection and quantification of modifications of the collagen fibers in the uterine cervix due to the development of a precancerous lesion using changes in the polarity indices of light. It is a noninvasive technique in which wide-field images (up to 20 cm^2) are obtained without tissue contact and use of chemical products and low-cost white-light sources are used such as LEDs or halogen lamps [33]. In CIN, thick tissue causes scattering of light and increased absorption and hence decreases depolarization power [34]. It has only one in vivo study in normal cervix and large studies are still awaited. Ex vivo studies have shown optimized values of sensitivity and specificity of about 83% for HSIL diagnosis [35].

33.4.2 Confocal Endomicroscopy

Confocal endomicroscopy technique utilizes optical sectioning for acquiring high-resolution images with depth selectivity [36]. When images are viewed at such depth, the morphology of the tissue can be seen clearly, and dysplastic changes can also be appreciated with high sensitivity (approximately 97%). Training required for confocal endomicroscopy is greater than that required for conventional colposcopy. The specificity for predicting low-grade lesions is 80% and for CIN2/3 is 93% [37].

33.5 Portable Point of Care Colposcopes

These are simple, handheld, user-friendly portable devices that need minimal technical maintenance.

33.5.1 AV Magnivisualizer

It is a low-cost illumination and magnifying device which was indigenously developed at the Institute of Cytology and Preventive Oncology, Delhi, and launched by Indian Council of Medical Research [38]. The instrument has an inbuilt light source using halogen bulb of 100 W with interchangeable magnifying lenses (1+, 2+, 3+ diopter) (Fig. 33.1). It uses a 12 V rechargeable battery and can be used by both physicians and paramedics. Parashari et al. compared magnivisualizer with histology and concluded that the sensitivity of AV Magnivisualizer was 57.7% to detect low-grade lesions vs. 75.3% for cytology but similar for high-grade lesions. The specificity of the magnivisualizer was 94.3% vs. 99% with cytology [39]. Singh et al. compared the magnivisualizer with colposcope in 659 symptomatic women and concluded that sensitivity to detect CIN2 and higher lesions was 88.3% versus 86.7% that of colposcopy, while the specificity to detect CIN2 and higher lesions was significantly higher with the colposcope (90.4% versus 55.8%) [40]. Aggarwal et al., in their study, found higher sensitivity (95% versus 86%) and comparable specificity (78% versus 79%) of magnivisualizer versus colposcope to detect high-grade lesions [41].

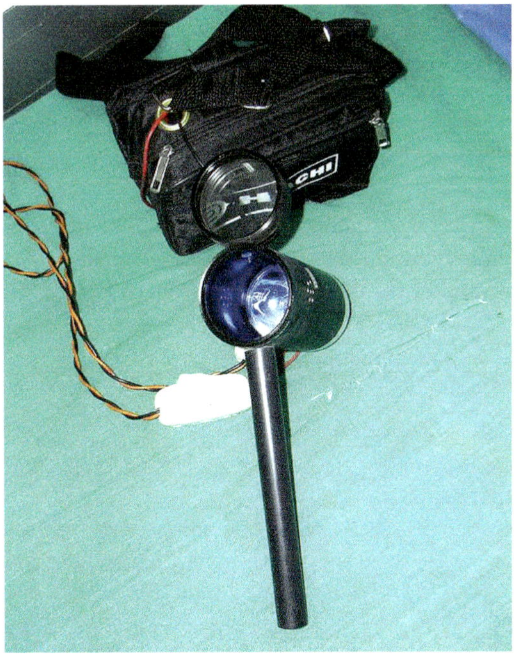

Fig. 33.1 AV Magnivisualizer

33.5.2 Gynocular

Gynocular is a pocket-size monocular colposcope, handheld, lightweight (480 gm), and measures 50 × 33 × 166 mm (Fig. 33.2a, b). The magnifications are of 5×, 8×, and 12× and focal distance of 300 mm. It uses warm white LED illumination and has a green filter. It is powered by a rechargeable lithium-ion battery and has a smartphone adapter (T2D) software for recording the results. Various studies have shown the moderate to good agreement between colposcope and Gynoculars (weighted kappa 0.65–0.998) [42, 43].

33.6 Conclusion

Traditional colposcopy has its limitations of operator dependence and inter- and intraobserver variability. To counteract these, new technologies using spectroscopy (reflectance, electrical impedance, and fluorescence), digital imaging, etc. have been introduced to improve the accuracy of traditional colposcopy. Moreover, to increase the availability of screening and diagnosis in remote areas, portable devices like Gynoculars and Magnivisualizer have been developed.

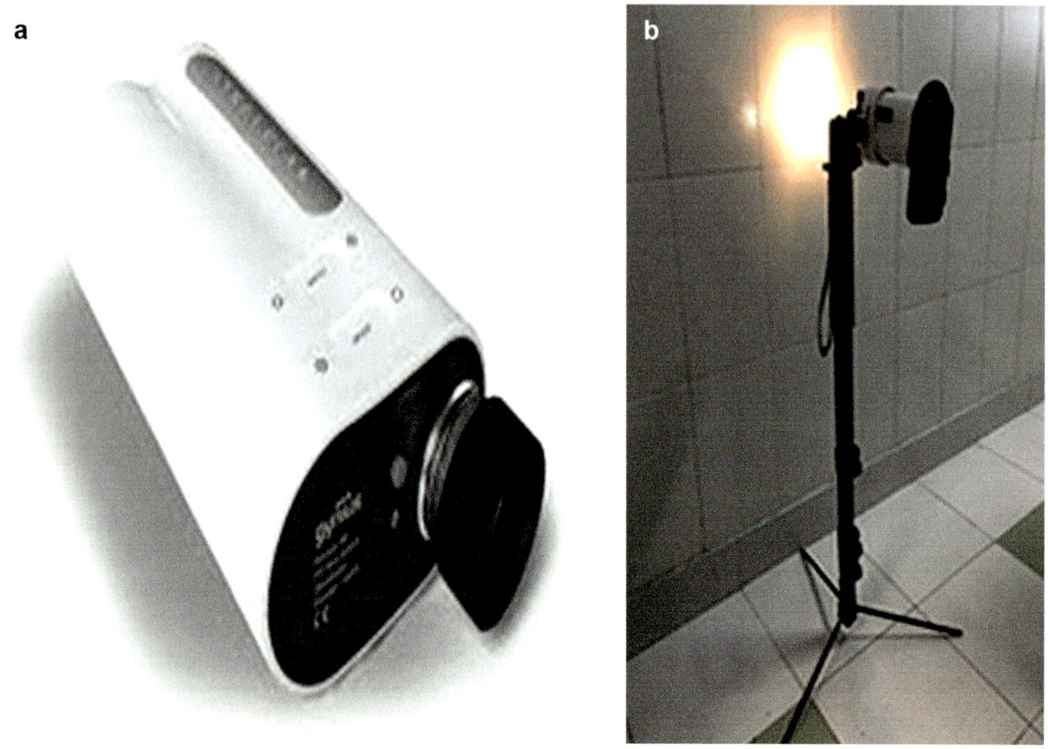

Fig. 33.2 Gynoculars. (**a**) Device. (**b**) Gynocular mounted on a tripod

Key Points

- The sensitivity and specificity of colposcopy for CIN2+ disease are 96% and 48%, respectively, and have interobserver and intraobserver variability. Hence newer devices that use advance technologies of spectroscopy, etc. are being developed to overcome these limitations.
- DySIS (DySIS Medical Ltd., Livingston) is a digital video colposcope that measures the rate, extent, and duration of acetowhitening of cervical epithelium to guide the colposcopist to the site of biopsy by using dynamic spectral imaging.
- LuViva Advanced Cervical Scan (Guided Therapeutics, Norcross) uses multimodal hyperspectroscopy (MHS) and identifies metabolic alterations in dysplastic tissue. It provides a real-time objective result obviating the need for a tissue biopsy.
- LUMA Cervical Imaging System scans tissue with a combination of fluorescence spectroscopy, white-light diffuse reflectance spectroscopy, and video imaging.
- Zedscan provides an objective assessment of the impedance profile of cervical epithelium at the point of measurement and guides the colposcopist to the site of biopsy, while TruScreen is a hybrid optoelectronic device.
- Digital imaging colposcopy has been developed to characterize colposcopic features that predict histological grade. The specific areas can be enlarged, enhanced, or measured using image processing techniques.
- Simple, handheld, user-friendly portable devices like Gynoculars and AV Magnivisualizer have been developed as an alternative to colposcopes that need minimal technical maintenance.

References

1. Nazeer S, Shafi MI. Objective perspective in colposcopy. Best Pract Res Clin Obstet Gynaecol. 2011;25(5):631–40.
2. Mitchell MF, Schottenfeld D, Tortolero-Luna G, et al. Colposcopy for the diagnosis of squamous intraepithelial lesions: a meta-analysis. Obstet Gynecol. 1998;91:626–31.

3. Hopman EH, Voorhorst FJ, Kenemans P, et al. Observer agreement on interpreting colposcopic images of CIN. Gynecol Oncol. 1995;58:206–9.
4. ALTS group. Results of a randomized trial on the management of cytology interpretations of atypical squamous cells of undetermined significance. Am J Obstet Gynecol. 2003;188:1383–92.
5. Underwood M, et al. Accuracy of colposcopy-directed punch biopsies: a systematic review and meta-analysis. BJOG. 2012;119:1293–301.
6. Balas C. A novel optical imaging method for the early detection, quantitative grading, and mapping of cancerous and precancerous lesions of cervix. IEEE Trans Biomed Eng. 2001;548:96–104.
7. Balas C, Papoutsogglou G, Potirakis A. In vivo molecular imaging of cervical neoplasia using acetic acid as biomarker. IEEE J Sel Top Quantum Electron. 2008;14:29–42.
8. Louwers JA, Zaal A, Kocken M, et al. Women's preferences of dynamic spectral imaging colposcopy. Gynecol Obstet Invest. 2015;79:239–43.
9. Soutter WP, Diakomanolis E, Lyons D, et al. Dynamic spectral imaging: improving colposcopy. Clin Cancer Res. 2009;15:1814–20.
10. Louwers JA, Zaal A, Kochen M, et al. Dynamic spectral imaging colposcopy: higher sensitivity for detection of premalignant cervical lesions. BJOG. 2011;118:309–18.
11. Roensbo MT. Can dynamic spectral imaging system colposcopy replace conventional colposcopy in the detection of high-grade cervical lesions? Acta Obstet Gynecol Scand. 2015;94(7):781–5.
12. Coronado PJ, Fasero M. Correlating the accuracy of colposcopy with practitioner experience when diagnosing cervical pathology using the dynamic spectral imaging system. Gynecol Obstet Invest. 2014;78(4):224–9.
13. Zaal A, Louwers J, Berkhof J, et al. Agreement between colposcopic impression and histological diagnosis among human papillomavirus type 16-positive women: a clinical trial using dynamic spectral imaging colposcopy. BJOG. 2012;119:537–44.
14. Wade R, Spackman E, Corbett M, Walker S, Light K, Naik R, et al. Adjunctive colposcopy technologies for examination of the uterine cervix--DySIS, LuViva Advanced Cervical Scan and Niris Imaging System: a systematic review and economic evaluation. Health Technol Assess. 2013;17(8):1–240, v–vi.
15. Leeson S. Advances in colposcopy: new technologies to challenge current practice. Eur J Obstet Gynecol Reprod Biol. 2014;182:140–5.
16. Ferris DG, Lawhead RA, Dickman ED, et al. Multimodal hyperspectral imaging for the noninvasive diagnosis of cervical neoplasia. J Low Genit Tract Dis. 2001;5:65–72.
17. DeSantis T, Chakhtoura N, Twiggs L, et al. Spectroscopic imaging as a triage test for cervical disease: a prospective multicenter clinical trial. J Low Genit Tract Dis. 2007;11:18–24.
18. Twiggs LB, Chakhtoura NA, Ferris DG, et al. Multimodal hyperspectroscopy as a triage test for cervical neoplasia: pivotal clinical trial results. Gynecol Oncol. 2013;130:147–51.
19. Flowers LC, Ault KA, Twiggs LB, et al. Preliminary assessment of cervical spectroscopy for primary screening of moderate and high grade cervical Dysplasia. In: ASCCP conference; 2012. Available at: http://www.guidedinc.com/Pub%20data/ASCCP%20 2012%20Poster.pdf. Accessed 03 Feb 2018.
20. Tan JH, Wrede CD. New technologies and advances in colposcopic assessment. Best Pract Res Clin Obstet Gynaecol. 2011;25(5):667–77.
21. Imaging system helps detect precancerous cervical abnormalities. FDA Consum. 2006;40:4.
22. Alvarez RD, Wright TC. Effective cervical neoplasia detection with a novel optical detection system: a randomized trial. Gynecol Oncol. 2007;104:281–9.
23. Georgakoudi I, Sheets EE, Muller MG, et al. Trimodal spectroscopy for the detection and characterization of cervical precancers in vivo. Am J Obstet Gynecol. 2002;186:374–82.
24. Tidy JA, Brown BH, Healey TJ, et al. Accuracy of detection of high-grade cervical intraepithelial neoplasia using electrical impedance spectroscopy with colposcopy. BJOG. 2013;120:400–9.
25. Abdul S, Brown BH, Milnes P, Tidy JA. The use of electrical impedance spectroscopy in the detection of cervical intraepithelial neoplasia. Int J Gynecol Cancer. 2006;16(5):1823–32.
26. Balasubramani L, Brown BH, Healey J, et al. The detection of cervical intraepithelial neoplasia by electrical impedance spectroscopy: the effects of acetic acid and tissue homogeneity. Gynecol Oncol. 2009;115(2):267–71.
27. Brown BH, Milnes P, Abdul S, Tidy JA. Detection of cervical intraepithelial neoplasia using impedance spectroscopy: a prospective study. BJOG. 2005;112(6):802–6.
28. Barrow AJ. Wu SM. Impedance measurements for cervical cancer diagnosis. Gynecol Oncol. 2007;107(Suppl. 1):S40–3.
29. Singer A, Coppleson M, Canfell K, et al. A real time optoelectronic device as an adjunct to the Pap smear for cervical screening: a multicentre evaluation. Int J Gynecol Cancer. 2003;13:804–11.
30. Escobar PF, Rojas-Espaillat L, Tisci S, et al. Optical coherence tomography as a diagnostic aid to visual inspection and colposcopy for preinvasive and invasive cancer of the uterine cervix. Int J Gynecol Cancer. 2006;16:1815–22.
31. Liu Z, Belinson SE, Li J, et al. Diagnostic efficacy of real-time optical coherence tomography in the management of preinvasive and invasive neoplasia of the uterine cervix. Int J Gynecol Cancer. 2010;20:283–7.
32. Park SY, Follen M, Milbourne A, et al. Automated image analysis of digital colposcopy for the detection of cervical neoplasia. J Biomed Opt. 2008;13:014029.
33. Vizet J, Rehbinder J, Deby S, Roussel S, Nazac A, Soufan R, et al. In vivo imaging of uterine cervix

with a Mueller polarimetric colposcope. Sci Rep. 2017;7(1):2471.
34. Novikova T, Pierangelo A, Manhas S, Benali A, Validire P, Gayet B, et al. The origins of polarimetric image contrast between healthy and cancerous human colon tissue. Appl Phys Lett. 2013;102:241103.
35. Rehbinder J, Haddad H, Deby S, Teig B, Nazac A, Novikova T, et al. Ex vivo Mueller polarimetric imaging of the uterine cervix: a first statistical evaluation. J Biomed Opt. 2016;21(7):71113.
36. Inoue H, Kudo S, Shiokawa A. Technology insight: laser scanning confocal microscopy and endocytoscopy for cellular observation of the gastrointestinal tract. Nat Clin Pract Gastroenterol Hepatol. 2005;2:31–6.
37. Tan J, Quinn MA, Pyman JM. Detection of cervical intraepithelial neoplasia in vivo using confocal endomicroscopy. BJOG. 2009;116:1663–70.
38. Parashari A, Singh V, Sehgal A, Mehrotra R. BMJ Innov. 2015;1:99–102.
39. Parashari A, Singh V, Sehgal A, et al. Low-cost technology for screening uterine cervical cancer. Bull World Health Organ. 2000;78:964–7.
40. Singh V, Parashari A, Gupta S, et al. Performance of a low cost magnifying device, Magnivisualizer, versus colposcope for detection of pre-cancer and cancerous lesions of uterine cervix. J Gynecol Oncol. 2014;25:282–6.
41. Aggarwal P, Batra S, Gandhi G, et al. Can visual inspection with acetic acid under magnification substitute colposcopy in detecting cervical intraepithelial neoplasia in low-resource settings? Arch Gynecol Obstet. 2011;284:397–403.
42. Nessa A, Roy JS, Chowdhury MA, Khanam Q, Afroz R, Wistrand C, et al. Evaluation of the accuracy in detecting cervical lesions by nurses versus doctors using a stationary colposcope and Gynocular in a low-resource setting. BMJ Open. 2014;4(11):e005313.
43. Nessa A, Wistrand C, Begum SA, Thuresson M, Shemer I, Thorsell M, Shemer EA. Evaluation of stationary colposcope and the Gynocular, by the swede score systematic colposcopic system in VIA positive women: a crossover randomized trial. Int J Gynecol Cancer. 2014;24(2):339–45.

Update on HPV Vaccination

34

Anshul Grover

34.1 Introduction

Human papillomavirus is a sexually transmitted virus responsible for cancer of the cervix, vagina, vulva, anus, penis, oral cavity, and oropharynx. It also is the causative agent for anogenital warts [1]. There are about 40 different serotypes of HPV, which are further divided into high-risk and low-risk types. The high-risk HPV serotypes include 16, 18, 31, 33, 45, 52, and 58. HPV types 16 and 18 are responsible for 70% of all cervical cancer, 90% of anal cancer, 40% of vaginal and vulvar cancers, 50% of penile cancer, and 35% of oropharyngeal cancers [2]. Ninety percent of anogenital warts are caused by low-risk HPV serotypes 6 and 11 [1].

Vaccines against HPV were developed with the aim to reduce the burden of HPV-related diseases and to provide protection from cervical cancer. The vaccine development was initiated in parallel, by researchers at Georgetown University Medical Center and the University of Rochester in the United States, the University of Queensland in Australia, and the US National Cancer Institute. Since its advent and FDA approval in 2006 [3, 4], the HPV vaccine has emerged as a game changer in the prevention of cervical cancer. As of the year 2017, it has been approved for use in the routine immunization program for girls in 71 countries [5].

34.2 Human Papillomavirus Vaccine

The HPV vaccines are composed of hollow virus-like particles commonly referred to as virus-like particles (VLP). These are recombinant HPV coat proteins known to generate a virus-neutralizing antibody response that is claimed to prevent initial infection with HPV types. The HPV virus is a double-stranded DNA virus, which has an outer shell made up of 72 capsomeres; these capsomeres are made up of L1 and L2 protein molecules which provide it the capability to affect the skin and the mucous membranes. The vaccines are developed using recombinant DNA technology to produce L1 major capsid protein of HPV in yeast *Saccharomyces cerevisiae*. These empty shells lack the genetic material essential for expression of the virus in the cells. The vaccine uses these VLPs as antigens to produce a strong antigenic response [5].

The two vaccines available before 2014 were the bivalent and quadrivalent HPV vaccine. The bivalent vaccine is made up of a combination of L1 proteins of HPV serotypes 16 and 18 with ASO4 as adjunct. It has shown to have an effi-

A. Grover (✉)
Specialist, Department of Obstetrics and Gynaecology, Babu Jagjivan Ram Memorial Hospital, New Delhi, India

S. Mehta, A. Singla (eds.), *Preventive Oncology for the Gynecologist*,
https://doi.org/10.1007/978-981-13-3438-2_34

cacy of 90% in HPV type 16- and 18-related CIN 2/3 and AIS at 15-month follow-up in various clinical trials [6]. Whereas the quadrivalent vaccine is a combination of L1 proteins of HPV serotypes 6, 11, 16, and 18 with an aluminum-containing adjunct. Clinical trials have reported a 100% efficacy at a median follow-up at 1.9 years against HPV serotype 16- and 18-related CIN 2/3 and AIS. It also provides protection against genital warts associated with HPV serotypes 6 and 11 [7]. Since its approval by the FDA, reports published as early as 3 years of its use have shown a beneficial effect in reducing the incidence of anogenital warts and the prevalence of the vaccine HPV types in high-grade lesions [8–11].

34.3 Nonavalent Vaccine (9-Valent Vaccine)

Studies on invasive cervical cancer conducted all over the world have reported that the HPV types responsible for it other than the 16 and 18 serotypes are HPV types 31/33/45/52/58. These high-risk HPV types are responsible for 90% of invasive cervical cancer and intermediate precursor lesions of cervical cancer classified as CIN 2 and AIS. Persistent infection with these serotypes is responsible for the maximum risk of developing CIN 3 or cervical cancer. After the success of the quadrivalent vaccine, the next task was to prevent the development of cervical cancer by the next common oncogenic HPV serotypes—HPV 31/33/45/52/58 [12–14]. On December 10, 2014, the FDA licensed the 9-valent vaccine for use in girls 9–26 years and boys aged 9–15 years. The second generation of vaccine is also prepared from purified L1 structural proteins that self-assemble to form HPV type-specific empty shells or virus-like particles.

In the phase III trial of the vaccine, it was inferred that the efficacy of the vaccine was 96%. The trial also commented on non-inferiority of the quadrivalent vaccine against HPV serotype 6/11/16/18 [15]. The French EDiTH studies showed that the nonavalent vaccine provides an additional benefit of preventing 33% of CIN 2/3, invasive cervical cancer by 15%, LSIL by 12%, and anal cancer by 10% [16–19]. There was no additional benefit in the prevention of genital warts and oropharyngeal cancer. The limited benefit to oropharyngeal cancer and genital warts is explained by the fact that these are exclusively associated with HPV types which are also targeted by bivalent and quadrivalent vaccine. The study conducted by Riethmuller et al. published in 2015 suggested that development of nonavalent vaccine could target 77% and up to 90% of all CIN 2/3 cases. This would directly reduce the cost related to management of these lesions and reduce the number of conization procedures [20]. An international manufacturer funded clinical trial of >14,000 women aged 16–26 years who received three doses of 9-valent vaccine and were followed up for 6 years. This trial inferred that the incidence of cervical, vulval, and vaginal disease associated with additional HPV types was reduced by 97% in those who received this vaccine. There was also decline in the number of cervical biopsies performed in this subgroup of women [21].

The Advisory Committee on Immunization Practices recommends similar dosing schedules for nonavalent vaccine as is for the quadrivalent vaccine. In individuals already vaccinated with either bivalent or quadrivalent vaccines, revaccination with nonavalent vaccine is not recommended.

34.4 Rationale for Vaccination

34.4.1 Rationale for Female Vaccination

Female vaccination against HPV has shown to have a direct benefit in protecting against cancers and anogenital warts. As previously discussed HPV types 16 and 18 are responsible for 70% of all cervical cancer, 90% of anal cancer, 40% of vaginal and vulvar cancers, and 35% of oropharyngeal cancers [2]. HPVs 31/33/45/52/58 are responsible for another 20% of cervical cancer.

Ninety percent of anogenital warts are caused by low-risk HPV serotypes 6 and 11 [1]. The National Health and Nutrition Examination Survey compared HPV prevalence data from prevaccine years (2003–2006) to post initiation of vaccine (2007–2010). Even though the three-dose vaccine coverage was only 32% among 13–17 years' young females in 2010, a 56% decline in the vaccine type prevalence was noted. The decline in the vaccine type HPV was more than expected probably due to herd immunity [22]. In Australia, there was a dramatic decline in the prevalence of genital warts in young females after the three-dose HPV vaccination program was introduced. This decline was also observed in males due to generation of herd immunity [10, 23]. The preventive effect of HPV vaccination is best evaluated for cervical cancer which is one of the most common cancers in females. A 97% reduction in cervical, vulvar, and vaginal cancers has been reported with the newly introduced 9-valent HPV vaccination. It has been proven through research that vaccinating preadolescent girls in comparison to boys is more cost-effective in reducing the burden of cervical cancer. Taking into consideration the disease burden of cervical cancer and the cost-effectiveness of the vaccine, WHO recommends that the HPV vaccination for preadolescent girls may be introduced in the National Immunization Program of all countries worldwide [24]. More than 71 countries have already approved HPV vaccine for preadolescent girls in their National Immunization Program by 2017 [5]. Global Alliance for Vaccine and Immunization (GAVI) is offering financial assistance to countries who have not begun HPV vaccination on a national level [25].

34.4.2 Rationale for Male Vaccination

Persistent HPV infection in males is responsible for 90% of anal cancers, 50% of penile, and 35% of oropharyngeal cancers by serotypes 16 and 18. Low-risk HPV types 6 and 11 are responsible for 90% of anogenital warts. Vaccination in males provides direct benefit of protection against all the above. The incidence of HPV-related cancers in males is less than the incidence of cervical cancer in females due to which the HPV vaccination for males has not been included in any vaccination program worldwide [26, 27]. At present Australia is the only country with a vaccination program for adolescent boys [24].

A Dutch study conducted by Bogaards et al. [28] demonstrated that an uptake of 60% vaccination in females would result in protection by one third of HPV vaccine-preventable cancers in men. If the vaccine uptake increases to 90% in females, this would translate into 66% reduction in HPV-related cancers in men barring anal cancer, which shows a decline only by 32%. This disproportionate decline in anal cancer rates is due to the fact that herd immunity generated by female vaccination brings about a reduction in mainly penile and oropharyngeal cancers. The burden of anal cancer is high in men having sex with men (MSM) who do not benefit with female vaccination. UK Joint Commission on Vaccination and Immunization (JCVI) has recommended a targeted vaccination in MSM in the age group of 16–40 years through genitourinary clinics and HIV clinics [29]. This targeted vaccination may have fallacies as demonstrated by a study conducted by Zou et al. [30]. The study suggested that most MSM will have multiple sexual partners and may have acquired HPV infection before they visit the health clinic. Also, many MSM who are bisexual or gay may not visit such clinics or disclose their sexual behavior, so as to be offered vaccination. Therefore, even if high herd protection is attained with greater vaccine coverage of females, men will remain at risk when they move out of the herd. Associations with unvaccinated females from other countries or other men make them susceptible.

Therefore, a universal HPV vaccination for both boys and girls should be recommended for reducing the burden of HPV preventable cancers and to provide protection to heterosexual men who move outside the herd, MSM and unvaccinated women. The cost versus benefit of a male HPV vaccination program is still under debate, and therefore not universally advocated at present.

34.5 Changes in HPV Vaccine Schedule: CDC Recommendations

CDC has updated its recommendations for HPV vaccination schedule in October 2016 in consultation with the Advisory committee on Immunization Practices (ACIP) [31, 32].

34.5.1 Recommended Age Group

HPV vaccine is recommended for routine vaccination at the age 11 or 12 years. It can be given starting at 9 years of age.

- ACIP also recommends vaccination for females aged 13 through 26 years and males 13 through 21 years not adequately vaccinated previously.
- Vaccination is also recommended through age 26 years for gay, bisexual, and other men who have sex with men, transgender people, and immunocompromised persons (including those with HIV infection) not adequately vaccinated previously.

The above recommendations are also supported by the American Academy of Physicians, American Academy of Family Physicians, American College of Obstetrics and Gynecology, American Cancer Society, and International Papillomavirus Society. WHO recommendations for HPV vaccination for resource-limited countries are to vaccinate females 9–14 years old. Older females may be vaccinated if found to be affordable and cost-effective by that country.

The above age recommendations are aimed to reach out to the adolescents prior to their sexual debut. Clinical trials for vaccine efficacy suggest that none of the available HPV vaccine can treat or clear already existing virus. The HPV vaccine can be administered without any special evaluation. HPV DNA testing or pregnancy testing is not recommended prior to vaccination. There is no recommendation for measurement of postvaccination antibody titers for assessment of immunity by ACIP.

34.5.2 Dosing Schedule

Two doses of HPV are recommended for most persons, starting the vaccination before the age of 15:

- The ideal interval between the two doses is 6–12 months.
- In situations where the adolescent receives the second dose <5 months apart, a third dose is recommended.
- There is no recommendation for any maximum interval between two doses. It is recommended that the interval should not exceed 12–15 months so as to complete the schedule as soon as possible before the female becomes sexually active.
- The need for a booster dose is not yet established.

Three-dose schedule is recommended for:

- Adolescents, young adults who begin the dosing schedule after the age of 15 and before the age of 26 years.
- All immunocompromised persons including persons with HIV infection, aged 9–26 years.

The dose schedule for three doses is 0, 1–2, and 6 months.

In case of missed doses, the ACIP recommends that the vaccination schedule can be resumed without restarting the series, even if interrupted for any length of time.

34.6 Rationale for Two-Dose Regimen

It was observed by the Centers for Disease Control and Prevention in the United States in 2012 that only 53.8% of girls aged 13–17 years had initiated HPV vaccine and that only 33.4% of them had received all three doses [33]. The three-dose regimen was found to be expensive and difficult to complete. The Costa Rica trial and PATRICIA trial showed that the vaccine efficacy against HPV 16/18 infections 4 years after vaccination among women was the same whether they received one dose, two doses, or three doses. The high efficacy of the vaccine against HPV 16/18 was replicated in a cohort of women who had never been previously infected with the HPV 16/18 strains. This suggests that the two-dose benefit of vaccine was relevant in girls who received the vaccine in the preferred age that is 11–12 years (before sexual debut) [34]. The advantage of the two-dose schedule is retained only if the doses are given at least 6-month intervals. Comparison of the two dosage schedules in two separate RCTs suggested that a 6-month interval between the doses resulted in superior GMC (geometric mean concentration) when compared to a 2-month interval in all age groups [35]. Safaeian et al. in their study inferred that the titers after one dose were lower than that after two doses. It was also inferred that one dose or two doses of vaccine separated by a short interval (1–2 months) may not produce adequate cross protection [36]. Kreimer et al. in his study concluded that there is evidence to suggest that HPV vaccination program using two-dose regimen instead of the recommended three-dose schedule could vaccinate 50% more women and could reduce the incidence of cervical cancer significantly using the same number of doses, thus making it more cost-effective [37].

34.6.1 Special Populations

- Pregnant women: Not recommended during pregnancy due to limited data available regarding its safety profile. Women should delay the initiation of vaccine schedule if they are aware of their pregnant status. If women are found to be pregnant during the vaccination schedule, further doses may be deferred until delivery. As the vaccine has not been associated with any harmful effects on the fetus till now, therefore no intervention is required. Pregnancy testing prior to vaccination is not recommended.
- Lactating women: Can be given vaccination as per schedule as the vaccine is not known to affect the safety of breastfeeding.
- Pre-existing HPV-associated disease: Vaccination is recommended in the prescribed age group even in the presence of prior HPV infection such as genital warts and abnormal cervical, vulvar, vaginal, or anal cytology. They have to be told that this vaccine will not treat the already existing infection but will provide protection from other HPV types [31, 32].
- Immunocompromised individuals: A vaccination schedule of three dose regimen is recommmended for individuals in the age group 9–26 years with B-lymphocyte antibody deficiency, complete or partial T-lymphocyte defects, HIV infection, malignant neoplasm, autoimmune disease, who are transplant recipients, and on immunosuppressive therapy [38].

34.7 Contraindications

An allergic reaction to the vaccine or its component is a contraindication to administration of the vaccine. In the presence of any acute severe or moderately severe illness, vaccination may be deferred till the illness is recovered from, but may be given in any minor illness like diarrhea or upper respiratory tract infection without fever. Latex allergy is a contraindication to bivalent vaccine as its prefilled syringe may contain a tip cap made of natural rubber latex. Allergy to yeast will deter the use of quadrivalent and 9-valent vaccine which are produced in *Saccharomyces cerevisiae*.

34.8 Vaccine Safety Profile

As per the report of GACVS meeting in June, 2017, HPV vaccines are considered extremely safe. The risk of anaphylaxis was found to be 1.7 per million doses. Local reactions such as injection site pain, redness, or swelling were reported by 20–90% recipients. Syncopal attack, which may be experienced during any medical procedure, is a stress-related reaction that might be experienced by some. Therefore, it is recommended that the adolescents are seated or in lying position for 15 min after the vaccination to avoid injuries due to fall [39].

34.9 Efficacy

All these three vaccines are prophylactic and not therapeutic. They do not provide protection against vaccine HPV types to which the subject has acquired infection prior to vaccination. This forms the basis of administering the vaccine to girls below the age of 15 years, that is prior to initiation of sexual activity. The antibody response rises with every dose and then plateaus by 24 months. At 36 months the vaccine-generated antibody response is higher than the response generated by natural infection. Various studies demonstrated that the highest immune response of the vaccine was seen in girls of the age group of 9–15 years with three dose schedules [5]. Both the bivalent and quadrivalent vaccines had consistent high antibody titer for at least 8 years with 100% seropositivity [40].

The vaccines do not protect against all HPV types; hence they will not prevent all cases of cervical cancer. Approximately 30% of cervical cancers will not be prevented by vaccination, and so screening for cervical cancer should continue as per guidelines even in vaccinated women.

34.10 Choice of Vaccine

Nine-valent vaccine ideally should be preferred for females as it provides a wider HPV coverage as compared to quadrivalent or bivalent vaccine in protection against cervical cancer. Availability and cost are the two important factors due to which its use is limited. In the United States, since 2017, only 9-valent vaccine is available. As recommended the same vaccine once started should be used to complete the schedule. But in the event that the initial formulation used is unavailable or not known, the schedule may be completed using 9-valent vaccine.

In males, further research is required to conclude if there is any additional benefit of 9-valent vaccine over the quadrivalent vaccine to prevent male cancers. The possible benefit may be to reduce the risk of cervical cancer in females by generating herd immunity.

34.11 Therapeutic Vaccines

All the available vaccines at present are preventive in nature. A humoral immune response is generated by antibody production against the capsid protein of the virus. This response is ineffective in treating an already established HPV infection. There is an ongoing research to develop vaccines which will generate an immune response in an already established HPV infection and HPV-induced cancers. These vaccines are being developed to target HPV oncogenes E6 and E7, which are essential for expression of virus-infected cells.

34.11.1 MEL-1

This vaccine is also known as MVA −2. It is a recombinant vaccinia virus Ankara (MVA) containing bovine papillomavirus E2 protein. It has shown to stop human tumor growth in mice and tumor regression in rabbits. It contains an immunogenetic peptide pool containing epitopes which act against all the high-risk HPV strains and 14 conserved immunogenic peptide fragments from E1, E2, E6, and E7 proteins of 16 high-risk HPV types. These proteins generate a CD8+ response. Phase I and phase II trials in patients of CIN 2/3 have shown a positive reduction in eliminating the virus. This vaccine at present is undergoing phase III clinical trial [41].

34.11.2 VGX-3100

This is a therapeutic DNA vaccine being manufactured by Inovio Pharmaceuticals. It is a genetically engineered vaccine which consists of two DNA plasmids pGX 3001 and pGx 3002 which target HPV-16 and HPV-18 E6 and E7 oncoproteins responsible for CIN 2/3. The vaccine generates a specific CD8 T-cell to act on virus-infected premalignant and malignant cells. The vaccine has shown to have clinical efficacy comparable to surgical excision but devoid of side effects in the trials conducted till now. It has entered the phase III clinical trial called REVEAL-1 for treatment of HPV-associated high-grade squamous intraepithelial lesions [42].

34.12 Conclusion

A new 9-valent vaccine has been FDA approved to the already existing two prophylactic vaccines. There have been changes in the vaccination dosage schedule with two doses being recommended now instead of the earlier three doses. This recommendation is based on many RCTs which have shown that two-dosage schedule could vaccinate 50% more women and could reduce the incidence of cervical cancer significantly using the same number of doses. Therapeutic HPV vaccines are the latest addition to the fight against HPV infection and are currently undergoing phase III trials.

Key Points

- FDA licensed the 9-valent vaccine for use in girls 9–26 years and boys aged 9–15 years in 2014. It protects against HPV 31/33/45/52/58 in addition to HPV 6/11/16/18.
- Two doses of HPV are recommended for most girls, starting the vaccination before the age of 15, and the ideal interval between the two doses is 6–12 months.
- 9-valent vaccine ideally should be preferred for females as it provides a wider HPV coverage as compared to quadrivalent or bivalent vaccine in protection against cervical cancer.
- Screening should continue as per recommendations after immunization.
- Therapeutic vaccines MEL 1 and VGX-3100 are the newer developments currently undergoing phase III trials.

References

1. National Advisory Committee on Immunization. Update on human papillomavirus (HPV) vaccines. An advisory committee statement. Commun Dis Rep. 2012;38:1–62.
2. Muñoz N, Bosch FX, Castellsagué X, Díaz M, de Sanjose S, Hammouda D, et al. Against which human papillomavirus type shall we vaccinate and screen? The international perspective. Int J Cancer. 2004;111(2):278–85.
3. World Health Organization. Human papillomavirus vaccines. WHO position paper, May 2017 [PDF]. Wkl Epidemiol Rec 19. 12 May 2017;92:241–68.
4. World Health Organization. The immunological basis for immunization series. Module 19: human papillomavirus infection [PDF]. May 2011.
5. Kaarthigeyan K. Cervical cancer in India and HPV vaccination. Indian J Med Paediatr Oncol. 2012;33(1):7–12.
6. Harper DM, Franco EL, Wheeler C, Ferris DG, Jenkins D, Schuind A, et al. Efficacy of a bivalent L1 virus-like particle vaccine in prevention of infection with human papillomavirus types 16 and 18 in young women: a randomised controlled trial. Lancet. 2004;364:1757–65.
7. Villa LL, Costa RL, Petta CA, Andrade RP, Paavonen J, Iversen OE, et al. High sustained efficacy of a prophylactic quadrivalent human papillomavirus types 6/11/16/18 L1 virus-like particle vaccine through 5 years follow up. Br J Cancer. 2006;95:1459–66.
8. Baldur-Felskov B, Dehlendorff C, Munk C, Kjaer SK. Early impact of human papillomavirus vaccination on cervical neoplasia—nationwide follow-up of young Danish women. J Natl Cancer Inst. 2014;106(3):djt460.
9. Giuliano AR, Palefsky JM, Goldstone S, Moreira ED Jr, Penny ME, Aranda C, et al. Efficacy of quadrivalent HPV vaccine against HPV infections and disease in males. N Engl J Med. 2011;364(5):401–11.
10. Read TR, Hocking JS, Chen MY, Donovan B, Bradshaw CS, Fairley CK. The near disappearance of genital warts in young women 4 years after commencing a national human papillomavirus (HPV) vaccination programme. Sex Transm Infect. 2011;87(7):544–7.
11. Crowe E, Pandeya N, Brotherton JM, Dobson AJ, Kisely S, Lambert SB, et al. Effectiveness of quadrivalent human papillomavirus vaccine for the prevention of cervical abnormalities: case-control study nested within a population based screening programme in Australia. BMJ. 2014;348:g1458.
12. de Sanjose S, Quint WG, Alemany L, Geraets DT, Klaustermeier JE, Lloveras B, et al. Human papillomavirus genotype attribution in invasive cervical cancer: a retrospective cross-sectional worldwide study. Lancet Oncol. 2010;11:1048–56.
13. Joura EA, Ault KA, Bosch FX, Brown D, Cuzick J, Ferris D, et al. Attribution of 12 high-risk human papillomavirus genotypes to infection and cervical disease. Cancer Epidemiol Biomark Prev. 2014;23:1997–2008.
14. Tjalma WA, Fiander A, Reich O, Powell N, Nowakowski AM, Kirschner B, et al. Differences in human papillomavirus type distribution in high-grade cervical intraepithelial neoplasia and invasive cervical cancer in Europe. Int J Cancer. 2013;132:854–67.

15. Joura EA, Giuliano AR, Iversen OE, Bouchard C, Mao C, Mehlsen J, et al. A 9-valent HPV vaccine against infection and intraepithelial neoplasms in women. N Engl J Med. 2015;372:711–23.
16. Pretet JL, Jacquard AC, Carcopino X, Charlot JF, Bouhour D, Kantelip B, et al. Human papilloma virus (HPV) genotype distribution in invasive cervical cancers in France: EDITH study. Int J Cancer. 2008;122(2):428–32.
17. Pretet JL, Jacquard AC, Carcopino X, Monnier-Benoit S, Averous G, Soubeyrand B, et al. Human papilloma virus (HPV) genotype distribution in high grade lesions in France: EDITH study. Int J Cancer. 2008;122(2):424–7.
18. Abramowitz L, Jacquard AC, Jaroud F, Haesebaert J, Siproudhis L, Pradat P, et al. Human papillomavirus distribution in anal cancer in France: the EDITH V study. Int J Cancer. 2011;129(2):433–9.
19. St Guily JL, Jacquard AC, Prétet JL, Haesebaert J, Beby-Defaux A, Clavel C, et al. Human papillomavirus genotype distribution in oropharynx and oral cavity cancer in France – the EDITH study. J Clin Virol. 2011;51(2):100–4.
20. Riethmuller D, Jacquard AC, St L, Gully J, Aubin F. Potential impact of a nonavalent HPV vaccine on the occurrence of HPV-related diseases in France. BMC Public Health. 2015;15:453.
21. Huh WK, Joura EA, Giuliano AR, Iversen OE, de Andrade RP, Ault KA, et al. Final efficacy, immunogenicity, and safety analysis of a nine valent vaccine in women aged 16-26 years: a randomized, double blind trial. Lancet. 2017;390(10108):2143–59.
22. Markowitz LE, Hariri S, Lin C. Reduction in human papillomavirus (HPV) prevalence among young women following HPV vaccine introduction in United States, National Health and Nutrition Examination Survey, 2003-2010. J Infect Dis. 2013;208(3):385–93.
23. Tabrizi SN, Brotherton JM, Kaldor JM, Skinner SR, Cummins E, Liu B, et al. Fall in human papillomavirus prevalence following national vaccination program. J Infect Dis. 2012;206:1645–51.
24. World Health Organization. Comprehensive cervical cancer prevention and control: a healthier future for girls and women. Geneva: World Health Organization; 2013.
25. Global immunization data: WHO 2015. Available from: https://www.who.int/immunization/monitoring_surveillance/en/. Accessed 15 Nov 2015.
26. Kim JJ, Goldie SJ. Health and economic implications of HPV vaccination of men who have sex with men in the USA: a cost-effectiveness modelling analysis. Lancet Infect Dis. 2010;10:845.
27. Chesson HW, Ekwueme DU, Saraiya M, Dunne EF, Markowitz LE. The cost-effectiveness of male HPV vaccination in the United States. Vaccine. 2011;29:8443.
28. Bogaards JA, Wallinga J, Brakenhoff RH, et al. Direct benefit of vaccinating boys along with girls against oncogenic human papillomavirus: Bayesian evidence synthesis. BMJ. 2015;350:h2016.
29. Department of Health and Public Health England. JVCI interim position statement on HPV vaccination of men who had sex with men. 2014. Available from: https://www.gov.uk/government/uploads/system/uploads/attachment-data/fil.
30. Zou H, Tabrizi SN, Grulich AE, Garland SM, Hocking JS, Bradshaw CS, et al. Early acquisition of anogenital human papillomavirus among teenage men who have sex with men. J Infect Dis. 2014;209:642–51.
31. Kim DK, Riley LE, Harriman KH, Hunter P, Bridges CB, Advisory Committee on Immunization Practices. Recommended immunization schedule for adults aged 19 years or older, United States, 2017. Ann Intern Med. 2017;166:209.
32. Markowitz LE, Dunne EF, Saraiya M, Chesson HW, Curtis CR, Gee J, et al. Human papillomavirus vaccination: recommendations of the advisory committee on immunization practices (ACIP). MMWR Recomm Rep. 2014;63:1.
33. Printz C. One HPV vaccine dose may prevent cervical cancer. Cancer. 2014;120:772–3.
34. Kreimer AR, Struyf F, Del Rosario-Raymundo MR, Hildesheim A, Skinner SR, Wacholder S, et al. Efficacy of fewer than three doses of an HPV-16/18 ASO4-adjuncted vaccine: combined analysis of data from the Costa Rica vaccine and PATRICIA trials. Lancet Oncol. 2015;16:775–86.
35. Romanowski B, Schwarz TF, Ferguson LM, Peters K, Dionne M, Schulze K, et al. Immunogenicity and safety of the HPV-16/18 ASO4-adjuvanted vaccine administered as 2 dose schedule compared to the licensed 3 dose schedule: results from a randomised study. Hum Vaccin. 2011;7:1374–86.
36. Safaeian M, Porras C, Pan Y, Kreimer A, Schiller JT, Gonzalez P, et al. Durable antibody responses following one dose of the bivalent human papillomavirus L1 virus like particle vaccine in the Costa Rica Vaccine Trial. Cancer Prev Res (Phila). 2013;6:1242–50.
37. Kreimer AR, Rodriguez AC, Hildesheim A, Herrero R, Porras C, Schiffman M, et al. Proof-of-principal evaluation of efficacy of fewer than three doses of a bivalent HPV 16/18 vaccine. J Natl Cancer Inst. 2011;103:1444–51.
38. Rubin LG, Levin MJ, Ljungman P, Davies EG, Avery R, Tomblyn M, et al. 2013 IDSA clinical practice guideline for the vaccination of the immunocompromised host. Clin Infect Dis. 2014;58:309.
39. World Health Organization. Global advisory committee on vaccine safety statement on the continued safety of HPV vaccination. 12 March 2014. http://www.who.int/vaccine_safety/committee/topic/hpv/GAVC_statement_HPv_12_March_2014.pdf.
40. Schiller JT, Castellsague X, Garland SM. A review of clinical trials of human papillomavirus prophylactic vaccine. Vaccine. 2012;30(suppl 5):F123–38.
41. Rosales R, Lopez-Conteras M, Rosales C, Magallanes-Molina JR, Gonzalez-Vergara R, Arroyo-Cazarez JM, et al. Regression of human papillomavirus intraepithelial lesions is induced by MVA E2 therapeutic vaccine. Hum Gene Ther. 2014;25(12):1035–49.
42. REVEAL 1 (evaluation of VGX-3100 and electroporation for the treatment of cervical HSIL). Clinicaltrials.gov. https://clinicaltrial.gov

Printed by Printforce, the Netherlands